The Physics & Technology
of Radiation Therapy

The Physics & Technology of Radiation Therapy

Patrick N. McDermott
Staff Physicist
William Beaumont Hospital
Troy, Michigan

and

Colin G. Orton
Professor Emeritus
Wayne State University
Grosse Pointe, Michigan

MEDICAL PHYSICS PUBLISHING
Madison, Wisconsin

20 19 18 17 16 15 14   3 4 5 6 7 8 9 10 (soft cover)

Library of Congress Cataloging-in-Publication Data

McDermott, Patrick N.
  The physics & technology of radiation therapy / by Patrick N. McDermott and Colin G. Orton.
      p. cm.
   ISBN-13: 978-1-930524-32-3 (alk. paper)
   ISBN-10: 1-930524-32-3 (alk. paper)
   ISBN-13: 978-1-930524-44-6 (sc :alk. paper)
   ISBN-10: 1-930524-44-7 (sc :alk. paper)
   1. Medical physics. 2. Radiotherapy. 3. Cancer--Radiotherapy. 4. Radiation dosimetry. I. Orton, Colin G. II. Title.
   R895.M335 2010
   616.99'40642--dc22
                              2010278039

ISBN 13: 978-1-930524-44-7 (soft cover)
ISBN 10: 1-930524-44-6 (soft cover)

Medical Physics Publishing
4513 Vernon Boulevard
Madison, WI 53705-4964
Phone: 1-800-442-5778, 608-262-4021
Fax: 608-265-2121
Web: www.medicalphysics.org

This book is printed on acid-free paper.

Printed in the United States of America

Dedication

Kenneth J. McDermott, M.D.
(1915–2001)

My father. He is a big influence on my life.
He "was real."

Patricia S. McDermott
(1921–2009)

My mother. She taught me right from wrong.

And now reader,—bestir thyself—for though we will always lend thee proper assistance in difficult places, as we do not, like some others, expect thee to use the arts of divination to discover our meaning, yet we shall not indulge thy laziness where nothing but thy own attention is required; for thou art highly mistaken if thou dost imagine that we intended when we began this great work to leave thy sagacity nothing to do, or that without sometimes exercising this talent thou wilt be able to travel through our pages with any pleasure or profit to thyself.

HENRY FIELDING

Contents

Chapter 1   Mathematics Review

Chapter 2   Review of Basic Physics

Chapter 3   Atomic Nuclei and Radioactivity

Chapter 4   X-Ray Production I: Technology

Chapter 5   X-Ray Production II: Basic Physics and Properties of Resulting X-Rays

Chapter 6 The Interaction of Radiation with Matter

Chapter 7 Radiation Measurement Quantities

Chapter 8   Radiation Detection and Measurement

Chapter 9   External Beam Radiation Therapy Units

Chapter 10   Central Axis Dose Distribution

Chapter 11   Calibration of Megavoltage Photon Beams

Chapter 12   Calculation of Monitor Unit/Timer Setting
for Open Fields

Chapter 13   Shaped Fields

Chapter 14   Dose Distributions in Two and Three Dimensions

Chapter 15   Electron Beam Dosimetry

Chapter 16   Brachytherapy

Chapter 17   Radiation Protection

Chapter 18   Physical Quality Assurance and Patient Safety

Chapter 19   Imaging in Radiation Therapy

Chapter 20   Special Modalities in Radiation Therapy

Preface

This book is the outgrowth of a course taught to residents in radiation oncology at Wayne State University and at William Beaumont Hospital. Over the years the residents have repeatedly urged that the lecture notes for the course be turned into a book. This is a result of frustration stemming from the lack of a text that is set at the correct mathematical level, is technically accurate, and pedagogically effective.

This book is aimed at the reader who has taken one year of college physics, perhaps years ago (and may not have been terribly thrilled about it). The reader may or may not have taken college calculus or precalculus years ago and may only dimly recall natural logs and the exponential function.

There are a number of excellent texts on the physics of radiation therapy including those by Khan and Johns and Cunningham. We recommend these as good secondary texts for those who wish to go beyond the basics. Both of these texts seem to be a compromise between the needs of graduate students in medical physics and the rest of the radiation therapy community. This book is specifically for the rest of the radiation therapy community. This includes radiation therapy technologists and dosimetrists as well as radiation oncologists; however, it may also be useful to the novice physicist who is looking for a quick qualitative overview. Do not be misled, however; this is not a "watered down" text. Every effort has been made to make explanations clear and simple without *oversimplifying*. If you seek erudite and obfuscating verbiage, find another text. To get the most out of this book we suggest that you "work" your way through it: follow along with pen in hand and work through the example problems and derivations with us (see the quote, page vi).

We are mindful of the fact that people have professional exams that they must study for and pass. This book has been written with a close eye on the requirements for these exams—the ABR boards for physicians, the CMD exam for dosimetrists, and the ARRT for therapists. We make no apology to purists for this. If these exams are good exams, then they reflect what practitioners really need to know to be effective clinicians. Teaching for the exam is simply teaching what people need to know.

It is one of the goals of this book to be interesting so that you will want to read it. We have attempted to accomplish this in two ways: by making the material as directly relevant to clinical activity as possible and by adding some interesting sidelights here and there, such as a brief discussion of atomic bombs, the discovery of x rays, and grand unified theories (GUTS) of particle physics, to name a few. You will have to be the judge as to whether we have succeeded in this.

Whenever possible we have endeavored to explain where results come from and to emphasize principles. In some cases this means simple derivations, in other cases plausibility arguments. Otherwise one is left to blindly memorize facts and rules. Simple memorization leaves one lost when the circumstances change slightly. On the other hand, we don't want this book to be overly "theoretical." For this reason we have included the "clinical example" boxes and "rules of thumb" in the chapters that are more theoretical.

There has not been any attempt to cover treatment planning. It is "beyond the scope of this book," as they say. We recommend the excellent books by Bentel and Khan et al. We do however explain some of the basic principles that determine dose distributions in patients. It is our opinion that the basic foundational material in this book should be covered first, before learning treatment planning.

A word about the use of mathematical symbols and equations. We know that the rather extensive use of mathematical symbols may be foreign to our readers (unless they have majored in mathematics, physics, engineering, or Greek). We have endeavored to choose symbols very carefully for the many quantities referred to in this book. We have tried to make these symbols as simple as possible. As a result of the large number of quantities involved in the study of radiation therapy physics, there are simply not enough Latin letters and we resort to Greek letters and or subscripts. We have tried to conform to standard usage where we believe it to be sensible. Unfortunately there are some symbols that are used for more than one quantity even in standard usage. The meaning of duplicate symbols is generally clear from the context.

Each chapter has a complete summary and a full problem set. Answers to selected problems may be found in appendix D. Clinically realistic dosimetry data for a fictitious linear accelerator may be found in appendix C.

We have made every effort to provide accurate data and information; however the information in this book should not be used for treating patients without first consulting a qualified medical physicist.

We welcome your comments and suggestions. We will try to answer e-mail questions whenever possible.

Patrick N. McDermott, Ph.D.
Email: Patrick.McDermott@beaumonthospitals.com

Colin G. Orton, Ph.D.
Email: ortonc@comcast.net

Acknowledgments

Thanks to all of the residents that we have taught over the years. We have learned much from all of you. In particular, thanks to Charles Lee, M.D., Kim Hart, M.D., Tanya Powell, M.D., Raj Patel, M.D., for detailed comments and corrections to the text. Thanks to Jay Burmeister, Ph.D., for reviewing the section on BNCT and for many helpful corrections and suggestions. Thanks to Tony He, Ph.D., for reviewing the section on Monte Carlo calculations.

Thanks to Sharon Carter for reviewing chapter 1. Thanks to Cheryl Culver-Schultz for her expert, meticulous, and extensive review of the chapter on radiation safety. Thanks to Wenzheng Feng for reviewing the chapter on imaging. Thanks to Ann Maitz for reviewing the section on stereotactic radiosurgery. Thanks to Arthur T. Porter, M.D., for suggesting the clinical example boxes. Thanks to Betsey Phelps, our editor at Medical Physics Publishing, for her tireless efforts.

Patrick McDermott thanks his wife Monica and his children Sean and Shayla for just being there. He also thanks Angela Tapley for her steady encouragement. PND would also like to thank all of his colleagues in medical physics, especially his mentors Gary Ezzell, Ph.D., Carmen Mesina, Cathy Alektiar, Susie Garzon, Suzanne Chungbin, Richard Maughan, Ph.D., Mark Yudelev, Ph.D., and last, but by no means least, his coauthor Colin G. Orton, Ph.D.

We apologize to anyone we may have left out; so many people made suggestions over the years.

Any errors in the text are solely our responsibility.

1 Mathematics Review

This chapter is intended to be a review of some of the basic mathematics frequently used to plan and deliver radiation therapy. You will have encountered this material in high school and early college level mathematics courses. Please do not be insulted if you find this material especially elementary. Over the years we have found that people come to the study of radiation oncology with diverse backgrounds. If your mathematics background is strong, you may be able to move through this chapter very quickly, perhaps just by glancing at the pages. Do not fool yourself however—if you cannot do the problems at the end of the chapter, then you do not have a *working* knowledge of this material.

    This chapter will also help you to learn how to use your calculator (see box "Purchasing a Scientific Calculator") to solve not only the problems in this book but real problems in the clinic.

Purchasing a Scientific Calculator[1]

To do the homework problems in this book, you will need a scientific calculator. These can be purchased inexpensively (under $20) in drug stores, discount stores, and office supply stores.

---

[1] American Board of Radiology (ABR) examinees are currently required to use the PC-based Microsoft electronic calculator, which is an accessory to the Windows® operating system. It can be accessed by clicking on Start, then Programs, then Accessories, then Calculator. Click on View, then Scientific to get to the scientific calculator. ABR examinees are advised to spend time becoming familiar with this calculator.

1.1 Exponents

We shall frequently need to use exponents (or powers) in the study of radiation therapy physics.

Using the terminology, a^r, where a is the **base** and r is the **exponent** (sometimes called a *power*), the quantity a^r is sometimes referred to as an **exponential.** When the exponent is a positive integer (i.e., a counting number), it provides a shorthand notation to show repeated multiplication of a number. For example,

$$a^n = a \cdot a \cdot a \cdot \ldots \cdot a \cdot a \cdot a \ (n \text{ times}), \tag{1.1}$$

where n is a positive integer. Suppose the exponent is not an integer, for example, $r = \frac{1}{2}$. In this case,

$$a^{1/2} = \sqrt[2]{a} = \sqrt{a} . \tag{1.2}$$

An example of this is: $\sqrt{9} = 3$, because $3 \cdot 3 = 9$. The index "2" in equation (1.2) is usually omitted from the root symbol—it is understood to be there. Another example of a non-integer exponent is provided by the cube root, i.e.,

$$a^{1/3} = \sqrt[3]{a} . \tag{1.3}$$

An illustration of this is $\sqrt[3]{8} = 2$, because $2 \cdot 2 \cdot 2 = 2^3 = 8$.

The exponent r can be negative or zero. Any non-zero number raised to the zero power is defined to be 1, i.e.,

$$a^0 = 1 \qquad (a \neq 0). \tag{1.4}$$

Also $1^r = 1$ for any value of r.

Negative exponents have the following meaning:

$$a^{-n} = \frac{1}{a^n}. \tag{1.5}$$

One example is $a^{-3} = 1/a^3$.

Suppose that the exponent r is not a nice "neat" (rational) fraction. For example: $2^{1.71}$. We would expect the value of this quantity to be between $2^1 = 2$ and $2^2 = 4$. A more exact value can be found using a calculator with a $\boxed{Y^x}$ key (Microsoft key $\boxed{x^y}$). To three significant digits, $2^{1.71} = 3.27$. See if you can verify this on your calculator. Press the keys: $\boxed{2}$ $\boxed{Y^x}$ $\boxed{1}$ $\boxed{.}$ $\boxed{7}$ $\boxed{1}$ $\boxed{=}$.[2]

---

[2] If the calculator does not have an "equals" key, it may use RPN (Reverse Polish Notation) logic and the correct keystrokes will be different from the ones given here.

There are various rules for manipulating and combining expressions involving exponents.

1.1.1 Multiplication

An example of multiplication of exponentials is:

$$2^3 \cdot 2^2 = (2 \cdot 2 \cdot 2)(2 \cdot 2) = 2^5 = 2^{3+2}.$$

When two exponentials are multiplied, the exponents are *added:*

$$a^p \cdot a^q = a^{p+q}. \tag{1.6}$$

Note that the base (i.e., a) in both factors must be the same; otherwise the exponents cannot be added.

1.1.2 Division

An example of division of exponentials is:

$$2^3 / 2^2 = (2 \cdot 2 \cdot 2) / (2 \cdot 2) = 2^1 = 2^{3-2}.$$

When two exponentials are divided, the exponents are *subtracted:*

$$a^p/a^q = a^{p-q}. \tag{1.7}$$

Note that the base in the numerator and the denominator must be the same; otherwise the exponents cannot be subtracted.

1.1.3 An Exponential Raised to a Power

An example of an exponential raised to a power is:

$$(2^3)^2 = (2^3)(2^3) = 2^6.$$

When an exponential is raised to a power, the exponents are *multiplied:*

$$(a^p)^q = a^{pq}. \tag{1.8}$$

Note that when an exponential is *raised* to a power, we multiply powers, but when two exponentials are multiplied, we *add* the powers [see equation (1.6)].

1.1.4 A Product Raised to a Power

An example of a product raised to a power is:

$$(2 \cdot 3)^2 = 6^2 = 36 = 2^2 \cdot 3^2 = 4 \cdot 9 = 36.$$

When a product is raised to a power, the result is:

$$(ab)^q = a^q \, b^q. \tag{1.9}$$

1.1.5 Base e

There are some values of the base a that are particularly useful. One of these is $a = 10$; another is a value that mathematicians denote by the letter "e." The value of this important constant is $e = 2.71828\ldots$. This number is so important in mathematics that it rivals the significance of pi ($\pi = 3.1415\ldots$). To many people the number e seems very mysterious. Actually, it is not that much different from π. The number π seems less mysterious because we have been hearing about it since we were in elementary school. It seems old and familiar.

Pi also has simple geometric applications that e does not have: The circumference of a circle of radius r is $C = 2\pi r$ and the circle's area is $A = \pi r^2$.

Both π and e are examples of *irrational* numbers. These are numbers that *cannot* be expressed either as simple ratios or as repeating or terminating decimals. The number e comes up again and again in mathematics, particularly in applications concerning rates of change. In radiological science, e appears in the radioactive decay equation, in the equation for radiation attenuation, in ultrasound, in equations for cell survival in radiobiology, etc. These are very diverse applications!

Most scientific calculators have a button for $\boxed{e^x}$. On some calculators you may need to press the $\boxed{\text{2nd}}$ key first. Be careful to distinguish the $\boxed{e^x}$ key from the power of 10 exponent key, which frequently looks like this: $\boxed{10^x}$. If there is any doubt, enter the number 1.0 and press the key. If the result is 2.718, you have the right key.

It is often possible to make a quick, rough prediction of the value of e^x given x (Microsoft, click Inv option first, then click the $\boxed{\text{ln}}$ key). We know that $e^0 = 1$ because $a^0 = 1$ for any value of a, provided that a is not zero. Can you guess the approximate value of $e^{+0.02}$ or $e^{-0.02}$? Since 0.02 is small compared with 1.0, we expect $e^{+0.02}$ to be slightly larger than 1.0 and $e^{-0.02} = 1/e^{+0.02}$ to be slightly less than 1.0. You may wish to evaluate these on your calculator to check this. The value of e^{10} is expected to be quite large since $e^{10} \approx (2.72)^{10}$ and the value of e^{-10} is expected to be quite small.[3] Figure 1.1 shows graphs of e^x and e^{-x}.

---

[3] The symbol "$\approx$" means approximately equal to.

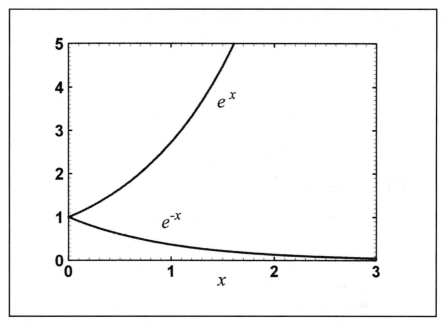

Figure 1.1: Graphs of e^x and e^{-x}. The value of e^x grows rapidly, whereas the value of e^{-x} declines toward zero very rapidly. Note that $e^0 = 1$.

An interesting application of the number e involves interest that is compounded continuously (see Examples 1.1 and 1.2). It is amazing how good people become at mathematics when the problems involve money! Suppose you deposit a certain amount of money (principal) P in an interest-bearing bank account with an *annual* interest rate r ($r = 10\%$/year $= 0.10$/year $= 0.10$ year^{-1}). The interest could be compounded annually, quarterly, monthly, or even daily. Clearly, the more frequently the interest is compounded, the more advantageous it is to you. We can carry this further and imagine that the interest is compounded every second, every millisecond, etc. Let us carry this process to the limit and say that the interest is compounded *continuously*.

In the case of interest that is compounded continuously, the amount A in the account after t years is (stated without proof):

$$A = Pe^{rt}, \tag{1.10}$$

where P is the principal, r is the annual interest rate, and t is the time in years.

Exponents must always be unitless; that is, they must be without units. For interest compounded continuously, the quantity rt is the exponent of e. This combination must be unitless. If r is an annual interest rate (e.g., $r = 10\%$ per year or 0.10/year), the time **must** be given in years (e.g., $t = 2$ years) so that the combination $rt = 0.10$/year $\times$ 2 years $=$

0.20 is unitless. The unit years cancel when multiplying r and t. Always make sure when you are doing problems using exponents that you use a consistent set of units and that the overall units of any expression appearing in an exponent cancel one another, leaving the exponent unitless.

You cannot mix units. As an example, suppose that you express t in months and the interest rate as 5% per year = 0.05/year. The quantity rt will not be unitless because (assume $t = 1$ month) $rt = 0.05$/year $\times$ 1 month = 0.05 month/year. Here, one remedy is to convert t to years by writing $t = 1/12$ year, then

$$rt = \frac{1}{12}\text{year} \times \frac{0.05}{\text{year}} \approx 0.0042. \qquad (1.11)$$

In doing any numerical calculation, always verify that the exponent is unitless. If it is not, then convert the units so that all units are consistent; then they will cancel one another.

Example 1.1

a.   An amount ($2,000) was placed in an Individual Retirement Account (IRA) on January 2, 1997. The interest rate is 10% per year compounded continuously. What will the IRA be worth on January 2, 2017?

$$A = Pe^{rt} = \$2,000\; e^{(0.10)(20)} = \$14,778.11$$

b.   Suppose the interest is compounded annually?

At the end of the first year: $A = P + Pr = P(1 + r)^1$.

At the end of the second year: $A = [P(1 + r)] + [P(1 + r)]r$
                                                          $= P(1 + r)(1 + r)$
                                                          $= P(1 + r)^2$.

You can see that there is a pattern here.

After 20 years:

$$A = P(1 + r)^{20} = \$2,000\;(1 + 0.10)^{20} = \$13,455.00.$$

As expected, the ending balance in the account is less when it is compounded annually rather than continuously.

Example 1.2

An amount ($1,000) is invested for 18 months in an interest-bearing account paying 5% annually and compounded continuously. What is the account balance at the end of 18 months?

$$A = Pe^{rt}, \quad P = \$1,000, \quad r = 0.05/\text{year}, \quad t = 18 \text{ months}$$

If you substitute $rt = 0.05/\text{year} \times 18$ months $= 0.90$ month/year into the equation for A, the result is $2,459.60. Upon brief reflection, it is clear that this answer is nonsense. The correct calculation requires conversion. This can be accomplished in either of two ways. The easiest method is to convert months to years: 18 months is equal to 1.5 years, and $rt = 1.5$ year $\times 0.05/\text{year} = 0.075$. The value of A then becomes $1,077.88. An equivalent method is to convert the interest rate as follows:

$$r = 0.05 \frac{1}{\cancel{\text{year}}} \times \frac{1 \cancel{\text{year}}}{12 \text{ months}} = 0.00417 \frac{1}{\text{month}},$$

then $rt = 0.00417/\text{month} \times 18$ months $= 0.075$, the same as before. The slashes indicate cancellation of units.

1.2 Logarithms

Consider the exponential equation $10^x = 100$. The value of x is 2 because $10^2 = 100$. The value of x is said to be the logarithm or *log* of 100 to the base 10. It is the value of the exponent of 10, which gives 100. We say that the log of 100 (base 10) is 2 or $\log_{10}(100) = 2$. Another equation of this type is $10^x = 0.01$. The value of x that satisfies this equation is –2 because $10^{-2} = 1/10^2 = 1/100$. We say that the log of 0.01 (base 10) is –2 or $\log_{10}(0.01) = -2$. Yet another example is $2^x = 8$. Now the base is 2. The value of x that satisfies this equation is 3 because $2^3 = 8$. We say that log (base 2) of 8 is 3 or $\log_2(8) = 3$.

We can generalize this discussion by examining the exponential equation

$$a^x = y, \tag{1.12}$$

where a and y are positive real numbers and $a \neq 1$. It is often useful to determine the value of the exponent x, given the values of y and a. Another way of stating this is: to what value does a have to be raised in order to get y? This value is called the *logarithm* of y with the base a and it is usually written as follows:

$$x = \log_a(y). \tag{1.13}$$

As an example, $\log_2 (4) = \log_2 (2^2) = 2$.

Some additional examples are:

- if $10^3 = 1000$, then $\log_{10} (1000) = 3$
- if $10^{-3} = 0.001$, then $\log_{10} (0.001) = -3$
- if $10^0 = 1$, then $\log_{10} (1) = 0$
- if $3^2 = 9$, then $\log_3 (9) = 2$.

There is one fundamental fact about logarithms that you should repeat to yourself frequently:

The log is the exponent.

The log of any number y is the exponent to which the base must be raised to get the value of y. If you examine the equations and examples above, you will see that this is indeed true. Remembering this one fact will carry you a long way in your work with logarithms.

When the base is 10, we usually do not write it—it is understood to be there. Log base 10 is referred to as the *common* log. As an example: $\log_{10} (1000) = \log (1000) = 3$. A more difficult case is presented in Example 1.3.

Example 1.3

We have looked at simple cases such as log (1000). Suppose we have something a bit more complex, such as log (5). We know that log (10) = 1 and log (1) = 0, so log (5) must have a value between 0 and 1. Use your calculator to evaluate this log. Look for a key [LOG] (you may have to press a [2nd] function key first). Try this with your calculator to see whether you get log (5) ≈ 0.699.

There is a special type of log that has e for its base. It is called the *natural log*. A shorthand notation is often used,

$$\log_e(M) = \ln(M), \tag{1.14}$$

so that

$$e^x = M \Rightarrow x = \log_e(M) = \ln(M). \qquad (1.15)$$

Most scientific calculators have a button for natural logs; look for a key $\boxed{\text{LN}}$ or $\boxed{\ln x}$.

In Example 1.4, whatever the value of ln 2 is, it is the exponent to which e must be raised to give 2, therefore $e^{\ln 2}$ must be 2.

Example 1.4

$$\log_e e^1 = \ln e = 1$$
$$e^{\ln 2} = 2$$
$$\ln e^{½} = ½$$
$$\ln e^{\star} = \star$$

A list of useful properties of logarithms is shown in Figure 1.2. You should study these properties. An example is

$$\log (1000/10) = \log(1000) - \log(10)$$
$$= 3 - 1 = 2 = \log(1000/10 = 100).$$

In some applications we are given the numerical value of $\log_a (y)$ and we need to find the value of y. If $\log_a (y) = x$, then $y = a^x$ [see equations (1.12) and (1.13)]. A simple example is $\log y = 2$; in this case, we know that $y = 10^2 = 100$. A somewhat more complex example is $\log y = 2.5$. In this instance, $y = 10^{2.5}$. This can be evaluated on a calculator using the $\boxed{10^x}$ key (Microsoft, click Inv option first, then click the $\boxed{\log}$ key). You may have to press the $\boxed{\text{2nd}}$ key first. Try it. The value is $y = 316$. Some problems may involve base e. An example is $\ln y = -2.30$, the value of y is $e^{-2.30} = 0.100$.

Properties of Logs

$$\log_a (1) = 0 \quad \log_a a = 1$$
$$a^{\log_a M} = M \quad \log_a a^r = r$$

$$\log_a (M N) = \log_a M + \log_a N$$
$$\log_a (M/N) = \log_a M - \log_a N$$
$$\log_a M^n = n \log_a M$$
$$\log_a (1/M) = -\log_a M$$

Figure 1.2: Properties of logs.

It is sometimes necessary to solve equations in which the unknown is in an exponent. This is illustrated in Examples 1.5 and 1.6.

Example 1.5

Find n if $(0.5)^n = 0.1$.

We can bring the exponent down by taking the log of both sides of this equation:

$$\log [(0.5)^n] = \log [0.1]$$

$$\log [(0.5)^n] = n \log [0.5] \text{ (see Figure 1.2)}$$

so

$$n \log [0.5] = \log [0.1].$$

Now divide both sides by log [0.5]: $n = \dfrac{\log[0.1]}{\log[0.5]} = \dfrac{-1.000}{-0.301} = 3.32.$

Check the answer by evaluating $(0.5)^{3.32} = 0.100$.

Example 1.6

You invest \$1,000 in an account bearing an annual interest rate of 5% per year *compounded continuously*. How long will it take the balance to reach \$5,000?

$$A = Pe^{rt}$$
$$5000 = 1000 \, e^{0.05t}$$

We need to solve this equation for t, i.e., to get t alone on one side of the equation.

a. Divide both sides by 1000.
$$5000/1000 = e^{0.05t}$$

b. The quantity t is in the exponent; we can bring it down by taking the log (base e) of both sides (remember, **the log is the exponent**).
$$\ln 5 = \ln [e^{0.05t}]$$
$$\ln 5 = 0.05t$$

c. Isolate t by dividing both sides by 0.05.

$$\frac{\ln 5}{0.05} = t \qquad\qquad t = 32 \text{ years.}$$

1.3 Geometry

Do you remember the Pythagorean theorem? It gives a mathematical relationship between the lengths of the sides of a right triangle (any triangle containing a 90° angle). The hypotenuse is the longest side of the triangle. It is always opposite the 90° angle. Figure 1.3 shows a right triangle. The hypotenuse is the side with length c. If a, b, and c represent the lengths of the sides, the Pythagorean theorem states that

$$c^2 = a^2 + b^2. \tag{1.16}$$

Note that this relationship does not hold unless the triangle has a 90° angle.

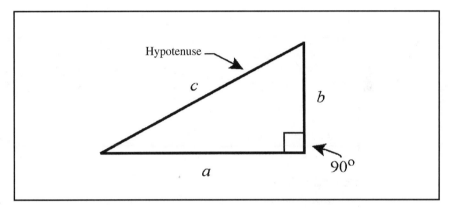

Figure 1.3: A right triangle with the hypotenuse (the side with length c opposite the 90° angle).

Similar triangles are triangles that have the same "shape" but different sizes. To have the same shape, two triangles of different size must have the corresponding angles equal. The lengths of the sides of similar triangles are in proportion to one another, as shown for the similar triangles in Figure 1.4:

$$\frac{a}{A} = \frac{b}{B} = \frac{c}{C}. \tag{1.17}$$

Note that the triangles do not need to be right triangles. Similar triangles have many direct applications in radiation therapy. Probably the best example is the calculation of the necessary gap on the skin so that adjacent edges of two radiation fields meet at depth (see chapter 14). An application of similar triangles to diverging radiation beams is presented in Example 1.7.

Formulas for the circumference and area of a circle are frequently useful in radiation therapy. The area of a circle of radius r is $A = \pi r^2$, and the circumference is $C = 2\pi r$. Likewise, the formulas for the surface area and volume of a sphere are handy to know. The surface area of a sphere of radius r is $S = 4\pi r^2$, and the volume is $V = 4/3\pi r^3$.

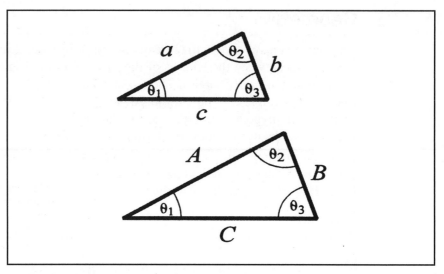

Figure 1.4: Example of similar triangles. Both triangles have the same shape and their corresponding angles are equal. The lengths of their sides are in proportion to one another.

Example 1.7

A radiation beam spreads out (diverges) with increasing distance from the source, as shown in the diagram. At a distance of 100 cm from the source the radiation beam is 15 cm wide. What is the width of the radiation beam at a distance of 120 cm?

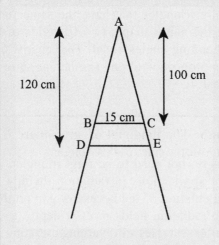

Triangle ADE is similar to triangle ABC and therefore the sides of these triangles are in proportion. The heights measuring 100 cm and 120 cm are also in proportion.

$$\frac{DE}{BC} = \frac{120}{100}$$

$$DE = 1.2 \times BC$$

$$DE = 1.2 \times 15 \text{ cm} = 18 \text{ cm}$$

Clinical Example 1.1

A patient's leg is to be treated with a radiation beam using a linear accelerator. The total length of the portion of the leg to be treated must be 40 centimeters (cm). The largest square radiation field size available is 30 × 30 cm². To achieve the necessary treatment length, the radiation therapist proposes rotating the field so that the patient's leg lies along the diagonal of the 30 × 30 cm², as shown at right.

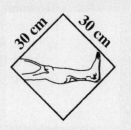

Treatment portal with patient's leg along the diagonal of the field.

Will this field be large enough to treat the patient?

The diagonal of the square field forms the hypotenuse of a right triangle. We need to determine whether the hypotenuse is 40 cm or larger. Both a and b = 30 cm; therefore

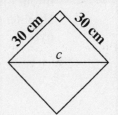

$$c^2 = 30^2 + 30^2 = 900 + 900 = 1800;$$

and

$$c = \sqrt{1800} = 42.4 \text{ cm.}$$

Yes, the field will be large enough to treat the patient's leg.

Note that in Clinical Example 1.1 the length of the diagonal of the square is equal to $30\sqrt{2} = 42.4$ cm.

Rule of thumb: The diagonal of any square is $\sqrt{2}$ (≈ 1.4) times the length of a side or 40% longer.

1.4 Trigonometry

Trigonometric functions—sine, cosine, and tangent—are used to determine angles and sides of triangles. Trig functions are directly applicable in the radiation therapy clinic for field matching calculations and for calculating the necessary shift for isocentric breast treatments, just to name two applications.

Definitions (refer to Figure 1.5):

These definitions are only valid for right triangles. There are numerous mnemonic tricks for remembering the definitions of the terms sine, cosine, and tangent. We like the one that refers to the venerable (but fictitious) Native American chief **SOH-CAH-TOA** (**S**in = **O**pposite over **H**ypotenuse, **C**os = **A**djacent over **H**ypotenuse, and **T**an = **O**pposite over **A**djacent).

$$\sin\theta = \frac{b}{c} = \frac{opposite\ side}{hypotenuse}$$

$$\cos\theta = \frac{a}{c} = \frac{adjacent\ side}{hypotenuse} \tag{1.18}$$

$$\tan\theta = \frac{b}{a} = \frac{opposite\ side}{adjacent\ side}$$

Values of the trigonometric functions can be obtained from a scientific calculator. Look for keys $\boxed{\text{SIN}}$, $\boxed{\text{COS}}$, and $\boxed{\text{TAN}}$. It is useful to know a few special values of the trig functions:

sin 0° = 0	cos 0° = 1	tan 0° = 0
sin 30° = 0.5	cos 60° = 0.5	tan 45° = 1
sin 90° = 1	cos 90° = 0	tan 90° → ∞

Note that sine and cosine *never* have values greater than 1.00.

When evaluating trig functions on a calculator, it is important to know whether the calculator is operating in degree mode or radian mode.[4] We will use degrees here. To check your calculator, try computing sin 30°. If the result is 0.5, then your calculator is operating in degree mode.

---

[4]We will not review radian angular measure here. Suffice it to say that radians are an alternative to degrees for measuring angles. You may recall that 360° is equal to 2π radians.

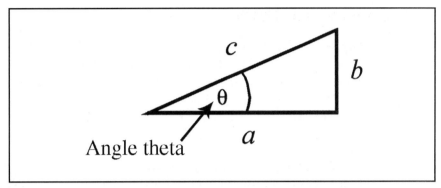

Figure 1.5: Triangle used to define the trigonometric functions [see equation (1.18)].

Example 1.8

It is possible to determine the height of a radio tower (or any other structure for that matter) by measuring the angle of elevation of the top of the tower as shown in figure (a) at right. The angle of elevation is measured at a distance of 300 meters (m) from the base of the tower and at a height of 2 m above the surface of the level ground.

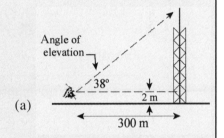

(a)

Determine the height of a radio tower by measuring the angle of elevation of the top of the tower at a distance of 300 meters from the base of the tower. Trigonometry can then be used to find the height of the tower.

The essential geometry is shown in (b). We know an angle (38°) and the length of one side (a side adjacent to the angle, 300 m) and we wish to know the length of the opposite side x. The height of the radio tower is the length of the side of the triangle x **plus** 2 m

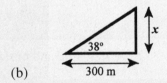

(b)

The essential geometry for this example.

since the angle of elevation was measured at a height of 2 m above the surface of the ground [see figure (a)]. The trig function that involves both opposite and adjacent sides is the tangent function,

and therefore: $\tan 38° = \dfrac{opposite}{adjacent} = \dfrac{x}{300 \text{ m}}$,

$x = 300 \tan 38° = 300 \, (0.781) = 234$ m.

The tower is $234 + 2 = 236$ meters tall.

In many problems it is useful to be able to determine the angle given the value of the sine, cosine, or tangent of the angle. As an example, if $\sin \theta = 0.5$, then the angle is 30°. Given the value of a trig function, the angle can be found by using inverse trig functions: $\sin^{-1}$, $\cos^{-1}$, and $\tan^{-1}$. The example in the previous sentence can be rewritten as $\theta = \sin^{-1} 0.5 = 30°$. Note that $\sin^{-1} 0.5$ is not equal to $(\sin 0.5)^{-1}$. In the first expression the superscript symbol, $(^{-1})$, is an abbreviation that tells us that we want the angle whose sine is 0.5. The second expression is equal to $1/\sin 0.5$.

Try evaluating some inverse trig functions on your calculator. (See Example 1.9.) On some calculators this requires that you press $\boxed{\text{2nd}}$ and then the inverse trig function that you want. On other calculators you press an inverse button first: $\boxed{\text{INV}}$ and then $\boxed{\text{SIN}}$, $\boxed{\text{COS}}$, or $\boxed{\text{TAN}}$ (Microsoft, click Inv option first, then click the desired trig function key.) Try evaluating $\cos^{-1} 0.5$ and $\tan^{-1} 1$. Are the results what you expect?

Example 1.9 illustrates the use of inverse trig functions.

Example 1.9

Determine the angle θ shown in the triangle at right.

The lengths of the opposite and the adjacent sides are given, therefore use the tangent

$$\tan \theta = \frac{10}{100},$$

and

$$\theta = \tan^{-1} 0.1 = 5.7°.$$

100

10

Problems

1. Using a calculator with a $\boxed{Y^x}$ key, evaluate the following expressions and give the answer to three significant digits.
    a. $3^{2.2}$
    b. $5^{1.73}$
    c. $3.14^{2.71}$
    d. π^e

2. Simplify each expression (by hand).
    a. 3^0
    b. $(-3)^2$
    c. $3^{-6} \cdot 3^4$
    d. $\left(\dfrac{2}{3}\right)^{-2}$
    e. $\dfrac{3^{-2} \cdot 5^3}{3 \cdot 5}$

3. Simplify each expression and make sure that all exponents are positive.
    a. $x^0 y^2$
    b. $x^{-1} y$
    c. $\left(\dfrac{4x}{5y}\right)^{-2}$
    d. $\dfrac{(-2)^3 x^4 (yz)^2}{3^2 xy^3 z^4}$

4. a. Use the $\boxed{Y^x}$ key of a calculator to find e^5 to three significant digits. Use the $\boxed{e^x}$ key to check your answer.
    b. Evaluate ln 2 using your calculator. Use the numerical value that you obtain and evaluate $e^{\ln 2}$. Does the result have the expected value?

5. Use your calculator to evaluate a through j (to three significant digits).
    a. $e^{-0.1}$ f. e^1
    b. $e^{-0.01}$ g. e^{10}
    c. $e^{-0.001}$ h. e^{-1}
    d. e^{-0} i. e^{-10}
    e. $e^{0.01}$ j. e^{π}

    In each case, look at your answer. Does it make sense?

6. An amount of $1,000 is invested for 16 months in an interest-bearing account paying 5% annually and compounded continuously. What is the account balance at the end of the 16 months?

7. The fraction of tumor cells that survive a radiation dose D (in Gy) is given by $e^{-(\alpha D + \beta D^2)}$ where $\alpha = 0.3$ Gy^{-1} and $\beta = 0.03$ Gy^{-2}. The gray (Gy) is a unit of radiation dose. Calculate the fraction of cells that survive a radiation dose of 2.0 Gy.

8. Evaluate a through h by hand.
    a. $\log_e 1$
    b. $\log_2 8$
    c. $\log_3 (1/3)$
    d. $e^{\ln x}$
    e. $\ln (e^{2x})$
    f. $\ln\left(e^{\sqrt{\pi}}\right)$
    g. $e^{\ln 3}$
    h. $\log_9 3$

9. This exercise should be performed without the use of a calculator.
    a. What is the value of $\log (100,000)$? What is the value of $\log (100) + \log (1000)$?
    b. What is the value of $\log (10^3)$? What is the value of $3 \log (10)$?
    c. What is the value of $\log (1/1000)$? What is the value of $-\log (1000)$?

10. Find the value of x in a–c.
    a. $\log_8 x = 2$
    b. $\log_x 8 = 3$
    c. $\log_\pi x = 3$

11. Solve for x: $e^{x+3} = \pi$.

12. If $(0.5)^n = 0.01$, what is the value of n?

13. How long does it take an investment to double in value if it is invested at 8% per annum compounded continuously? Repeat assuming the interest rate is 8% per *month*.

14. What is the side length b of the right triangle shown?

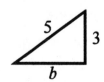

15. For the right triangle shown below:
    a. Find the value of x.
    b. Find the value of sin θ, cos θ, and tan θ.
    c. Find the value of θ three different ways: by taking the inverse sine, the inverse cosine, and the inverse tangent of the values found in part b.

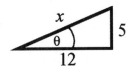

16. Use your calculator to find the approximate values (to three significant digits) of the following expressions:
    a. cos 48°
    b. tan 48°
    c. sin 48°
    d. tan 90°

    Do your answers have approximately the values that you expected?

17. A 20-ft extension ladder leans up against a building making a 65° angle with the ground. How far up the building does the ladder reach?

18. The radiation beam shown below has a width of 24 cm at a distance of 100 cm from the source.
    a. What is the width of the beam at a distance of 140 cm from the source?
    b. What is the value of the angle θ?

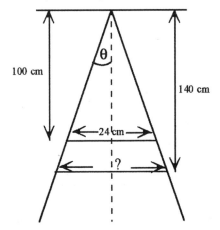

19. A radiosurgery case involves a tumor volume of 1 cm³. If the tumor is approximately spherical, what is its *diameter*?

2

Review of Basic Physics

This review of physics is cast in such a way as to make direct contact with the subject of radiation therapy.

2.1 Units for Physical Quantities

The standard metric system in use worldwide for scientific purposes is the International System of Units (Système International d'Unités), or SI. Scientific journals are becoming increasingly strict that papers submitted for publication contain only SI units. Table 2.1 lists the fundamental quantities of the SI. We will consider quantities related to radiation measurement separately in chapter 7.

Any true SI unit is a combination of the fundamental units listed in Table 2.1. A combination of the fundamental units is called a *derived unit*. An example is the SI unit of force, the newton (as in Isaac, not fig): 1 newton = 1 N = 1 kg m/s^2. Unit abbreviations are capitalized when they refer to a proper name, thus the abbreviation for newton is "N", whereas the abbreviation for meter is "m". Examples of non-SI units are: electron volts, ergs, rads, roentgens, etc. Even though the electron volt is a non-SI unit, its use with the SI is considered acceptable. Do not mix different systems of units when doing calculations or you will get a

Table 2.1: Fundamental SI Units

Quantity	Name	Symbol
length	meter	m
mass	kilogram	kg
time	second	s
electric current	ampere	A
thermodynamic temperature	Kelvin	K
amount of substance	mole	mol
luminous intensity	candela	cd

nonsensical result. Always make sure that your units are consistent before combining them in a calculation.

In this book the units of a quantity will be represented by square bracket notation, [ ]. As an example, consider the SI unit of force, F: $[F] = N$. Some standard SI prefix multipliers are listed in Table 2.2.

2.2 Mechanics

Mechanics is a very broad subject. It is not about fixing your car, but rather, in essence, it is the study of the motion of material objects. This topic is important for radiation therapy because some forms of radiation consist of high-energy elementary particles. The motion of these particles is governed by the laws of mechanics. As an example, the laws of mechanics describe the motion of electrons in the waveguide of a linear accelerator (linac), a device often used in the treatment of cancer.

We start with a review of the definition of a vector and a scalar. A **vector** is any physical quantity that has a direction associated with it as well as a size or *magnitude*. To specify a vector, you must give two quantities: a size or magnitude and a direction. Arrows are often used to symbolically represent vectors. Vectors are written as a character with an arrow over it such as $\vec{a}$. When one of the authors travels home on Route 75 northbound, his velocity, $\vec{v}$, is 88 ft/s (magnitude) due north

Table 2.2: SI Prefixes

Prefix	Symbol	Example	Prefix	Symbol	Example
kilo = 10^3	k	1 km = 10^3 m	centi = 10^{-2}	c	1 cGy = 10^{-2} Gy
mega = 10^6	M	1 MHz = 10^6 Hz	milli = 10^{-3}	m	1 mm = 10^{-3} m
giga = 10^9	G	1 GBq = 10^9 Bq	micro = 10^{-6}	μ	1 μs = 10^{-6} s
tera = 10^{12}	T	1 THz = 10^{12} Hz	nano = 10^{-9}	n	1 nC = 10^{-9} C
			pico = 10^{-12}	p	1 pA = 10^{-12} A

(direction).[1] Examples of vector quantities are velocity, acceleration, force, and electric field. A **scalar** is any physical quantity that does not have a direction associated with it. Examples of scalar quantities are temperature, speed, and mass. Note that speed is the magnitude of the velocity, $\vec{v}$. The magnitude of a vector quantity is denoted by writing the symbol without the arrow above it. For example, speed is denoted as v.

Acceleration is the rate of change of velocity. This can be expressed mathematically as

$$\vec{a} = \frac{\Delta \vec{v}}{\Delta t} = \frac{\vec{v}_2 - \vec{v}_1}{t_2 - t_1}, \qquad (2.1)$$

where the Greek letter Δ (upper case delta) preceding a quantity usually indicates a change in that quantity. In equation (2.1), $\vec{v}_1$ is the velocity at time t_1 and $\vec{v}_2$ is the velocity at time t_2. Acceleration is a measure of how fast the velocity is changing. The units of acceleration are the units of velocity divided by the units of time:

$$[\vec{a}] = \left[\frac{v}{t}\right] = \frac{m/s}{s} = m/s^2. \qquad (2.2)$$

Note that an acceleration can result from a change in speed or *direction* or both [see equation (2.1) and Figure 2.1]. An example of acceleration is provided by an object that is falling without hindrance (free fall) toward the surface of the earth. In this case, the acceleration is 9.8 m/s^2 (near the surface of the earth) toward the center of the earth. The magnitude of this acceleration (due to gravity) is sufficiently important that it is given its own symbol: $g = 9.8$ m/s^2. Another example of acceleration, which we shall encounter later, is the case of a body in uniform circular motion. This is an object that moves in a circular path with constant *speed* (see Figure 2.1). Even though the speed is constant, the object is accelerating because the *velocity* (specifically the direction of motion) is changing. As it turns out, for uniform circular motion the acceleration always points from the body toward the center of the circle and its magnitude is given by

$$a = \frac{v^2}{r}, \qquad (2.3)$$

where v is the speed and r is the radius of the circle. This is called *centripetal* (which means center seeking) *acceleration*.

---

[1] In physics, certain technical terms are used that have a common or colloquial meaning in English. This can be very confusing because the words are often used differently. Although we frequently use terms like "velocity" and "work" in everyday language, these terms have very specific technical definitions in physics that are somewhat different from common usage.

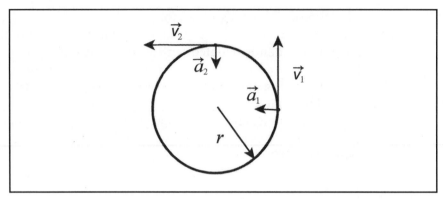

Figure 2.1: A particle in uniform circular motion at two separate instants in time denoted by subscripts 1 and 2. Although the speed of the particle remains constant as it moves around the circle, the direction of motion, and therefore the velocity, is constantly changing. This implies that the particle is undergoing an acceleration. A detailed analysis shows that the acceleration always points from the particle toward the center of the circle as shown. This is called *centripetal acceleration.*

2.2.1 Newton's Second Law[2]

Newton's second law states, in essence, that forces cause accelerations. This corresponds to our common sense. If there is a net force on an object, it will experience an acceleration. This is embodied in one of the most important equations in physics:

$$\vec{F} = m\vec{a},$$ (2.4)

where $\vec{F}$ is the net force on the object and m is its mass. You may take this equation as a definition of force. This may surprise you but unless we formulate an independent definition of force, we are compelled to accept this equation as *the* definition. The unit of force is named after Sir Isaac:

$$\left[\vec{F}\right] = \left[m\vec{a}\right] = \left(1\text{ kg}\right)\left(1\text{ m/s}^2\right)$$
$$= 1\text{ kg} \cdot \text{m/s}^2 = 1\text{ newton} = 1\text{ N}.$$ (2.5)

The gravitational force exerted by the earth on an object is called the weight of the object. We can compute the weight of an object of mass m using Newton's second law:

$$Weight = mg.$$ (2.6)

The SI units of weight are newtons. The older, English units of weight are pounds. It is technically incorrect to refer to the weight of an object in kilograms (or grams for that matter) since the kilogram is a unit of mass.

---

[2] We will not discuss the first and third laws here, although they are very important in any systematic development of mechanics.

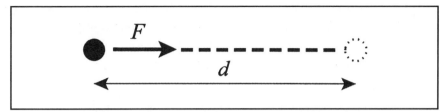

Figure 2.2: Illustration of the work done on an object traveling in a straight line and acted on by a constant force. The object moves through a distance *d*. In this case, the work done on the object can be calculated using equation (2.7).

2.2.2 Work

Work is related to energy. We can give an object energy by doing work on it. We can dissipate an object's energy by allowing it to do work on its surroundings—the object will then give up energy.

Let us examine the simplest possible case in which the force and the direction of motion of a particle lie along the same line and the force is constant (i.e., it does not change from moment to moment). In this very specialized case (see Figure 2.2), the work can be calculated using the formula:

$$W = Fd, \tag{2.7}$$

where *d* is the distance through which the force acts.

The units of work are the units of force times distance: $[W] = [F][d]$. In SI, the units are $[W] = \text{N} \cdot \text{m}$. This combination of fundamental units is sufficiently important that it is given a special name: $1\ \text{N} \cdot \text{m} = 1\ \text{joule} = 1\ \text{J}$ (after the physicist James Joule). We will meet the joule unit again when we discuss the unit of absorbed dose, the gray, as 1 gray = 1 joule/kg. Work is one of those quantities that has a technical meaning that is different from its common meaning. According to the common usage of this word, you would be working very hard if you were to stand stationary holding a 100-lb weight (motionless). According to the technical definition of the word "work," the work done by you on the 100-lb weight would be zero because you have not moved the weight through any distance (i.e., the quantity *d* is zero).

2.2.3 Work Energy Theorem and Energy Conservation

When work is done on an object, its energy changes. Energy is found in various forms: kinetic, potential, heat, light, chemical, etc. Kinetic energy is the energy associated with motion. A particle of mass *m* traveling with speed *v* has kinetic energy equal to

$$T = \frac{1}{2}mv^2. \tag{2.8}$$

The connection between work and energy is provided by the work-energy theorem, which states: the work done on an object in going from an initial state i to a final state f is equal to the change in the kinetic energy,

$$W = T_f - T_i = \Delta T. \tag{2.9}$$

If the object starts from rest, then $T_i = 0$ and $W = T_f = \frac{1}{2}\, mv^2$, where v represents the final speed of the object. The units of kinetic energy are the same as those of work; that is, $[T] =$ joule.

The total energy of an isolated system must have the same value after an event or process as before that event or process. Energy can be transformed from one type to another, but the total amount must be the same before and after. This principle is known as the *conservation of energy*.

2.2.4   Power

Power is the rate at which work is done. If the symbol t represents the time interval over which the work is done, then the power is given by the equation

$$P = \frac{W}{t}. \tag{2.10}$$

The units of power can be determined from the defining equation: $[P] = [W]/[t] =$ joule/s. This unit has a special name: 1 watt = 1 W = 1 joule/s.

When you pay your "power" bill, what you are really paying for is energy or work, *not* power. The power company expresses your usage in kilowatt-hours (kW-h). This is a nonstandard quantity that has the units of work because it is a power multiplied by a time.

2.3   Electricity and Magnetism

2.3.1   Charge and the Coulomb Force

The standard SI unit of electrical charge is the coulomb (C).[3] The electrical force between charged objects is referred to as the electrostatic or Coulomb interaction. The force between two charged *particles* separated by a distance r is given by Coulomb's law:

$$F = k\frac{Q_1 Q_2}{r^2}, \tag{2.11}$$

---

[3] You will notice that we have evaded a definition of electrical charge.

where Q_1 and Q_2 are the charges on the two particles and k is a constant of nature with the approximate value $k = 9.0 \times 10^9$ N · m²/C². This force is sometimes called the Coulomb force or Coulomb interaction. If the charge of both particles has the same algebraic sign, either both positive or both negative, the particles will repel one another. If the charge on each particle has a different sign, one negative and one positive, then the particles will attract one another. Coulomb's law is important in the study of atomic physics. The force between negatively charged electrons and the positive atomic nucleus is given by equation (2.11). The Coulomb force holds electrons in atoms.

Electrical charge is said to be *conserved*. Total net electrical charge can neither be created nor destroyed. An equal amount of positive and negative charge can be combined to give zero net charge. In any given process the total algebraic sum of the charge must be the same before and after the process.

Note that equation (2.11) only applies to point-like particles; that is, both charged objects must be small in size compared to the distance r between them. Consider the following illustration: suppose someone rubs a balloon against your sweater on a dry, winter day. If conditions are right, the balloon may then stick to your sweater. The reason, of course, is that some electrical charge has been transferred between the balloon and your sweater. Both the sweater and the balloon started out uncharged. The charge on your sweater and the charge on the balloon must be equal and opposite in algebraic sign because of the principle of charge conservation. As a result of this there is a force of attraction between them. This force cannot be directly calculated from equation (2.11), however, because neither the balloon nor your sweater is small compared to the distance between them.

The smallest amount of electrical charge is the so-called "elementary" charge. This is the amount of charge carried by a single electron or proton:

$$Q = e = 1.60 \times 10^{-19} \text{ C.}^4 \tag{2.12}$$

This number is very important in radiation physics. It is the smallest amount of free charge that has ever been detected. All measurable charges come in integer multiples of this fundamental quantity of charge. Elementary particles called *quarks* may have charges of $(1/3)\,e$ or $(2/3)\,e$, depending on the type of quark. Single quarks have never been observed in isolation. They are always found in bound aggregates in which the total charge is $\pm e$. In fact, the "standard model" of elementary particle physics forbids the existence of isolated quarks.

A device called an electrometer is used frequently in radiation therapy departments to measure small charges (see Figure 2.3). A typical electrometer, as used in the clinic, can measure charges as small as 1 pC.

---

[4]The symbol e used here to denote the charge on an electron can be distinguished from the base of the natural logarithm by context.

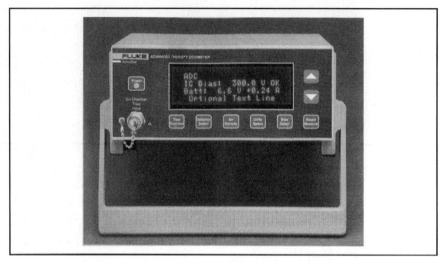

Figure 2.3: An electrometer of the type used in radiation therapy clinics to measure electrical charge. (Courtesy of Fluke Biomedical, Everett, WA)

2.3.2 Electric Fields

We know that charges exert forces on one another. The modern conception of the mechanism for this is that charges establish electric fields in space and that these electric fields exert forces on other charges. The force is mediated by the electric field. Electric field configurations are represented on paper by drawing lines of force. Arrows drawn on the lines of force show the direction of the force exerted on a small positive test charge placed at that location. The closer the lines of force are in a given region, the stronger the electric field (see Figures 2.4 and 2.5).

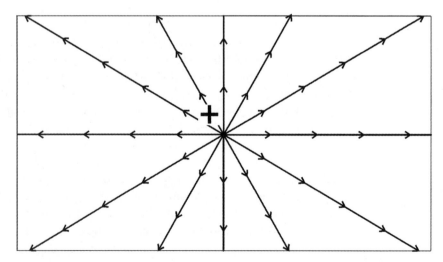

Figure 2.4: Electric field lines for a positive source charge. The arrows point in the direction of the force that would be exerted on a tiny positive test charge if it were placed in this field. The lines of force are closer together near the source charge where the electric field is stronger.

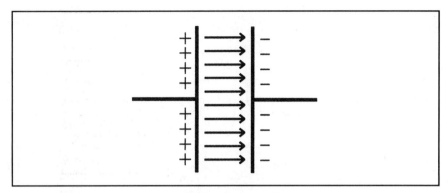

Figure 2.5: The electric field lines between two charged parallel plates. The plate on the left is charged positively and the one on the right is charged negatively. Note that the field lines go away from the positive charge and toward the negative charge. The field is uniform (constant) throughout the region between the plates. At every location between the plates the electric field points in the same direction and the distance between field lines is constant.

2.3.3 Current

Electrical current is the amount of charge Q per unit time that flows through an electrical device. The equation for current is

$$i = \frac{Q}{t} .$$

(2.13)

The unit of current is $[i] = [Q]/[t] =$ coulomb/s = C/s. This combination of units has a special name: 1 ampere = 1 A = 1 C/s.

There are two possible directions of current flow in a thin wire. There is a convention, established before the discovery of the electron, that the current flows in the direction in which positive charge would move. We now know that it is the electrons that carry the charge. Nevertheless, the convention has persisted and the current is always drawn in the direction opposite to the motion of the electrons.

Figure 2.6 shows a very simple electrical circuit in which current flows from the positive terminal of a battery, through a light bulb, and back into the negative terminal of the battery. The schematic diagram of this circuit is shown in the same figure. The symbol for a battery is shown and the light bulb is represented as a generic device called a *resistor*. A resistor is any device that dissipates electrical energy. The resistance R of the resistor is a measure of the amount of current that flows through the resistor when it is connected to a battery. The larger the value of the resistance, the smaller the current that will flow through the resistor when connected to the same battery.

An ammeter is a device that is used to measure electric current. The circuit symbol for an ammeter is shown in Figure 2.7. An ammeter must be placed in series in the portion of the circuit in which current is to be measured. An ammeter should have a low resistance so that it does not

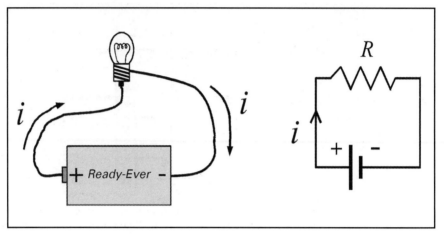

Figure 2.6: A battery connected to a light bulb and a schematic diagram for this circuit. The light bulb is represented by a resistor, R. Note that by convention the current always flows away from the positive terminal and toward the negative terminal, even though the electrons actually move in the opposite direction.

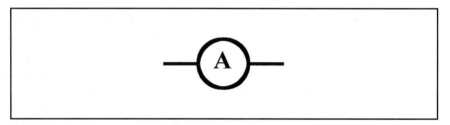

Figure 2.7: The circuit symbol for an ammeter, a device that measures electrical current.

affect the current that you are trying to measure. An important parameter that must be set on an x-ray machine prior to exposure is the current through the x-ray tube. This is usually expressed in milliamps (mA).

2.3.4 Potential Difference

The potential difference between point a and point b in an electrical circuit is the work per unit charge necessary to move a charge Q from a to b. The formula for the potential difference is

$$V = \frac{W}{Q}, \qquad (2.14)$$

where W is the work necessary to move the charge from a to b. The SI unit of potential difference is $[V] = [W]/[Q] = $ J/C. This combination of units has a special name: 1 J/C = 1 volt = 1 V. Do not confuse volts and amps; they are very different quantities. Potential differences can be measured with a voltmeter as shown in Figure 2.8.

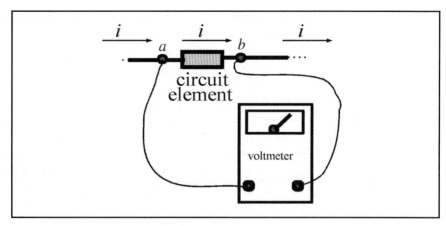

Figure 2.8: A voltmeter is used to measure the potential difference (in units of volts) between points *a* and *b*. A current *i* is flowing through this portion of the circuit. Note that the voltmeter is connected in "parallel" with the circuit element for which the voltage is to be measured. The voltmeter should have a high internal resistance so that very little current is "drained" off through it.

There is a good analogy between charge flow in a wire and the flow of water in a pipe. Current is analogous to water flow rate (say in liters/minute) and voltage difference is analogous to the pressure difference between the ends of the pipe. If the difference in pressure between one end of a pipe and the other end is low, then the rate of flow of water will be relatively low. Conversely, if the pressure difference is high, then the rate of flow will be high. If the voltage difference across a circuit element (say a resistor) is high, then the charge flow (current) through that element can be high.

A current will flow through an electrical conductor when a potential difference (usually measured in volts) is applied across the material. The potential difference may be supplied by a battery or by the electric power company. In a normal material the current drops rapidly to zero when the potential difference is removed. This is because of electrical resistance to charge flow (current). In 1911 the Dutch physicist H. Kamerlingh-Onnes made the stunning discovery that some materials lose all electrical resistance when cooled to very low temperatures. Such materials are called *superconductors*. A current established in a ring of superconducting material can persist for years with no measurable reduction. The temperature below which a material becomes a superconductor is called the *critical temperature*. Solid mercury becomes a superconductor at a critical temperature of 4.2 K. The need for very low temperatures makes superconductivity difficult and expensive to achieve. A common method for attaining the necessary low temperatures is to use liquid helium. The boiling temperature of liquid helium at atmospheric pressure is 4.2 K. Until 1985 the highest known critical temperature was 23 K (Nb_3Ge). In 1987 a new class of superconductors was discovered having a critical temperature of about 90 K. Such temperatures can be reached by using liquid nitrogen (boiling temperature 77 K) rather than liquid helium. Liquid nitrogen is much cheaper and is easier to work with than liquid helium. As of this writing, liquid helium costs about $5.00 per liter whereas liquid nitrogen costs $0.35 per liter (for large amounts), cheaper than bottled water! Unfortunately the new high critical temperature superconductors are ceramics and as such they are not easily fashioned into wires. This has limited the technological applications of these materials.

High voltages are generally but not always dangerous. The amount of danger presented to a human being is related to the amount of work that the electricity can do. From equation (2.14) we can see that this depends on the amount of charge that moves through the potential difference. Static electricity is associated with high voltages but very low currents. If the current is low, then very little charge moves across the potential difference. When you receive a shock from a doorknob on a dry, winter day, there may be a readily visible spark. The voltages associated with such static discharges are quite large, perhaps several thousand volts. Compare this to the voltage supplied by a household battery, 1.5 V, or to the line voltage at your electrical outlet, which is usually 110/120 volts (in North America). Very little charge is transferred between your hand and the doorknob when you receive a static electric shock and therefore little harm is done. Your electrical outlet is much more dangerous even though the voltage is far lower. The outlet is connected to wires that lead into your home, and the power company can supply large amounts of charge through these wires!

The linear accelerators which are used in radiation therapy clinics make use of high voltages that are extremely dangerous—high currents can be delivered. You should never "monkey around" inside the gantry stand or modulator cabinet of a linac without careful guidance from service personnel or a physicist.

2.3.5 The Electron Volt: A Unit of Energy, *Not* Voltage

The SI unit of energy, the joule, is very unwieldy for a discussion of atomic and nuclear physics; it is far too large. Therefore we introduce a special unit of energy that is quite natural for the atomic and nuclear scale: the electron volt (eV).

Imagine two parallel charged plates as in Figure 2.9, one positively charged and one negatively charged. Let us suppose that the potential difference between the plates is 1 volt. If an electron is placed at the surface of the negative plate, it will be accelerated toward the positive

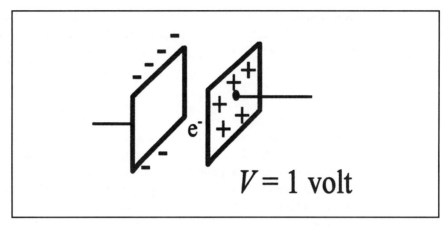

$V = 1$ volt

Figure 2.9: An electron is accelerated from a negatively charged metal plate to a positively charged plate. If there is a potential difference of 1 volt between the plates, the electron will acquire an amount of energy equal to 1 electron volt = 1 eV.

plate. Work will be done on the electron and therefore its kinetic energy will change by an amount ΔT given by equations (2.9) and (2.14):

$$\Delta T = W = QV = (1.6 \times 10^{-19} \text{ C}) \, (1 \text{ volt})$$
$$= 1.6 \times 10^{-19} \, (\text{C} \cdot \text{volt}), \tag{2.15}$$

but 1 volt = 1 joule/C, so $\Delta T = 1.6 \times 10^{-19}$ joule and we define:

$$1 \text{ eV} = 1.6 \times 10^{-19} \text{ J.} \tag{2.16}$$

An electron volt is the amount of energy gained by a particle (it does not have to be an electron) with one elementary unit of charge ($Q = e$), which is accelerated through a potential difference of 1 volt. The amount of kinetic energy T (in units of electron volts) acquired by a charged particle accelerated through a potential difference V (in units of volts) is:

$$T \, (\text{eV}) = \frac{|Q|}{e} \times V \, (\text{volts}) \,. \tag{2.17}$$

Notice that the mass of the particle does not affect the change in kinetic energy—only the charge on the particle affects the energy. The mass does however affect the final speed of the particle: a more massive particle will have a lower speed than a less massive particle. Be careful to distinguish between an electron volt and a volt, they are not the same; it is incorrect to refer to "volts of energy." In radiation therapy it is common to deal with particle energies on the order of thousands or millions of electron volts. The shorthand nomenclature is 1 keV = 10^3 eV and 1 MeV = 10^6 eV. Example 2.1 illustrates the use of electron volts.

Example 2.1

a.   An alpha particle of mass 6.64×10^{-27} kg and charge $+2e$ is accelerated from rest through a potential difference of 1000 volts. Calculate the final kinetic energy and speed of this particle.

$$T(\text{eV}) = \frac{|Q|}{e} \times V \,(\text{volts}) = \frac{2e}{e} \times 1000 = 2000 \text{ eV}$$

$T = \frac{1}{2}\,mv^2$. Solving this for v, we obtain $v = \sqrt{2T/m}$. The kinetic energy units must be converted to joules before substituting into this equation:

$$2000 \text{ eV} \times 1.60 \times 10^{-19} \text{ J/eV} = 3.20 \times 10^{-16} \text{ J.}$$

Therefore

$$v = \sqrt{2\left(3.20 \times 10^{-16}\right) / \left(6.64 \times 10^{-27}\right)} = 3.1 \times 10^{5} \text{ m/s}$$

b.   Repeat part a for an electron of mass 9.11×10^{-31} kg.

$$T(\text{eV}) = \frac{|Q|}{e} \times V \,(\text{volts}) = \frac{1e}{e} \times 1000 = 1000 \text{ eV}$$

Converting this to joules, we obtain 1.60×10^{-16} J, and therefore

$$v = \sqrt{2\left(1.60 \times 10^{-16}\right) / \left(9.11 \times 10^{-31}\right)} = 1.9 \times 10^{7} \text{ m/s}$$

Notice that the final speed of the electron is much higher than the final speed of the alpha particle because of its low mass.

2.3.6   Magnetism

A moving charge (i.e., a current) will produce a magnetic field. In magnets such as those found holding papers on a refrigerator or a filing cabinet, the currents are microscopic in nature and involve the motion of electrons in atoms. These "permanent" magnets are made from materials that retain their magnetism more or less permanently. Permanent magnets generally contain *ferromagnetic* elements—iron, cobalt, and nickel. A current-carrying wire can also produce a magnetic field. This is the basis for the electromagnet.

The vector quantity $\vec{B}$ describes the strength and direction of a magnetic field. The strength is related to how hard the magnet "pulls on things" and the direction can be determined by use of a compass needle or iron filings. The SI unit of magnetic field strength, [B], is the tesla (T). The earth's magnetic field strength is about 2.5×10^{-5} T. A very strong permanent magnet might have a field strength as high as 0.5 T. Permanent magnets are incapable of producing field strengths much larger than this. To produce higher field strengths, electromagnets are required. An electromagnet can be made by winding a coil of wire around a piece of iron. When a current passes through the wire, a magnetic field is generated. An electromagnet made with superconducting wire, such as used in an MRI (magnetic resonance imaging) machine, can produce field strengths of 4 T. This requires liquid helium to reach the critical temperature. A 4T magnetic field is very strong, strong enough to tear a wrench out of your hand at close range (not to speak of erasing the magnetic information encoded on all your credit cards). Whenever entering an MRI room, be sure to divest yourself of all metallic objects and credit cards!

A charged particle *at rest* in a magnetic field experiences no force due to the magnetic field. If the particle moves however, it will experience a force as illustrated in Figure 2.10. The notation used in this book for a magnetic field perpendicular to the page is: ⊙, for a magnetic field pointing out of the page, and ⊕, for a magnetic field pointing into the page. A way to remember the symbolism: for a magnetic field out of the page you see the tip of the arrow which is pointing right at you inside a circle, for a magnetic field pointing into the page you see the tail of the

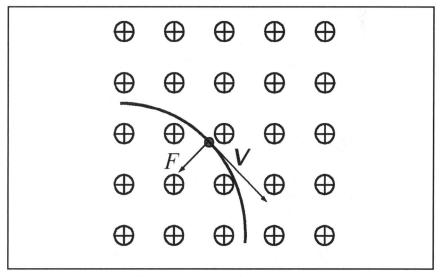

Figure 2.10: An electron enters a region in which there is a uniform magnetic field pointing into the page. The circular symbols with the crosses represent the backside of the magnetic field arrows that are entering the page. At the instant the electron is at the position shown, its velocity is toward the lower right. At that moment it experiences a force toward the lower left. It will follow the path shown.

arrow. When a charged particle moves with a constant speed, v, perpendicular to a constant uniform magnetic field, B, the force on the particle is given by[5]:

$$F = QvB. \qquad (2.18)$$

A magnetic field can be used to deflect charged particle beams as shown in Figures 2.10 and 2.11.

2.4 Electromagnetic Spectrum

We start this section by posing a question: What is the physical nature of light? We will give two answers to this question.

Up until the mid 1800s the nature of light was a mystery. Experiments revealed that light very definitely has wavelike properties, but exactly what is "waving"? The speed of transmission of light, 3×10^8 m/s in vacuum, was also known at this time. In the 1860s James Clerk Maxwell, a Scottish theoretical physicist, developed a set of differential equations, known as Maxwell's equations, that summarize all of our basic knowledge of electricity and magnetism. Maxwell noticed that these equations have a solution that is wavelike. The waves are undulations of perpendicular electric and magnetic fields that propagate through space. Curious,

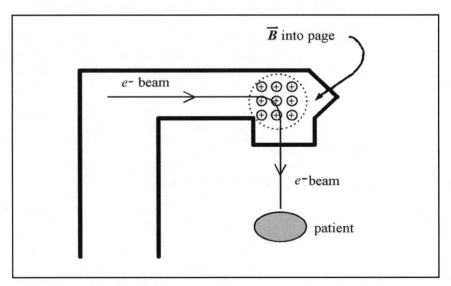

Figure 2.11: A side view of a linear accelerator that produces an electron beam for patient treatment. The electron beam is generated so that it is initially traveling in a horizontal direction. It must be redirected so that it will travel down and irradiate the patient lying below. To accomplish this, a magnetic field is produced in the region shown. This causes a deflection of the beam in the desired direction.

---

[5]The direction of the force is given by the so-called "right-hand rule." A description of this can be found in any elementary physics textbook.

Maxwell calculated the speed of these "electromagnetic" waves from basic constants of electricity and magnetism, including the constant in equation (2.11). He found their speed to be 3×10^8 m/s, the same as the speed of light. This was an unexpected and dramatic demonstration that light is an electric and magnetic wave that travels through space at a speed of 3×10^8 m/s! This marked a major triumph in theoretical physics. To our knowledge no one had previously suspected that light had anything whatever to do with electricity and magnetism. Furthermore, this breakthrough led to the discovery of radio waves by Heinrich Hertz in 1890.

Electromagnetic waves are generated by accelerated charges. You can see radio broadcast aerials (or towers) throughout the countryside. These aerials produce radio waves by sending (oscillating) currents up and down.

Light is just one example of an electromagnetic wave, and it is only a small part of the whole spectrum of electromagnetic waves, which includes radio, infrared, and ultraviolet rays and x-rays. All electromagnetic waves travel at the same speed, $c = 3 \times 10^8$ m/s in vacuum. The type of electromagnetic wave, whether visible, radio, etc., is determined by the **wavelength.** The wavelength, denoted by the Greek letter λ (lambda), is the distance between adjacent crests or troughs, as shown in Figure 2.12. The wavelength of light determines its color. Visible light ranges in wavelength from 400 nanometers (nm) (4×10^{-7} m) for violet up to 700 nm for red. Green light is in the middle of the visible spectrum with a wavelength of about 500 nm.

The **frequency** of a wave is the number of troughs or crests that go by an observer per second. The standard symbol for frequency is the Greek letter ν (lower case nu). Be careful to distinguish this from the symbol for speed, v. The units of frequency are crests per second. Since the number of crests is unitless, $[\nu] = s^{-1}$. This unit, as applied to frequency measurements, is called a hertz (Hz, after the physicist Heinrich

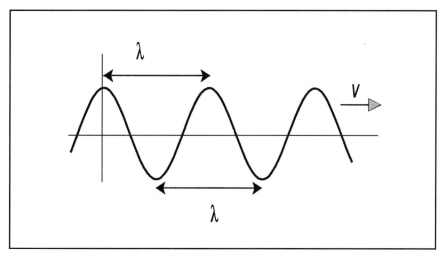

Figure 2.12: A wave traveling to the right with a speed v. The wave has a wavelength, λ, which is the distance between adjacent crests or troughs.

Hertz). As an example, if a wave has a frequency of 5 Hz, you will count 5 crests per second as it passes you. This applies to all types of waves, including water waves, sound waves, and electromagnetic waves.

There is a relationship between frequency, wavelength, and speed:

$$\nu\lambda = c. \tag{2.19}$$

The value of c, the speed of the wave, is roughly constant in any given medium; and therefore if ν increases, then λ must decrease and vice versa. The quantities λ and ν are inversely related to one another. Equation (2.19) applies to all types of waves, not just electromagnetic waves. It is applicable to sound waves as well, including ultrasound, provided that the proper value is substituted for c, the speed of the wave.

To get a better feel for the variety of electromagnetic waves that exist, let's discuss different portions of the spectrum (see Figure 2.13). We will switch back and forth between wavelength and frequency as we discuss different types of waves. Radio waves have a wide range of wavelengths and frequencies. If you look at the AM radio display in your car, you will see that AM radio waves have frequencies of about 1000 kHz. In contrast, FM radio waves are much higher in frequency. A typical FM frequency is about 100 MHz. Microwaves, such as those generated in your microwave oven (and in a medical linear accelerator) have a wavelength of about 10 cm. Microwaves that accelerate electrons in a conventional medical linear accelerator have a frequency of 3000 MHz.

Infrared radiation has wavelengths that are somewhat longer than those of visible light, about 10,000 nm or 10^{-5} m. Although you cannot see infrared radiation, you can feel it if it is strong enough. It is the infrared radiation component of sunlight that makes your skin feel warm.

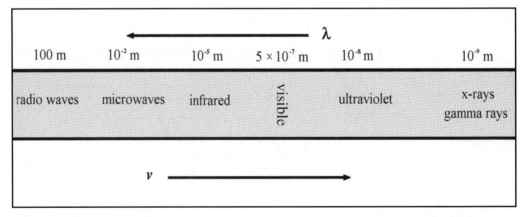

Figure 2.13: The electromagnetic spectrum. Wavelength increases toward the left and frequency toward the right. The diagram does not accurately depict the size of the different bands of the spectrum. For example, the extent of the visible portion of the spectrum is tiny in comparison to the range in wavelengths of radio waves.

The wavelength of ultraviolet (UV) radiation lies between approximately 200 and 400 nm. The ultraviolet spectrum is divided into three bands: UVA (320–400 nm), UVB (290–320 nm), and UVC (<290 nm).[6] There is no physical distinction between these bands other than their slightly different wavelengths. The difference lies in the biological effect. Human skin is relatively insensitive to UVA but very sensitive to UVB and UVC. Fortunately the earth's atmosphere filters out all the UVC. It is UVB that causes sunburn and promotes skin cancer. UVA is used to produce tanning in tanning salons. It is now believed that exposure to UVA is not as harmless as previously thought. UVA is deeply penetrating; it easily penetrates the epidermis to reach the dermis. Excessive exposure to UVA is likely to produce prematurely sun-aged skin.

X-rays have very short wavelengths. X-rays that are used for medical diagnostic purposes have a wavelength of roughly 0.1 nm—about the size of an atom! The distinction between gamma rays (γ rays) and x-rays is one of origin, not energy. To qualify as gamma rays, electromagnetic waves must originate in an atomic nucleus or from positron annihilation (see chapter 3).

It is important to emphasize that there are no gaps in the electromagnetic spectrum. It is a continuous spectrum from the very shortest wavelengths to the very longest wavelengths. The divisions between various types of electromagnetic waves, such as radio waves and microwaves, is somewhat arbitrary because of the continuous nature of the spectrum. The electromagnetic spectrum spans an enormous range in wavelengths from hundreds of meters for radio waves to fractions of a nanometer for x-rays. It is no wonder that these different types of electromagnetic waves have very diverse properties.

At the beginning of this section we promised to give two answers to the question: What is the physical nature of light? The first answer is that light is an electromagnetic wave. Experiments conducted in the late 1800s and early 1900s led Albert Einstein to speculate that light sometimes acts like a particle. In this picture, light (as well as ultraviolet, x-rays, etc.) consists of massless particles called *photons*. It took Einstein's bold genius to assert that an entity can act like both a wave and a particle. The photon is a neutral (i.e., uncharged) particle. The modern picture of light is that it is an entity that can sometimes act like a wave and sometimes like a particle. In any given experiment it acts like either a wave or a particle but never both simultaneously. There is now ample evidence for both the wavelike and particlelike natures of light. Due to the brief nature of this review, we are unable to discuss the many experiments that provide this evidence.

The energy of a photon is proportional to the frequency of the associated wave:

$$E = h\nu, \tag{2.20}$$

---

[6]There is no widespread agreement on the numerical division between these bands. The values given are fairly typical.

where h is Planck's constant (the value of Planck's constant is $h = 6.63 \times 10^{-34}$ J s). We know that $\lambda \nu = c$ and we can therefore write the energy of a photon as given by equation (2.20) in terms of the wavelength of the associated wave:

$$E(\text{eV}) = \frac{1.24 \times 10^{-6}}{\lambda(\text{m})}, \tag{2.21}$$

where the energy E is in units of electron volts and the wavelength is given in units of meters. Note that x-ray photons are considerably more energetic than visible light photons because of their much smaller wavelength. An x-ray photon with $\lambda = 0.1$ nm has an energy of 12.4 keV. Can you verify this by putting numbers into equation (2.21)?

2.5 The Special Theory of Relativity

In 1905 Albert Einstein published a paper with a technical and rather innocent sounding title: "On the Electrodynamics of Moving Bodies." This is one of the most famous papers ever published in physics, for it was in this paper that Einstein laid out, in remarkably complete form, the special theory of relativity. The paper showed that at speeds comparable to the speed of light ($c = 3 \times 10^8$ m/s) the laws of mechanics as established by Newton and those who followed him are no longer valid. Einstein developed a new theory of mechanics called *special relativity*. Newton's laws emerge as a special, limiting case when speeds are small compared to the speed of light ($v \ll c$, or $v/c \ll 1.0$).[7] The theory could not possibly be correct otherwise. Newton's laws of mechanics had been tested at speeds small compared to the speed of light for about 200 years prior to Einstein's publication. These laws were found to be highly accurate. This low-speed limiting case covers our everyday experience. Examples of the highest speeds that we ordinarily encounter: (1) a jet aircraft traveling at 600 mph, which is about 270 m/s; (2) the speed of the earth in its orbit around the sun is considerably faster than a jet—it is about 3×10^4 m/s. Both of these speeds, however, are minuscule compared to the speed of light. For the speed of the earth in its orbit, $v/c = (3 \times 10^4)/(3 \times 10^8) = 10^{-4} \ll 1.0$.

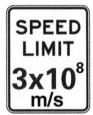

Probably no theory in physics has generated more interest among the public than the special theory of relativity. This is certainly due to the fascinating and bizarre effects such as time dilation and the universal speed limit. The prediction of time dilation says that moving clocks run slow. An example of this is provided by young twins, one of whom leaves earth in a rocket ship at high speed (close to the speed of light)

---
[7]The symbol, $\ll$, means much less than.

and returns many earth years later having aged only a few days. The twin that stayed behind is now an old man, many years older.

We know that this is not just speculation; it is a fact. Experiments have been conducted in which two atomic clocks are synchronized. One of them is then taken in a jet aircraft and flown around. When the two clocks are brought together again, the one flown on the jet reads less elapsed time than the clock that stayed at home. The difference is small because the speed of a jet is small compared to the speed of light. The amount of the difference agrees very well with what the formulas of special relativity predict.

Many people do not seem to like this theory because it is difficult to understand, appears to fly in the face of common sense, and because they believe that it limits the possibilities for space travel. Every physics professor is approached from time to time by people who wish to refute this theory. Anyone attempting to do so must have an alternative that (1) makes quantitative predictions which are as good as, or better, than special relativity; (2) reduces to Newtonian mechanics in the limit of small speeds; (3) is consistent with the theory of electricity and magnetism as embodied in Maxwell's equations, etc. This is a tall order since the special theory makes predictions that have been verified to a high degree of accuracy. In fact, the design of linear accelerators for the radiation therapy clinic is based on the special theory because the electrons in a linac travel at very close to the speed of light. Every time a linac produces a beam, the special theory is put to the test. The special theory is fact.

A systematic discussion of the theory of relativity would occupy a whole course. Here we shall simply cite some of the key results of the theory. We wish we could tell you more (see the bibliography)—it is so interesting!

1. The speed of light in a vacuum is a universal speed limit. No material object can travel at or faster than this speed. Material objects can and do however travel arbitrarily close to this speed.
2. An object's mass increases with its speed. We do not notice this effect at everyday speeds because the effect is so small under these circumstances ($v \ll c$). Crudely speaking, this provides an explanation of 1. above. As an object's speed increases, its mass increases; and it then becomes more difficult to accelerate. As an object's speed approaches c, its mass increases without bound; and it becomes impossible to accelerate further. The mass of an object at rest is called its rest mass and the symbol m_0 is often used to denote this.
3. Mass can be converted into energy. Mass is a concentrated form of energy. This is embodied in the famous equation:

$$E = mc^2, \tag{2.22}$$

where E is the amount of energy that is equivalent to the mass m. A small amount of mass is equivalent to a large amount of energy because c^2 is such a very large number. There are many examples of processes in which mass is converted into energy. In the interior of the sun thermonuclear fusion reactions convert 4×10^9 kilograms (kg) of the sun's mass into energy every second! This provides the radiant energy without which life as we know it would be impossible. In nuclear reactors, nuclear fission slowly converts small amounts of the mass of uranium into energy. Finally, nuclear weapons are so destructive because they convert a small amount of matter into an enormous amount of energy—energy that is released so quickly that it is explosive. Both mass and energy are interchangeable. Energy can be converted into matter. In the next chapter we will study the process of pair production in which some energy disappears to be replaced by an electron and a positron.

The *rest mass* of a particle can be expressed in terms of energy since mass and energy are equivalent. The rest mass of an elementary particle is an important characteristic. We can work out the rest mass of an electron in terms of energy, given that $m_0 = 9.11 \times 10^{-31}$ kg: $E = m_0 c^2 = (9.11 \times 10^{-31}$ kg$) \times (9 \times 10^{16}$ m^2/s$^2) = 8.20 \times 10^{-14}$ J. This energy is more conveniently expressed in terms of electron volts:

$$8.20\times10^{-14}\,\text{J}\times\frac{1\,\text{eV}}{1.6\times10^{-19}\,\text{J}}=5.11\times10^5\,\text{eV}=0.511\,\text{MeV}. \quad (2.23)$$

(The slashes indicate units that cancel each other.) The rest mass energy of an electron is an important number; it should be committed to memory. Although a photon can never be brought to rest (as it always travels at the speed of light), its rest mass in the equations of special relativity is always given the value zero.

4. The total energy of a particle is the sum of its rest mass energy and its kinetic energy, T:

$$E = T + m_0 c^2 = mc^2. \quad (2.24)$$

Note that $T \neq \frac{1}{2} mv^2$ (the Newtonian limit) unless $v \ll c$ and that m_0 is the rest mass. We do not need to be concerned with the relativistic expression for T. If the kinetic energy of a particle is a significant fraction of its rest mass energy, or if it exceeds its rest mass energy, then the particle must be traveling close to the speed of light.

2.6 Review of Atomic Structure

By the year 1900, electrons had been discovered and the existence of atoms had been fairly conclusively established. The prevailing model of the atom at that time was due to J. J. Thomson, the discoverer of the electron. This model is known as the "plum pudding" model. Thomson speculated that positive charge is distributed smoothly throughout the atom and that electrons are embedded within this charge distribution much like plums (or perhaps raisins) in a pudding. The total positive charge and the total negative charge of all the electrons balance to leave the atom with a net charge of zero (i.e., neutral).

This model of the atom was shown to be incorrect by a landmark experiment in physics carried out in 1909 by Hans Geiger and Ernest Marsden under the direction of Ernest Rutherford (a former student of Thomson's). Geiger and Marsden bombarded thin foils made out of various substances with alpha particles (doubly ionized helium atoms or helium nuclei). Most of the alpha particles passed through the foil and were deflected through small angles, as shown in the Figure 2.14. This is consistent with an explanation based on the plum pudding model. If the positive charge is smoothly distributed throughout the atom and the electrons are very low in mass compared to the alpha particle, one would not expect large deflections in the trajectories of the alpha particles—in the same way one does not expect a running elephant to be deflected by a mosquito. On occasion, however, very large angle deflections, up to 180°, were observed. This was completely unexpected. To quote Rutherford: "It was quite the most incredible event that ever happened to me in my life. It was as incredible as if you fired a 15″ shell at a piece of tissue paper and it came back and hit you."

Rutherford developed the nuclear model of the atom in 1911 based on the data collected from alpha scattering experiments. In this model all the positive charge, and almost all the mass, is concentrated in a small dense region in the center called the *nucleus* (yes, this term was

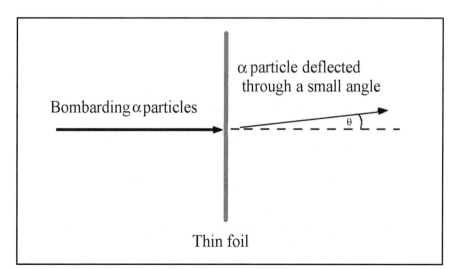

Figure 2.14: Alpha particles incident from the left on a thin metallic foil. As the alpha particles pass through the foil, they are usually only deflected through a small angle θ, but on occasion they are deflected through a very large angle, sometimes 180°.

borrowed from biology). The electrons are of comparatively little mass and are distributed around the nucleus. Within the framework of this model, occasional large angle scattering of alpha particles occurs when an alpha particle passes close to a small, relatively massive atomic nucleus. Since the nucleus is very small in comparison to the size of the atom, this happens infrequently.

It is now known that atoms typically have a size of 10^{-10} m and that the nucleus is 10^{-14} m (ten thousand times smaller). This has prompted one cynical physicist to remark: "Most of humanity is empty space." Nuclei are composed of protons and neutrons, which are collectively referred to as nucleons. The proton has a single unit of positive elementary charge ($Q = +1e$). The neutron is neutral. The number of protons in the nucleus is called the **atomic number** and the symbol used for this number is Z. Examples are hydrogen with $Z = 1$ and uranium with $Z = 92$. The total number of nucleons (neutrons + protons) is called the *mass number, A*.

In 1912 the Danish physicist Neils Bohr was a visitor in Rutherford's laboratory in Manchester, England. He published a model of the hydrogen atom in 1913 based on his research in Manchester. This model has since become known as the *Bohr model* of the atom. In the Bohr model the electron "orbits" the atomic nucleus. The Coulomb attraction between the positively charged nucleus and the electron provides the force necessary to keep the electron in its orbit. The Bohr model explained some features of the hydrogen atom but left many aspects unexplained. Furthermore, it could not explain the properties of multi-electron atoms.

A complete theory of atomic phenomena had to await the development of quantum mechanics in the 1920s. It was discovered that Newtonian mechanics is not valid in the microscopic world of the atom. In the larger macroscopic world that we normally inhabit, Newtonian mechanics emerges as a special limiting case of quantum mechanics. All of modern atomic, nuclear, and elementary particle physics is based on quantum mechanics. Quantum mechanics provides the framework for a very detailed analysis of atomic structure. It can be used to calculate the structure and properties of multi-electron atoms. The description that follows is very superficial.

A simplified picture describes electrons as orbiting the atomic nucleus. This depiction undoubtedly originates from the observed structure of our solar system in which planets orbit the sun. One must not take this picture too literally in the case of the atom—the atom is not a miniature solar system.

Electrons are said to occupy "shells" or "orbits" around the nucleus. The shells are characterized by the quantum number n or equivalently by letters beginning with K:

$$n = \quad 1 \quad 2 \quad 3 \quad 4$$
$$ \quad K \quad L \quad M \quad N$$

Each shell can only hold a certain number of electrons. Generally shells are filled in turn by electrons as we go up through the periodic table to higher values of atomic number (see Figure 2.15). The K shell can hold 2 electrons, the L shell can hold 8 electrons, the M shell 18, etc. Each shell can hold a maximum number of $2n^2$ electrons. For example, the M shell ($n = 3$) can hold a maximum of $2 \times 3^2 = 18$ electrons.

Electrons residing in an atom cannot have just any old value of energy. Electrons can only have specific discrete energies. Electrons in different shells have different energies that are unique to each element. The energies are represented by negative numbers to indicate that the electrons are bound to the atom; that is, a positive amount of energy must be given to an atomic electron to free it (ionization) from the atom. As an example of this, the K shell electrons in tungsten have an energy of approximately –70 keV. To free such an electron from a tungsten atom requires an amount of energy equal to +70 keV. After the electron receives this amount of energy, it will have zero kinetic energy—it will be free from the atom, but it will be motionless. If the electron were to receive +90 keV, it would be freed from the atom and it would be left with a kinetic energy of 20 keV.

Electrons in inner shells are more tightly bound to the atom than electrons in outer shells. An atom can be thought of as a little like a water well. Those electrons occupying inner shells are deep in the well and it takes more energy to remove them from the atom (lift them out of the well). The higher the atomic number, Z, the more tightly bound the inner electrons are. Binding energies are roughly proportional to Z^2. Physicists use energy level diagrams such as in Figure 2.16 to illustrate this. The ground state of an atom is the lowest possible energy configuration of electrons—all electrons are in the lowest energy states possible. An excited state occurs when one or more electrons occupy a higher energy state than they would if the

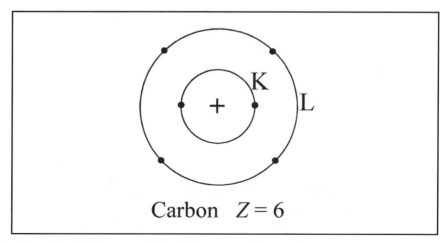

Figure 2.15: A "comic book" depiction of the shell structure of a carbon atom. The K shell can hold a maximum of two electrons and the L shell a maximum of eight.

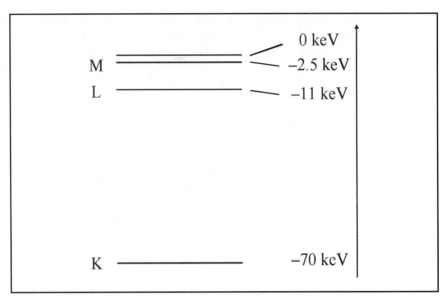

Figure 2.16: An energy level diagram for a tungsten atom shows the energy of each shell. It requires 70 keV to remove a K shell electron from a tungsten atom. Shells with energy higher than M are not shown. Every element has its own unique energy levels.

atom was in the ground state. Ionization occurs when one or more electrons receive so much energy that they are removed from the atom. The atomic binding energy of an electron in a given shell is the amount of energy necessary to completely remove that electron from the atom. Each of the energy levels represents the binding energy of an electron in that shell.

Electrons can make transitions between shells. A transition from a lower energy state to a higher energy state occurs if the atom absorbs an amount of energy equal to the difference between the energy levels. This could happen as the result of a collision between the atom and another particle or by the absorption of a photon with an energy equal to the difference in energy between the two levels. This is illustrated in Figure 2.17. After this process the atom is left with excess energy and is said to be in an excited state.

Electrons can make transitions to lower energy states if there is a vacancy in a lower energy shell (see Figure 2.18). A vacancy can be the result of the excitation process described in the previous paragraph or the consequence of an ejection (ionization) of an inner shell electron from the atom. Ionization can happen as the result of a collision or the absorption of a high-energy photon. Once a vacancy in an inner shell becomes available, an electron in a higher energy shell will rapidly "drop" down and fill the vacancy. Energy is released in the form of photon emission when an electron goes to a lower shell. The photon has a frequency given by $\Delta E = h\nu$, where ΔE is the energy difference between the shells.

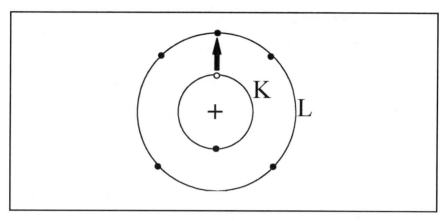

Figure 2.17: An electron makes a transition from the K to the L shell in carbon. The atom is left with excess energy and is said to be in an "excited" state.

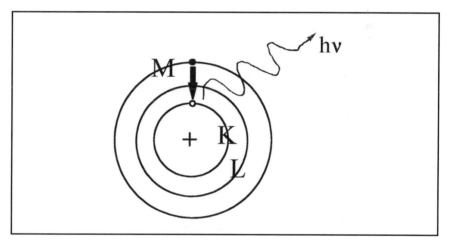

Figure 2.18: Transition from the M shell to the K shell. When an electron makes a downward transition a photon is emitted with an energy equal to the difference in energy between the two levels.

The number of electrons and their configuration determines the chemical properties of an element. Chemical reactions involve the sharing or exchange of outer electrons between atoms. Energies associated with atomic processes such as chemical reactions are on the order of a few electron volts, whereas energies associated with nuclear processes are on the order of millions of electron volts.

Example 2.2

An electron makes a transition from the M shell of a tungsten atom to a vacancy in the K shell.

a.   What is the energy of the emitted photon?

Figure 2.16 shows that the energy of the K shell in tungsten is −70 keV and the energy of the M shell is −2.5 keV. The emitted photon must have an energy of 70.0 − 2.5 = 67.5 keV.

b.   What is the wavelength of this photon and in what portion of the electromagnetic spectrum does it reside?

From equation (2.21):

$$E(\text{eV}) = \frac{1.24 \times 10^{-6}}{\lambda(\text{m})},$$

and therefore

$$\lambda(\text{m}) = \frac{1.24 \times 10^{-6}}{E(\text{eV})} = \frac{1.24 \times 10^{-6}}{67,500} = 1.84 \times 10^{-11} \text{m}.$$

This is in the x-ray part of the spectrum.

In example 2.2, once the M shell electron drops down to the K shell, there becomes a vacancy in the M shell. An electron in a higher shell will drop down to occupy the vacancy in the M shell. This leads to a cascade of downward transitions. Each transition will be accompanied by the emission of a photon with an energy equal to the difference in the energy levels. These photon energies will be characteristic of the particular element.

Problems

1. Use the standard prefixes listed in Table 2.2 to express:[8]
   a. 10^6 phones
   b. 10^{-6} phones
   c. 10^9 los
   d. 10^{-2} pedes
   e. 10^{-12} boos
   f. 2×10^3 mockingbirds

2. To how many milliseconds is a 1/10 s radiographic exposure equivalent?

3. How fast does a 1-kg object have to move to have a kinetic energy of 1 joule?

4. Water has a density of 1.0 g/cm³. Express this density in units of kg/m³.

5. A current of 0.01 mA is equivalent to _____ μA?

6. a. An alpha particle of mass: 6.64×10^{-27} kg is accelerated from rest through a potential difference of 10,000 volts. Calculate the final kinetic energy (in electron volts) and the final speed of this particle (in m/s).
   b. Repeat part a for an electron of mass 9.11×10^{-31} kg.
   c. Is the neglect of special relativity justifiable in part a? In part b? Why?

7. a. Calculate the rest mass energy (in MeV) of a proton ($m_0 = 1.67 \times 10^{-27}$ kg).
   b. What is the ratio of the mass of a proton to an electron?

8. A charge of 10 nC is collected from an ion chamber that is irradiated in a linear accelerator beam.
   a. To how many electrons does this charge correspond?
   b. If the 10 nC is collected over 1.0 min, what is the current in units of nA?

9. a. Derive the formula $\lambda = hc/E$ for the wavelength associated with a photon of energy E.
   b. From this, derive equation (2.21).
   c. What wavelength is associated with a 10 keV photon (diagnostic energy)?
   d. How does this wavelength compare to the size of an atom?

---

[8] Question 1 taken from Halliday, D., and R. Resnick. *Fundamentals of Physics*. (Part I). New York: John Wiley & Sons, 1978.

10. Give the SI units for the following quantities:
    a. frequency
    b. wavelength
    c. power
    d. energy

11. a. Write the following list of types of electromagnetic radiation in order of *decreasing* wavelength: radio, x-rays, visible light, ultraviolet, infrared, microwaves.
    b. Is the energy increasing or decreasing?

12. a. Describe briefly, in words, the nature of an electromagnetic wave.
    b. Compute the frequency and wavelength of a 100 keV photon.

13. a. What is the frequency, expressed in MHz, of an electromagnetic wave with a wavelength of 6.0 cm?
    b. What band of the electromagnetic spectrum is this in?

14. a. An electron makes a transition from the L to the K shell in tungsten. What is the energy of the emitted photon?
    b. What is the wavelength of the photon and in what part of the electromagnetic spectrum does it reside?

Bibliography

Epstein, L. C. *Relativity Visualized.* San Francisco, CA: Insight Press, 1985.

Gardner, M. *Relativity Simply Explained.* Mineola, NY: Dover Publications, 1997.

Halliday, D., and R. Resnick. *Fundamentals of Physics.* (Part I). New York: John Wiley & Sons, 1978.

Pais, A. *Inward Bound: Of Matter and Forces in the Physical World.* New York: Oxford University Press USA, 1986.

3 Atomic Nuclei and Radioactivity

Radioactive materials are commonly used to deliver radiation for therapeutic purposes. It is therefore essential to have a detailed understanding of radioactivity. Placement of the radioactive material inside or on the surface of a patient's body is called *brachytherapy*. Commonly used radioactive materials for brachytherapy are cesium-137, iridium-192, iodine-125, iodine-131, palladium-103, and strontium-90. Using radioactive material to produce a beam of radiation that is applied externally to the patient is called *external beam therapy* or *teletherapy*. A commonly used material for external beam therapy is cobalt-60.

3.1   Basic Properties of Nuclei

Let us briefly review some of the basic properties of atomic nuclei. The nucleus is a dense, positively charged body that consists of neutrons and protons. Neutrons and protons together are called *nucleons*. The mass of a neutron and the mass of a proton are roughly comparable. The mass of a nucleon is approximately 2000 times that of an electron. Atomic nuclei are represented by the notation $_Z^A X$, where A is the atomic mass number, Z is the atomic number, and X is the chemical symbol. The number of protons is equal to Z and the number of nucleons is equal to A. Examples are: $_1^1 H$, $_2^4 He$, $_{27}^{60} Co$. Sometimes nuclei are denoted by the chemical symbol followed by a dash and the atomic mass number, such as Co-60. We will use both notations interchangeably. The number of neutrons can be written: $N = A - Z$. An example is provided by the nucleus $_2^4 He$ (alpha particle) for which $N = A - Z = 4 - 2 = 2$ neutrons.

The chemical identity of an element is determined by the number of protons in the nucleus. Under normal conditions an atom is electrically neutral and therefore the number of electrons will equal the number of protons. It is the number of electrons in an atom that determines its chemical behavior (i.e., which particular element it is). There are approximately 100 known elements. Two atoms that have the same number of protons in the nucleus and a different number of neutrons will be chemically identical, but the atom with more neutrons will have a somewhat larger mass. Two atomic nuclei with the same number of protons but a different number of neutrons are called *isotopes*. There are hundreds of known isotopes. Some examples of isotopes are described in the following paragraph.

Hydrogen has three isotopes: $_1^1 H$ is ordinary *light* hydrogen and is the predominantly occurring isotope; deuterium ($_1^2 H$) and tritium ($_1^3 H$) are considered heavy hydrogen. Deuterium has one proton and one neutron. The nucleus of a deuterium atom is called a "deuteron." Deuterium occurs naturally in water in low concentration. When two deuterium atoms combine with an oxygen atom, the product is a type of water that is slightly heavier than normal and is therefore called "heavy water." Tritium has one proton and two neutrons. Tritium is radioactive and does not occur naturally. $_{27}^{59} Co$ is a nonradioactive, naturally occurring isotope of cobalt. $_{27}^{60} Co$ is a radioactive isotope of cobalt, which is used in radiotherapy. The uranium that is found naturally in the mineral pitchblende is a mixture of isotopes. $_{92}^{235} U$ is the isotope that readily undergoes nuclear fission (see section 3.15.1). $_{92}^{238} U$ is the predominantly occurring isotope and does not readily undergo fission.

Definitions

Isobar: Same A value (number of nucleons) but different Z value (number of protons). The nuclei $_{15}^{32} P$ and $_{16}^{32} S$ are examples of isobars.

Isomer: Same A and Z values, but the nucleus is in a different energy state—an excited state. An example of an isomer is Tc-99*m*. Tc-99*m* is an isomer of Tc-99 and is widely used in nuclear medicine; decay is by gamma emission. The *m* indicates that the nucleus is an isomer. The nucleus is in a metastable state, i.e., an excited state that has a relatively long lifetime (see section 3.12.2).

Isotone: Same number of neutrons.

Memory Aid	
isoto**p**e	same number of **p**rotons *(Z)*
isob**a**r	same number of nucleons *(A)*
isoto**n**e	same number of **n**eutrons
iso**m**er	**m**etastable state

The terms "isobar" and "isotone" are only mentioned here because they occasionally appear on standard exams. We will have no further need for these terms in this book.

The *atomic mass unit* (denoted *u*) is one-twelfth (1/12) the mass of a $^{12}_{6}C$ *atom* (not nucleus, as some books state) (1.66×10^{-27} kg). This corresponds to an energy of 931 MeV. One *u* is roughly the mass of a single nucleon; the mass of the proton is 1.00727 *u,* and the mass of the neutron is 1.00866 *u.*

3.2 Four Fundamental Forces of Nature

How does an atomic nucleus composed of protons (along with neutrons) that repel one another remain intact? Why doesn't it fly apart? There must be another force, which is stronger than the electrical repulsion, that holds the nucleus together. This force is called the *strong nuclear force*. Its range only extends over a short distance and therefore especially large nuclei are unstable and will (under the right conditions) break apart (fission). The positively charged fragments will be repelled from one another and gain a large amount of energy.

It is surprising to most people to learn that there are only four fundamental forces known in nature. In order of increasing strength, they are:

1. gravitational
2. weak nuclear
3. electric/magnetic
4. strong nuclear

strength increasing

The gravitational and electric/magnetic forces are familiar from every-day life, but the weak and the strong nuclear forces are not familiar because they only manifest themselves on a microscopic scale. The weak nuclear force is responsible for certain types of radioactive decay (beta decay).

Every force that you can think of can be put into one of these cate-gories. As an illustration, consider the force that holds you up against gravity when you stand on the floor. Your weight causes the material from which the floor is made to compress very slightly. This compres-sion forces the atoms in the material closer to one another. The elec-trons in the atoms resist by repelling one another and thus the force that holds you up is ultimately electric in nature.

The "holy grail" of physics is to find an all encompassing unified theory that describes all four forces within a single framework. It is thought that there may be a single force that, under different circum-stances, manifests itself as one of the four forces in the list. This theory is sometimes called the "theory of everything," as it would describe all known forces in the universe.

Our list lumps electric and magnetic forces together, but there was no known connection between electricity and magnetism prior to the 1800s, when it was shown that electrical currents can produce magnetic fields and that changing magnetic fields can produce electric fields. This is described by Maxwell's equations of electromagnetism, which form the basis for a unified theory of electricity and magnetism. The culmination came in Einstein's theory of special relativity, which shows that electric and magnetic fields are deeply interconnected.

The modern theory of gravitation is the general theory of relativity developed by Einstein in the early 1900s. Einstein did everything! Einstein spent his later years in a futile quest for a unified theory of gravitation and electromagnetism, and since his death in 1955 some progress has been made in the quest for unification. There is now a successful unified theory of electromagnetism and the weak force, called the *electroweak theory*. The theory of the strong nuclear force is called *quantum chromodynamics*. The electroweak theory, together with quantum chromodynamics, is referred to by physicists as the "standard model."

There have been attempts over the past 20 years to move beyond the standard model by combining electroweak theory and quantum chromodynamics into a single theory. The theories put forward as can-didates are called *grand unified theories,* or *GUTs* for short. Early ver-sions of GUTs predicted that the proton is an unstable particle that can decay into other particles with an average lifetime of 10^{31} years. Labori-ous searches have shown that if the proton is unstable, its average lifes-pan is greater than 10^{31} years. For this reason, the early versions of GUTs cannot be completely correct.[1]

---

[1] What? You say you don't care if the life span of the proton is 10^{31} years! Would you care if it was 10^8 seconds? You probably would, because you would be dead by now!

Grand unified theories do not incorporate gravitation. In recent years a class of quantum theories, called *string theory,* has emerged that do include gravitation. The equations of general relativity arise quite naturally from the equations of string theory. In string theory elementary particles, such as the electron, are viewed as one-dimensional structures (like strings) rather than as point objects. The mathematics of string theory is horrendously difficult and it has not yet been possible to work out the full implications of the equations. Although string theory seems promising, it is not yet known whether it will turn out to be the long sought "theory of everything."

3.3 Nuclear Binding Energy: Mass Defect

Consider a deuterium nucleus (called a deuteron): ^2_1H consists of a proton and a neutron. It is the simplest composite nucleus. Let us add the mass of the free neutron and the mass of the free proton and then compare it to the mass of a deuteron.

$$\begin{array}{ll} 1.00727 \ u & \text{mass of proton} \\ +1.00866 \ u & \text{mass of neutron} \\ \hline 2.01593 \ u & \end{array}$$

The mass of a deuteron is known to be 2.01355 u. It is less than the mass of the free neutron plus the mass of the free proton. There is a mass deficit or *defect* Δm. This suggests that some energy, ΔE, is necessary to separate a deuteron into independent free particles. This energy is called the *binding energy* of the nucleus. Let us compute this binding energy for the deuteron by first determining the difference in mass between the deuteron and a free proton + neutron:

$$\Delta m = -0.00238 \ u,$$

and since 1 u corresponds to 931 MeV:

$$\Delta E = -2.3 \ \text{MeV}.$$

The minus sign signifies that energy has to be absorbed by a deuteron to separate it into a free neutron and a free proton. This is the amount of energy that you can get out when you combine a neutron and a proton to make a deuteron or, conversely, this is the amount of energy that you must put in to separate a deuteron into a free neutron and a free proton.

This demonstrates that energies associated with nuclei are on the order of megaelectron volts (MeV). Compare this with energies that are associated with atomic electrons, which are on the order of electron volts (eV). Chemical reactions involve transfer or sharing of electrons between atoms. The energies associated with chemical reactions are on the order of electron volts. Energies associated with nuclear reactions are approximately a million times larger than the energies associated with chemical reactions! This accounts for the fact that nuclear weapons have approximately a million times the explosive energy of chemical explosives.

3.4 Stability of Nuclei

We can generalize our previous discussion of the binding energy of the deuteron. Let $m(A,Z)$ equal the mass of an atomic nucleus of nuclear number A and atomic number Z; m_p, the mass of a free proton; and m_n, the mass of a free neutron. In general, the binding energy of a nucleus characterized by A and Z with $(A - Z)$ neutrons is:

$$\Delta E = \left\{ m(A,Z) - Zm_p - (A-Z)m_n \right\} c^2. \tag{3.1}$$

Note that ΔE will have a negative value.

It is instructive to make a graph of $|\Delta E|/A$, the average binding energy per nucleon, versus the mass number A. This graph (shown in Figure 3.1) is called the *curve of binding energy*. Most nuclei have an average binding energy of approximately 8 MeV per nucleon. Very light elements such as lithium have a low average binding energy and $|\Delta E|/A$ increases rapidly with increasing mass number. The curve reaches a

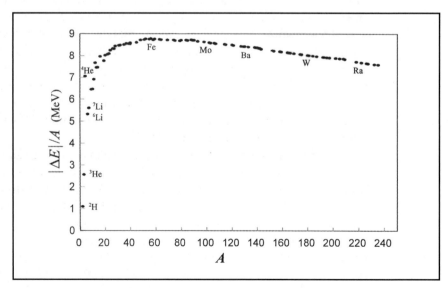

Figure 3.1: A graph of the binding energy per nucleon vs. atomic number is called the curve of binding energy. Most nuclei have a binding energy of about 8 MeV per nucleon. Light nuclei have lower than average binding energy. If two light nuclei combine (fuse) into a heavier nucleus, energy is released. The binding energy per nucleon reaches a peak for Fe-56 and declines for larger values of A. When heavy nuclei split into two parts (fission), the lighter nuclei have a higher average binding energy per nucleon and energy is released.

peak for Fe-56 and then slowly declines as A increases. The peak is due to the short range of the nuclear force. For light nuclei, each nucleon "feels" the nuclear force from all the other nucleons. As nucleons are added to the nucleus, the nucleus becomes larger and eventually becomes large enough that each nucleon can no longer feel the nuclear force from all the other nucleons in the nucleus but only from nearby neighbors. This is a consequence of the very short range of the strong nuclear force. When this occurs a sort of saturation results and the average energy per nucleon no longer rises with the addition of more nucleons. For very large nuclei the long range Coulomb repulsion between protons becomes increasingly important and $|\Delta E|/A$ declines slowly with increasing A.

If light nuclei could be made to combine, the average binding energy of the resulting nucleus would be greater, leaving excess energy to be released. This process, called *nuclear fusion*, does occur in nature. To combine two nuclei in this way requires them to come close enough for the nuclear force to provide the "glue" to hold the nucleons together. As nuclei are positively charged, they repel one another and therefore high speeds are required to overcome the Coulomb repulsion. The nuclei in a high temperature gas travel at high speeds. If the temperature is sufficiently high, the nuclei can approach each other closely enough that there is a significant chance that the short range strong nuclear force can overcome the long range Coulomb repulsion and fusion will occur. This process provides the energy source for stars.[2] In the sun, a series of fusion reactions combines hydrogen to form helium. This energy has been released here on earth in the form of a hydrogen bomb.

If a nucleus with an atomic number beyond 56 were to split into two smaller nuclei, the two smaller nuclei would have a higher average binding energy per nucleon and therefore energy would be released. This process is called *nuclear fission*. Energy from nuclear fission is released from uranium in a nuclear reactor under controlled conditions. Energy is released explosively from fission in an atomic bomb. This will be discussed in more detail in section 3.15.1.

Nature attempts to minimize ΔE, i.e., to make it as negative as possible. This sometimes manifests itself as the spontaneous transformation of one nucleus into another with lower (more negative) binding energy. The excess energy is emitted as radiation. This process is called *radioactive decay*. The resulting nucleus, called the *daughter*, is more tightly bound. Nuclei that do not undergo radioactive decay are said to be stable.

---

[2] In massive stars, a series of fusion reactions over the lifetime of the star culminate in the production of Fe-56. This spells doom for the star because no further energy release is possible in fusion reactions beyond Fe-56. Lacking a ready source of fuel, the star collapses until atomic nuclei "touch," causing a rebound explosion called a *supernova*. A small part of the explosive energy is absorbed to produce all of the elements with $A > 56$.

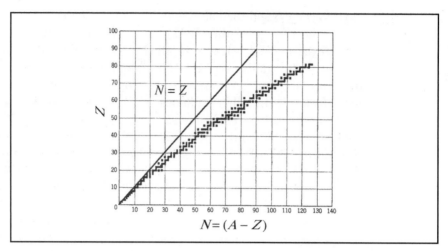

Figure 3.2: Atomic number Z versus neutron number N for the stable nuclides. It is apparent that for Z greater than ~20, the number of neutrons exceeds the number of protons for stable nuclei. For reference purposes the line $Z = N$ has been drawn. (From *Quantum Physics of Atoms, Molecules, Solids, Nuclei, and Particles* by R. Eisberg and R. Resnick, © 1985. Reproduced with permission from John Wiley & Sons, Inc.)

The stability of nuclei depends on the relative number of neutrons and protons:

- for low atomic number $N \approx Z$ for stable nuclei;
- for $Z \gtrsim 20$; $Z < N$ for stability. Too many protons make a nucleus unstable.

This is illustrated in Figure 3.2. Any individual nucleon in a large nucleus feels the strong nuclear force exerted by only nearby nucleons. The Coulomb force, however, makes itself felt throughout the nucleus. All protons exert repulsive forces on other protons. For this reason nature favors an imbalance in which, for large, stable nuclei, the number of neutrons exceeds the number of protons.

There is a tendency for stable nuclei to have an even number of protons and an even number of neutrons. It is rare for stable nuclei to have an odd number of protons and an odd number of neutrons. The reason for this is based on quantum effects, which are beyond the scope of this discussion. Table 3.1 shows the number of stable nuclei having various combinations of even and odd numbers of neutrons and protons.

Table 3.1: Stable Nuclei

N	Z	Number of Stable Nuclei
Even	Even	166
Even	Odd	57
Odd	Even	53
Odd	Odd	8

3.5 Antimatter

In 1928 the English physicist Paul Dirac formulated a relativistic theory of quantum mechanics. The "Dirac equation" seemed to suggest the existence of positively charged electrons. It was not clear what this meant until the discovery of a new type of matter, called *antimatter,* in 1932. In that year positrons were discovered by the American physicist Carl D. Anderson. The discovery was made while Anderson was studying cosmic rays, which are high-energy charged particles that bombard the earth. Cosmic rays interact with atomic nuclei in the earth's atmosphere, producing a "shower" of secondary particles. It is among these secondary particles that positrons are found. The positron can be described as an "antielectron." Its mass is identical to the mass of the electron and its charge is exactly equal in magnitude but opposite in sign. When a positron meets an electron, they both disappear, or annihilate, leaving behind two gamma-ray photons. The symbol for an electron is e^- or β^- and for a positron e^+ or β^+. The annihilation reaction can be written: $e^+ + e^- \rightarrow 2\gamma$. This is an example of the complete conversion of matter into energy as described by Einstein's equation $E = mc^2$. Charge is conserved in this reaction because the net charge both before and after is zero. Each gamma ray has an energy of 0.511 MeV. The total energy of the two gamma photons is equal to the rest mass energy of the positron plus electron. This gamma radiation is called *annihilation radiation*. The gamma photons travel in opposite directions.[3] It is now known that every particle has an antiparticle. If a particle has an electrical charge, its antiparticle has a charge of the opposite sign. When a particle meets its antiparticle, they annihilate to form gamma photons. There are antiprotons, antineutrons, etc. A photon is considered to be its own antiparticle. Astronomical observations suggest that the existence of large amounts of antimatter, in the form of stars and galaxies made of antimatter, is unlikely. The reason for the prevalence of matter over antimatter is the subject of research at the forefront of physics.

3.6 Properties of Nuclei and Particles

Table 3.2 contains a summary of some of the particles and nuclei that are commonly encountered in radiation therapy.

---

[3] Two photons are emitted traveling in opposite directions because the emission of a single 1.02 MeV photon would violate conservation of momentum.

Table 3.2: Properties of Selected Elementary Particles and Nuclei

Name	Symbol	Charge (in units of e)	Rest Mass (kg)	Rest Energy (MeV)	Comments
Electron	e^- or β^- or ${}^{0}_{-1}\beta$	−1	9.11×10^{-31}	0.511	Used in radiotherapy for treatment of shallow anatomical structures
Positron	e^+ or β^+ or ${}^{0}_{+1}\beta$	+1	9.11×10^{-31}	0.511	Antimatter, sometimes produced in therapy beams when a high energy photon interacts with a nucleus
Proton	p or ${}^{1}_{1}H$	+1	1.672×10^{-27}	938.3	Nucleon, sometimes used in radiotherapy
Neutron	n or ${}^{1}_{0}n$	0	1.675×10^{-27}	939.6	Nucleon, sometimes used for radiotherapy; contaminant of linac photon beams with energy above 10 MV
Deuteron	d or ${}^{2}_{1}H$	+1	3.34×10^{-27}	1880	Neutron + proton; a form of heavy hydrogen (isotope)
Alpha particle	α or ${}^{4}_{2}He$	+2	6.65×10^{-27}	3730	Helium nucleus; often emitted during radioactive decay
Neutrino	ν	0	0 ?	0 ?	Emitted during certain types of radioactive decay, interacts very weakly with matter but does carry energy away
Pi-mesons or pions	π^+, π^0, π^-	+1, 0, −1	$\approx 2.5 \times 10^{-28}$	≈ 140	Associated with the strong nuclear force; have been experimentally used for radiotherapy

3.7 Radioactivity

Radioactivity results when unstable nuclei attempt to minimize their energy (make it as negative as possible) and thus become more tightly bound. The "parent" nucleus undergoes a spontaneous transformation into a "daughter" nucleus.

All elements with $Z > 83$ (bismuth) are radioactive. There are three main types of radiation that are emitted when a nucleus undergoes radioactive decay:

1. Gamma rays (γ rays). These are high-energy photons (neutral). Any photons emitted by nuclei or in electron-positron annihilation are called gamma rays. High-energy photons from other sources are

called *x-rays*. Note that the distinction is one of origin, not energy. An x-ray photon may have more energy than a gamma-ray photon or vice versa.

2. Alpha (α) particles: helium nuclei ($_2^4\mathrm{He}$). These particles travel only a short distance in matter.
3. Beta (β) particles: either electrons (β^-) or positrons (β^+).

Protons and neutrons are generally not spontaneously emitted from nuclei.

Radioactive nuclei can occur naturally or they can be produced artificially in a particle accelerator or nuclear reactor. Most natural radioisotopes generally belong to one of three "decay" series. All of these series stop at one or another stable isotope of lead (Pb).

1. Uranium Series

$$_{92}^{238}\mathrm{U} \to \cdots \to {}_{88}^{226}\mathrm{Ra} \to {}_{86}^{222}\mathrm{Rn} + {}_2^4\mathrm{He} \to \cdots \to {}^{206}\mathrm{Pb}$$

The dots indicate intermediate isotopes, not shown. The half-life for the decay of U-238 is 4.5×10^9 years and the half-life for the decay of Ra-226 is 1600 years.

2. Actinium Series

$$_{92}^{235}\mathrm{U} \to \cdots \to {}^{207}\mathrm{Pb}$$

The half-life of U-235 is 7.13×10^8 years. Note that this is considerably less than the half-life of U-238, which may explain why U-235 is relatively rare by comparison.

3. Thorium Series

$$^{232}\mathrm{Th} \to \cdots \to {}^{208}\mathrm{Pb}$$

The half-life of Th-232 is 1.39×10^{10} years.

These decay series explain the natural existence of shorter-lived radioisotopes such as Ra-226. The shorter-lived isotopes are constantly being produced by the decay of parent isotopes.

3.8 Mathematics of Radioactive Decay

Radioisotopes are used extensively as therapeutic agents. It is therefore essential to understand the mathematics of radioactive decay. It is not possible, even in principle, to predict when a specific nucleus in a radioactive sample will decay. The branch of physics known as quantum mechanics can be used in some cases to predict the probability that a given nucleus will decay in a given time period. Usually the probability of decay per unit time for a particular radioisotope is measured rather than calculated.

Suppose that we have a radioisotope X that decays to D:

$$X \rightarrow D.$$

We would like to know the number $N(t)$ of nuclei X at any time t. Our physical expectation is that we start out with some initial number of nuclei N_0 and that number decreases with time until, after some long period of time, there will be no nuclei left ($N = 0$).

Assume that we know the number of nuclei initially present at $t = 0$ (which can be whenever we start our clock). We can write the initial condition mathematically as

$$N(t = 0) = N_0. \tag{3.2}$$

It seems reasonable that if we have two samples of a radionuclide, with one sample having twice as many nuclei as the other, the number of decays per second will be twice as large in the larger sample. This suggests that the number of decays per second is proportional to the number of nuclei present in the sample; that is:

$$\frac{\text{number of decays}}{\text{sec}} \propto N. \tag{3.3}$$

It is also true that

$$\frac{\text{number of decays}}{\text{sec}} = -(\text{rate of change of } N)$$
$$= -\frac{\Delta N}{\Delta t}, \tag{3.4}$$

where ΔN equals the final minus the initial value of N and Δt is the elapsed time. The minus sign is necessary because the rate of change of N is negative; that is, N is decreasing.

If we combine equations (3.3) and (3.4):

$$\frac{\Delta N}{\Delta t} \propto -N. \tag{3.5}$$

Let's put in a proportionality constant λ, then we can write:[4]

$$\frac{\Delta N}{\Delta t} \approx -\lambda N. \tag{3.6}$$

The proportionality constant λ is called the decay constant and it is characteristic of the particular radionuclide (i.e., it is different for

---

[4]The symbol $\approx$ means approximately equal to. Equation (3.6) is only valid when ΔN is small compared to N. For those readers familiar with calculus, $\Delta N/\Delta t$ should be replaced by the derivative dN/dt.

different radioisotopes). The rate of decay is governed by the constant λ. The larger the value of λ, the more rapid the decay. The units of λ are $[\lambda] = 1/$time, expressed in whatever units of time are convenient such as $\sec^{-1}$, hr^{-1}, yr^{-1}, etc. As $\left|(\Delta N/N)/\Delta t\right| \approx \lambda$, the decay constant can be thought of as the fractional amount of decay per unit time for *small fractional decay*.

We would like to know N as a function of time t. Without derivation we will write down the solution to equation (3.6):

$$N = N_0 e^{-\lambda t}. \tag{3.7}$$

We can verify, at least qualitatively, that this equation gives the expected behavior. For time $t = 0$, $N = N_0 e^{-0} = N_0$ and for $t \to \infty$, $N \to 0$, as expected.

3.9 Activity

Generally we are not really interested in the number of atoms remaining in the sample. There is no easy way to measure N anyway. Of greater interest is the rate of decay or, equivalently, the number of decays per second. Note that the number of decays per second is not necessarily the same as the number of particles emitted per second, as each decay may cause the emission of more than one particle.

The number of decays per second is called the *activity*:

$$A = \left|\frac{\Delta N}{\Delta t}\right| = \left|-\lambda N\right| = \lambda N$$

$$A = \lambda N_0 e^{-\lambda t}. \tag{3.8}$$

The quantity λN_0 is simply the initial activity, A_0. The equation for the activity as a function of time can therefore be written:

$$A = A_0 e^{-\lambda t}. \tag{3.9}$$

This equation for the decrease in activity is mathematically of the same form as the equation for the number of remaining nuclei [equation (3.7)]. The SI unit of activity is decay/sec, 1 decay/sec = 1 becquerel = 1 Bq (after the physicist who discovered radioactivity). The old unit of activity is the curie (Ci).[5] 1 Ci is approximately the activity of 1 gm of radium and 1 Ci = 3.7×10^{10} Bq. The curie is a large unit; instead millicuries (mCi) and microcuries (μCi) are often used. Although the becquerel is the standard SI unit of activity, it is still common to see activities quoted in curies. Typical values of activity in radiation therapy are mCi for low dose rate (LDR) brachytherapy; A ~ 10 Ci for a high dose rate (HDR)

---

[5] At Marie Curie's request, the curie was actually named after her late husband Pierre.

brachytherapy afterloader; A ~ 10,000 Ci for a Co-60 teletherapy source—this is a hot tamale!

 Rule of thumb: 1 mCi = 37 MBq.

A sample containing a radioactive isotope may contain a stable isotope of that particular element as well. When stable isotopes are present, they are called "carriers." When no stable isotope is present, the sample is said to be "carrier free." The *specific activity* is defined as the radioisotope activity divided by the total mass of the element present, including any carriers. The specific activity of radium is about 1 Ci/g. Ir-192 sources, which are prepared for HDR use, have a specific activity of about 450 Ci/g. This is a very high specific activity and it makes this isotope well suited for a remote afterloader (discussed in chapter 16) because the source can be made small and still retain a fairly high absolute activity.

3.10 Half-Life

The half-life, $T_{1/2}$, is the amount of time that it takes for half of the original sample to decay or, equivalently, for the activity to become half of its initial value. The half-life is an intrinsic property of a radionuclide. It is independent of external temperature, pressure, chemical bonding, etc., because none of these have any effect on the atomic nucleus.

The rate of decay of a radioisotope is related to the decay constant, λ. The larger the value of λ, the more rapid the decay and hence the smaller the value of $T_{1/2}$. We expect that $T_{1/2}$ and λ are inversely related. Let us now determine the exact relationship by substituting $t = T_{1/2}$ when $A = \frac{1}{2} A_0$ in equation (3.9):

$$A = A_0 e^{-\lambda t}$$

$$A = \frac{1}{2} A_0 = A_0 e^{-\lambda T_{1/2}}$$

$$\frac{1}{2} = e^{-\lambda T_{1/2}}$$

$$\ln \frac{1}{2} = \ln\left(e^{-\lambda T_{1/2}}\right)$$

$$\ln 1 - \ln 2 = -\lambda T_{1/2}$$

$$0 - \ln 2 = -\lambda T_{1/2}.$$

(3.9a)

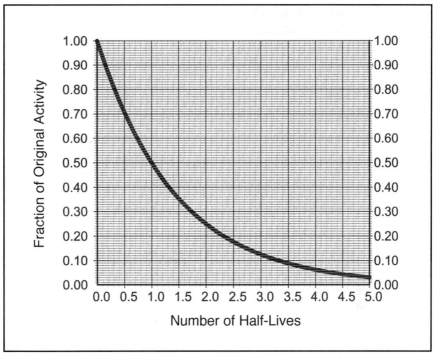

Figure 3.3: The fraction of the original activity (A/A_0) as a function of the number of half-lives ($t/T_{1/2}$, where $T_{1/2}$ is the half-life). This graph can be used to solve radioactive decay problems.

We note that $\ln 1 = 0$ and $\ln 2 \approx 0.693$. We may now determine $T_{1/2}$ by solving for it in the last equation in (3.9a) above:

$$T_{1/2} = \frac{\ln 2}{\lambda} \approx \frac{0.693}{\lambda}. \tag{3.10}$$

After one half-life, the activity of the radioisotope will be $(\frac{1}{2})^1$ of the original activity, after two half-lives, the activity will be $(\frac{1}{2})^2$ of the original activity, and after n half lives the activity will be $(\frac{1}{2})^n$ of the original activity. We can express this in the form of an equation by writing:

$$A = A_0 \left(\frac{1}{2}\right)^n = \frac{A_0}{2^n} = A_0 (0.5)^n, \tag{3.11}$$

where $n = t/T_{1/2}$ is equal to the number of half-lives. Equation (3.11) is mathematically equivalent to equation (3.9) and it is easier to use to solve radioactive decay problems. A graph of the fraction of the original activity remaining (A/A_0) as a function of the number of half-lives is shown in Figure 3.3. The use of this graph can make radioactive decay problems very easy.

Example 3.1

The isotope I-125 (commonly used for radioactive implants) has a half-life of 60 days and an initial activity of 10 mCi. What is its activity after 30 days?

Solution No. 1 (the hard way): $T_{1/2} = 60$ d;

therefore

$$\lambda = \frac{\ln 2}{T_{1/2}} = 0.0116 \, \text{d}^{-1},$$

and

$$A = A_0 e^{-\lambda t}$$
$$A = (10 \, \text{mCi}) e^{-(0.0116)(30)}$$
$$A = 7.1 \, \text{mCi}.$$

Note that the units cancel in the exponent.

Solution No. 2 (easier): Use equation (3.11):

$$n = \frac{30}{60} = 0.5,$$

and therefore

$$A = \frac{A_0}{2^n} = \frac{10}{2^{0.5}} = 7.1 \, \text{mCi}.$$

Solution No. 3 (easiest): Consult Figure 3.3; when $t / T_{1/2} = 0.5$, $A/A_0 = 0.71$; and therefore $A = 10 \times 0.71 = 7.1$ mCi.

This is the easiest method provided that Figure 3.3 is available for use (it may not be when taking exams). This method is only accurate to two significant digits.

Example 3.2

A source has a half-life of 12 hours and an initial activity of 10 mCi. What is the activity after 3 days?

Three days is equal to 6 half-lives; therefore, $n = 6$:

$$A = A_0 \left(\frac{1}{2}\right)^n = 10\left(\frac{1}{2}\right)^6 = 0.16 \text{ mCi}.$$

In this case the number of half-lives exceeds the limit of the graph shown in Figure 3.3.

Example 3.3

The radioisotope Ir-192 decays at the rate of 0.94% per day. What is the half-life of this isotope?

$$\left|\frac{\Delta N/N}{\Delta t}\right| \approx \lambda = 0.0094 \text{ d}^{-1} \quad \left(\text{valid only when } \Delta N/N \text{ is small}\right)$$

and

$$T_{1/2} = \frac{0.693}{\lambda} = \frac{0.693}{\left(0.0094 \text{ d}^{-1}\right)} = 73.7 \text{ days}.$$

Clinical Example 3.1

A patient is treated on a Monday with a radioactive Ir-192 source using a high dose rate (HDR) remote afterloader treatment unit. The treatment duration to deliver a given dose is 289 seconds.

The patient is to be treated again on Wednesday at the same time of day. The dose to be delivered is the same as on Monday. The activity of the iridium will be lower on Wednesday; therefore the treatment time must be increased. What should the treatment duration be for the Wednesday treatment? The half-life of Ir-192 is 74 days.

The decay of the activity of the iridium is $A = A_0 (0.5)^n$, where $n = 2/74 = 0.0270$; therefore $A/A_0 = (0.5)^{0.0270} = 0.981$.

The activity of the iridium on Wednesday is 98.1% of what it was on Monday; therefore the treatment time needs to be *increased* by the factor $1/0.981 = 1.019$, an increase of 1.9%, for a total treatment time of 295 seconds.

3.11 Mean-Life

The concept of mean-life is useful for determining the radiation dose delivered by radionuclides for permanent implants (see Example 3.4). A permanent implant is a radioisotope that is placed in a patient's body and left there permanently (see chapter 16). If the initial activity were constant, how long would it take a sample to completely decay? Let us denote this time by the Greek symbol τ (tau) and call it the "mean-life." Let's work out an expression for τ:

$$\left(\frac{\text{decays}}{\text{sec}}\right)\tau = N_0$$

$$(\lambda N_0)\tau = N_0 \tag{3.12}$$

$$\tau = \frac{1}{\lambda} = \frac{T_{1/2}}{\ln 2}.$$

The value of $1/(\ln 2) \approx 1.44$ and therefore

$$\tau = \frac{1}{\lambda} \approx 1.44\, T_{1/2}. \tag{3.13}$$

A useful equation for solving problems is:

$$A_0 \tau = N_0. \tag{3.14}$$

Example 3.4

A patient receives a permanent I-125 implant. The total dose received by the patient (at some specified anatomic location) is proportional to the total number of disintegrations. Given that the half-life of I-125 is 59.5 days, calculate the total number of disintegrations if $A_0 = 0$ mCi.

The total number of disintegrations is $N_0 = A_0\tau$.

$$\tau \approx 1.44\, T_{1/2} = \ 85.7 \text{ days} = 7.40 \times 10^6 \text{ seconds}$$

$$A_0 = 10 \text{ mCi} = 10^{-2} \text{ Ci, but 1 Ci} = 3.7 \times 10^{10} \text{ decays/sec,}$$

so

$$10^{-2} \text{ Ci} = 3.7 \times 10^8 \text{ decays/sec.}$$

$N_0 = 3.7 \times 10^8$ decays/~~see~~ $\times$ 7.40 $\times$ 10^6 ~~see~~ $= 2.74 \times 10^{15}$ decays.

3.12 Modes of Decay

There are various ways in which an unstable nucleus can undergo radio-active decay. Some isotopes decay by more than one mode. The three principal modes we shall discuss are alpha decay, electromagnetic decay, and beta decay.

3.12.1 Alpha Decay

The equation for alpha decay is:

$$^A_Z X \to ^{A-4}_{Z-2}D + ^4_2 He.$$

An example is the decay of Ra-226 to Rn-222. The alpha particles emitted by radium emerge with a single kinetic energy of about 4.5 MeV. The range in kinetic energies of the alpha particles emitted in alpha decay of various radionuclides is approximately 4 to 9 MeV. It is important to emphasize that for any given radioisotope the energy of the emitted alpha particle is always the same. Alpha particles are not usually used for therapeutic purposes in radiation therapy because their range in tissue is so small.

In any radioactive decay (or nuclear reaction) certain quantities must have the same value both before and after the process. For example, charge must be conserved. For this reason the sum of the subscripts must be the same on the left and the right sides of the reaction equation. In the equation for alpha decay we have Z on the left side and $(Z - 2) + 2 = Z$ on the right side. In addition to charge conservation, it has been found that the number of nucleons must be conserved. This implies that the sum of the atomic numbers on the left side must be equal to the sum of the atomic numbers on the right side. In the alpha decay reaction we have A on the left hand side and $(A - 4) + 4 = A$ on the right side.

3.12.2 Electromagnetic Decay

Atomic nuclei have energy levels just as atoms do, although the levels are much more complicated. When a nucleus undergoes alpha or beta decay, the daughter is often left in an excited state. There are various ways in which a nucleus can rid itself of this excess energy.

1. **Nuclear de-excitation:** By emitting a gamma ray. This process is called "gamma emission." Note that during gamma emission there is no change in either A or Z.
2. **Internal conversion (IC):** By ejecting an electron from the atom. Note that this electron is an atomic electron and does not reside in the nucleus (electrons do not reside in nuclei). It is incorrect, as some texts state, to interpret this as emission of a gamma by the nucleus, which

then ejects an electron from the atom. Instead, the excess energy of the nucleus is transferred *directly* to the atomic electron. It is important to understand that this process competes with nuclear de-excitation. In a sample of a radioisotope in which the nuclei are in an excited state, some fixed percentage will decay by gamma emission and the remainder will decay by internal conversion. Usually the ejected electron (sometimes called a "conversion electron") is a K shell electron, although L and M shell electrons can be ejected with lower probability. Conversion electrons have discrete energies. Once an atomic electron is ejected, the atom is now missing an electron. The missing electron causes one of two possible consequences:

i.   *Fluorescence or characteristic x-rays:* Electrons cascade "down" to lower-energy unoccupied shells emitting x-rays with well-defined discrete energies; these x-rays have wavelengths that are characteristic of that element (see section 2.6).

ii. *Auger (pronounced* o'zhay*) electron emission:* A vacancy in an inner shell is filled by an electron in an outer shell, and another outer shell electron is ejected from the atom. As an example, suppose that there is a K shell vacancy as a result of internal conversion decay. This vacancy could be filled by an L shell electron and an M shell electron could be ejected from the atom. The energy difference between the K and L shells will be delivered to the ejected M shell electron, providing the energy to eject it and endow it with residual kinetic energy. There are now vacancies in both the L and M shells. These will be filled by electrons from higher-energy states leading to photon emission or further Auger emission.

3.   **Isomeric transition:** Most nuclei in excited states lose energy immediately by gamma emission or internal conversion. In some cases, however, the excited nucleus has an appreciable lifetime. Such a nucleus is said to be *metastable*. An example is Tc-99m (technetium):

$$^{99m}\text{Tc} \rightarrow {}^{99}\text{Tc} + \gamma.$$

The energy of the gamma is 0.141 MeV. This isotope is widely used in nuclear medicine imaging studies.

3.12.3 Beta Decay

There are three processes that we will discuss that fall under the general heading of beta decay and which are governed by the weak nuclear force: β^- decay, positron emission, and electron capture.

β^- Decay

In β^- decay the atomic nucleus emits an electron. It is important to understand that electrons do not exist as independent particles in nuclei.

When a nucleus undergoes beta decay, the electron is created just prior to its ejection.

When a radioisotope decays by beta emission, each individual nuclear decay may result in a beta of different energy. Thus, in a sample of a radioisotope that decays by beta emission, the betas emerge with a spectrum or range of energies (see Figure 3.4). There is a maximum energy, T_{max}, of the emitted betas. No betas are observed to have a kinetic energy greater than T_{max}. The average kinetic energy of the beta particles is approximately $T_{avg} \approx 1/3\ T_{max}$.

When a parent nucleus decays to a daughter by beta emission, an amount of energy, T_{max}, is available. When a beta is emitted with an energy less than T_{max}, where does the rest of the energy go? Some energy is unaccounted for; it appears as if energy is not conserved.

The apparent lack of conservation of energy led to an "energy crisis" in physics in the 1930s. At that time, energy conservation was already a long and well-established principle. Physicists resorted to very extreme and creative ideas in an attempt to account for the missing energy. Neils Bohr suggested that perhaps energy is simply not conserved in some quantum phenomena. The famous physicist Wolfgang Pauli said: "Rubbish!"—that there must exist a new particle that carries off the excess energy. To meet the constraints of experimental evidence, Pauli hypothesized that the new particle is neutral (to conserve electrical charge in beta decay), that it interacts exceedingly weakly with matter (which explains why it had not yet been discovered), and that it carries

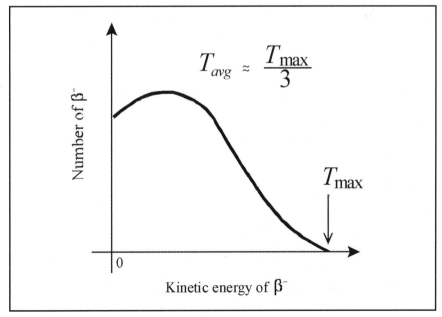

Figure 3.4: The energy distribution or spectrum of electrons emitted in beta decay. There is a maximum energy, T_{max}. The average energy is approximately $T_{max}/3$.

off the excess energy. Saying that the particle interacts very weakly with matter is equivalent to stating that it is extremely penetrating. This is, in fact, quite an understatement: the average distance that one of these particles can travel through lead before interacting is four *light years*![6] This particle was named the neutrino by Enrico Fermi (it means "little neutral one" in Italian). The symbol for a neutrino is the Greek letter nu: ν. At first it was believed that the neutrino had a rest mass of zero. Today, there are some indications that the neutrino may have a small non-zero rest mass. Various lines of evidence rapidly convinced physicists that neutrinos really do exist. However, it was not until 1956 that neutrinos were actually detected in the laboratory. The nuclear reactions occurring in the core of the sun produce copious neutrinos. You are constantly bombarded by these neutrinos. During the day they come from overhead. At night they come from below because they pass through the entire earth with almost no attenuation!

The generic equation for beta decay is:

$$_Z^A X \rightarrow {}_{Z+1}^A D + {}_{-1}^0 \beta + {}_0^0 \bar{\nu}.$$

The bar over the ν denotes an antiparticle. Even though neutrinos are neutral, like photons, the neutrino is not its own antiparticle. In the equation for beta decay, charge is conserved because $Z = (Z + 1) - 1$ (the neutrino is neutral). The number of nucleons is conserved because $A = A + 0$.

Examples of beta (β^-) decay are:

$$_{15}^{32} P \rightarrow {}_{16}^{32} S + {}_{-1}^0 \beta + {}_0^0 \bar{\nu}$$

$$_{38}^{90} Sr \rightarrow {}_{39}^{90} Y + {}_{-1}^0 \beta + {}_0^0 \bar{\nu}$$
$$\llcorner \; {}_{40}^{90} Zr + {}_{-1}^0 \beta + {}_0^0 \bar{\nu}.$$

The beta that is emitted in the decay of Sr-90 has a low energy and is absorbed in the sample. The beta that results from the yttrium decay is used therapeutically in ophthalmic applicators for the treatment of pterygium, a rare eye condition. This beta has an energy of $T_{max} = 2.27$ MeV.

Unstable nuclei that are neutron rich usually undergo beta decay. Beta decay is a way of getting rid of a neutron. Inside the atomic nucleus a neutron decays to a proton, a beta, and an antineutrino. The decay equation is:

$$_0^1 n \rightarrow {}_1^1 p + {}_{-1}^0 \beta + {}_0^0 \bar{\nu}.$$

Neutron deficient nuclei undergo positron (β^+) emission or electron capture.

---

[6]McGervey, John D. *Introduction to Modern Physics,* 2nd ed., 1983.

Positron Decay

In positron decay (sometimes called β^+ decay) the nucleus emits a positron (β^+) and a neutrino:

$$_Z^A X \rightarrow {}_{Z-1}^A D + {}_{+1}^0 \beta + {}_0^0 \nu.$$

The positron goes on to annihilate with an electron generating, in turn, two 0.511 MeV photons. The photons travel in opposite directions (angle of 180°); this is exploited for positron emission tomography (PET). Charge and mass number are conserved as always; note that the other particle emitted is a neutrino, not an antineutrino. Positron emission occurs in nuclei that are proton rich or, equivalently, neutron deficient. In the nucleus a proton is converted to a neutron: $_1^1 p \rightarrow {}_0^1 n + {}_{+1}^0 \beta + {}_0^0 \nu$. Note that a free proton cannot decay to a heavier particle such as a neutron.

Examples of positron decay are:

$$_{11}^{22} Na \rightarrow {}_{10}^{22} Ne + {}_{+1}^0 \beta + {}_0^0 \nu$$

$$_8^{15} O \rightarrow {}_7^{15} N + {}_{+1}^0 \beta + {}_0^0 \nu.$$

Electron Capture

The process of electron capture is an alternative to positron emission. The two processes compete with one another: a nuclide might decay by both processes. Both processes have the same end point; that is, they both reduce Z by 1. Positron decay is more prevalent among lighter elements, whereas electron capture is more common for heavier elements. In electron capture, an inner shell electron, usually from the K shell, is captured by the nucleus and combines with a proton to become a neutron: $_1^1 p + {}_{-1}^0 \beta \rightarrow {}_0^1 n + {}_0^0 \nu$. If the capture is indeed from the K shell, the process is called *K-capture*. The equation for electron capture is:

$$_Z^A X + {}_{-1}^0 \beta \rightarrow {}_{Z-1}^A D + {}_0^0 \nu.$$

An example is provided by Na-22, in which 90% of the atoms decay by positron emission and the remaining 10% by electron capture. Another example is I-125, which has a half-life of 59.5 days:

$$_{53}^{125} I + {}_{-1}^0 \beta \rightarrow {}_{52}^{125} Te + {}_0^0 \nu + \gamma \left(35.5 \text{ keV} \right).$$

Following the electron capture, characteristic x-rays are emitted with energies of 27 and 31 keV. The Te-125 is formed in an excited state; 93% of the time it decays by internal conversion and the other 7% by the emission of a 35.5-keV gamma ray. I-125 does not decay by positron emission for reasons explained below.

Example 3.5

Consider the beta decay: $^{210}_{83}\text{Bi} \rightarrow {}^{A}_{Z}\text{D} + {}^{0}_{-1}\beta + \bar{\nu}$. Find the value of A and Z.

Conservation of nucleon number requires that $210 = A + 0$ and thus $A = 210$. Conservation of charge requires $83 = Z - 1$ and thus $Z = 84$. Consulting a periodic table shows that this element is polonium and we can therefore write $^{A}_{Z}\text{D} = {}^{210}_{84}\text{Po}$.

3.13 Decay Diagrams

It is useful to draw diagrams to illustrate the various modes of decay that a nuclide undergoes. In these diagrams arrows are drawn to the left when Z decreases and to the right when it increases. The spacing between levels is proportional to the energy difference between the neutral atoms of the parent and daughter species (see diagram numbers 1–4).

The vertical line in the decay diagram (number 2) for positron emission represents the threshold for this decay. The difference between the amount of mass-energy of the parent neutral atom and the daughter neutral atom must be at least two times the electron mass energy (1.02 MeV) for this decay to occur. This is because the parent atom emits a positron and it must also rid itself of an atomic electron to become a neutral atom. This is not seen in β^- decay because the beta emitted from the nucleus of the parent atom is compensated for by an extra electron that the daughter must capture to remain a neutral atom. Every isotope that undergoes positron emission can also decay by electron capture but not vice versa because of the threshold. An example is I-125, which decays by electron capture. This isotope cannot decay by positron emission because the difference in mass between the neutral I-125 atom and the neutral Te-125 atom is less than 1.02 MeV.

1. β^- decay:

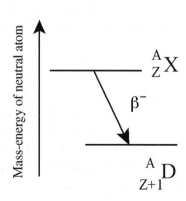

2. β^+ decay (positron emission):

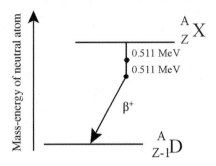

3. Electron capture (EC):

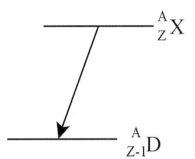

4. Internal conversion (IC):

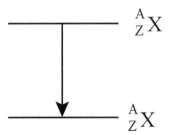

Figure 3.5 shows an example of diagrams 2 and 3 above where Na-22 decays by positron emission or electron capture to $^{22}_{10}$Ne. Positron emission occurs 90.5% of the time and electron capture, the remaining 9.5%. $^{22}_{10}$Ne * is an excited state of Ne-22, which decays to the ground state by gamma emission.

Figure 3.6 illustrates the decay of Cs-137, an isotope that has been widely used in brachytherapy, particularly for the treatment of gynecological cancers. Its half-life is 30.0 years. Approximately 95% of the time it decays to a metastable, excited state of Ba-137; the other 5% of the time it decays by beta emission directly to the ground state of Ba-137. The excited state of Ba-137 decays to the ground state either by emission of a 660 keV gamma (85%) or by K, L, or M shell internal conversion.

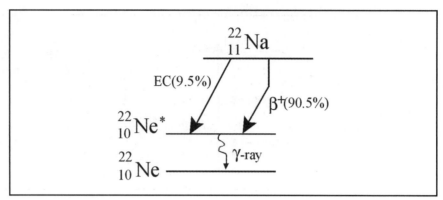

Figure 3.5: Na-22 decays by positron emission or electron capture to $^{22}_{10}$Ne.

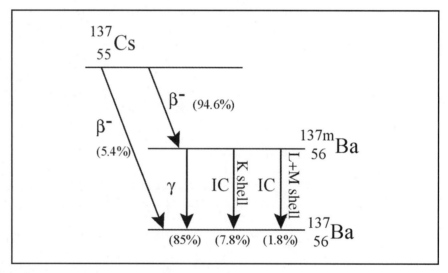

Figure 3.6: The decay scheme for Cs-137, an isotope commonly used for radiation therapy. The gamma ray has an energy of 0.660 MeV.

3.14 Radioactive Equilibrium

Suppose that a radioactive parent isotope X decays to a daughter product D with a half-life T_p. Further suppose that D in turn decays to G with a half-life T_d. This is the situation for the various intermediate isotopes in the decay series discussed in section 3.7 and shown here in Figure 3.7. In some cases, X can decay to more than one species of daughter. The apparent decay rate of the daughter will depend on its rate of production (from the decay of X) and its rate of decay to G.

We will state certain results without proof. If $T_p > T_d$, then after some period of time the ratio of the activity of D to the activity of X (A_D/A_X) will approach a constant value. This is called **radioactive equilibrium.**

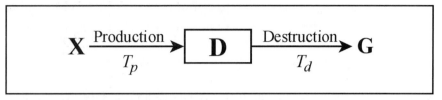

Figure 3.7: Radioisotope **D** is produced by the decay of **X**. In turn, **D** decays into **G**. The amount of **D** present as a function of time depends on both the rate of production and the rate of destruction. The rate of production of **D** depends on the half-life T_p and the rate of destruction of **D** depends on T_d.

The net rate of accumulation of daughter nuclei, R_d, is equal to the rate of decay of the parent minus the rate of decay of the daughter:

$$R_d = \lambda_p N_p - \lambda_d N_d,\tag{3.15}$$

where λ_p and λ_d are the decay constants for the parent and the daughter, respectively; N_p and N_d are the number of atoms of parent and daughter, respectively.

There are two types of radioactive equilibrium:

- Secular: $T_p \gg T_d$
- Transient: $T_p \gtrsim T_d$

Note: The symbol $\gtrsim$ means somewhat greater than, and the symbol $\gg$ means much greater than. We shall consider each case in turn below.

3.14.1 Secular Equilibrium

Secular equilibrium occurs when the half-life of the daughter is much shorter then the half-life of the parent. One example is provided by the decay of Sr-90 (see section 3.12.3) into daughter product Y-90. This isotope is sometimes used for brachytherapy treatment of the eye. The half-life of Sr-90 is 28.0 years and the half-life of Y-90 is 64 hours. The prime example of secular equilibrium is the decay of radium into radon:

$$^{226}_{88}\text{Ra} \rightarrow\ ^{222}_{86}\text{Rn} + ^{4}_{2}\text{He}$$
$$\downarrow$$
$$^{218}_{84}\text{Po} + ^{4}_{2}\text{He}.$$

The radon in turn decays to Po-218. Radon is a noble gas (any of the elements found in Group VIII at the far right of the Periodic Table). The half-life of radium is 1600 years and the half-life of radon is 3.8 days.

The decay of radium is accompanied by the emission of gamma rays. In the early days of radiation therapy these gamma rays were used for therapeutic purposes.

Imagine placing some pure radium in a sealed container in which radon can accumulate. Over an interval of, say, a few years, the rate of production of radon remains constant because radium decays so slowly. Another way of stating this is to say that $\lambda_p N_p$ in equation (3.15) remains almost constant. As the amount of radon builds up, its decay rate ($\lambda_d N_d$) increases because the amount of radon present increases. Eventually the rate of decay becomes equal to the rate of production and the amount of radon present thereafter remains constant; that is, each time a radium atom decays to produce a radon atom, a radon atom also decays. This condition is called **secular equilibrium.** In secular equilibrium the activity of the radon will be equal to the activity of the radium. If 1.00 mCi of Ra-226 is sealed in a closed container at time $t = 0$, after about 30 days, it will be accompanied by 1.00 mCi of Rn-222 (within about 0.5%). See Figure 3.8 for an illustration of the approach to secular equilibrium.

3.14.2   Transient Equilibrium

Transient equilibrium occurs when the half-life of the daughter is somewhat less than the parent. In the limit in which $T_d \ll T_p$, transient equilibrium becomes secular equilibrium. An important example of transient equilibrium is provided by the decay of $^{99}_{42}\text{Mo}$. This isotope undergoes beta decay to $^{99}_{43}\text{Tc}$ (technetium-99) with a half-life of 66.7 hours. The daughter, which 86% of the time is the isomer $^{99\text{m}}_{43}\text{Tc}$, decays by

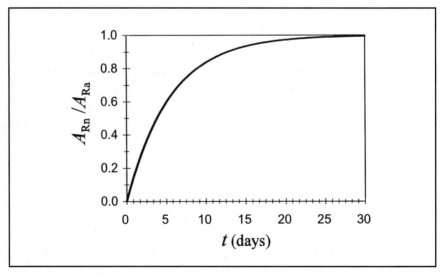

Figure 3.8: The ratio of the activity of radon to that of its parent, radium. The radium is placed in a sealed container at $t = 0$. After about 30 days the activity of the radon becomes equal to the activity of the radium. This is called secular equilibrium.

gamma emission to the ground state of $^{99}_{43}$Tc with a half-life of 6.03 hours. The remaining 14% of the time the Mo-99 (sometimes called "molly") decays to other (nonmetastable) excited states of Tc-99. These excited states decay virtually instantaneously to the ground state, emitting a gamma in the process.

Tc-99m is widely used for diagnostic scans in nuclear medicine. It has a convenient half-life: not too short—there is sufficient time to scan patients after they are administered Tc-99m; and not too long—the activity in the patient's body will decline quickly after the procedure so that the patient does not pose a radiation hazard. The gamma ray emitted has an energy of 140 keV. This energy can easily escape the body and be detected with a device called a gamma camera, which forms an image of the distribution of Tc-99m in the patient's body. Mo-99 is used in hospital nuclear medicine departments to generate Tc-99m, which is then "milked" from the generator "cow". The term describing this process is *elution*.

Suppose we start with a pure sample of Mo-99. At first there is no Tc-99m. After a short while the amount of Tc-99m will increase as the Mo-99 decays. As time progresses, the amount of Mo-99 decreases and, therefore, the rate of production of Tc-99m decreases. The amount of Tc-99m must therefore reach a maximum value and then begin to decline as less and less is produced (see Figure 3.9). The maximum activity is reached after 23 hours. After a long time the decay curves become almost parallel to one another and the apparent half-life of the Tc-99m becomes the same as the half-life of the Mo-99 and the ratio of the activities reaches a constant value of 0.945. When this occurs, it is called **transient equilibrium.**

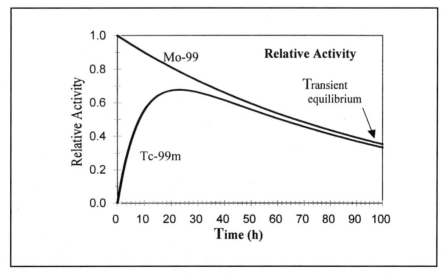

Figure 3.9: Relative activity of Mo-99 and one of its daughters, Tc-99m. It is assumed that there is no Tc-99m to begin with. The activity of the Tc-99m reaches a maximum after 23 hours. After a long period of time has elapsed, the ratio of the activity of Tc-99m to Mo-99 reaches a constant value of 0.945. This is called transient equilibrium.

The activity of the Tc-99m is always less than the activity of the Mo-99 because there are other daughters for Mo-99.

3.15 Production of Radionuclides

There are four main sources of radioisotopes: (1) naturally occurring, (2) produced as a byproduct of nuclear fission, (3) produced in a nuclear reactor by deliberate exposure to intense bombardment by neutrons, and (4) produced by exposing a material to a charged particle beam from a particle accelerator such as a cyclotron. A list of isotopes that are commonly used in radiation therapy appears in Table 3.3.

3.15.1 Fission Byproducts

Large atomic nuclei (high Z values) contain a large number of protons that must be held together by the strong nuclear force. This force, which acts only over very short distances, has difficulty holding large nuclei together. Some large nuclei, if given a slight push will break apart into two fragments. The fragments are smaller nuclei, which are more tightly bound (see section 3.4). At the same time several neutrons will be emitted. The smaller nuclei do not "want" these. This process is called **nuclear fission.** The "push" that can send a heavy nucleus over the threshold is the absorption of a neutron. A neutron can easily enter the nucleus because it is not repelled by the positively charged protons.

Probably the best-known example of nuclear fission is provided by U-235. In natural uranium, the predominantly occurring isotope is U-238 (99%), which does not readily undergo fission. An example of uranium fission is given by the reaction:

$$_{92}^{235}\text{U} + _{0}^{1}\text{n} \rightarrow _{92}^{236}\text{U} \rightarrow _{56}^{141}\text{Ba} + _{36}^{92}\text{Kr} + 3_{0}^{1}\text{n}.$$

Note that both charge and nucleon number are conserved in this process. The fission products in this reaction, Ba-141 and Kr-92, are just two of

Table 3.3: Commonly Used Isotopes in Radiation Therapy

Isotope	Half-Life	Therapeutic Radiation	Production
Co-60	5.26 years	1.25 MeV (average) γ	Neutron activation
Cs-137	30.0 years	0.662 MeV γ	Fission product
I-125	59.5 days	0.028 MeV (average) x-rays	Neutron activation
I-131	8.0 days	0.364 MeV γ	Fission product
Ir-192	73.8 days	0.38 MeV (average) γ	Neutron activation
Pd-103	17.0 days	0.021 MeV characteristic x-rays	Neutron activation
Sr-90	28.1 years	0.7 MeV β^- (average)	Fission product

the many possible products of the fission of U-235. Others include Cs-137 and Sr-90, which are widely used in radiation therapy. In general:

$$^{235}_{92}\text{U} + ^{1}_{0}\text{n} \rightarrow \text{FP}_1 + \text{FP}_2 + 2.5\,^{1}_{0}\text{n} + 200 \text{ MeV},$$

where FP_1 and FP_2 are specific fission product nuclides ("fragments"). On average, 2.5 neutrons are emitted and 200 MeV of energy is released. The 200 MeV appears in the form of kinetic energy of fission fragments, neutrons, and gamma rays.

Some of the emitted neutrons are lost to the fission process. They either go on to interact in different ways or they actually fly out of the material. Suppose that two neutrons, on average, go on to cause other fissions. This is illustrated in Figure 3.10. You can see that this can have a multiplying effect and a chain reaction will ensue. If the chain reaction proceeds rapidly enough, the energy released by the fission reactions will be explosive. The result is an atomic bomb. In a nuclear reactor the fission process occurs slowly under controlled conditions.

If the sample of U-235 is physically small, many neutrons will escape through the surface and will not cause additional fission reactions. Unless the sample of U-235 is larger than some minimal mass, a chain reaction will not be possible. The minimum amount of fissionable material necessary for a chain reaction is called the *critical mass*. The critical mass depends on the shape of the sample. The critical mass for a sphere of U-235 is roughly 50 kg, which is about the size of a cantaloupe.

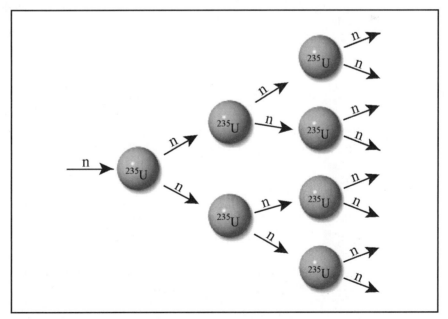

Figure 3.10: The development of a chain reaction. In this example each fission releases two neutrons that each subsequently cause another fission. Very rapid multiplication occurs, which can be explosive.

Fission fragments are generally radioactive and have many uses, including medical applications. These nuclei are separated from the fuel rods in a nuclear reactor when these rods are removed for replacement. Fission fragments usually have a high neutron-to-proton ratio. They are therefore neutron rich—and neutron rich nuclei often decay by β^- emission. An example of a fission byproduct that is used for medical purposes is Cs-137. Any radioactive material that is produced as a byproduct of nuclear fission is regulated by the U.S. Nuclear Regulatory Commission (NRC) (or by an Agreement State; see chapter 17).

The main impediment to the production of atomic weapons is the manufacture of material that can readily undergo fission—99% of naturally occurring uranium is U-238, which does not readily undergo fission. The actual design and the construction of an atomic weapon are much less of a technical hurdle. Construction of a uranium atomic bomb requires significant enhancement of natural uranium in the isotope U-235. This is quite a challenge as U-235 and U-238 are chemically identical: no chemical process will separate them. The only way to do so is by exploiting the very small mass difference between them. A colossal factory was constructed in Oak Ridge, TN, during World War II to accomplish this task.

3.15.2 Neutron Activation

A material can be made radioactive by exposure to neutrons. If a material is placed inside a nuclear reactor, it will be subject to intense neutron bombardment. The neutrons may react with the nuclide placed in the reactor to produce a useful radioactive material via the reaction:

$$_Z^A X + {}_0^1 n \rightarrow {}_Z^{A+1} X + \gamma.$$

The production of I-125 is an example of this process:

$$_{54}^{124} Xe + {}_0^1 n \rightarrow {}_{54}^{125} Xe + \gamma$$

$$_{54}^{125} Xe + {}_{-1}^0 \beta \rightarrow {}_{53}^{125} I \quad (EC).$$

The first reaction is a result of the neutron exposure; the second is an electron capture, which gives the desired I-125.

Another example is the production of P-32:

$$_{15}^{31} P + {}_0^1 n \rightarrow {}_{15}^{32} P + \gamma.$$

P-32 decays by β^- emission. The product isotopes of neutron activation are neutron rich and will usually decay by β^- emission.

Let us take Xe-124 as an example of neutron activation. When a large amount of Xe-124 is first placed inside a reactor, there is no I-125. Slowly the amount of I-125 builds up and as it does, it begins to decay.

Eventually the amount of I-125 becomes large enough that the rate of decay becomes equal to the rate of production. A steady state develops in which no additional I-125 will be accumulated. This occurs after several half-lives of the I-125. This situation is analogous to secular equilibrium (see Figure 3.8). In this case the isotope is produced by neutron bombardment (at a constant rate) rather than decay from a parent. Once steady state has been reached, there is no further gain to be made by leaving the isotope in the reactor any longer.

Many of the neutrons inside a nuclear reactor have low energies. They are said to be *thermal neutrons*. Atoms and molecules in a sample of gas at room temperature move randomly with an average kinetic energy of 1/40 eV. When neutrons with high energy (MeV) penetrate matter, they may undergo many collisions with nuclei. Some of these collisions result in immediate absorption of the neutrons into the nucleus. Many other collisions, however, result in a simple transfer of energy, the energetic neutron giving up some of its energy. Eventually those neutrons that do not react will slow down until they have the same random thermal energy as the atoms in the sample. This process is called *moderation*. Slow (thermal) neutrons usually react much more readily with a target nucleus than fast neutrons do.

Cancer researchers are always attempting to find the "magic bullet" that targets malignant cells only and not normal cells. As early as 1936, shortly after the discovery of neutrons, an intriguing idea was proposed called *boron neutron capture therapy* (BNCT).[7] It was discovered that B-10 has a very high probability of capturing thermal neutrons. When B-10 captures a thermal neutron, it briefly becomes B-11, which then disintegrates into Li-7 and an alpha particle. The reaction is:

$$^{10}_{5}B + ^{1}_{0}n \rightarrow ^{11}_{5}B \rightarrow ^{7}_{3}Li + ^{4}_{2}He.$$

Both the Li-7 recoil nucleus and the alpha particle are highly ionizing radiation (and thus very biologically damaging). The range of these particles is quite small; for the Li-7 the range is about 4 μm and for the alpha the range is about 8 μm. A mammalian cell is roughly 10 μm across. Thus the damage done by the Li-7 and alpha particle is highly localized. Boron compounds have been found that are preferentially absorbed by malignant cells. If the region encompassing a tumor is irradiated with thermal neutrons, the dose enhancement in the tumor (over that of surrounding normal tissue) can be substantial. Difficulties in BNCT are in finding boron compounds that are significantly preferentially absorbed by malignant cells and in delivering thermal neutrons to the tumor. Thermal neutrons, by their very nature, are not

[7]Zamenhof, R. G., P. B. Busse, O. K. Harling, and J. T. Corley. "Boron Neutron Capture Therapy," chapter 24 in *The Modern Technology of Radiation Oncology*, J. Van Dyk (Ed.), Madison, WI: Medical Physics Publishing, pp. 981–1020, 1999.

very penetrating. BNCT applications include brain tumors and melanoma. Even after all these years, BNCT is considered experimental therapy. Many researchers are actively working on developing the promise of this form of therapy.

3.15.3 Particle Accelerators

A particle accelerator is a device that will accelerate charged particles to high energies. The charged particles are electrons, protons, or other nuclei (such as deuterons). Particle accelerators rely on electric fields to provide the accelerating force. There are many different types of particle accelerators, such as linear accelerators (linacs), cyclotrons, betatrons, microtrons, synchrotrons, etc. Each of these works by somewhat different principles and each has advantages and disadvantages for different applications. The common feature is that they all rely on an electric field to exert a force on the charged particles to be accelerated.

For the production of radionuclides, heavy (relative to the electron) positively charged particles (protons, deuterons, etc.) can be used to bombard nuclei and cause nuclear reactions. For a nuclear reaction to occur, the particle must approach the nucleus closely enough so that the nuclear force can act between them. For this to happen, a charged particle must have a very high energy because it must overcome the long range Coulomb repulsion between itself and the nucleus.

An example of the production of a radionuclide by a cyclotron is the bombardment of N-14 by deuterons:

$$^{14}_{7}\text{N} + ^{2}_{1}\text{H} \rightarrow ^{15}_{8}\text{O} + ^{1}_{0}\text{n}.$$

When positive charge is added to a stable nucleus, the product tends to decay by either electron capture or positron emission. O-15 decays by positron emission and is used in PET. PET facilities require a cyclotron on site (or close by) to produce the needed short-lived positron emitters.

Chapter Summary

- **Radionuclides** (sometimes called radioisotopes) are characterized by their atomic number, Z, which determines their chemical properties, and by their atomic mass number, A, which indicates the number of *nucleons* (neutrons plus protons) in the nucleus. The notation used for radionuclides is $^A_Z X$, where X is the chemical symbol of the element. The number of neutrons, N, in a nucleus is $N = A - Z$.

- **Isotopes** are chemically identical; they have the same Z but different A; they differ only by the number of neutrons in the nucleus.

- **Memory Aid**

Memory Aid	
isoto*pe*	same number of *p*rotons *(Z)*
isob*ar*	same number of nucleons *(A)*
isoto*ne*	same number of *n*eutrons
iso*m*er	*m*etastable state

- **Atomic mass unit:** u is one-twelfth the mass of a $^{12}_6 C$ *atom* $= 1.66 \times 10^{-27}$ kg. This corresponds to a rest mass energy of about 930 MeV.

- The **rest mass energy** of an electron is approximately 0.5 MeV, whereas the rest mass energy of a neutron or proton is about 940 MeV—about 2000 times larger.

- **Strong nuclear force:** A very-short-range force between nucleons that holds the atomic nucleus together against the mutual repulsion of the positively charged protons.

- **Nuclear binding energy:** Energy necessary to completely separate all protons and neutrons in a nucleus from one another. Equivalently, the energy released when free neutrons and protons come together to form a nucleus. Average binding energy per nucleon is about 8 MeV for most nuclei. Light nuclei have a lower than average binding energy.

- **Nuclear stability:** For low atomic number $N \approx Z$ for stable nuclei. For $Z \gtrsim 20$, $Z < N$ for stability.

- When a radionuclide X decays to another species D, X is called the **parent** and D is called the **daughter.** When radioisotopes decay, radiation is emitted. This radiation is in the form of either beta particles (also called beta rays: either electrons or positrons), alpha particles (helium nuclei), or gamma or x-rays.

- Let N be the **number of atoms** of species X in a radioactive sample at time t and let ΔN be the change in the number of atoms in this sample in a time interval Δt. The rate of decay of species X can then be written as $\Delta N/\Delta t$. The rate of decay of a radioisotope at any given time is proportional to the number of atoms, N, present at that time:

$$\frac{\Delta N}{\Delta t} \approx -\lambda N.$$

(This equation is only correct for time intervals in which ΔN is much smaller than N.) The proportionality constant, λ, is called the **decay constant.** It is characteristic of the specific radionuclide X.

- The **activity,** A, is the rate of radioactive decay:

$$A = \left| \frac{\Delta N}{\Delta t} \right| \approx \lambda N.$$

- The activity declines with time as the number of atoms, N, decreases:

$$A = A_0 e^{-\lambda t}.$$

where A_0 is the activity at time $t = 0$. This equation is always valid.

- **SI units of activity:**

$$1 \text{ decay/sec} = 1 \text{ becquerel} = 1 \text{ Bq.}$$

- The old unit of activity is the curie (Ci). 1 Ci is approximately the activity of 1 gm of radium.

$$1 \text{ Ci} = 3.7 \times 10^{10} \text{ Bq} \qquad 1 \text{ mCi} = 37 \text{ MBq}$$

- Typical therapy activities:
  - Brachytherapy
    - Low dose rate: mCi
    - High dose rate: ~10 Ci

  - Teletherapy
    - Co-60 unit: ~10,000 Ci

- The **half-life,** $T_{1/2}$, is the amount of time it takes the activity to fall to one-half of its initial value. The half-life is an intrinsic property of a specific radionuclide and is independent of external conditions such as temperature, pressure, chemical bonding, etc.
  The half-life is inversely proportional to λ:

$$T_{1/2} \approx \frac{0.693}{\lambda}.$$

- **Radioactive decay problems** can be solved using the equation:

$$A = A_0 \left(\frac{1}{2}\right)^n = A_0 \left(0.5\right)^n.$$

where n is the number of half lives: $n = t/T_{1/2}$ (t is the amount of time elapsed). This equation is equivalent to the exponential equation above, but it is easier to use.

- The mean-life, τ, of a radioisotope is the time that it would take the sample to decay completely if the decay rate (or, equivalently, the activity) were to remain constant:

$$\tau = \frac{1}{\lambda} \approx 1.44\, T_{1/2}.$$

- An equation that is sometimes useful is:

$$A_0 \tau = N_0,$$

where N_0 is the initial number of atoms in the sample and the activity A_0 is in units of becquerel (Bq).

- There are three principle modes of **radioactive decay:**

  - **Alpha decay:**

$$^A_Z X \rightarrow\ ^{A-4}_{Z-2} D + ^4_2 He.$$

  An example of alpha decay is the decay of radium:

$$^{226}_{88} Ra \rightarrow\ ^{222}_{86} Rn + ^4_2 He.$$

  All alpha particles from a given radioisotope emerge with the same energy.

  - **Electromagnetic decay:** There are different ways in which the energy can be emitted:

    ◦ *Nuclear de-excitation:* Emission of a gamma

    ◦ *Internal conversion (IC):* An atomic electron is ejected from the atom. Consequences of missing atomic electron are:
      - Characteristic x-ray emission
      - Auger electron emission: Vacancy in inner shell is filled by an outer shell electron and another outer shell electron is ejected

    ◦ *Isomeric transition:* A special type of electromagnetic decay, where the parent is in a long-lived excited state, emission of a gamma. An example is the decay of technetium:

$$^{99m} Tc \rightarrow\ ^{99} Tc + \gamma,$$

    where the m indicates a long-lived or metastable state.

– Beta Decay

- Emission of an electron (also called a beta minus; β^-) by the atomic nucleus:

$$^A_Z X \rightarrow ^A_{Z+1}D + ^0_{-1}\beta + ^0_0\bar{\nu}.$$

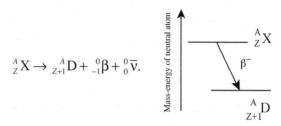

Beta particles emerge with a spectrum of energies ranging from 0 to some maximum value, T_{max}. The average energy of an emitted beta is approximately $T_{max}/3$. During beta decay antineutrinos ($\bar{\nu}$) are also emitted. These neutral particles carry away energy but do not deposit dose. Neutron rich nuclei undergo beta decay.

- Emission of a positron (also called a beta plus, β^+) by the atomic nucleus:

$$^A_Z X \rightarrow ^A_{Z-1}D + ^0_{+1}\beta + ^0_0\nu.$$

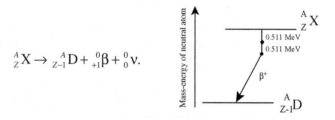

The positron will subsequently annihilate with an electron, producing a pair of 0.5 MeV annihilation photons that travel in opposite directions. These photons can be used for PET imaging. A neutrino is also emitted during the process of beta decay. Neutron deficient nuclei decay either by positron emission or by electron capture.

- Electron Capture: This is a process in which the nucleus captures an atomic electron (usually K-shell). This process competes with positron emission:

$$^A_Z X + ^0_{-1}\beta \rightarrow ^A_{Z-1}D + ^0_0\nu.$$

- **Radioactive equilibrium:** X decays to D with half-life T_p and D in turn decays to G with half-life T_d. If $T_p > T_d$, then A_D/A_X will approach a constant value after some interval of time.

- **Secular equilibrium:** $T_p \gg T_d$; an example is:

$$_{88}^{226}\text{Ra} \rightarrow {}_{86}^{222}\text{Rn} + {}_{2}^{4}\text{He};$$

$A_D = A_X$ occurs after about 30 days for radium sealed in a container.

- **Transient equilibrium:** $T_p \gtrsim T_d$; an example is:

$$_{42}^{99}\text{Mo} \rightarrow {}_{43}^{99}\text{Tc} + {}_{-1}^{0}\beta + {}_{0}^{0}\overline{\text{v}}. \quad A_D/A_X = 0.945 \text{ at equilibrium.}$$

- **Sources of radionuclides:**

  – Naturally occurring.

  – Fission byproducts: radioisotope fragments from fission process of U-235; examples are Cs-137 and Sr-90. These are neutron rich and therefore often decay by β^- emission.

  – Neutron activation: material is placed in nuclear reactor and bombarded by neutrons; examples are I-125, P-32. These are neutron rich and therefore often decay by β^- emission.

  – Particle accelerators (e.g., cyclotron): material is bombarded with charged particles, usually protons; example is production of O-15. This material usually decays by positron emission or electron capture; used for PET.

Problems

1. Compare I-131 with I-125 in terms of their chemical properties, Z values, and the number of neutrons.

2. a. What is the atomic mass unit (u) and how is it defined?
   b. Which of the following have an atomic mass near 1 u?
      i.   Electron
      ii. Proton
      iii. Neutron
      iv. Hydrogen nucleus
      v.   Deuterium nucleus

3. a. Compute the binding energy for an alpha particle ($^4_2$He nucleus). Express your answer in units of MeV. Consult the table below.

Particle	Mass (u)
Proton	1.00727
Neutron	1.00866
Electron	0.00055
Deuteron	2.01355
Alpha particle	4.00151

   b. Compute the average binding energy per nucleon for $^4_2$He. Does the value agree with Figure 3.1?
   c. Determine whether energy would be required or released if an alpha particle were produced by fusion of two deuterons ($^2_1$H). Compute the energy released or required and express your answer in units of MeV.

4. Define activity and define two commonly used units for activity.

5. a. The activity of a source is 298 Bq. Estimate its activity in units of nanocuries (nCi).
   b. Give the range of activities used in radiation therapy.

6. Convert 15 mCi to MBq.

7. Calculate how much the activity of Co-60 decreases in one month. State the answer as a percentage. The half-life of Co-60 is 5.25 years.

8. A 4.0-mCi source with a 2.69-day half-life is implanted into a patient. The prescribed emitted radiation is 2.80×10^{13} disintegrations. Estimate the length of time after which the source has to be removed.

9. A source has a half-life of 12 hours and an initial activity of 10 mCi. After 4 days what is its activity?

10. Calculate the percentage of activity remaining in a source after 10 half-lives.

11. a. A radionuclide decays 1% in one day. Calculate the half-life.
    b. A radionuclide decays 70% in one day. Calculate the half-life.

12. A sample of 10.0 mCi of a radioisotope decays 1.2% in a single day.
    a. What is the activity after one day?
    b. What is the activity after 30 days?

13. A sample of Cs-137 initially contains 1000 atoms.
    a. What is the value of the decay constant for this isotope?
    b. How many Cs-137 atoms does the sample contain after 2 years? Use equation (3.7).
    c. What is the change ΔN in the number of atoms over this time period?
    d. Verify the equation $(\Delta N/\Delta t) \approx -\lambda N$ by substituting the values from parts a through c above, on both sides of the equation.

14. A radioactive source has a half-life of 74 days and an activity of 370 MBq. What was the activity 30 days ago?

15. A radioactive source has a half-life of 60 days. What is the relative activity after one week?

16. An 11-Ci Ir-192 source is received on August 20. Regulatory requirements do not allow use of the source until its activity is 10 Ci or less. On what date will the source reach this activity?

17. A patient had a 25-mCi I-125 permanent seed implant 3 years ago. What is the activity now?

18. For a prostate "seed" implant, I-125 seeds with an activity of 0.350 mCi are needed on the day of the implant. The seeds are to be delivered one week prior to the implant. What activity should the seeds have on the day of delivery?

19. Describe the beta decay process. Explain the energy spectrum of the emitted beta rays. Write down the general equation for β^+ and β^- decay processes and give one example for each case.

20. Describe the processes of electron capture and internal conversion.

21. Explain how a radioactive isotope such as I-125 can emit x-rays as the therapeutic agent along with or instead of gamma rays.

22. The isotope $^{18}_{9}F$ is widely used for PET imaging. It decays by positron emission with a half-life of 110 minutes. What isotope does it decay to? Write the decay equation. You will need to consult a periodic table.

23. What is the predominant decay mode of radioisotopes created by bombarding an element with neutrons? Give an example.

Bibliography

Attix, F. H. *Introduction to Radiological Physics and Radiation Dosimetry*. New York: Wiley InterScience, 1986.

Eisberg, R., and R. Resnick. *Quantum Physics of Atoms, Molecules, Solids, Nuclei, and Particles*. New York: John Wiley and Sons, 1985.

Greene, B. *The Elegant Universe: Superstrings, Hidden Dimensions, and the Quest for the Ultimate Theory*. New York: W. W. Norton & Company, 1999.

Greene, B. *The Fabric of the Cosmos: Space, Time, and the Texture of Reality*. New York: Knopf, 2004.

Johns, H. E., and J. R. Cunningham. *The Physics of Radiology*, Fourth Edition. Springfield, IL: Charles C Thomas, 1983.

Khan, F. M. *The Physics of Radiation Therapy*, Fourth Edition. Philadelphia: Lippincott Williams & Wilkins, 2009.

McGervey, J. D. *Introduction to Modern Physics*, Second Edition. San Diego, CA: Academic Press, 1983.

Pais, A. *Inward Bound: Of Matter and Forces in the Physical World*. New York: Oxford University Press USA, 1986.

Zamenhof, R. G., P. B. Busse, O. K. Harling, and J. T. Corley. "Boron Neutron Capture Therapy," Chapter 24 in *The Modern Technology of Radiation Oncology*, J. Van Dyk (Ed.). Madison, WI: Medical Physics Publishing, pp. 981–1020, 1999.

4 X-Ray Production I: Technology

4.1 Introduction

X-rays were discovered by Wilhelm Conrad Röntgen in November 1895 while he was studying electrical discharges in evacuated tubes. See the section at the end of chapter 5 for the story of the discovery.

There are two main purposes for the production of x-rays in medicine: diagnosis and therapy. The role of diagnostic x-rays is to produce an image that can be interpreted for signs of disease or injury. X-ray photons generated for diagnostic imaging studies typically have average energies in the range of approximately 10 to 50 keV. The purpose of therapeutic x-rays is to treat disease, principally cancer. Therapeutic x-ray photons have energies in the range of approximately 50 keV up to 25 MeV. It should not be surprising that there are differences in the technology used to produce low-energy x-rays and high-energy x-rays. This chapter will concentrate on the technology used to generate low-energy x-rays for both diagnosis and therapy. High-energy (megavoltage) therapeutic x-rays are produced by linear accelerators and these machines will be discussed later in chapter 9. Chapter 5 covers the basic physics of x-ray production, and details pertaining to radiation therapy simulators are discussed in chapter 19.

An x-ray machine has two major components: the x-ray tube and the generator. The x-rays are produced inside the tube and exit the tube through a "window" (see Figure 4.1); the generator supplies voltage and current to the tube. X-rays are created when a beam of electrons, accelerated inside the evacuated x-ray tube, strikes a target at the end of the tube. When the electrons strike the target, a fraction of their kinetic energy is converted to x-rays and the remaining kinetic energy is converted to heat. A vacuum is necessary because otherwise the electrons would be slowed down and deflected by collisions with gas molecules, thus interfering with their acceleration. The electrons must be accelerated through a large potential difference (tens of thousands of volts) because they must gain an amount of kinetic energy sufficient to produce energetic x-ray photons (see section 2.4, *Electromagnetic Spectrum*).

4.2 X-Ray Tubes

X-ray tubes are made out of glass or, in some cases, metal, and they have a window through which the x-rays may easily escape. Electrodes are sealed inside the x-ray tube (see Figure 4.1) and a high potential difference is applied between them. Electrons emitted by one of the electrodes

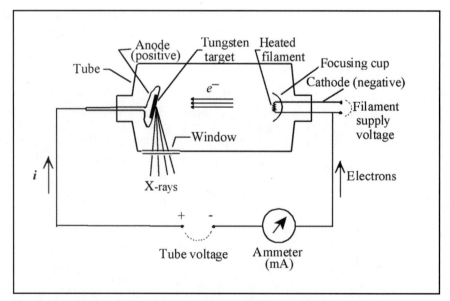

Figure 4.1: A schematic diagram of an x-ray tube and simplified circuitry. A sealed, evacuated tube contains two electrodes: a cathode, which is negative, and an anode, which is positive. Electrons emitted by the cathode filament are accelerated across the tube and strike a target embedded in the anode. As the electrons lose energy in the target, they produce x-rays which escape from the tube through a window.

are accelerated across the tube. The positive electrode is called the *anode* and the negative electrode is called the *cathode*. The x-ray target is embedded in the anode. It is common to call the potential difference between the electrodes in the tube the *tube voltage.*

The anode is commonly made of copper with an embedded tungsten (W) target. The narrow electron beam striking the target produces intense local heating. Copper (Cu) is a good heat conductor and it efficiently conducts heat away from the target. The target is usually tungsten (molybdenum [Mo] is used for mammography). Tungsten is a good choice because of its high melting temperature (3370 °C) and its high atomic number ($Z = 74$). X-ray production efficiency is higher for high Z target materials.

In modern x-ray tubes a filament is used to produce the electrons which are to be accelerated. The filament is electrically heated (like a toaster wire). This causes electrons to "boil off" the surface of the filament in a process called *thermionic emission.* A filament is not absolutely essential (Röntgen didn't have one) but it does give much higher efficiency. The tube current can be increased enormously with a filament.

The work-energy theorem (see section 2.2.3) provides a quantitative relation between the work done, *W*, on the electron of charge *e* in accelerating it between the electrodes, final kinetic energy, *T*, of the electrons striking the target, and the potential difference, *V*, across the tube (see section 2.3.4):

$$W = QV = eV = T. \tag{4.1}$$

If an electron gives up all of its energy in a single event to produce one photon, then that photon will have the maximum possible energy and the minimum possible wavelength:

$$eV = h\nu_{max} = \frac{hc}{\lambda_{min}}, \tag{4.2}$$

where $h\nu_{max}$ is the maximum photon energy and λ_{min} is the corresponding minimum wavelength. If the potential difference, *V*, across the tube is too small, then λ_{min} will not be in the x-ray range of the electromagnetic spectrum.

The number of x-ray photons created in the target is proportional to the number of electrons striking the target. This is, in turn, proportional to the electrical current through the tube. Twice the current will lead to twice the number of x-ray photons. The current must be sufficiently high to produce an x-ray beam of adequate intensity.

The potential difference across the tube may not be constant in time. This depends on the details of the design of the x-ray generator. The electrical current supplied by the power company is alternating current (ac), where the current and the voltage oscillate back and forth in the wires with a frequency of 60 Hz (in the United States). This contrasts with direct current (dc) in which the current always travels in the same direction in the wire. X-ray machine generators have a circuit called a *rectifier*, which converts ac to dc, and there may be some residual ripple in the voltage applied to the electrodes in the x-ray tube. Newer x-ray machines have high-frequency generators that produce minimal ripple. The potential difference across the tube is usually quoted in terms of the maximum value in units of 1000 volts. This is called *kVp*, short for kilovolts-peak.

The kVp is the maximum or peak voltage across the tube. The kVp available may range from 20 to 300 kVp. It is important to understand that kVp is *not* the same as keV; they do not even have the same units. The maximum voltage across the tube is given by the kVp. Electrons cross the tube almost instantaneously. At the instant that the voltage is at its maximum, those electrons accelerated across the tube will have the maximum possible energy. The maximum energy of the electrons, $(keV)_{max}$, is numerically equal to the kVp. Even though they *do* have the same numerical value, they *are not equal* because they do not have the same units.

Diagnostic x-ray machines utilize a potential difference ranging from 20 kVp up to about 120 kVp. There are three classes of therapeutic x-ray beams: superficial, orthovoltage, and megavoltage. Superficial x-ray beams have tube potentials between 50 and 150 kVp and are used to treat skin conditions (see Figure 4.2). Orthovoltage beams are produced by tube potentials between 150 and 300 kVp. Megavoltage beams are produced by linear accelerators. Linear accelerators produce

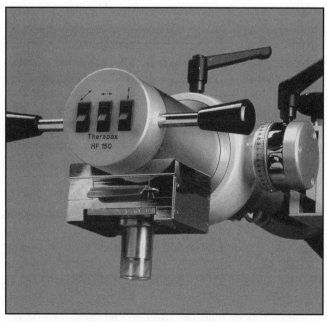

Figure 4.2: The Pantak HF150 superficial therapy x-ray machine. The beam emerges from the cylindrical applicator at the bottom. The tube is inside the housing at the top. (Reprinted from chapter 9 "Kilovoltage X-rays" by P. Biggs et al., Figure 9.3, p. 290, in *The Modern Technology of Radiation Oncology*, J. Van Dyk, Editor. © 1999, with permission.)

x-ray beams by accelerating electrons through the equivalent of a potential difference of one million volts (1 MV) or higher. In this chapter we shall concentrate our attention on the technology of production of diagnostic, superficial, and orthovoltage x-rays.

The region of the target from which x-rays are emitted is called the *focal spot*. To obtain sharp images, it is desirable to have a small focal spot. A large focal spot will lead to blurry images as shown in Figure 4.3. An x-ray radiograph is a "shadow" picture. If the x-ray source is large, the shadow will be fuzzy. The ideal situation would be to have a point source of x-rays.

A trade-off is necessary because a small focal spot produces intense heating, and this leads to a heat dissipation problem. If the heating is sufficiently intense, it can cause melting and damage the target, which can ruin the tube. Modern x-ray tubes can cost about \$15,000.

There are two technical tricks that are used to decrease the target heating and to reduce the apparent size of the focal spot.[1] First, the "apparent" focal spot size can be made smaller than the actual focal spot size by tilting the target at an angle, as shown in Figure 4.4. The "apparent" focal spot size is the size of the focal spot "seen" by the film. This is called the *line focus principle*. If the actual focal spot size is S and the target angle is θ, then the apparent focal spot size is

$$s = S \sin \theta. \tag{4.3}$$

---

[1] Note that the size of the focal spot may depend on the tube current.

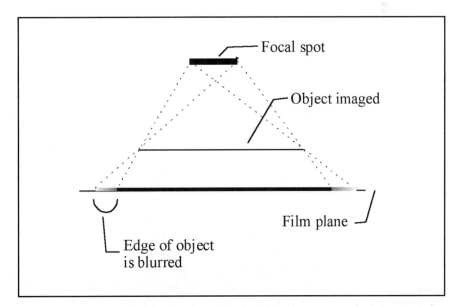

Figure 4.3: A source of x-rays (focal spot) is used to image an object by casting a shadow onto radiographic film. The dotted lines depict x-rays originating from different locations within the focal spot. A large focal spot will lead to significant blurring of the edges.

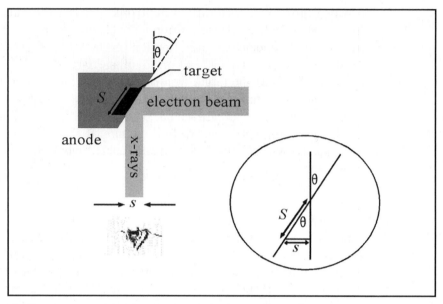

Figure 4.4: The line focus principle. The "apparent" focal spot size *s* can be made smaller than the actual focal spot size *S* by tilting the target at an angle θ. The inset (circle) shows the geometry used to find the relationship between *s* and *S*.

Diagnostic tubes use an angle of between 6 and 17 degrees. Superficial therapy tubes use an angle of about 30 degrees. For diagnostic applications the apparent focal spot size ranges from 0.1×0.1 mm^2 (for mammography) and up to 2×2 mm^2, depending on the design of the tube. A particular x-ray machine may have two focal spot sizes available. The two focal spots are produced by the use of two different filaments. The operator chooses the focal spot based on the image detail needed and the expected heat loading of the tube. For therapy applications a small focal spot size is not as important and focal spot sizes range from 5×5 mm^2 to 7×7 mm^2.

Second, the heat dissipation problem presented by a small focal spot size can be overcome by making the anode in the shape of a disk (as shown in Figure 4.5) and then rotating the disk. The assembly that rotates the disk is called the *rotor*. The tilting of the target is retained by beveling the edge of the disk. The electron beam strikes the edge of the disk and the heat is distributed over the circumference of the disk. Rotor speeds can range from 3000 to 9000 revolutions per minute (rpm). The sound of the spinning rotor can sometimes be heard as a whine from the tube housing (although do not confuse it with fan noise).

There is a variation or gradient in x-ray intensity in going from the anode to the cathode side of the x-ray tube, as illustrated in Figure 4.6. This is called the *heel effect*. The reason for this has to do with absorption of x-rays that are produced in the target. These x-rays must escape from the target. Figure 4.6 shows that the x-rays traverse a smaller amount of target material when escaping toward the cathode. Fewer x-ray photons are absorbed by the target in this case.

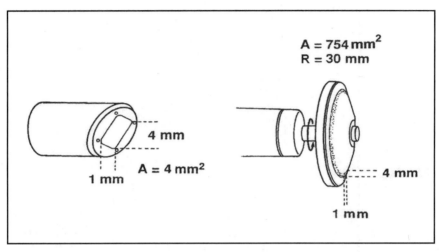

Figure 4.5: The difference between a stationary and a rotating anode. Both anodes have the same apparent focal spot size. The stationary anode has a target area of 4 mm², whereas the rotating anode has a radius of $R = 30$ mm and a target area of 754 mm². The heat energy is spread over an area 200 times larger than for the stationary anode. (Adapted from Figure 10-13, p. 130, *Radiologic Science for Technologists,* Seventh ed., Stewart C. Bushong. © 2001 Mosby, Inc., with permission from Elsevier.)

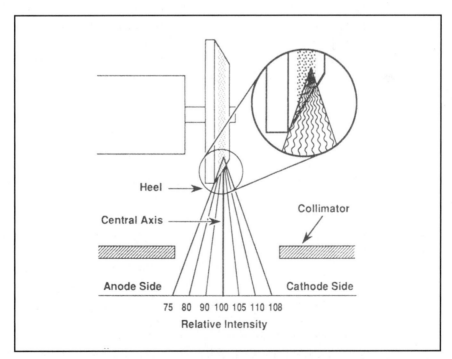

Figure 4.6: The heel effect. The intensity is lower on the anode side than on the cathode side because the x-rays traverse more target material in escaping toward the anode side. (Adapted from Figure 10-20, p. 133, *Radiologic Science for Technologists,* Seventh ed., Stewart C. Bushong. © 2001 Mosby, Inc., with permission from Elsevier.)

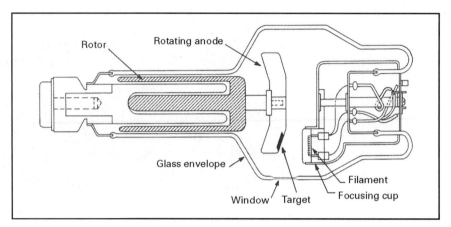

Figure 4.7: A rotating anode x-ray tube. Electrons are emitted from the filament by thermionic emission. These electrons are accelerated across the tube and strike the target. A small fraction of the energy of the electrons is converted to x-rays, which exit the tube through the window at the bottom. Note the angled target used to take advantage of the line focus principle. (Adapted from Figure 10-3, p. 125, *Radiologic Science for Technologists,* Seventh ed., Stewart C. Bushong. © 2001 Mosby, Inc., with permission from Elsevier.)

Figure 4.7 shows a modern rotating anode x-ray tube. The x-ray tube is contained in a protective housing (see Figures 4.8 and 4.9). This housing serves a number of functions. It protects the tube against mechanical shock. It provides some shielding against stray or leakage radiation. The x-rays produced in the target are emitted in almost all directions. A well-channeled or collimated beam of x-rays, which is sometimes called the "useful" beam, is desired for either diagnosis or therapy. X-rays traveling in other directions pose a radiation safety hazard. Appropriately

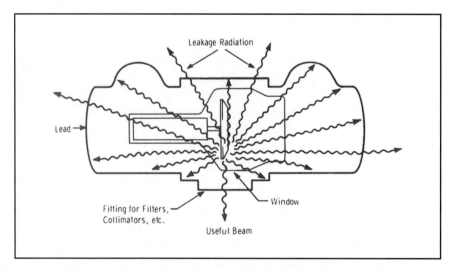

Figure 4.8: Protective housing reduces leakage radiation. (After from Figure 10-2, p. 124, *Radiologic Science for Technologists,* Seventh ed., Stewart C. Bushong. © 2001 Mosby, Inc., with permission from Elsevier.)

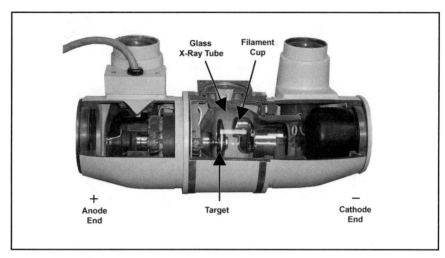

Figure 4.9: X-ray tube inside its housing. (Photo courtesy of Dunlee, © Philips Medical Systems. Modified and printed with permission from Dunlee, a Division of Philips Medical Systems.)

designed housing can help to absorb these unwanted x-rays. The housing can also help to protect the operator from the high voltages applied across the tube. Protective housings sometimes contain oil, which serves two purposes: to provide electrical insulation (oil is a good electrical insulator) and to dissipate heat (the oil absorbs heat and carries it away from the tube).

4.3 Therapy X-Ray Tubes

The design considerations for an x-ray tube for superficial or orthovoltage therapy are different from those for diagnostic x-ray machines. Therapy tubes do not have a rotating anode. Focal spot size is not critical for therapy and therefore these tubes have a larger spot size—5 mm is typical. The instantaneous heating rate is lower; these tubes are designed to be run continuously for a relatively long period of time. Newer therapy tubes are compact, water-cooled, and constructed from metal and ceramic (see Figure 4.10). Therapy tubes with electron beams having energy above 200 keV have a hooded anode. At these energies the primary electrons that strike the target eject secondary electrons from the target material. These secondary electrons could reach the wall and accumulate there. These charges would distort the electric field that accelerates the primary electrons and interfere with the focus of primary electrons on the target. The secondary electrons would also produce unwanted x-rays when they strike the wall of the tube. The copper of the hooded anode stops the secondary electrons and any x-rays produced by them. In summary, therapy tubes have: (1) a larger focal spot size; (2) no rotating anode; and (3) a hooded anode.

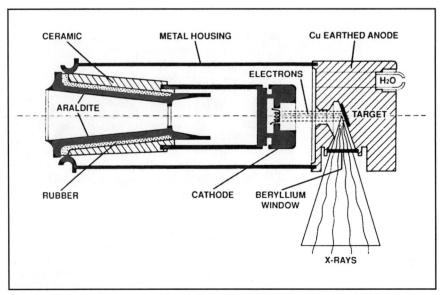

Figure 4.10: A metal ceramic x-ray tube for kilovoltage radiation therapy. The high-voltage cable (not shown) enters at the left. The Araldite®, rubber, and ceramic materials provide electrical insulation. The target is tungsten embedded in copper. The anode, which is grounded, is water cooled. Note that the copper forms a hood around the target. (Reprinted from *Radiotherapy Physics: In Practice,* Second edition, J. R. Williams and D. I. Thwaites, Editors. Figure 6.1, p. 100, © 2000 Oxford University Press, with permission from Oxford University Press, USA.)

4.4 X-Ray Film and Screens

When radiographic film is exposed to x-rays and processed, the film is blackened. It is important to understand that radiographs are negative images. Dark regions are regions that have been exposed to a lot of x-rays, and the light regions are regions that have been exposed to relatively few x-rays. This means that a film that is too black is overexposed.

X-ray film consists of a film base that is coated on one or both sides with an emulsion (see Figure 4.11) of silver halide crystals (grains). The film base is made from a blue-tinted translucent plastic. It is designed to be flexible and relatively transparent. The emulsion is a silver halide (silver bromide is common) compound 3 to 5 μm thick. The film used in radiation therapy departments is typically 14 × 17 in.

Film is not an efficient means for detecting x-rays. When a piece of film is exposed to x-rays, most of the x-rays go right through the film without making any change to the film. Film is, however, very sensitive to visible light. For this reason, diagnostic x-ray films are usually used with an intensifying screen. The intensifying screen converts some of the x-ray energy to light, which in turn exposes the film. The film is placed inside a light-tight cassette (see Figure 4.12) which has an intensifying screen built into it. The film type must be matched to the screen used in the cassettes. The use of a screen reduces the radiation dose to

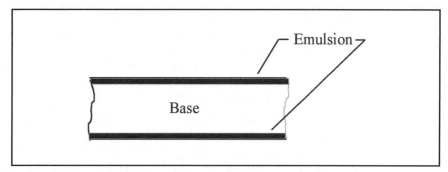

Figure 4.11: The construction of radiographic film. A light-sensitive emulsion is coated on one or both sides of a plastic film base. The relative thickness of the emulsion has been highly exaggerated for illustration purposes.

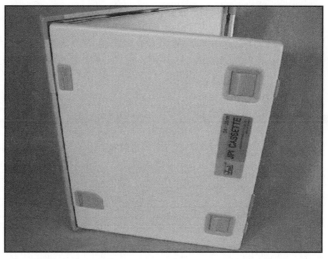

Figure 4.12: An x-ray film cassette. The cassette opens on the right and the film is placed inside. The cassette is "light tight." The screen can be seen inside the cassette (white area at the top of the photograph). (Courtesy of Radco Imaging Technologies, Inc., Midland, TX)

the patient and shortens the exposure time (reducing any blurring from patient motion). The purpose of a screen for megavoltage therapy portal imaging is somewhat different. This will be discussed in chapter 19.

It must be noted that digital imaging is having the same effect on radiography as it is in the world of photography. Digital cameras are rapidly replacing cameras that use film. It is anticipated that digital x-ray imaging will eventually supersede the use of film as well.

Radiographic films are shadow pictures. We have already seen one way in which the shadow can be blurred, due to non-zero focal spot size. In addition, image contrast is degraded by radiation scattering inside the patient. Radiation scattering occurs whenever the direction of travel of an x-ray photon changes as a result of an interaction with matter. Radiation that is not scattered is called *primary radiation*. We will discuss the details of this in chapter 6, but for now it is enough to know that this process occurs and that it leads to a loss of contrast in the radiographic image. This is illustrated in Figure 4.13, which shows a point source of radiation. Most of the rays emanating from the point source are either absorbed (and therefore cast a shadow) or travel straight through the patient to expose the film. It is easy to see that the scattered radiation will lead to a loss of image quality.

One way of reducing the amount of scatter is with the use of a grid, as shown in Figure 4.13. The grid is made of thin lead strips separated by x-ray–transparent spacers. The thickness of the strips is highly exaggerated in the figure. Typically the distance between the grid strips is 0.25 to 0.30 mm and the height of the strips is approximately 2.0 mm (see Figure 4.14). The lead strips intercept and absorb most of the scatter radiation. The grid can be placed above the film cassette or inside the cassette. If the grid is inside the film cassette, the cassette must be oriented with the proper side facing the focal spot of the tube. If the cassette is upside down, the grid will not function as intended. The price that is paid for the use of a grid is that some of the radiation is blocked from reaching the film. Therefore, the radiation dose to the patient must increase somewhat. If the strips are thin, this may not present a serious problem. If you carefully examine a film taken with a grid, you can see fine lines on the film caused by the grid strips.

Different types of arrangement of the grid pattern are possible. The illustration in Figure 4.13 shows a focused grid and Figure 4.14 shows a parallel grid. Sometimes a crossed pattern or some other arrangement

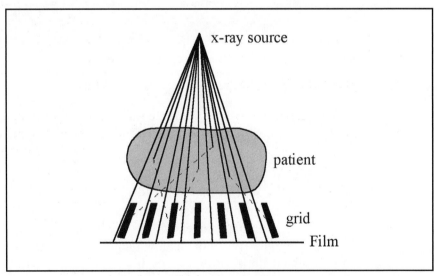

Figure 4.13: The use of a grid minimizes the amount of scatter radiation reaching the film. Scatter is illustrated by the dashed lines. This is a "focused" grid. The dimensions of the grid are highly exaggerated for illustration purposes. The thickness of each strip is typically 0.05 mm. Note that a focused grid must be properly oriented with respect to the focal spot.

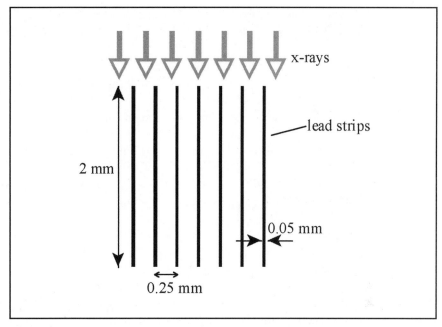

Figure 4.14: Cross section of a portion of a parallel (unfocused) radiographic grid designed to increase contrast. The diagram shows typical dimensions for the lead strips.

will be used. The ideal grid would remove all the scattered radiation but no primary radiation. This would result in the best film contrast with no increase in patient exposure. In reality, the grid will not remove all of the scatter and it will remove some of the primary radiation, requiring some increase in exposure to the patient to make up for the loss of primary radiation.

4.5 X-Ray Generator

In this section we will concentrate on diagnostic x-ray units and radiotherapy simulators; however, many of the comments also pertain to superficial and orthovoltage generators. The x-ray generator supplies the needed voltages and currents to the x-ray tube; it must supply enough voltage to accelerate electrons between the cathode and the anode. The generator has to supply enough current to ensure that a sufficient number of electrons cross the tube, so that the intensity of the x-ray beam will be adequate. The generator also must supply the voltage to the filament for thermionic emission.

To make a radiographic exposure, there are three fundamental quantities that must be set at the generator console: the tube voltage (measured in kVp), the tube current (measured in milliamperes [mA]), and the time of the exposure (usually measured in seconds [s]). We will consider each of these parameters in more detail shortly. A good-quality radiograph depends on the proper choice of these values. This combination of settings is often referred to as the *technique*. As an example, for an anterior-posterior (AP) abdominal film on a particular x-ray unit, using a specific screen-film combination, the technique might be 80 kVp, 200 mA, and 0.4 s. The technique generally varies somewhat from one x-ray machine to another.

The current through the tube (*i,* as in Figure 4.1) is usually specified in units of milliamperes, and is directly related to the number of electrons that cross the tube and strike the target.

The length of time that the tube emits x-rays is set at the generator console. The units are expressed in seconds. A typical radiograph may only require a few tenths of one second. Longer time exposures risk image blurring from patient motion. The time settings available can range from 2 ms to 5 s.

The x-ray "output" is proportional to the number of x-ray photons produced by the use of a particular technique. The degree to which film is blackened by x-rays is related to the output. For a given radiographic exposure, the number of electrons crossing the tube, N_e, is equal to the charge that is accelerated across the tube divided by the charge of a single electron: $N_e = Q/e$. The charge Q is equal to the tube current multiplied by the time for the exposure: $Q = i\,t$ and thus $N_e = i\,t/e$. The important point to note here is that the total number of electrons striking the target (and hence the total number of x-ray photons emitted) is directly proportional to the product of the tube current and the time of the exposure. This product is often measured in mA $\times$ s and is often written "mAs". The mAs for the abdominal film mentioned above is 200 mA $\times$ 0.4 s = 80 mAs. The current and the time can be changed independently of one another; however, if the product remains the same, the x-ray output will remain the same.

The above discussion assumes that the kVp stays the same. How does the output change when the kVp changes? Unfortunately, there is no simple answer to this question. The number of x-ray photons emitted by the target is sensitive to the kVp value. A small increase in the kVp leads to a large increase in output. It is approximately true that the x-ray output is proportional to a power of the kVp:

$$\text{x-ray ``output''} \propto (\text{kVp})^a \times \text{mAs} \quad \text{(Approximate)},$$

where the value of a ranges from 2 to 3 and depends on the specific tube.

The appropriate kVp, mA, and time settings depend on the body part to be imaged, the distance of the focal spot from the film, the type of screen-film combination in use, etc. The factors involved in choosing a proper technique are complex and are part of the art and science of radiography. Repeat films are necessary when the choice of technique is suboptimal. An alternative to completely manual settings is the use of automatic exposure control (AEC). In AEC the x-ray machine measures the amount of radiation passing through the film and terminates the exposure when the amount is sufficient to produce an acceptable degree of darkness on the film. When using AEC the technologist sets the kVp and mA, and the x-ray machine terminates the exposure when the film has received sufficient radiation for an acceptable image. The radiation is sensed by x-ray–detecting ionization chambers (see chapter 8) behind the film cassette. AEC can automatically compensate for differences in patient thickness and film distance.

With heavy use, overheating of the anode, tube, and tube housing become a threat. An x-ray tube can be ruined by overheating. There is a limit on the heat deposited in the anode by a single exposure. If this limit is exceeded, the heat production can be sufficiently high to cause some melting of the target material at the focal spot. This may produce a pitting in the target. A typical example of the limit for a single exposure is: at 120 kVp the current should not exceed 400 mA for the large focal spot. The anode cools rapidly after an exposure, but the tube and the housing do not. The tube and the housing can overheat depending on the number of exposures, the time between exposures, and the technique. Charts and graphs (called "tube rating charts") are available that provide guidance to the technologist regarding the limits of heating.

Chapter Summary

- **X-rays** are produced when electrons are accelerated between the cathode (negative electrode) and anode (positive electrode) in an evacuated metal or glass tube and strike the anode at the end of the tube. When the electrons strike the target (embedded in the anode), a large fraction of their energy is dissipated as heat; the remainder is converted to x-rays. The cathode has a heated filament that gets very hot like a toaster wire. The electrons are boiled off (thermionic emission) the cathode filament and are accelerated toward the anode.

- **kVp** (kilovolts-peak) is the peak potential difference across the tube in units of 1000 volts. Diagnostic x-rays are produced with kVp in the range between 20 to 120 kVp. Radiation therapy simulators utilize diagnostic x-ray tubes.

- **Diagnostic X-rays** (therapy simulator)

  – 20 kVp to 120 kVp

- **Therapy X-rays**

  – Superficial: 50 to 150 kVp (treat skin conditions)

  – Orthovoltage: 150 to 300 kVp

  – Megavoltage: 1 MV and above

- **Target:** Most diagnostic tubes use tungsten for the target material (molybdenum is used for mammography)

  – Tungsten (W):

    1. High melting point (3370 °C); electron beam produces high heating rate.

    2. High $Z = 74$; high efficiency for x-ray production.

- **Focal Spot:** The spot on the target from which x-rays are emitted. An x-ray image is a "shadow" picture. If the x-ray source is large, the shadow will be fuzzy. The ideal situation would be to have a point source of x-rays:

  – Small focal spot for sharp images (not so important for therapy)

  – Small focal spot produces intense heating, heat dissipation problem, can cause melting and damage target

    ○ Two tricks used to reduce heating: (1) anode rotation and (2) line focus principle

    ○ Apparent focal spot sizes:
      – Diagnostic: 0.1×0.1 mm^2 (mammography) to 2×2 mm^2
      – Therapy: 5×5 mm^2 to 7×7 mm^2

- **Rotating Anode:** Heat dissipation problem presented by small focal spot size can be overcome by making the anode in the shape of a disk and then rotating the disk (see Figure 4.5). The x-ray beam strikes the edge of the disk and the heat is distributed over the circumference of the disk. Rotation speeds range from 3000 to 9000 rpm.

- **Line Focus Principle:** The "apparent" focal spot size = size of focal spot "seen" by the film. The apparent focal spot size can be made smaller than the actual focal spot size by tilting the target at an angle (see Figure 4.4). Diagnostic tubes use an angle of 6 to 17 degrees. Therapy tubes use an angle of about 30 degrees. The apparent focal spot size is given by $s = S \sin \theta$, where S is the actual spot size and θ is the angle between the face of the target and the vertical.

- **Heel Effect:** There is a gradient in intensity in going from the anode to the cathode side of the x-ray tube; the intensity is higher on the cathode side of the tube.

- **Therapy tubes compared to diagnostic tubes:**

  1. Larger focal spot size.

  2. No rotating anode necessary.

  3. Hooded anode: Absorbs secondary electrons ejected from anode by primary electron beam.

- **X-ray film** consists of a plastic base coated on one or both sides with a silver halide emulsion, 3 to 5 µm thick. X-ray film is usually placed inside a light-tight cassette. The cassette contains an intensifying screen in close contact with the film. The screen converts x-rays to visible light. Film is more sensitive to visible light.

- **Screen:**

  1. Reduces radiation dose to patient.

  2. Shortens exposure time.

- **Grid:** Thin lead strips used to minimize scatter radiation reaching the film. Scatter results in a loss of image contrast.

- **X-Ray Generator:** Supplies the needed voltages and currents to the x-ray tube.

  1. Supplies voltage to accelerate electrons across the tube.

  2. Supplies voltage to the filament to "boil off" electrons.

- **Technique:** Combination of kVp, mA, and time (or mA × time = mAs) suitable for a high-quality image. Technologists sometimes adjust these settings manually or they use automatic exposure control (AEC).

- X-ray "output" $\propto (kVp)^a \times$ mAs (Approximate), where the value of a is between 2 and 3.

Problems

1. What is a rotating anode and why is it used in some x-ray tubes?

2. What is the ratio between the apparent size and actual size of the focal spot in a tube with a target angle of _____ ?
    a. 6°
    b. 17°
    c. 30°

3. What is the heel effect and why does it occur?

4. What is the purpose of the x-ray tube filament found in an x-ray circuit? How does it work?

5. What are the benefits of the use of an intensifying screen for diagnostic x-ray film imaging?

6. What is the maximum energy photon emitted by an x-ray tube having a tube potential of 100 kVp?

7. What material is usually used for the target of an x-ray tube? Why is this material a good choice?

8. An x-ray technologist makes an exposure at 100 kVp, 100 mA, 0.5 s. The film darkness is acceptable, but the image is blurry because the patient is fidgeting. The technologist decides to reduce the time to 0.2 s. What mA should be chosen to keep the film darkness the same?

9. Draw a diagram like Figure 4.13 showing the effect of orienting a film cassette with the grid upside down. Why is it important to orient the grid properly?

10. Carefully examine an x-ray film taken with the use of a grid. Can you see the grid lines? A magnifying glass may help.

11. If you have access to an x-ray unit (a conventional radiation therapy simulator will do fine), take an image of an interesting object of your choice. You may need to ask for help from an x-ray technologist or a physicist. Ask someone to show you how the film is processed. Record the technique on the film (kVp, mA, and time). If you are in a classroom setting, take the film to class and ask the other students to guess what it is. Discuss the features of each student's film as they relate to the object x-rayed.

Bibliography

Bushong, S. C. *Radiologic Science for Technologists,* Eighth Edition. New York: Mosby, Inc. 2004.

Curry, T. S. III, J. E. Dowdey, and R. C. Murray, Jr. *Christensen's Physics of Diagnostic Radiology,* Fourth Edition. Philadelphia: Lippincott Williams and Wilkins, 1990.

Johns, H. E., and J. R. Cunningham. *The Physics of Radiology,* Fourth Edition. Charles C Thomas, 1983.

Pizzutiello, R. J., and J. E. Cullinan. *Introduction to Medical Radiographic Imaging.* Rochester, NY: Eastman Kodak Company, 1993.

5 X-Ray Production II: Basic Physics and Properties of Resulting X-Rays

5.1 Production of X-Rays: Microscopic Physics

When an electron strikes the target of an x-ray tube (or the target in a linear accelerator), it interacts with the matter in the target. On a microscopic level there are only two entities that the electron can interact with: atomic electrons or the atomic nucleus.[1] We will consider each of these two interactions in turn.

---

[1] Very high-energy electrons can interact with individual nucleons, but that process does not play an important role in this context.

5.1.1 Characteristic X-Rays

When a high-energy electron interacts with atomic electrons in the target of an x-ray–producing device, there are two broad categories of subsequent events, which depend on whether the incoming electron interacts with an outer or an inner shell electron.

Outer shell electrons can be excited to higher-level energy states. They will subsequently drop back to their original states and emit low-energy photons in the process. These low-energy photons will be absorbed very quickly inside the target material. The energy of these photons will be converted into random motion of the atoms in the target; i.e., heat. Another possibility is that an outer shell electron can be ejected from the atom (i.e., the atom is ionized). The ejected electron will move through the target material; it may collide with other atoms giving up some of its energy to the random motion of these atoms—heat again. Eventually it will find another atom that is missing an outer shell electron and it will "recombine" with that atom emitting a low-energy photon in the process. The energy of this photon will ultimately be absorbed, contributing once again to heat production.

Occasionally a high-energy bombarding electron will eject an inner shell electron (e.g., K or L shell). There will then be a vacancy that can be filled by outer shell electrons dropping down (see Figure 5.1). Inner shell electrons are very tightly bound. The energy released when outer shell electrons drop down to fill an inner shell vacancy will be high, particularly for a material with a high atomic number. Many of the photons emitted in the downward cascade will be of sufficiently high energy to be classified as x-rays. Some of the higher energy x-rays may be able to escape from the target without being absorbed. These x-rays will have discrete energies (monoenergetic spectral lines), which are

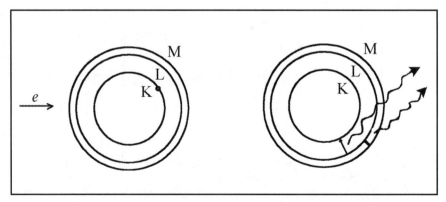

Figure 5.1: On the left, a high-energy bombarding electron ejects an electron from the K shell of an atom. On the right, an L shell electron drops down to occupy the vacancy in the K shell. This in turn leaves a vacancy in the L shell, which is now filled by an M shell electron and so on. The result of this downward cascade of electrons is the emission of x-rays with discrete energies that are *characteristic* of the particular element.

characteristic of the atomic species from which they are emitted and are unique for each element. The emission of characteristic x-rays is sometimes called *x-ray fluorescence*.[2] In order for the emission of characteristic x-rays to occur, the bombarding electrons must have sufficient energy to eject an inner shell atomic electron, usually a K or L shell electron. For tungsten the K shell binding energy is 69.5 keV. The emission of characteristic x-rays may also occur following radioactive decay by electron capture or internal conversion. The photoelectric effect (see chapter 6) can also lead to characteristic x-ray emission. Figure 5.2 shows the discrete spectrum for transitions to the K shell in tungsten. The energies of transition to the K shell are listed in Table 5.1 (see Figure 2.16). Transitions from the L shell have the lowest energy because this shell is the "closest" to the K shell. Transitions from higher shells have progressively higher energies. The *probability* of transitions from higher shells is lower and therefore these lines have lower amplitudes.

In the event of an L shell vacancy, emission of fluorescence is less likely than for the K shell and the energy of those transitions is considerably less than for the K shell. Therefore, L shell lines are of little importance.

Only a small fraction (<<1%) of the bombarding electron energy appears in the form of characteristic x-rays. Most of the energy is dissipated either as heat or as bremsstrahlung x-rays, which are discussed in the next section.

---

[2] An alternative possibility is Auger electron emission.

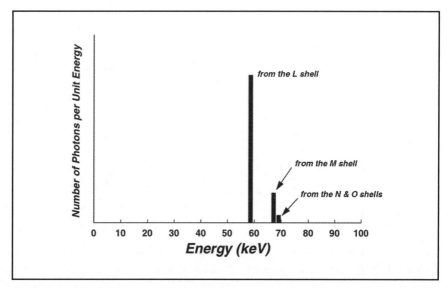

Figure 5.2: Characteristic x-ray spectrum (line spectrum) from transitions to the K shell in tungsten. The transitions from the N and O shells are so close together in energy that they have been combined into a single line.

Table 5.1: Characteristic K Shell X-Rays from Tungsten

Transition From	Average Energy[a] (keV)	Relative Number of Photons
L	58.6	100
M	67.2	20
N, O	69.1	5

[a]This is an average over the different subshells that the electron initially occupies.

5.1.2 Bremsstrahlung Emission

If a bombarding electron passes closely enough to the atomic nucleus, it may interact directly with the nucleus rather than the atomic electrons in the atom (see Figure 5.3). In this case the electron will be deflected in its motion by the nucleus. The velocity vector of the electron will change. The electron will therefore be subject to an acceleration (actually a deceleration). The theory of electricity and magnetism says that an accelerated electrical charge will radiate electromagnetic waves. An example of this is provided by a radio transmission antenna. You have probably seen radio transmission towers, which are often visible from the roadway. An electrical charge or current oscillates back and forth in these towers and produces a relatively long wavelength electromagnetic wave that you can detect with your radio receiver. An electron that has a close encounter with an atomic nucleus also emits electromagnetic radiation. This radiation is called *bremsstrahlung,* which means "braking radiation" in German. This radiation can be of very short wavelength, i.e., x-rays.

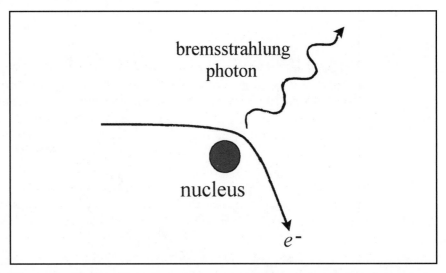

Figure 5.3: When a bombarding electron passes close to an atomic nucleus, it is deflected and a bremsstrahlung (or braking radiation) photon is emitted.

Let us call the initial kinetic energy of the electron as it enters the target T_0. The energy loss by the electron, ΔT, is equal to the energy of the photon emitted in the bremsstrahlung process. The photon energy is $h\nu = hc/\lambda$ and therefore

$$\Delta T = \frac{hc}{\lambda}. \tag{5.1}$$

Usually in any one encounter with a nucleus, an electron loses only a fraction of its kinetic energy. An electron may have many encounters with a nucleus before losing all of its kinetic energy and therefore any given electron may emit many bremsstrahlung photons.

The electrons that strike the target may have an energy that varies with time if the voltage across the tube varies with time. Let us denote the maximum kinetic energy of electrons striking the target as $(T_0)_{max}$. The numerical value of $(T_0)_{max}$ in keV is the same as the numerical value of the kVp. Note that we do not say that $(T_0)_{max}$ is *equal* to the kVp because they are different physical quantities.

The maximum possible x-ray photon energy emitted as bremsstrahlung will be produced by electrons that strike the target with maximum kinetic energy *and* which come to rest in a *single* interaction. The maximum photon energy is $\Delta T = (T_0)_{max} = hc/\lambda_{min}$ and therefore $\lambda_{min} = hc/(T_0)_{max}$. The value of the minimum possible wavelength, λ_{min}, can be expressed in nanometers by inserting the value of h and by substituting the numerical value of the kVp for $(T_0)_{max}$:

$$\lambda_{min} = \frac{1.24}{kVp} \, nm. \tag{5.2}$$

5.2 X-Ray Spectrum

The x-rays produced by the bremsstrahlung process can have any energy between 0 and $(T_0)_{max}$. This is in contrast to characteristic x-rays, which can have only discrete energies. The spectrum resulting from bremsstrahlung is a *continuous* spectrum. In an x-ray target both bremsstrahlung and characteristic x-ray production can occur. The x-ray spectrum produced by both of these processes is shown in Figure 5.4. The horizontal axis is the photon energy and the vertical axis represents the number of photons per unit energy interval. The number of photons emitted over some energy interval is simply the area under the curve over that energy interval. The dashed line labeled "Unfiltered" is the theoretical bremsstrahlung spectrum expected if none of the x-rays were absorbed in escaping from the target. The maximum photon energy corresponds to the kVp across the tube. In a real target some x-rays will be absorbed before they can escape. The lowest energy x-rays are the least penetrating and therefore

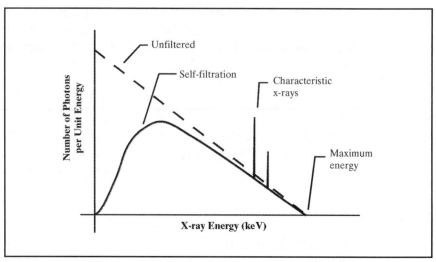

Figure 5.4: An x-ray spectrum showing filtered and unfiltered bremsstrahlung and characteristic x-rays. The filtered spectrum results from preferential absorption of low-energy photons as the x-rays escape from the target material. The unfiltered spectrum is what would be observed in the absence of any filtration.

we expect these to be absorbed more strongly than higher-energy x-rays. The lower-energy x-rays are preferentially absorbed. This is called *self-filtration* or inherent filtration. The effect of self-filtration is to preferentially remove low-energy photons. The x-ray spectrum that emerges from the target is shown in Figure 5.4 and is labeled "self-filtration." Note that the x-rays also must escape from the tube; some may be absorbed in the window. The filtered spectrum follows the unfiltered spectrum at high energy because high-energy photons have little difficulty escaping. As the energy decreases, the filtered spectrum reaches a maximum and then turns over and declines as more photons are absorbed before they can escape. At very low energy no photons are able to escape. The average energy of the x-rays in the continuous spectrum is much less than the maximum energy (perhaps about one-third).

Systematic Dependencies

It is helpful to understand how the x-ray spectrum changes as various parameters are altered. These parameters include tube current, tube voltage, target material, applied tube voltage waveform, and filtration, which is deliberately added to the beam.

Recall that in the previous chapter we found that the number of x-rays emitted is proportional to the total current (mA). Therefore, we expect that the effect of raising the current (keeping time constant) on the spectrum is simply to raise the height of the spectrum. It will not affect the maximum x-ray energy nor will it affect the relative distribution of photons of different energies. Only the area under the curve will change. For example, referring to Figure 5.5, the area under the curve for a tube current of 400 mA (assuming the time remains the same) is exactly double the area under the 200 mA curve. We say that the "intensity" or "output" at 400 mA is double that at 200 mA.

The tube voltage determines the maximum x-ray photon energy emitted by the bremsstrahlung process. The tube voltage also strongly affects the amplitude of the spectrum. We do not expect it to affect the characteristic spectrum *provided* that the bombarding electrons have sufficient energy to eject inner shell electrons. The effect of increasing the kVp is shown in Figure 5.6. The average beam energy is roughly one-third the maximum x-ray energy.

If the target material is changed, then the energies of the characteristic x-rays (if any) emitted by the new target will be different. When the atomic number Z increases, the energy of the characteristic lines will increase. Bremsstrahlung x-ray production is somewhat more efficient at higher Z values and the amplitude of the continuous spectrum will therefore rise as Z goes up. This is illustrated in Figure 5.7.

In chapter 4 we discussed the possibility that the voltage applied to an x-ray tube may vary in time because current supplied by the power company is alternating current. The x-ray generator circuitry smooths out the variations in the voltage and current supplied to the x-ray tube. There may however remain some residual ripple in the applied voltage,

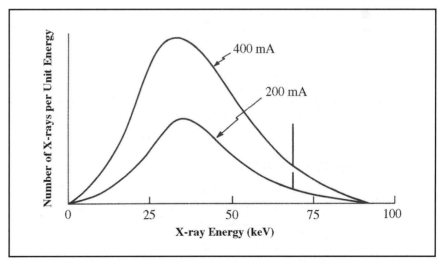

Figure 5.5: The effect of changing the tube current on the x-ray emission spectrum. When the tube current doubles (assuming constant exposure time), the area under the curve doubles. The maximum x-ray energy remains unchanged, as does the average energy of the x-rays. (Adapted from Figure 11-11, p. 149, *Radiologic Science for Technologists,* Seventh ed., Stewart C. Bushong. © 2001 Mosby, Inc., with permission from Elsevier.)

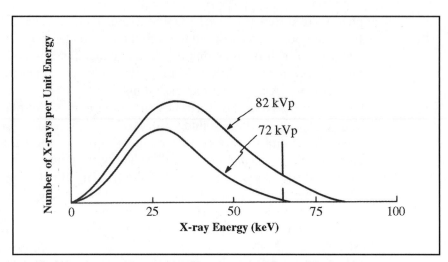

Figure 5.6: The effect on the x-ray spectrum of changing the tube voltage. As the tube voltage increases, the maximum x-ray energy rises and the amplitude of the spectrum increases. (Reprinted from Figure 11-12, p. 149, *Radiologic Science for Technologists,* Seventh ed., Stewart C. Bushong. © 2001 Mosby, Inc., with permission from Elsevier.)

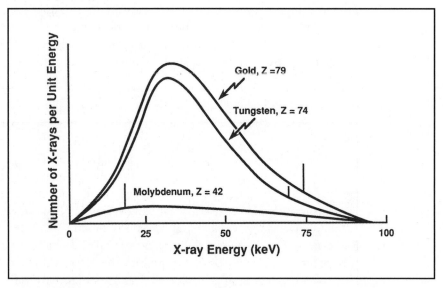

Figure 5.7: The effect on the x-ray spectrum of the target composition. The characteristic x-ray lines shift to higher energy as the atomic number (Z) of the target material increases. The amplitude of the bremsstrahlung spectrum increases with increasing Z. The maximum x-ray energy remains the same since the kVp is fixed. (Adapted from Figure 11-14, p. 151, *Radiologic Science for Technologists,* Seventh ed., Stewart C. Bushong. © 2001 Mosby, Inc., with permission from Elsevier.)

depending on the design of the generator. Figure 5.8 shows the effect of the ripple on the spectrum. There are three spectra shown, each of which has a different degree of ripple. The applied kVp is the same for all three spectra and therefore they all have the same maximum bombarding

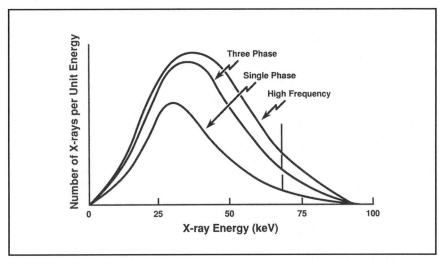

Figure 5.8: The effect on the x-ray spectrum of different voltage waveforms. All waveforms have the same kVp and thus the maximum x-ray energy is the same for all of the spectra. The single-phase waveform has the most ripple followed by the three-phase waveform. The high-frequency waveform is almost dc. The single-phase waveform has the lowest *average* energy, followed by three phase and high frequency. This explains why the amplitude of the single-phase spectrum is the lowest. (Adapted from Figure 11-16, p. 152, *Radiologic Science for Technologists,* Seventh ed., Stewart C. Bushong. © 2001 Mosby, Inc., with permission from Elsevier.)

electron energy. The single-phase curve has the most ripple, followed by the three-phase curve. The high-frequency waveform has almost no ripple and is almost like direct current. As all of the applied voltage waveforms have the same maximum energy, the one with the most ripple must have the lowest average bombarding electron energy. It is for this reason that the single-phase spectrum has the lowest amplitude.

As we learned in section 5.2, self-filtration preferentially reduces low-energy x-rays emerging from the target of an x-ray tube. Self-filtration is unavoidable and cannot be eliminated. For some applications external filters are deliberately placed in the x-ray beam to alter the spectrum of the x-rays. For diagnostic energy x-rays, aluminum is usually used for this purpose. You can probably predict the effect of added beam filtration from the discussion in section 5.2. This is shown in Figure 5.9.

Added filtration reduces the overall intensity of the x-ray beam but increases the average energy of the photons that pass through the filter. This is because many more low-energy photons are absorbed than high-energy photons. This is sometimes referred to as *beam hardening*. Beam hardening can be of importance in radiation therapy with the use of wedges (see section 14.4.2).

Added filtration is sometimes deliberately introduced in diagnostic x-ray beams to eliminate low-energy x-ray photons. The lowest energy x-rays in an x-ray beam without added filtration may not be nearly energetic enough to penetrate a patient and to reach the radiographic film. As

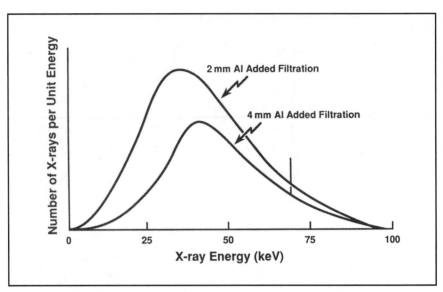

Figure 5.9: The effect on the x-ray spectrum of adding filtration to the x-ray beam. Increased filtration reduces the amplitude of the spectrum at all energies but more so at lower energies
than at higher energies. While the overall intensity of the x-ray beam is reduced by
added filtration, the average beam energy will increase. (Adapted from Figure 11-13,
p. 150, *Radiologic Science for Technologists*, Seventh ed., Stewart C. Bushong. © 2001
Mosby, Inc., with permission from Elsevier.)

these x-rays do not reach the film, they contribute nothing to the diagnostic value of the image. These low-energy x-rays do however contribute to the radiation exposure that the patient receives since they are
all absorbed in the patient. It is usually possible to reduce the radiation
exposure of the patient without compromising the quality of the radiographic image by inserting filters in the beam. The U.S. Food and Drug
Administration (FDA) regulates the design and manufacture of x-ray
machines (among its many other regulatory functions). The FDA
requires a certain amount of filtration in diagnostic x-ray beams to avoid
unnecessary radiation exposure to patients.

5.3 Efficiency of X-Ray Production

When electrons penetrate a thick x-ray target, they eventually lose all of
their kinetic energy and come to rest. One mechanism of electron energy
loss is bremsstrahlung emission. All other energy loss mechanisms
(except the small fraction leading to characteristic x-rays) ultimately
lead to heat production. Even some fraction of bremsstrahlung photons
will contribute to heat production because low-energy photons will be
absorbed before they can escape the target. The energy absorbed from
these low-energy photons will appear as heat.

Figure 5.10 shows a graph of the efficiency of photon production
for a beam of electrons incident upon thick tungsten and molybdenum
targets. The term "thick" in this context means that the electrons lose

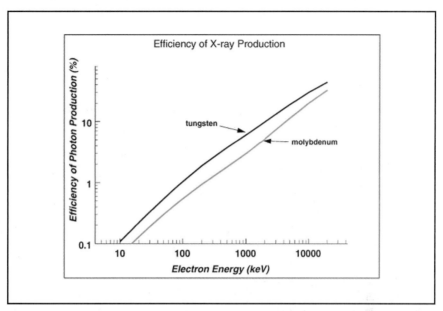

Figure 5.10: The efficiency of bremsstrahlung photon production as a function of the electron energy for an electron beam incident on a thick tungsten or molybdenum target. Note that both the horizontal and vertical scales are log scales. The efficiency is the percentage of the initial electron kinetic energy that is converted to photons. The remaining energy appears as heat except for a small fraction in the form of characteristic x-rays. For tungsten the efficiency of x-ray production is less than about 1% in the diagnostic energy range (20 to 150 keV). In the therapy range ($T_0 > 1000$ keV) the efficiency is much higher, perhaps as much as 50%. Molybdenum has $Z = 42$ in comparison to tungsten with $Z = 74$ and thus x-ray production in molybdenum is less efficient.

all of their kinetic energy in the target. A thin target would be one in which the electrons pass through the target, emerging with some remaining kinetic energy. The *efficiency* is the fraction (as a percentage) of the bombarding electron kinetic energy that is converted to photons as the electrons are brought to rest in the target. The remaining kinetic energy is dissipated as heat except for that small fraction that appears in the form of characteristic x-rays. These graphs represent an upper limit on the efficiency of x-ray production because not all photons are x-ray photons and because low-energy x-ray photons are absorbed in the target. At diagnostic energies x-ray production is very inefficient. For electron energies between 10 and 100 keV the efficiency is less than 1%. This means that approximately 99% of the electron kinetic energy is dissipated as heat! At therapy energies (above 1 MeV) the efficiency is much higher and can approach 50% for thick tungsten targets.

The efficiency of x-ray production depends on the atomic number of the target as well as the electron energy. For an unfiltered bremsstrahlung spectrum at low energy, the efficiency is proportional to both Z and the kinetic energy of the bombarding electron. Figure 5.10 shows the efficiency of bremsstrahlung photon production for tungsten and molybdenum as a function of the electron energy. Figure 5.7 shows that

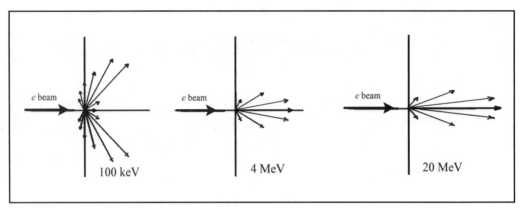

Figure 5.11: A qualitative illustration of the directional nature of bremsstrahlung x-rays produced by electron beams of differing energy coming in from the left. The length of the arrows represent the intensity of the x-rays. At low energies the emission is predominantly at an angle to the bombarding electron beam. At high energies the emission is highly peaked in the forward direction. We are ignoring absorption in escaping from the target, which leads to the heel effect for diagnostic x-rays.

the amplitude of the entire spectrum for tungsten ($Z = 74$) is much higher than for molybdenum ($Z = 42$). This is one of the reasons that tungsten is widely used as a target material in x-ray tubes.

5.4 Directional Dependence of Bremsstrahlung Emission

At low-incident electron energies the bremsstrahlung emission from a target is primarily at a large angle to the direction defined by the incident electron beam. This is illustrated in Figure 5.11. At high energies, however, most of the x-rays are emitted in the forward direction (the direction in which the electrons are traveling). This forward peaking at high energy has important implications for linear accelerator design, as we shall discuss in a later chapter.

5.5 X-Ray Attenuation

X-ray intensity is related to the number of x-ray photons passing through a given area in a given time (see Figure 5.12). The intensity is the amount of energy carried by the photons per unit time per unit area across an area perpendicular to the beam. The dimensions of the intensity in the SI system are J/(s · m^2).[3] For diagnostic x-ray application a quantity that is directly proportional to this is called the *exposure rate*. The exposure rate can be measured in units of milliroentgen per unit time (e.g., mR/h, mR/min, etc.). We will define the roentgen (R) later; it

---

[3] The intensity as defined here is technically known as the energy fluence rate (see section 7.4).

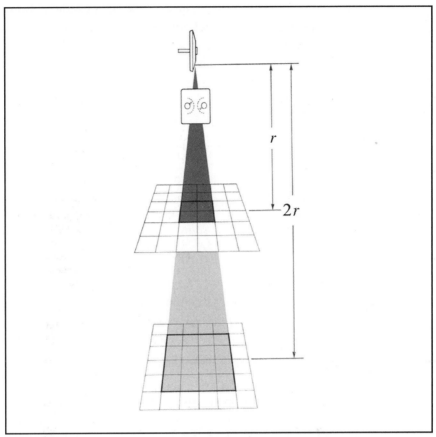

Figure 5.12: Demonstration of the Inverse Square Law. At a distance *r*, all of the photons go through an area comprising four squares. At a distance 2*r*, all of the photons go through an area consisting of 16 squares. (Adapted from Figure 2.14, p. 43, *Introduction to Medical Radiographic Imaging.* Pizzutiello, R. J., and J. E. Cullinan. © 1993, Health Sciences Division, Eastman Kodak Company, Rochester, NY.)

is not important to understand the exact definition of this now, only that this is a measure of intensity.

As an x-ray beam travels away from the source, its intensity can decrease by two mechanisms:

(1) *Spreading of the beam:* The beam spreads out or diverges, which spreads the same amount of energy over a broader area (see Figure 5.12). This "dilutes" the beam and reduces the intensity. This is a purely geometric effect and will occur regardless of whether or not any material is in the beam.

(2) *Absorption and scattering in a medium:* The second mechanism occurs when matter is placed in the beam. As x-rays traverse matter, photons can be removed from the useful beam by absorption or scattering. Photons can be absorbed by the matter. In this case, the photon ceases to exist and its energy is converted to some other form of energy. Scattering occurs when the photon

interacts with the electrons or nuclei in the matter and is deflected. This deflected or scattered photon leaves the useful beam, carrying its energy away with it.

Both beam divergence and attenuation due to the presence of matter in the beam can occur simultaneously. For simplicity we shall consider each of these effects separately.

5.5.1   Beam Divergence and the Inverse-Square Effect

We can quantitatively analyze the reduction in beam intensity due to beam divergence. We shall assume that the size of the source of the radiation is always small compared to the distance from the source. Such a source is called a *point source*. Many real sources of radiation can be treated as point sources. As an example, consider the x-rays originating from a diagnostic x-ray tube, where the size of the focal spot is on the order of 2 mm. This is very small compared to the distances from the source that we are usually concerned with, which may be tens of centimeters or even several meters.

Let us call I the intensity of the source at some distance, r, from the point source. Examine Figure 5.12. A certain amount of energy goes through four squares at a distance r from the source. At a distance $2r$, the same amount of energy goes through 16 squares, four times the area at distance r. Since intensity is the amount of energy per unit area per unit time and since the area increases by a factor of 4 in going from distance r to distance $2r$, the intensity must decrease by a factor of 4. The distance has doubled and the intensity has decreased by a factor of 4. This suggests that the intensity is inversely proportional to the square of the distance from the source:

$$I \propto \frac{1}{r^2}. \tag{5.3a}$$

Let us insert a proportionality constant k:

$$I = \frac{k}{r^2}. \tag{5.3b}$$

Let us now derive a relationship between the intensities at two different distances. This will be useful in the situation in which we know the intensity at one distance and we wish to calculate the intensity at a different distance. Let I_1 = intensity at distance r_1 and I_2 = intensity at distance r_2, then:

$$I_1 = \frac{k}{r_1^2}, \quad I_2 = \frac{k}{r_2^2}. \tag{5.3c}$$

Let us take the ratio of:

$$\frac{I_2}{I_1} = \frac{k/r_2^2}{k/r_1^2} = \frac{k}{r_2^2} \times \frac{r_1^2}{k} = \frac{r_1^2}{r_2^2} = \left(\frac{r_1}{r_2}\right)^2, \tag{5.4}$$

and finally

$$\frac{I_2}{I_1} = \left(\frac{r_1}{r_2}\right)^2.$$ (5.5)

This important result is a statement of the *Inverse Square Law*. The Inverse Square Law is a general property of any type of radiation for which beam intensity changes are due solely to beam spreading from a point source. This equation will find widespread application throughout this book.

Example 5.1

The output of a fluoroscopic x-ray unit is 10 mR/min at a distance of 50 cm from the focal spot. What is the output at a distance of 75 cm from the focal spot?

$$I_1 = 10 \text{ mR/min} \qquad\qquad r_1 = 50 \text{ cm}$$

$$I_2 = ? \qquad\qquad r_2 = 75 \text{ cm}$$

$$\frac{I_2}{I_1} = \left(\frac{r_1}{r_2}\right)^2 = \left(\frac{50}{75}\right)^2 = 0.44$$

$$I_2 = I_1 (0.44) = 10(0.44) = 4.4 \text{ mR/min}$$

Example 5.2

The radiation "output" of a medical linear accelerator at a distance of 100 cm from the source is 1.00 unit.

(a) What is the "output" at a distance of 101 cm?

$$I_1 = 1.00 \text{ unit at } r_1 = 100 \text{ cm, therefore}$$

$$\frac{I_2}{I_1} = \left(\frac{r_1}{r_2}\right)^2 = \left(\frac{100}{101}\right)^2 = 0.980.$$

Thus $I_2 = 1.00 \times 0.980 = 0.980$ units at a distance of 101 cm.

(b) What is the output at a distance of 99 cm?

$$\frac{I_2}{I_1} = \left(\frac{r_1}{r_2}\right)^2 = \left(\frac{100}{99}\right)^2 = 1.020.$$

Thus $I_2 = 1.00 \times 1.020 = 1.020$ units at a distance of 99 cm.

Notice that in both parts (a) and (b) of Example 5.2 a change in distance of 1% resulted in a change in intensity of 2%. For small changes in distance (<10%), the percent change in intensity will be approximately twice the percent change in distance. This is characteristic of the Inverse Square Law.

> **Rule of thumb:** If the percentage change in distance from the source is small, the percentage change in the intensity of a radiation beam is approximately twice the percentage change in distance.

5.5.2   Attenuation by Matter

Let us now consider attenuation of a photon beam by matter. As the beam traverses the matter, it will diverge and the intensity will decrease by the inverse-square effect. We will ignore this for now and consider only the effect of the material present. Later we can combine both effects.

When photons traverse matter, some are removed from the beam either by absorption or scattering (deflection). When a photon is absorbed, it disappears and ceases to exist. When a photon is scattered, it is deflected, possibly out of the beam. Both of these mechanisms result in a loss in intensity. The microscopic details of scattering and absorption will be considered in the next chapter.

Narrow Beam Attenuation of Monoenergetic X-Rays

We start with a source of x-rays that emits photons in all directions. All of the photons have a single energy. Such a beam is said to be *monoenergetic*. If we place a collimator in front of the source, as shown in Figure 5.13, the collimator restricts the x-rays to a well-defined narrow beam. This beam enters a material of specified composition and thickness, x. Some of the photons are scattered out of the beam as shown and some are absorbed. A radiation detector that can measure intensity is placed on the other side of the attenuating material, far enough away that no scattered photons reach it. No scattered photons can reach the detector because of the narrow beam geometry and the distance. The intensity of the beam prior to entering the material is I_0. The intensity measured by the detector will be a function of the thickness of the material and its composition. Let $I(x)$ be the intensity of the beam measured by the detector.

We expect the intensity to decrease with increasing thickness x of attenuating material and we also expect it to depend on the material

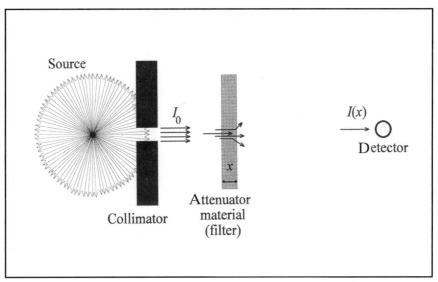

Figure 5.13: Narrow beam attenuation. The detector only detects photons that are not absorbed or scattered. The detector is placed far enough away from the attenuator material to obtain narrow beam geometry in which scattered photons do not reach the detector. We ignore loss of intensity due to beam spreading.

used and the beam energy. Experiments show (it can also be derived) that the intensity is given by the formula:

$$I(x) = I_0 e^{-\mu x}, \tag{5.6}$$

where μ is a constant called the *linear attenuation coefficient*. The linear attenuation coefficient depends on the composition of the material and the beam energy. The units of μ must be inverse distance (i.e., $[\mu]$ = cm^{-1}, mm^{-1}, or m^{-1}) so that the exponent of equation (5.6) is unitless. The larger the value of μ, the more strongly the beam will be attenuated. Note that equation (5.6) is exactly like the equation for radioactive decay; just substitute A for I, λ for μ, and t for x. Therefore you are already familiar with the properties of this equation!

Equation (5.6) only applies to monoenergetic beams with narrow beam geometry. The x-rays produced by the bremsstrahlung process are not monoenergetic, as we have seen; they are said to be *polyenergetic*. Equation (5.6) is not in general valid for such beams. It is sometimes possible to define an effective attenuation coefficient for a given material and a given polyenergetic beam, which enables approximate use of equation (5.6). If the effective attenuation coefficient for a particular beam and a particular material is denoted μ_{eff}, then equation (5.6) can be written $I = I_0 e^{-\mu_{eff} x}$.

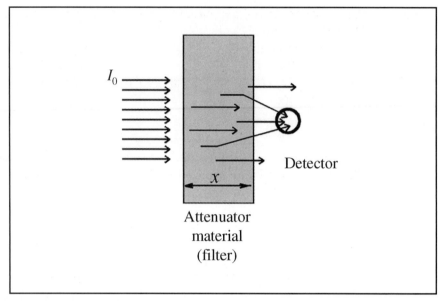

Figure 5.14: Broad beam geometry. Scattered photons can reach the detector. This type of geometry may be more relevant for shielding calculations than for narrow beam attenuation.

Broad Beam Attenuation

In broad beam attenuation some scattered radiation can reach the detector as shown in Figure 5.14. The geometrical arrangement shown in Figure 5.13 is sometimes called *narrow beam* or "good" geometry. In this arrangement photons can be scattered out of the beam, but they cannot be scattered into the detector as they can in the case of broad beam geometry.

Broad beam geometry is much more complex than narrow beam geometry because of the scattered photons. In general, it is not possible to write any simple equation for the intensity of the transmitted radiation. It is sometimes possible to use the approximate formula $I = I_0 e^{-\mu'x}$ where μ' is an effective attenuation coefficient for the broad beam geometry. If the beam is also polyenergetic, this further complicates the situation.

5.6 Half-Value Layer (HVL)

The half-value layer (HVL) is the thickness of a specified material (Al, Pb, Cu, etc.) that is necessary to reduce the intensity of a radiation beam to half its original value. The HVL depends on the energy or "quality" of the beam as well as the material that the beam traverses. Higher energy x-ray beams usually have higher values of the HVL. Conversely, a beam with high HVL is more penetrating than a beam with low HVL. Examples of the value of the HVL in Pb are 0.3 mm for 100 kVp x-rays and 1.2 cm for Co-60 radiation.[4]

For a monoenergetic beam, the relationship between the HVL and the linear attenuation coefficient, μ, is exactly analogous to the relationship between the radioactive half-life, $T_{1/2}$, and the decay constant, λ:

$$HVL = \frac{\ln 2}{\mu}. \tag{5.7}$$

The derivation of this equation is exactly the same as for half-life.

The second half-value layer (HVL_2) is the *additional* thickness necessary to reduce beam intensity by another factor of 2 (see Figure 5.15). As a polyenergetic beam penetrates the material, it usually becomes "hardened" (there are exceptions) and, therefore, it is generally true that $HVL_2 > HVL_1$. For a monoenergetic beam $HVL_2 = HVL_1$.

The energy distribution (beam "quality") of x-rays in a superficial or orthovoltage beam is often described in terms of the HVL for aluminum (Al) or copper (Cu), respectively. The HVL depends on the type of x-ray tube used, the kVp, and the amount of filtration deliberately introduced into the beam. Depending on the tube, kVp, and filtration, superficial x-ray beams have an HVL ranging from 1.0 to 4.0 mm Al. As an example, a glass window tube with 100 kVp and 1.0 mm Al added filtration has an HVL of about 2 mm Al. For orthovoltage beams the HVL is measured in terms of mm of Cu. At 160 kVp the HVL is about 0.5 mm Cu, and at 300 kVp it is about 4 mm Cu.

---

[4]This is why a lead apron for protection against Co-60 radiation is impractical. Such an apron would have to be made from a thickness of many centimeters of lead!

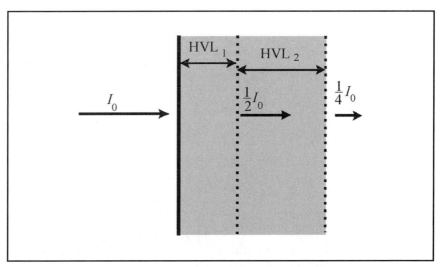

Figure 5.15: The first half-value layer (HVL₁) is the thickness necessary to attenuate the beam to one-half of its incident intensity, I_0. The second half-value layer (HVL₂) is the additional thickness necessary to reduce the intensity by an additional factor of 2.

5.7 Mass Attenuation Coefficient

The quantity μ is the *linear attenuation coefficient* and it has the units of $[\mu] = \text{cm}^{-1}$ or m^{-1}. Liquid water, steam, and ice have different μ values even though they all have the same atomic composition. The reason for this is that the densities of liquid water, of steam, and of ice are different. The mass density will be denoted by the symbol ρ. It is the mass per unit volume. The most common units are gm/cm^3 or kg/m^3 (the SI unit).

For attenuation, what really counts is the amount and the type of matter traversed. Let us consider a specific example. Liquid water has a value of $\mu = 0.267 \text{ cm}^{-1}$ for 40 keV x-rays. For ice, the value is $\mu = 0.245 \text{ cm}^{-1}$ and for steam (100 °C, 1 atmosphere pressure) $\mu = 0.000158 \text{ cm}^{-1}$. Suppose that the 40 keV x-rays traverse a column of liquid water of 1 cm^2 cross section that is $x = 1$ cm thick (see Figure 5.16, assume narrow beam geometry). The density of liquid water is 1.00 g/cm^3, ice is 0.917 g/cm^3, and steam (100 °C, 1 atmosphere pressure) is $5.90 \times 10^{-4} \text{ g/cm}^3$. The column of water has a mass of 1.00 g. The attenuation of the radiation

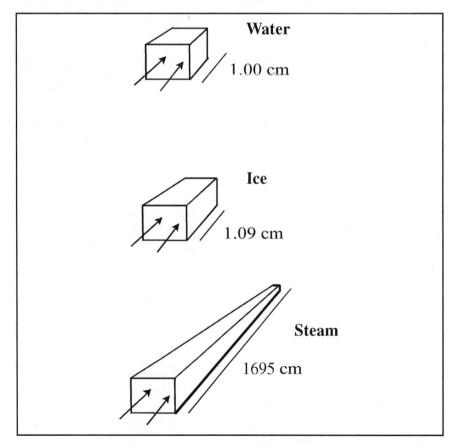

Figure 5.16: The attenuation of radiation in traversing each of these columns is the same because the mass and the composition of the matter are the same in each case.

in traversing this column is $e^{-\mu x} = e^{-(0.267)(1.00)}$. A column of ice having the same cross-sectional area and a mass of 1.00 g would have to be $1/0.917 = 1.09$ cm thick. The attenuation of the radiation in passing through this column of ice would be $e^{-\mu x} = e^{-(0.245)(1.09)} = e^{-0.267}$. A column of steam having the same cross-sectional area would have to be $1/5.90 \times 10^{-4}$ cm $= 1695$ cm. The attenuation of this column of steam would be $e^{-\mu x} = e^{-(0.000158)(1695)} = e^{-0.267}$. It can be seen that the value of $\mu/\rho = 0.267$ cm^2/g is the same for liquid water, ice, and steam. The quantity μ/ρ is called the *mass attenuation coefficient*. It is independent of the physical state of the material (e.g., solid, liquid, or gas) and it depends only on the composition and beam energy.

The units of the mass attenuation coefficient are:

$$\left[\frac{\mu}{\rho}\right] = \frac{cm^{-1}}{g/cm^3} = \frac{cm^2}{g} \text{ or } \frac{m^2}{kg}. \tag{5.8}$$

The factors affecting attenuation of photon radiation by matter appear in Table 5.2. The attenuation depends on the energy of the photons and the density of the matter. As we shall see in the next chapter, the attenuation also depends on the atomic number and the number of electrons per gram.

Table 5.2: Factors Affecting Attenuation of X-Rays

Property of Radiation	Property of Matter
energy	density
	Z
	electron density: electrons/gm

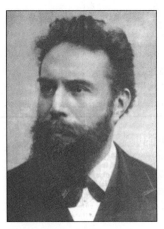

Röntgen circa 1895.

Appendix: Röntgen and the Discovery of X-Rays*

It is rare that a momentous discovery can be clearly attributed to a specific individual and to a definite date. Such is the discovery of x-rays. Late in the afternoon of Friday, November 8, 1895, Wilhelm Conrad Röntgen was conducting experiments on high-voltage discharges in evacuated glass tubes when he noticed that a nearby paper painted with a fluorescent material was glowing as though acted upon by some invisible agent.

In Röntgen's own words: "If the discharge of a fairly large Rühmkorff induction coil is allowed to pass through a Hittorf vacuum tube . . . and if one covers the tube with a fairly close fitting mantle of thin black cardboard, one observes in the completely darkened room that a paper screen painted with barium platinocyanide placed near the apparatus glows brightly or becomes fluorescent with each discharge, regardless of whether the coated surface or the other side is turned toward the discharge tube."

In 1895 there were virtually no telephones or automobiles, very little electrification and no airplanes. Grover Cleveland was the president of the United States. There were three great discoveries in physics in the years 1895–1897: x-rays, radioactivity, and the electron. Each one of these discoveries was linked to the other in some way. It is interesting that the discovery of x-rays led directly and swiftly to the discovery of radioactivity by Becquerel on March 1, 1896. After the discovery of x-rays it was thought that they might have something to do with phosphorescence, uranium-containing minerals are phosphorescent and it was therefore reasonable to investigate whether uranium minerals might produce x-rays.

The discovery of x-rays grew out of the investigation of cathode rays. When a high voltage is placed across electrodes which are sealed inside a highly evacuated glass tube, a greenish glowing discharge is produced. The glowing discharge is known as cathode rays because the rays emanate from the cathode or negative electrode. This phenomenon had been under fairly intensive investigation for a number of years before the discovery of x-rays. The study of electrical discharge in rarefied gases goes back at least to Michael Faraday in the 1830s. This was followed over the years by the research of Hittorf, Crookes, Lenard, and others. This work reached its culmination in 1897 after the discovery of x-rays when J.J. Thompson discovered the electron. It quickly became apparent that cathode rays consist of a beam of electrons and that x-rays are produced when energetic electrons strike a material target.

---

*Adapted from an invited talk "Fact, Fancy and Speculation about the Discovery of X-rays" given by PNM on January 25, 1995 at the meeting of the Great Lakes Chapter of the American Association of Physicists in Medicine (AAPM) in celebration of the 100th anniversary of the discovery of x-rays.

Röntgen was very much influenced by the earlier work of Lenard. In fact his intention was to initially reproduce Lenard's work. In that earlier work Lenard extracted cathode rays from the tube; so did Röntgen. Lenard encased his tube, so did Röntgen. Lenard even used phosphorescent materials to follow the progress of the cathode rays. Why is it, then, that Lenard did not discover x-rays first? The physicist Pais argues that the reason may well lie in the type of encasement used for the tube.[1] While Röntgen used thin black cardboard, Lenard used lead and "tinned iron." At an energy of 20 keV the half-value thickness of iron is 0.03 mm and for lead it is 0.007 mm. Unless the encasement was especially thin, it would have absorbed all the x-rays incident upon it. It is unclear why Röntgen did not follow Lenard on this particular detail, but such are the vagaries of history.

It is likely that Sir William Crookes was producing x-rays as early as 1879. It is known that Crookes was experimenting with cathode ray tubes with platinum anodes at that time. The x-rays generated by Röntgen were produced in the glass wall of the tube, primarily via the interaction of electrons with silicon in the glass. Platinum is about seven times more efficient for the production of x-rays.[2] Crookes stored photographic plates in his laboratory. On at least one occasion he returned plates to the manufacturer complaining that they were fogged!

Who was this man Röntgen and what was he like? It is unfortunate that his last will and testament stipulated that all his personal and scientific papers and letters be burned. Röntgen was born in Lennep in the Rhineland in 1845 and he died in 1923. Note that he was 50 when he made his seminal discovery. Reading the major biographies of Röntgen one gets the impression of a fussy, cranky man who must have things his own way.[3] When vacationing he apparently enjoyed playing cards although those people who knew him would prefer not to be his partner because he would get very angry if they played poorly. When jokes were played on him, he would often get very angry—he was not known for his sense of humor. No human being is one-dimensional, however, and there are many stories of warm friendliness. Furthermore, he refused to profit in any way from his discovery; he felt that it belonged in the public domain for the benefit of all humankind. It is staggering to imagine the profit that could have been reaped had Röntgen been granted a patent on the means to produce x-rays. He showed little interest in medical applications, preferring to leave that for others—his dedication to basic physics was total. In 1895 Röntgen was the director of the Physical Institute at the University of Wurzburg. As the director he and his wife resided on the upper floor of the institute in "commodious living

---

[1] Abraham Pais, *Inward Bound: Of Matter and Forces in the Physical World,* New York: Oxford University Press USA, 1986.

[2] This is estimated from the ratio of the radiation yield of platinum to glass.

[3] Otto Glasser, *Wilhelm Conrad Röntgen and the Early History of the Röntgen Rays,* Second Edition. San Francisco: Jeremy Norman Co., 1993.

quarters" which included "a well stocked wine cellar." The Röntgens' life was one "in which the social graces were not neglected."

Frau Röntgen described the days following Friday, November 8 as terrible. "Willi would come late for dinner in a state of bad humor. He ate little, did not talk at all, and returned to his laboratory immediately afterward." He said later that he was so astonished at what he discovered that he had to convince himself over and over again. He confided in no one, including his two laboratory assistants. To his wife he said that when people found out about it, that they would probably say: "Der Röntgen ist wohl verrückt geworden," or Röntgen has probably gone crazy.

One can well envision how this discovery captured the public imagination. It is not surprising that there was a great deal of misunderstanding of the capabilities of x-rays. Proper Victorians worried that the new rays might be exploited by licentious men to peer through ladies clothing. An advertisement from a London firm offered x-ray–proof underclothing for sale. In February 1896 a bill was introduced in the New Jersey legislature to "prohibit the use of X-rays in opera glasses in theaters." The Victorians were not totally without a sense of humor and there were many cartoons poking fun at the new discovery.

Röntgen shunned publicity to the point of being reclusive. He routinely turned down interviews and invitations to lecture. An invitation that could not be refused, however, was a request for a demonstration before Kaiser Wilhelm in January 1896. Röntgen was very anxious about this and said that he hoped he would have "Kaiser luck" with his tube.

Röntgen won the Nobel Prize in Physics in 1901, the first year in which the prizes were awarded. The prize was established as part of the last will and testament of Alfred Nobel. It is interesting to note that Nobel died on December 10, 1896, over one year after the discovery of x-rays. It seems likely that Nobel was actually aware of the discovery. During World War I Röntgen contributed his gold Nobel medal, which was melted down for the war effort.

One of the reasons for studying history is that it can provide useful lessons for today. Is there any lesson in the story of this discovery? We believe that there is. Since the late 1980s there has been increasing emphasis on "directed" research at the expense of fundamental or basic research. The discovery of x-rays is one example that shows that basic research in physics can result in the most profound discoveries which have extraordinary application. One can envision submitting a proposal to a federal funding agency for the investigation of "electrical discharges in rarefied gases." Of what possible use could that be? Can you imagine, even for a moment, where medicine would be without x-rays?

Chapter Summary

- **Characteristic x-rays:** X-rays with discrete wavelengths that are uniquely characteristic of the distinct energy levels of the atom from which they come. These result when a bombarding electron ejects an inner shell electron in the target medium.

- **Bremsstrahlung (continuous) x-rays:** When a bombarding electron passes close to an atomic nucleus in the target, it will be accelerated as a result of the electrical attraction between the electron and the nucleus. Accelerated charges generate electromagnetic radiation. Radiation will be emitted by the electron in this process over a wide range of energies. This radiation is called *bremsstrahlung,* which means "braking radiation" in German. The maximum energy of the emitted x-rays is equal to the total kinetic energy of the bombarding electron.

- In a typical x-ray target both characteristic x-rays and bremsstrahlung are produced.

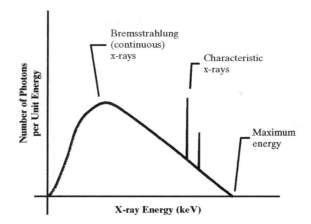

- An x-ray beam can be characterized by its intensity (the total number of x-ray photons emitted) and by the energy distribution (spectrum) of those x-rays. The settings of an x-ray generator will affect both of these characteristics in different ways:

  (1) **Tube current (mA):** The number of x-ray photons emitted is directly proportional to the tube current. The tube current has no effect on the energy distribution of the x-rays, only the intensity.

  (2) **Tube voltage (kVp):** This affects both the number of x-ray photons emerging (stronger than mA) and it affects the energy distribution (see Figure 5.6). The higher the kVp, the higher the average energy of the beam.

- **Target composition:**

  (1) Discrete spectrum (i.e., characteristic x-ray lines) are shifted to higher energies when Z is increased.

  (2) Bremsstrahlung (continuum) spectrum is more intense for higher Z because bremsstrahlung production is more efficient for higher Z materials.

- **Filtration:** Filtration reduces the intensity but usually *raises* average energy by preferentially removing low-energy x-rays.

  (1) *Self-filtration:* X-rays absorbed in escaping from the target material and x-ray tube.

  (2) *Added filtration:* Filter (usually aluminum) deliberately placed in beam to reduce patient dose during diagnostic radiographs.

- **Efficiency:** At diagnostic energies the efficiency of x-ray production is only about 1%; the rest of the energy (99%) dissipated by the bombarding electrons appears as heat. At therapeutic energies the efficiency of x-ray production is about 50%. As the Z value of the target material goes up, the efficiency rises. As the energy of the bombarding electrons goes up, the efficiency rises.

- **Directional dependence of bremsstrahlung emission:** At large angles with respect to electron beam for low-energy x-ray beams (diagnostic) but strongly peaked in the forward direction for therapeutic energies.

- **X-ray intensity:** Two factors reduce the intensity of x-rays:

  (1) *Spreading of the beam:* the beam spreads out as it travels becoming more "dilute".

  (2) *Absorption and scattering in a medium:* some x-rays are absorbed by a medium and some are deflected out of the beam (scattering).

- **Spreading of the beam:** Inverse Square Law

  I_1 is the intensity of the beam at distance r_1 from the source and I_2 is the intensity at distance r_2 from the source.

$$\frac{I_2}{I_1} = \left(\frac{r_1}{r_2}\right)^2 .$$

Rule of thumb: If the percentage change in distance is small, the percentage change in the intensity of a radiation beam is approximately twice the percentage change in distance.

- **Absorption and Scattering:**

  – Narrow beam attenuation: well-collimated beam, detector placed far from attenuating material so that no scattered photons may enter the detector (see Figure 5.13).

  – Narrow beam attenuation for monoenergetic x-ray beam (no spectrum)

  $$I(x) = I_0 e^{-\mu x},$$

  where I_0 is the incident intensity and $I(x)$ is the intensity after traversing a thickness x of material having a linear attenuation coefficient μ. The linear attenuation coefficient has units of inverse distance (e.g., cm^{-1}) and depends on the energy of the radiation and the attenuating medium.

  – Broad beam attenuation: scattered photons are allowed to enter detector (see Figure 5.14).

- **Mass attenuation coefficient:** μ/ρ (ρ is the mass density); independent of the phase of the material (liquid, solid, gas); has dimensions of m^2/kg.

- **Half-value layer (HVL)** (sometimes called first half-value layer): The thickness of specified material (Al, Pb, Cu, etc.) necessary to attenuate intensity of beam to half its original value for narrow beam geometry. Example: Co-60 radiation HVL = 1.2 cm for lead.

  $$HVL = \frac{0.693}{\mu}$$

- **Second half-value layer (HVL$_2$):** Additional thickness of material necessary to reduce the beam intensity by another factor of 2. For a polyenergetic beam usually $HVL_2 > HVL_1$ (beam hardening).

- **Superficial beams:** HVL = 1 to 4 mm Al; **Orthovoltage beams:** 0.5 to 4 mm Cu.

Problems

1. Consider an atom with a K shell binding energy of 30 keV. The binding energy of the M shell electron is 0.7 keV. An electron with a kinetic energy of 25.3 keV is ejected from the M shell as an Auger electron (see section 3.12.2) following an L to K transition. The binding energy of the L shell electron is _____ keV.

2. What is the approximate value of the efficiency of x-ray production for a 100 keV electron beam striking a thick tungsten target?

3. The dose rate in free space (intensity) of a Co-60 radiation therapy treatment unit is 12.1 cGy/min at a distance of 150 cm from the source. The dose rate in free space at a distance of 80 cm from the source is _____ cGy/min. (You do not need to know what cGy/min is to do this problem. It is sufficient to know that it is a measure of intensity.)

4. Name two effects on the spectrum of increasing the filtration of a diagnostic energy x-ray beam.

5. Draw a sketch of the graph of the spectrum from a diagnostic x-ray tube. Include bremsstrahlung continuum, characteristic lines, and the x-ray energy equivalent to the kVp of the tube. Label the graph.

6. a. The radiation emitted by Co-60 has an HVL of 1.2 cm in lead. What is the linear attenuation coefficient of lead for Co-60 radiation?
   b. If a 5.0 cm thick cast block is fashioned from lead, what percent of Co-60 radiation will be transmitted through this block?

7. Derive expression 5.2.

8. a. What is the maximum kinetic energy of electrons in an x-ray tube with a tube voltage of 120 kVp? Be sure to include the units along with your numerical answer.
   b. Approximately what fraction of the kinetic energy from part a is converted to photons as these electrons come to rest in a thick tungsten target?
   c. Where does the remaining energy go?
   d. What is the maximum energy of the bremsstrahlung photons in keV?
   e. What is the minimum wavelength of the bremsstrahlung photons in nm?

9. Is narrow beam geometry relevant to the transmission through a lead apron? Explain.

10. The intensity of a linear accelerator radiation beam is 1.00 unit at a distance of 100 cm from the source of radiation.
    a. Use the rule of thumb to estimate the intensity at a distance of 105 cm.
    b. Use the Inverse Square Law to calculate the intensity at a distance of 105 cm.

11. The linear attenuation coefficient for a material used to construct "compensators" for radiation therapy is 0.154 cm^{-1} for a 6 MV beam. What percentage of the radiation from this beam is transmitted through 15 mm of this material?

12. What is beam hardening and why does it occur?

Bibliography

Attix, F. H. *Introduction to Radiological Physics and Radiation Dosimetry.* New York: Wiley InterScience, 1986.

Bushong, S. C. *Radiologic Science for Technologists,* Eighth Edition. New York: Mosby, Inc., 2004.

Glasser, Otto. *Wilhelm Conrad Röntgen and the Early History of the Röntgen Rays,* 2nd edition. San Francisco: Jeremy Norman Co., 1993.

Johns, H. E., and J. R. Cunningham. *The Physics of Radiology,* Fourth Edition. Springfield, IL: Charles C Thomas, 1983.

Khan, F. M. *The Physics of Radiation Therapy,* Fourth Edition. Philadelphia: Lippincott Williams & Wilkins, 2009.

Pais, A. *Inward Bound: Of Matter and Forces in the Physical World.* New York: Oxford University Press USA, 1986.

Pizzutiello, R. J., and J. E. Cullinan. *Introduction to Medical Radiographic Imaging.* Rochester, NY: Eastman Kodak Company, 1993.

6

The Interaction of Radiation with Matter

6.1 **Photon Interactions with Matter**
6.2 **Interaction of Charged Particles with Matter**
6.3 **Neutron Interactions with Matter**
Chapter Summary
Problems
Bibliography

In the last chapter we discussed the attenuation of photons by matter and we introduced the linear and mass attenuation coefficients. In this chapter we shall discuss the microscopic details of radiation absorption and scattering of photons, neutrons, and charged particles. This is crucial for an understanding of how radiation acts on the human body. Human tissue is mostly water and therefore water is an important material to consider. From the point of view of radiation protection and shielding it is also important to understand how radiation interacts with matter. Materials that are frequently used for shielding are lead and concrete.

Radiation can be categorized as either *indirectly ionizing* or as *directly ionizing*. Fast charged particles are directly ionizing radiation. They deliver energy to matter directly by many small interactions, causing atomic excitation and ionization, which leads to biological damage. Examples of fast charged particles are electrons and protons. Neutral particles (photons, neutrons) are indirectly ionizing. They first transfer energy to charged particles; then the charged particles deliver energy directly to matter. Therefore the energy transfer is indirect, and it is a two-step process. Photons deliver their energy to electrons. Neutrons deliver their energy predominantly to protons.

6.1 Photon Interactions with Matter

It is important to distinguish between absorption and scattering. In absorption the photon is destroyed and ceases to exist, whereas in scattering the direction of travel of the photon is changed, and hence the photon may be effectively removed from the useful beam.

When a photon interacts with matter, there are only two microscopic entities with which it can interact: electrons or atomic nuclei. Highly energetic photons can, under the right circumstances, interact directly with individual nucleons; however this process is unimportant in the present context. For some interactions there is an energy threshold below which the interaction will not occur. For a given photon energy several interactions may be possible. Different interactions occur with varying probability depending on the photon energy and the composition of the matter. The dominant interaction mechanism is determined by the energy of the photon and the atomic number of the material.

When photons interact with electrons, there are three major types of interaction that need to be considered: (1) coherent or elastic scattering; (2) photoelectric effect; and (3) Compton scattering. When photons interact with nuclei, there are two major processes to be considered: (1) pair production and (2) photonuclear reactions.

In coherent scattering the photon is deflected (scattered) without any change in its energy. Coherent scattering is only important at low energies and for materials with low Z values. In the photoelectric effect the photon is absorbed and its energy is transferred to an atomic electron, which is ejected from the atom. The photoelectric effect is important in the diagnostic energy range and dominates at low energies and for high atomic number. Compton scattering is the process in which a photon interacts with an atomic electron, giving up some of its energy to the electron and changing direction in the process. The Compton effect is the predominant photon interaction in soft tissue in the therapy energy range. When a high-energy photon passes close to an atomic nucleus, the photon energy can be converted into matter. The energy of the photon appears in the form of an electron positron pair. This process is called *pair production*. We will discuss each of the different interaction processes in turn.

Figure 6.1 illustrates the conditions under which different interactions are predominant. The linear attenuation coefficient for the photoelectric effect (acting alone) is τ (tau). Likewise the linear attenuation coefficient for Compton scattering is denoted by the Greek letter σ (sigma) and for pair production by κ (kappa). Along the curve labeled $\sigma = \tau$, the Compton and photoelectric linear attenuation coefficients are equal. In the area to the upper left of the graph (low energy and high Z), the photoelectric effect dominates. The curve labeled $\sigma = \kappa$ is the curve along which the linear attenuation coefficient for Compton scattering is

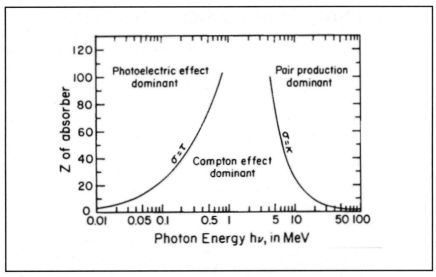

Figure 6.1: The way in which a photon interacts with matter depends on the energy of the photon and the atomic number, *Z*, of the material. For low-energy photons and large *Z* values the photoelectric effect dominates. For medium energy and low *Z*, the Compton effect dominates. Pair production is preeminent at high energy and high *Z* value. Note that in the therapy energy range Compton interactions predominate in tissue that has a low effective *Z*. (From Attix, F. H. *Introduction to Radiological Physics and Radiation Dosimetry,* Figure 7.1, p. 125. 1986. Copyright Wiley-VCH Verlag GmbH & Co., KGaA. Reproduced with permission.)

equal to that for pair production. In the middle region of the graph, the Compton effect dominates. In the region on the right (high energy and high Z value), pair production is dominant.

6.1.1 Coherent Scattering

In coherent scattering the photon interacts with an electron and simply changes its direction. There is no change in the energy of the photon, just a change in direction. This process is only important for photons of very low energy and for low-Z materials. It is of little interest for radiation therapy. There is however one interesting sidelight to this. Coherent scattering is the reason that the sky is blue! When you look at the sky away from the direction of the sun, the photons that reach your eye are photons that have been scattered by the O_2 and N_2 in the atmosphere. The probability of coherent scattering is inversely proportional to the fourth power of the wavelength of the radiation. Coherent scattering is therefore much more efficient for blue light than for any other color and that is the reason that you see a blue sky. This also implies that coherent scattering is efficient for ultraviolet radiation. Even if you are out of direct sunlight, you can be exposed to a considerable amount of UV if your skin is exposed to a large amount of the sky. You can get a sunburn under an umbrella!

6.1.2 Photoelectric Effect

In the photoelectric effect the photon interacts with an atomic electron and is totally absorbed by the atom and therefore ceases to exist. An atomic electron gains an amount of energy equal to the energy of the bombarding photon and is ejected from the atom. This electron is called a *photoelectron*. If E_γ represents the energy of the bombarding photon and E_b is the atomic binding energy of the ejected electron (here taken to be a positive number), then the kinetic energy of the photoelectron will be

$$T_e = E_\gamma - E_b. \tag{6.1}$$

As an example, for lead the K-shell binding energy is 88 keV. If a 90 keV photon is incident upon lead, it can be absorbed, ejecting a K-shell electron that will have a final kinetic energy of 2 keV.

The photoelectric effect cannot eject an electron from an atom unless $E_\gamma > E_b$. Once an electron is ejected from an atom, characteristic X-ray emission or Auger electron emission will follow. The photoelectric process is especially likely to occur when the photon energy just exceeds the electron binding energy. The electron binding energy depends on the atomic number of the atom and on the specific shell (K, L, M, etc.). There is a sharp rise in the linear attenuation coefficient when the photon energy just exceeds the binding energy of a shell. On a graph of the attenuation coefficient as a function of energy this sharp rise is called an *absorption edge* (see Figure 6.2).

The mass attenuation coefficient for the photoelectric effect (with no other absorption or scattering process operative) will be denoted as τ/ρ. The general dependence of this quantity on atomic number and energy is approximately:

$$\frac{\tau}{\rho} \propto \left(\frac{Z}{E_\gamma} \right)^3. \tag{6.2}$$

The photoelectric mass attenuation coefficient rises very rapidly with increasing Z and falls very rapidly with increasing E_γ. The strong dependence of τ/ρ on Z has important implications in diagnostic radiology. The ability to discern structures on a radiographic film depends on the relative opacity (contrast) of adjacent tissues. Most soft tissue consists predominantly of water. Bone, however, has a significant calcium content and therefore a relatively high effective Z value. For this reason, bone is very opaque to X-rays in the diagnostic energy range and bone will show up very clearly on a radiographic film, whereas soft tissues are not well differentiated. Equation (6.2) also forms the basis for the

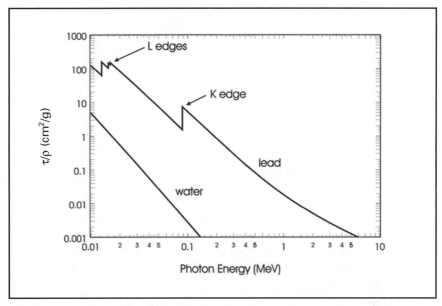

Figure 6.2: The mass attenuation coefficient for the photoelectric effect (τ/ρ in units cm^2/g) for lead and for water. The mass attenuation coefficient for lead is much larger than for water [see equation (6.2)] because lead has $Z = 82$ and water has an effective Z value of approximately 7.4. Note the rapid drop in τ/ρ with increasing energy as described by equation (6.2). As the energy of the bombarding photons increases above the threshold for L- or K-shell ionization, there is an abrupt rise in the mass attenuation coefficient. These features are referred to as absorption edges.

use of radiographic contrast agents such as barium and iodine compounds. Both barium and iodine have high values of Z (56 and 53, respectively) and therefore they are very radiopaque.

6.1.3   Compton Scattering

The most important photon interaction process in tissue at therapy energies is the Compton effect. The Compton effect is the dominant interaction in soft tissue in the range 25 keV (this corresponds approximately to 60 to 100 kVp) to 10 MeV. In the Compton effect the bombarding photon interacts with an atomic electron. The electron absorbs some of the photon energy and is ejected from the atom, often with substantial final kinetic energy. The photon therefore loses some of its energy, and it is also deflected in its path. The electron will have a significant amount of kinetic energy, and it is this electron that will deposit dose as it moves through the material. See Figure 6.3.

An expression can be derived relating the final energy of the photon $E_{\gamma'}$ to its initial energy E_γ and the angle θ through which it is scattered. This equation is derived by setting the total energy and the total momentum

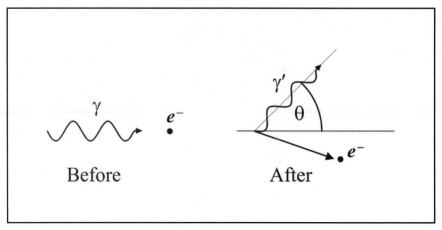

Figure 6.3: In the Compton scattering process a photon coming in from the left interacts with an atomic electron. The electron absorbs some of the photon's energy and is ejected from the atom. The direction of the motion of the photon changes by an angle θ with respect to its original direction of motion. The photon now has a lower energy because of the energy imparted to the electron.

before the interaction equal to the total energy and momentum after the collision.[1] The final photon energy is given by:

$$E_{\gamma'} = \frac{E_\gamma}{1+\alpha\left(1-\cos\theta\right)}, \tag{6.3}$$

where $\alpha = E_\gamma/m_0c^2$ and $m_0c^2 = 0.511$ MeV for an electron. This result is based on the assumption that the electron is initially unbound to an atom. This is a good approximation when the photon energy is much higher than the electron binding energy.

There are important limiting cases for equation (6.3) when the energy of the incident photon is much larger than the rest energy of the electron. This occurs when $\alpha \gg 1$.[2]

Case 1: $(\alpha \gg 1)$ and $\theta = 90° \Rightarrow \cos 90° = 0$

$$E_{\gamma'} = \frac{E_\gamma}{1+\alpha} \simeq \frac{E_\gamma}{\alpha} = \frac{E_\gamma}{\dfrac{E_\gamma}{m_0c^2}} = m_0c^2 = 0.511\,\text{MeV} \tag{6.4}$$

The maximum photon energy for a photon scattered at 90° is 0.511 MeV (also see Figure 6.4).

---

[1] See *Introduction to Radiological Physics and Radiation Dosimetry* by Frank Attix (Wiley 1986).
[2] The symbol >> means much greater than.

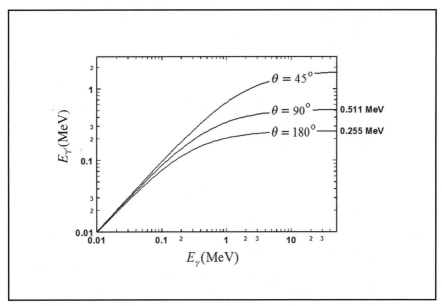

Figure 6.4: The energy of a Compton scattered photon $E_{\gamma'}$ as a function of the energy of the incident photon E_γ, for scattering angles of 45°, 90°, and 180°. Note the limiting energies for photons scattered through 90° and 180° when $E_\gamma \gg m_0c^2 = 0.5$ MeV.

Case 2: $(\alpha \gg 1)$ and $\theta = 180° \Rightarrow \cos 180° = -1$

$$E_{\gamma'} = \frac{E_\gamma}{1+2\alpha} \simeq \frac{E_\gamma}{2\alpha} = \frac{1}{2}m_0c^2 = 0.255 \text{ MeV} \qquad (6.5)$$

The maximum energy of a backscattered photon is 0.255 MeV (also see Figure 6.4). These limiting case relationships will be important later for the discussion of radiation shielding.

The energy given to the electron by the scattered photon is $E_\gamma - E_{\gamma'}$ as required by energy conservation. Note that a photon cannot give up all of its energy in a Compton interaction and therefore the energy of the recoil electron will always be less than the initial photon energy. The maximum possible energy is delivered to the recoiling electron when the photon is backscattered (i.e., $\theta = 180°$). In this case $E_\gamma - E_{\gamma'}$ $= 2\alpha E_\gamma/(1+2\alpha)$ and the electron will move in the direction of the bombarding photon. Example 6.1 illustrates an application of equation (6.3) and a calculation of the recoil electron energy.

Equation (6.3) gives us a relationship between the energy of the incident photon and the scattered photon as a function of the angle of scattering. This equation does not tell us the value of the angle however. It is not possible to predict with certainty the scattering angle for an incident photon of a given energy. It is however possible to predict the probability of scattering through any angle. Figure 6.5 shows the

Example 6.1

A gamma-ray photon from a Co-60 source ($E_\gamma = 1.25$ MeV) is scattered through an angle of 10°.

a.   What is the energy of the scattered photon?

The quantity $\alpha = E_\gamma/m_0 c^2 = 1.25/0.511 = 2.45$ and therefore:

$$E_{\gamma'} = \frac{E_\gamma}{1+\alpha\left(1-\cos\theta\right)} = \frac{1.25}{1+2.45\left(1-\cos 10°\right)} = 1.21 \text{ MeV}.$$

b.   What is the kinetic energy of the recoil electron?

The kinetic energy of the recoil electron is $E_\gamma - E_{\gamma'} = 1.25 - 1.21 = 0.04$ MeV.

probability of scattering as a function of angle. At low energies scattering is almost equally probable in all directions (isotropic). As the energy increases, scattering becomes more and more peaked in the forward direction.

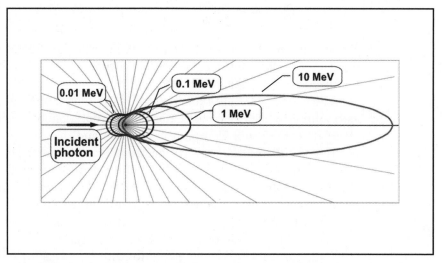

Figure 6.5: Polar graphs of the angular dependence of Compton scattering for a variety of energies ranging from 0.01 MeV to 10 MeV. The scattering angle is measured with respect to the origin of the polar coordinates. The distance from the origin to the graph is proportional to the probability of scattering at that angle. The most elongated curve is for 10 MeV. At high energies photons are predominantly scattered through small angles.

The mass attenuation coefficient for Compton scattering (with no other process operating) will be denoted by σ/ρ. As Compton scattering involves photon scattering with atomic electrons, we should not find it surprising that σ/ρ depends on the number of electrons per gram (electron density, n_e) of the scattering material. It turns out that σ/ρ is directly proportional to n_e. The electron density for chemical elements can be calculated from Avogadro's number, N_A, as follows. The number of atoms per gram is N_A/A_W, where A_W is the atomic weight of the element in grams per mole. Each atom has Z electrons, therefore:

$$n_e = N_A \frac{Z}{A_W}. \tag{6.6}$$

For all elements except hydrogen, $A_W \approx 2\,Z$, so $n_e \approx N_A/2$ (approximately 3.0×10^{23} electrons/g), which is independent of Z! For hydrogen, $A_W = Z$, and therefore $n_e = N_A$. We conclude that the Compton mass attenuation coefficient is roughly the same for all materials except for those rich in hydrogen.

The value of σ/ρ is approximately constant for photon energy less than about 1 MeV. For energies above 1 MeV, $\sigma/\rho \sim 1/E_\gamma$. The full energy dependence of σ/ρ is shown later in Figure 6.8 for lead.

6.1.4 Pair Production

When $E_\gamma > 2\,m_0c^2 = 1.022$ MeV, it becomes possible for the bombarding photon to disappear and be replaced by an electron positron pair. Note that charge is conserved in this process. If a single particle, either an electron or positron, were produced, charge would not be conserved. Pair production can occur when a photon with an energy above the threshold passes close to an atomic nucleus (see Figure 6.6). The presence of a nucleus is necessary for momentum conservation. Pair production is illustrated in Figure 6.7.

The positron created in pair production will eventually annihilate with another electron in the matter to produce two 0.511 MeV photons. These photons are sometimes called *annihilation radiation*. Two photons are produced traveling in opposite directions because otherwise momentum would not be conserved.

The mass attenuation coefficient for pair production with no other process operating will be denoted as κ/ρ.

Dependence on Z and E_γ:

1. $\kappa/\rho \propto Z$.
2. κ/ρ increases with increasing energy (see Figure 6.8).

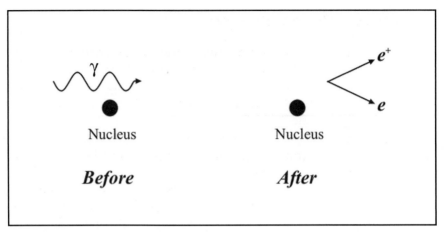

Figure 6.6: An incident photon is transformed into an electron-positron pair when passing close to an atomic nucleus. This pair production process demonstrates the conversion of energy to mass.

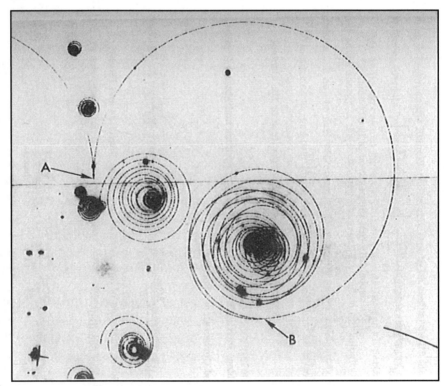

Figure 6.7: A photograph of the ionization tracks resulting from the pair production process. A photon comes in at the bottom and interacts with a nucleus at point A to produce an electron-positron pair. The track of the photon is not visible because it is a neutral particle and does not produce an ionization track. An applied magnetic field causes the electron and positron tracks to curve in opposite directions. The electron collides with a second electron at point B, losing about half of its energy in the process. The other tracks in the photograph are thought to be produced by Compton recoil electrons. (Reprinted from Kase, K. R., and W. R. Nelson, *Concepts in Radiation Dosimetry,* Fig. 3.1, p. 39. © 1978, with permission from Elsevier.)

6.1.5 Photonuclear Reactions

Photonuclear reactions are important in radiation therapy because they can produce unwanted neutrons via the reaction:

$$_{Z}^{A}X + \gamma \rightarrow \, _{Z}^{A-1}X + \, _{0}^{1}n. \tag{6.7}$$

This reaction is sometimes known as a (γ, n) reaction because a photon (γ) comes in and a neutron (n) goes out. This absorption mechanism does not contribute significantly to attenuation in patients. It does occur with some efficiency in the high Z jaws and collimator of a linear accelerator treatment machine. It can produce a significant amount of neutron radiation in the treatment room, although small compared to the dose that the patient receives in the direct (useful) beam. The treatment room and door must be shielded against this neutron radiation and that may impose special requirements. Neutrons can also cause activation of materials in the head of a linac (especially the X-ray target) so that they become radioactive. The threshold energy above which the (γ, n) reaction begins to become important is in the range 7 to 15 MeV. For linacs with beam energies higher than 10 MV there may be significant neutron production. This topic will be revisited when we discuss shielding for linacs.

6.1.6 Total Mass Absorption Coefficient

The total mass absorption coefficient is the sum of the mass absorption coefficients for the photoelectric effect, the Compton effect, and for pair production:

$$\frac{\mu}{\rho} = \frac{\tau}{\rho} + \frac{\sigma}{\rho} + \frac{\kappa}{\rho}. \tag{6.8}$$

Figure 6.8 shows the individual contributions to μ/ρ and the total value as a function of photon energy. Figure 6.9 shows the total mass attenuation coefficient for lead and for water as a function of energy. It is interesting to note that μ/ρ is about the same for lead and water at energies of a few MeV. This implies that, pound for pound, water and lead are approximately equally effective in attenuating photons with energies of a few MeV.

6.2 Interaction of Charged Particles with Matter

There are several reasons for studying the interactions of charged particles with matter. As we have seen, neutral particles (indirectly ionizing radiation) set charged particles in motion as they interact with matter. It

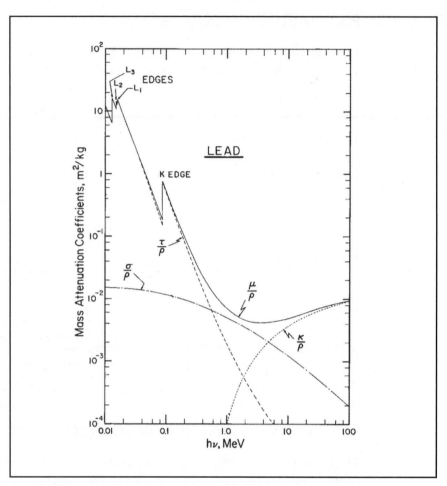

Figure 6.8: Contributions to the mass attenuation coefficient for lead (in units of m²/kg) as a function of the photon energy (in MeV). Note that both the horizontal and vertical scales are logarithmic. τ/ρ is the contribution from the photoelectric effect, σ/ρ from the Compton effect and κ/ρ is from pair production. Note how all the contributions add and which dominate in various regions. At low energies the photoelectric effect dominates. At intermediate energies the Compton effect is the most important interaction. At high energies the mass attenuation coefficient actually rises slightly with increasing energy as pair production becomes more important. (From Attix, F. H. *Introduction to Radiological Physics and Radiation Dosimetry*, Fig. 7.13, p. 141. 1986. Copyright Wiley-VCH Verlag GmbH & Co., KGaA. Reproduced with permission.)

is these secondary charged particles that deposit energy in the material. Therefore, the previous discussion of the interaction of photons with matter is only half the story! Secondly, charged particles themselves are sometimes the primary radiation. Electrons with energies ranging from 5 to 20 MeV are widely used in radiation therapy. The charged particle interactions we will consider here are Coulomb interactions with either atomic electrons or the positively charged nucleus.

There are two major categories of interactions between particles: elastic and inelastic. In an elastic collision the total kinetic energy of all

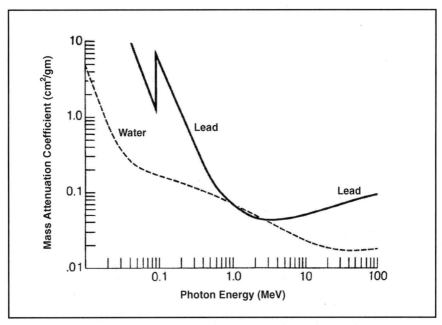

Figure 6.9: The total mass attenuation coefficient, μ/ρ as a function of photon energy for lead and for water. For low energies the photoelectric effect dominates and μ/ρ is much larger for lead than for water. At intermediate energies where the Compton effect is dominant μ/ρ is slightly less for lead than for water because lead has a somewhat lower number of electrons per gram than water. At high energies, pair production becomes important in lead leading to a rise in μ/ρ. (Reprinted from Khan, F. M. *The Physics of Radiation Therapy,* Third Edition, Fig. 5.12, p. 73 © 2003, with permission from Lippincott Williams & Wilkins; and in Johns, H. E., and J. R. Cunningham. *The Physics of Radiology,* 4th Edition. © 1983, with permission from Charles C Thomas.)

of the particles is the same before and after the collision. Individual particles may gain or lose kinetic energy, but the sum of all kinetic energies is the same before and after. In an inelastic collision some kinetic energy is lost. The lost kinetic energy appears as some other form of energy such as excitation energy, ionization energy, bremsstrahlung, etc.

The interaction of charged particles with matter is very different from the interaction of neutral particles. Photons undergo a small number of interactions (ranging from zero to a few dozen in patients) before they either exit the material or they are absorbed. Photons are exponentially attenuated as we have seen in chapter 5, section 5.5.2. Charged particles on the other hand, undergo a very large number of interactions before either exiting the material or losing all of their energy. Each of these interactions generally involves only a small loss of kinetic energy. As an example, a 1 MeV electron may undergo 10^5 interactions before losing all kinetic energy. Charged particles have a definite range. Beyond this range no particles are to be found. Charged particles form trails or tracks of ionization in the matter they traverse.

From the point of view of interaction with matter there are two types of charged particles: light charged particles and heavy charged

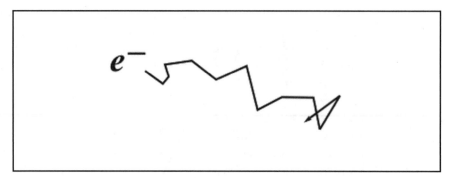

Figure 6.10: An example of the erratic path followed by an electron as it loses energy in matter.

particles. Light charged particles are electrons or positrons. Heavy charged particles are just about everything else: protons, alpha particles, pions, heavy nuclei, etc. There are distinct differences between light charged particles and heavy charged particles because of the large mass difference between them. Recall that a proton is about 2000 times more massive than an electron. Heavy charged particles follow relatively straight paths through matter. They are not easily deflected except in a close encounter with a nucleus and they are certainly no more bothered by electrons in the material than a charging elephant is bothered by a mosquito. Recall the discussion of Rutherford scattering in which the vast majority of the alpha particles were only scattered through small angles in traversing a gold foil. In contrast, electrons are easily scattered because of their low mass.

Electron paths are not straight—they follow a "zig-zag" or "tortured" path (see Figure 6.10). Electrons are easily scattered by high Z nuclei because of their relatively low mass. This is the reason that electron back scattering is of importance when high Z materials are used to block electrons (see chapter 15, section 15.5).

6.2.1 Electron Interactions with Matter

Electrons incident upon matter will interact either with atomic electrons or with the positively charged atomic nucleus. Let us consider each of these possibilities in turn.

As an electron traverses matter, it can interact over a long range with the atomic electrons in the medium. The electrons in these atoms are promoted to excited energy states. A small amount of energy is thus transferred from the incident electron to the electrons in the material. Such interactions are referred to as "soft collisions".[3] Because the Coulomb

---

[3]The word "collision" has a meaning in physics that is different from the common meaning. In everyday language, a collision implies physical contact between two objects. In physics, an interaction between two particles that results in energy transfer or scattering, even at a distance, is referred to as a collision.

force extends over a long range, a large number of such small energy losses can occur. If the incident electron should pass close to an individual atomic electron, it will interact primarily with that electron, transferring a large amount of energy. This is known as a hard or "knock on" collision. The electron will be ejected from the atom with considerable residual energy and the atom will be left in an ionized state. The ejected electron will form its own ionization track. This track is called a *delta ray* (see the interaction at point B in Figure 6.7). If an inner-shell electron is ejected, characteristic X-rays and or Auger electrons will be emitted as in the target of an x-ray tube. Energy loss via both hard and soft collisions is referred to as *collisional energy loss.*

When an incident electron interacts with an atomic nucleus, it is usually deflected with little energy loss. The deflection is expected to be larger for higher Z materials because of the higher charge on the nucleus. This is the main reason that electrons follow tortured paths. This scattering mechanism is put to use in the scattering foil of a linac (see chapter 9). In a few percent of the scattering events from atomic nuclei, bremsstrahlung emission will occur and the electron will lose a fraction of its kinetic energy in the process. This is an example of inelastic scattering in which some kinetic energy is lost. As we have seen in chapter 5, this possibility is much more likely for high Z materials. Energy loss by this mechanism is referred to as *radiative loss*. Bremsstrahlung emission does not occur for heavy charged particles because their accelerations in Coulomb interactions with nuclei are much smaller.

6.2.2 Stopping Power

The rate of energy loss by charged particles is described by a quantity called the stopping power. The stopping power is the kinetic energy loss ΔT per unit pathlength Δx, by a charged particle of type Y and kinetic energy T in a medium of atomic number Z:

$$S = \left(\frac{\Delta T}{\Delta x} \right)_{Y,T,Z}. \qquad (6.9)$$

This is actually only an approximate expression which becomes more exact in the limit in which $\Delta T \ll T$. The subscripts Y, T, and Z will be dropped from here on. It is important to understand that the stopping power changes with kinetic energy; as the particle slows down, the stopping power varies.

The units of stopping power are:

$$\left[S \right] = \left[\frac{\Delta T}{\Delta x} \right] = \frac{\text{MeV}}{\text{cm}}; \qquad (6.10)$$

these are not SI units, but they are convenient and frequently used.

It is more common to talk about the mass stopping power, which is defined as:

$$S_\rho = \frac{S}{\rho} = \frac{\Delta T}{\rho \Delta x}.$$

(6.11)

The units of mass stopping power are the units of stopping power divided by density:

$$\left[\frac{\Delta T}{\rho \Delta x} \right] = \text{MeV} \cdot \text{cm}^2 / \text{g}.$$

(6.12)

In section 6.2.1 the mechanisms by which electrons lose energy in matter were divided into two broad categories: (1) collisional and (2) radiative (i.e., bremsstrahlung). The mass stopping power can be written as the sum of these two components:

$$S_\rho = \left(S_\rho\right)_c + \left(S_\rho\right)_r ,$$

(6.13)

where subscript c denotes collisional losses and subscript r denotes radiative losses. Tables of values of stopping powers for various media can be found in reference compilations (e.g., Attix, 1986).

Figure 6.11 shows a graph of both the collisional and radiative mass stopping power as a function of electron energy for electrons incident on water and tungsten. The collisional mass stopping power is proportional to the number of electrons per unit mass of the medium. From equation (6.6), $n_e = N_A Z/A_W$. The atomic weight A_W is approximately equal to the atomic mass number A. We know that Z/A is relatively independent of Z for $Z > 1$ (because $A \propto 2 Z$), but it is not completely independent of Z. Figure 3.2 shows that nuclei become increasingly neutron rich as Z increases and therefore Z/A goes down slowly as Z rises. This is why the *mass* collisional stopping power is lower for tungsten than for water.

As an electron nears the end of its ionization track, the stopping power rises sharply. The qualitative explanation for this is that a slow electron has more time to interact with atomic electrons in its vicinity. At low energies (but not very low) $(S_\rho)_c$ is inversely proportional to the electron energy. At energies above the rest mass energy $(S_\rho)_c$ is roughly constant with increasing energy.

The radiative stopping power $(S_\rho)_r \propto Z^2$, and therefore radiative losses (i.e., bremsstrahlung) will be efficient for a high Z medium. This is one reason that high Z targets are used in x-ray tubes (see Figure 5.10). This also suggests that $(S_\rho)_r$ is not very important in tissue which has a relatively low effective value of Z. $(S_\rho)_r$ is independent of energy for small T ($T \ll m_0c^2$). For large values of T ($T \gg m_0c^2$) $(S_\rho)_r \propto T$ (see Figure 6.11). For electrons incident on water $(S_\rho)_c \approx (S_\rho)_r$ when $T_0 \approx 90$ MeV (see Figure 6.11). This discussion is for *electrons* only. Heavy particles have insignificant radiative losses.

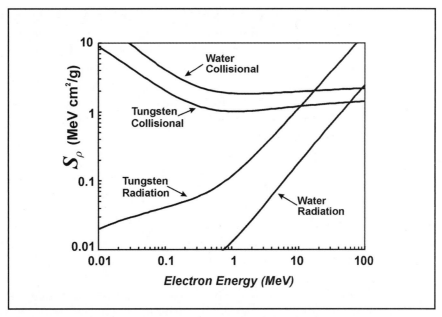

Figure 6.11: Mass collisional and mass radiative stopping power for water and for tungsten as a function of electron energy. Note that both the vertical and horizontal axes are logarithmic and that the collisional stopping power is roughly constant for energies above about 1 MeV. In water at therapeutic energies the radiative stopping power is significantly less than the collisional stopping power. (Data taken from http://www.nist.gov/physlab/data/radiation.cfm. Stopping Power Tables, M. J. Berger.)

The radiative mass stopping power gives the radiative energy loss rate for a particular energy. The radiation yield $Y(T_0)$ is the total fraction of the initial kinetic energy T_0 emitted as electromagnetic radiation as an electron slows down and comes to rest. The total energy radiated by each electron is $Y(T_0) \cdot T_0$.

Both delta rays and radiative interactions carry energy away from the main ionization "track." They do not deposit energy locally. To evaluate local energy deposition, interactions that produce δ-rays with energy above some cutoff value Δ should be excluded from the collisional stopping power.[4] Toward this end, we define the restricted mass collision stopping power, usually written as:

$$\frac{L}{\rho} = \left(\frac{\Delta T}{\rho \Delta x} \right)_{c, T_\delta < \Delta}. \tag{6.14}$$

The restricted stopping power is the mass collision stopping power from all soft collisions plus all hard collisions with $T_\delta < \Delta$, where T_δ is the kinetic energy of the delta ray. The cutoff energy is typically chosen as $\Delta = 100$ eV; beyond this energy the delta rays can travel far enough to

---

[4]Do not confuse the symbol Δ as used to denote a change (e.g., Δx) and the cutoff energy Δ: this may be a bit confusing, but it does correspond to standard usage of these symbols.

cause ionizations elsewhere. Note that when $\Delta \to \infty$, the restricted stopping power becomes equal to the mass collision stopping power. The restricted mass stopping power is important in beam calibration protocols and it forms the basis for the definition of linear energy transfer (LET), which is of great importance in the subject of radiobiology. Let us cite some numbers for a 2 MeV electron in water. For this case $(S_\rho)_c$ = 1.8 MeV cm^2/g, and if Δ = 100 keV, the restricted stopping power is 1.6 MeV cm^2/g; however if Δ = 100 eV, then L/ρ = 1.0 MeV cm^2/g.

Biological damage is related to the local energy deposition. A quantity that is frequently used to describe this is the linear energy transfer or LET. The LET is defined as:

$$L_\Delta \left(\text{keV}/\mu\text{m}\right) = \frac{\rho}{10}\left[\left(\frac{\Delta T}{\rho \Delta x}\right)_{c,T_\delta < \Delta} \text{MeV cm}^2/\text{g}\right]. \qquad (6.15)$$

Note that the density simply cancels in this definition. As the LET is a measure of local energy deposition, convenient units are keV/μm. The factor of 10 in the dominator of equation (6.15) is necessary for unit conversion. LET does not include energy losses due to delta rays above the cutoff or from radiative interactions. The LET for 1.00 MeV electrons is 0.25 keV/μm. When these electrons slow down and their energy drops to 1 keV, the LET rises to 12.3 keV/μm. The electrons set in motion by Co-60 radiation (1.25 MeV photons) have a range of initial kinetic energies and therefore the LET for these electrons has a range as well, from 0.2 to 2 keV/μm.[5]

6.2.3 Range

If the stopping power of a charged particle did not depend on its speed or kinetic energy, then we could easily calculate the distance it would travel by dividing the initial kinetic energy by the rate of loss of kinetic energy (i.e., the stopping power).[6] The distance that a charged particle travels before coming to rest is called its *range*. As an example, if the initial kinetic energy of a particle is T_0 = 5 MeV and its stopping power is a constant S = 2 MeV/cm (independent of its changing kinetic energy), the distance it would travel before coming to rest would be T_0/S = (5 MeV)/(2 MeV/cm) = 2.5 cm. An approximate expression for the range $\Re$ is:

$$\Re \approx \frac{T_0}{S}. \qquad (6.16)$$

---

[5] The LET values are from *The Physics of Radiology,* Fourth Edition, H.E. Johns and J. R. Cunningham, 1983.

[6] Assuming that the charged particle always continues to travel in the same direction. This is a dubious assumption for electrons.

This cannot be quite correct because S depends on T; that is, the stopping power changes as the particle slows down. The actual range is therefore expected to be somewhat different than given by this formula. Equation (6.16) also assumes what is known as the continuous slowing down approximation (CSDA), which presumes that energy loss is a continuous process rather than a discrete process due to abrupt collisions. The assumption of continuous energy loss is probably reasonable when the energy lost in any given collision $\Delta T \ll T$. This condition no longer holds at the end of a charged particle's path. Near the end of its path, the particle loses energy in abrupt steps, like a freely bouncing ball which loses energy each time it bounces. Example 6.2 illustrates the application of some of the quantities discussed in this and the previous section of the text.

Example 6.2

Electrons with energy 20 MeV are incident upon water and expend all of their energy in coming to rest. The radiation yield is $Y(20 \text{ MeV})$ = 0.0826 and the collisional and radiative stopping powers are:

$$(S_\rho)_c = 2.046 \text{ MeV cm}^2/\text{g and } (S_\rho)_r = 0.409 \text{ MeV cm}^2/\text{g}.$$

a. How much energy does each electron radiate (bremsstrahlung) in coming to rest?

Energy radiated = $T_0 \cdot Y(T) = 20 \times 0.0826 = 1.65$ MeV.

b. How much energy is lost due to collisional interactions?

Collision energy loss = $20.0 - 1.65 = 18.35$ MeV.

c. Estimate the range of the electrons.

$\mathfrak{R} \approx T_0/S$

$S_\rho = (S_\rho)_c + (S_\rho)_r = (2.046 + 0.409) \text{ MeV cm}^2/\text{g} = 2.454 \text{ MeV cm}^2/\text{g}$

$S = S_\rho \times \rho = 2.454 \text{ MeV cm}^2/\text{g} \times 1.00 \text{ g/cm}^3 = 2.454 \text{ MeV/cm}$

$\mathfrak{R} \approx (20 \text{ MeV})/(2.454 \text{ MeV/cm}) = 8.2$ cm

The actual CSDA range for 20 MeV electrons is 9.3 cm.

Figure 6.11 shows that the mass collision stopping power, which is the dominant contribution to S_ρ for electrons in water, is approximately constant with energy for energies of interest in radiation therapy.

Rule of thumb: At therapy energies, for electrons in water, $S \approx 2$ MeV/cm; that is, electrons lose about 2 MeV for every centimeter traveled. The approximate range of such electrons in centimeters is therefore: $\Re$(cm) $\approx T_0$ (MeV)/2.

6.2.4 Mean Energy To Produce an Ion Pair

The average energy lost by a charged particle (in a specified medium) in producing an ion pair is given by:

$$\overline{W} = \frac{T_0}{\overline{N}}, \tag{6.17}$$

where T_0 is the initial kinetic energy of the particle and $\overline{N}$ is the average number of ion pairs produced by a given type of particle stopping in a specified medium. The average energy necessary to produce an ion pair is almost totally independent of the initial electron energy.[7] For electrons stopping in dry air:

$$\overline{W}_{air} = 33.97 \text{ eV/ion-pair}$$

$$\frac{\overline{W}_{air}}{e} = 33.97 \text{ J/C}. \tag{6.18}$$

This value is roughly the same for electrons in tissue, as the effective Z of air and of tissue are roughly the same. An illustration of the application of equations (6.17) and (6.18) is given in Example 6.3.

Example 6.3

How many ion pairs does a 1 MeV electron produce (in air) along its track and the track of its δ-rays?

$$\overline{N} = \frac{T_0}{\overline{W}} = \left(10^6 \text{ eV}\right) / \left(34 \text{ eV/ion-pair}\right) = 2.9 \times 10^4 \text{ ion pairs}.$$

6.2.5 Heavy Charged Particle Interactions and the Bragg Peak

Heavy charged particles include protons, alpha particles, heavy ions, etc. As we have discussed in section 6.2, energy loss for heavy charged particles differs from electrons in that heavy charged particles tend to

---

[7]The reason for this is not expected to be obvious.

have straight ionization tracks because they are not as easily scattered as electrons, and radiation losses are negligible. The ionization tracks of heavy charged particles are dense and these particles have a high LET. For two heavy charged particles having the same speed, $(S_\rho)_c \propto z^2$, where z is the charge of the incident particle. For this reason, multiply charged particles (e.g., alpha particles) have a particularly high LET. The LET of 5 MeV protons is 8 keV/μm, and for 20 MeV alpha particles (which have the same speed as 5 MeV protons) the LET is 32 keV/μm.

At low energies, $(S_\rho)_c \propto 1/v^2$, where v is the speed of the particle.[8] This implies that the energy deposition rate rises rapidly as the particle slows down. Most of the energy (or dose, which we have not yet defined) will therefore be deposited at the end of the track. This results in a peak in the deposition of absorbed energy as a function of depth. This peak is called the *Bragg peak*. An example is shown in Figure 6.12 for a proton beam interacting with water.

The Bragg peak is very useful for certain types of localized therapy: the energy is preferentially deposited at larger depths where a tumor might be located and at the same time the absorbed energy is relatively small at smaller depths where normal tissue may reside. Most importantly, the dose beyond (distal to) the Bragg peak is essentially zero. There are a few centers in the United States (and elsewhere) that are exploiting this attribute of proton beams (see chapter 20). It is important to emphasize that only heavy charged particles exhibit a Bragg peak (protons, alpha particles, etc.). *Electrons do not exhibit a Bragg peak* because they are scattered very easily and they do not follow straight tracks like heavy charged particles. For the same reason, electrons do not have as distinct and well-defined a range as do heavy charged particles.

The Bragg peak is actually too narrow for the treatment of most tumors. The peak shown in Figure 6.12 extends only over a narrow range in depth of perhaps 20 mm. Many tumors are larger than this. The peak can be smeared out or spread out by inserting variable amounts of material into the beam to spread the beam energy. A single thickness of material would simply shift the Bragg peak toward the surface. A variable amount of material is inserted into the beam by using a rotating plastic propellor with varying thickness (see chapter 20). A range in incident particle energies leads to a plateau as shown in Figure 6.12. The "cost" of this is to raise the relative dose at smaller depths.

6.3 Neutron Interactions with Matter

Neutron interactions are of importance in radiation therapy for two reasons. First, high-energy linear accelerator beams have a neutron contaminant (see section 6.1.5). These neutrons do not contribute significantly to patient dose, but they do pose a radiation safety hazard. This is

---

[8]Clearly this dependence cannot extend all the way down to v = 0 or the stopping power would become infinite.

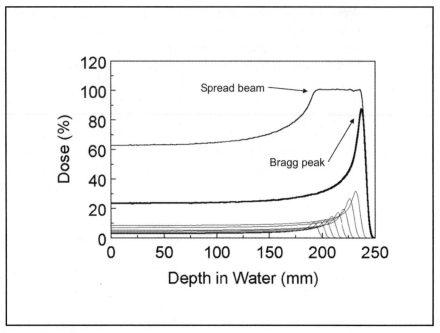

Figure 6.12: The relative absorbed energy per unit mass (dose) as a function of depth for a proton beam of energy 200 MeV. The sharp peak in energy deposition near the end of the track is called the Bragg peak. This distribution of dose with depth is quite different than for photons (chapter 10) and electrons (chapter 15). The peak is too narrow for treating most tumors and it is therefore "spread" out by interposing a varying amount of material in the beam. This creates the dose distributions shown at the bottom of the graph. These add to yield the spread beam plateau shown. (Courtesy of iThemba Labs, Faure, South Africa)

discussed in chapter 17, section 17.8. Second, there are a small number of facilities that treat patients directly with neutrons, either by external beam or brachytherapy.

We have already discussed neutron activation in chapter 3, section 3.15.2. Neutron activation is of importance for the production of medically useful radioisotopes and it is occasionally of relevance in radiation safety. It is not of importance in the treatment of patients with neutron beams. Activation of certain components (e.g., the flattening filter) of linear accelerators can be of significance during maintenance of these machines. The flattening filter of a decommissioned high-energy linear accelerator may have a significant amount of activity. In this case, the flattening filter cannot be simply discarded as trash.

Neutrons, like photons, are a form of indirectly ionizing radiation. As such, they must first transfer their energy to charged particles and then the charged particles in turn deposit their energy in the matter. Photons interact predominantly with electrons. Photon interactions are therefore dependent on the target material electron density. As shown in section 6.1.3, electron density is relatively independent of the elemental composition of the absorbing material. Neutrons interact primarily with nuclei in the absorbing material. Neutron interactions are therefore highly dependent on elemental composition. For this reason, neutron interaction with matter can be quite complex. In human tissue the predominant elements are hydrogen, oxygen, carbon, and nitrogen.

There are two major categories of neutron interactions. A neutron can scatter from a nucleus in the target material, changing direction and losing energy in the process, or the neutron can be absorbed by the nucleus and be replaced by secondary radiation. The secondary radiation can be a gamma ray, a proton, an alpha particle, and the nuclei of the absorbing material itself. The secondary particles can be produced by neutron-induced nuclear reactions.

For energetic neutrons the predominant energy transfer is elastic scattering with nuclei of the material itself. When a neutron collides with a nucleus, it transfers some of its kinetic energy to the nucleus, causing it to recoil. The most efficient energy transfer occurs with hydrogen. The proton has a mass that is nearly equal to that of the neutron. When a neutron collides with a proton, it can give up all of its energy to the proton in a single collision. When a neutron strikes a heavy nucleus, it can only transfer a portion of its kinetic energy in any single interaction. There is a good analogy between this and billiards. When the cue ball strikes another ball (with the same mass) head on, it can come completely to rest giving up all of its kinetic energy to the other ball. In contrast, when the cue ball strikes the side cushion, which is a part of the massive table, it rebounds losing only a small amount of its kinetic energy. When protons are set into motion by neutrons, they lose their associated atomic electron. They then traverse the absorbing material leaving a heavy ionization track.

Once neutrons have slowed down sufficiently, they can be captured by nuclei. When a neutron is captured by a nucleus. the nucleus can be left in an excited state and emit a gamma ray. This is the (n, γ) reaction: a neutron comes in, is absorbed, and a gamma goes out. This plays an important role in radiation shielding because when neutrons are absorbed by shielding material nuclei, those nuclei emit gammas, which must then be shielded for. The neutrons must be attenuated first, then the gammas released by the absorption of the neutrons must also be attenuated.

Efficient absorbers of neutrons are hydrogen-rich materials such as human fat, paraffin wax, polyethylene plastic, concrete, etc. Although lead is a good material for shielding photons, it is a poor shielding material against neutrons. The predominant mode of energy deposition from fast neutrons in tissue is due to recoil protons. The recoil protons have a much higher LET than electrons. This has important radiobiological implications.

Chapter Summary

- The type and strength of the interaction of radiation with matter depends on the kind of radiation, the energy of the radiation, and the composition of the material with which it interacts.

- Directly ionizing radiation: high-energy charged particles that directly cause ionization in the medium

- Indirectly ionizing radiation: neutral particles (photons or neutrons) that set charged particles in the medium into motion which then go on to cause ionization in the medium

Photon Interactions (incident photon energy is E_γ)

1. **Interaction with atomic electrons**
   a. *Coherent (elastic scattering):* photon changes direction without any change in energy. Only important at very low energy.
   b. *Photoelectric:* the photon is absorbed and its energy is transferred to an atomic electron (photoelectron), which is ejected from the atom. The photoelectric effect cannot eject an electron from an atom unless $E_\gamma > E_b$. The kinetic energy of the photoelectron will be $T_e = E_\gamma - E_b$. Dominates at low energies (diagnostic) and at high atomic number. The mass attenuation coefficient is approximately proportional to $(Z/E_\gamma)^3$. The photoelectric effect is especially likely to occur when the photon energy just exceeds the binding energy of a K, L, or M shell electron. As the energy of the bombarding photon just exceeds the binding energy, there is an abrupt rise in the mass attenuation coefficient because it suddenly becomes possible for the photon to be absorbed in a new way—referred to as a K, L or M shell edge, depending on which shell is affected. For water, the photoelectric effect dominates below about 25 keV. The strong Z dependence of the photoelectric effect forms the basis for the use of radiographic contrast agents such as iodine and barium because of the high Z value of these elements.
   c. *Compton scattering:* photon is scattered with reduced energy; that is, the photon changes its direction and its energy. The energy lost by the photon is transferred to an atomic electron that is ejected from the atom and deposits dose along its path. Compton scattering is the dominant interaction for photons in tissue at therapy energies. Mass attenuation coefficient is directly proportional to the electron density of the material, which is roughly independent of Z except for hydrogen-rich materials.

The maximum energy of a photon scattered through 90° is 0.511 MeV (equal to the rest mass energy of an electron). The maximum energy of a photon which is scattered at 180° is 0.255 MeV. At therapy energies, the angle of scattering is usually small. The value of σ/ρ is approximately constant for photon energy less than about 1 MeV. For energies above 1 MeV, $\sigma/\rho \sim 1/E_\gamma$.

2. **Interaction with atomic nucleus**
   a. *Pair production:* When $E_\gamma > 2\ m_0 c^2 = 1.022$ MeV, it becomes possible for the bombarding photon to disappear and be replaced by an electron positron pair. This process can occur when a photon passes close to an atomic nucleus. A positron will go on to annihilate with an electron producing a pair of 0.5 MeV photons. The mass attenuation coefficient for pair production is proportional to Z.
   b. *Photonuclear reactions:* High-energy photon reacts with a nucleus which then emits a neutron; (n, γ) reaction. High-energy linac beams contain a neutron contaminate which must be shielded.

Charged Particle Interactions with Matter

- Very different from photons.
  1. **Photons:** Perhaps a few dozen interactions (in traversing medium) or none—leads to exponential attenuation.
  2. **Charged particles:** Usually many small interactions, a small amount of kinetic energy is lost in each interaction—there is a definite range (beyond this range, no particles).

- A 1 MeV electron may undergo 10^5 interactions in tissue before losing all kinetic energy.

- High-energy electrons interact with matter either by "collisions" with electrons in the matter or via "radiative" interactions (bremsstrahlung radiation when an electron passes close to an atomic nucleus).

- There are distinct differences for electrons versus heavy charged particles such as protons, alpha particles, pions, etc. Electron paths are not straight—"tortured." Electrons have low mass and they are easily scattered.

- Mass stopping power: S_ρ = kinetic energy loss per unit length divided by the density of the material, typical units: MeV $\cdot$ cm^2/g.

- Delta rays: Electrons set in motion along the track of a high-energy bombarding electron, carry energy away from the main ionization track.

- Restricted stopping power: The collisional stopping power excluding the energy lost to delta rays above some specified cutoff energy value Δ.

- Linear Energy Transfer (LET): Restricted stopping power, except units are keV/µm; a direct measure of microscopic energy deposition, closely correlated with biological damage.

- The distance that a charged particle travels before coming to rest is called its **range**.

 Rule of thumb: The approximate range (in centimeters) for electrons in water at therapy energies is: $\Re(\text{cm}) \approx T_0 \,(\text{MeV})/2$, where T_0 is the initial energy of the electrons in MeV.

- Bragg Peak: A sharp rise in the deposition of energy (dose) at the end of the particle range—most of the energy is deposited at the end of the track. Electrons do not exhibit a Bragg peak because they are easily scattered. The Bragg peak can be very useful for radiation therapy (e.g., proton therapy) when the dose needs to be very localized.

Neutron Interactions with Matter

Neutrons, like photons, are indirectly ionizing radiation. They must first transfer their energy to charged particles, then the charged particles deposit dose. Neutrons interact with atomic nuclei in the target material. Neutron absorption is sensitive to elemental composition. There are two primary mechanisms of energy loss. High-energy neutrons scatter from nuclei losing some of their energy in the process. This mechanism is most efficient for hydrogen. When scattering occurs, the charged nucleus recoils carrying away some of the neutron energy. Once the neutrons have slowed down, they can be absorbed in the (n, γ) process. Efficient absorbers of neutrons are hydrogen-rich materials such as human fat, wax, plastics, etc. The predominant mode of energy deposition from fast neutrons in tissue is due to high LET recoil protons.

Problems

1. Why are barium and iodine chosen as contrast agents for medical x-ray imaging studies?

2. In the diagnostic energy range, if the atomic number of an absorbing material is doubled, how much will this change the number of photons absorbed per gram?

3. The K-shell binding energy of an electron in a lead atom is 88.0 keV and the L-shell energy is approximately 15.0 keV. A 100 keV photon ejects a K-shell electron.
   a. What is the energy of the photoelectron?
   b. An L-shell electron makes a transition to fill the K-shell vacancy. What is the energy of the photon emitted in this process?

4. Why is the mass attenuation coefficient for Compton scattering roughly independent of Z for all elements except hydrogen? Why is hydrogen an exception?

5. A 1.25 MeV photon undergoes Compton scattering by an electron through a 60° angle.
   a. What kinetic energy does the electron have after the scattering event?
   b. Roughly how far will electrons with this energy travel in water?

6. What is the maximum kinetic energy that can be imparted to an electron by a 1.25 MeV photon? What is the range of such an electron in water?

7. What is the threshold for pair production and why does it have the value that it does?

8. A 5 MeV photon undergoes pair production. What is the initial combined kinetic energy of the electron positron pair?

9. a. Under what conditions are the following interactions most probable? Discuss the dependence on E_γ and Z.
          i. photoelectric   ii. Compton   iii. pair
   b. Which of i through iii above has a threshold and what is the value of the threshold?

10. Which photon interaction mechanism is most probable for each of the following cases:
    a. 100 keV photon in soft tissue
    b. 5 MeV photon in muscle
    c. 5 MeV photon in lead
    d. 18 MeV photon in lead
    e. 50 keV photon in bone
    f. 200 keV photon in soft tissue

11. Identify the mechanisms by which electrons lose energy when moving through matter.

12. Estimate the range of 12 MeV electrons in soft tissue and in air if the density of air is approximately 0.0013 g/cm^3. Assume that S_ρ (2.0 MeV cm^2/g) is the same for soft tissue and air.

13. Calculate the average number of ion pairs produced along the entire paths of 12 MeV electrons that are brought to rest in air. Would the number of ion pairs produced in soft tissue be significantly different?

14. How does the fraction of kinetic energy of an electron that is converted to bremsstrahlung radiation vary with energy and atomic number of the medium?

15. Explain the nature of the Bragg peak. Why is there no Bragg peak for electrons?

16. a. Why is the mass collision stopping power for water higher than for tungsten (see Figure 6.11). Tungsten is far more dense than water. Wouldn't you expect it to be much more efficient at stopping electrons?
    b. In which material will electrons travel the furthest? The density of tungsten is 19 g/cm^3.

17. What is the approximate energy threshold for the production of neutrons via photonuclear reactions?

18. What is the predominant mode of energy transfer for fast neutrons in tissue?

Bibliography

Attix, F. H. *Introduction to Radiological Physics and Radiation Dosimetry.* New York: Wiley InterScience, 1986.

Johns, H. E., and J. R. Cunningham. *The Physics of Radiology,* Fourth Edition. Springfield, IL: Charles C Thomas, 1983.

Kase, K. R., and W. R. Nelson. *Concepts in Radiation Dosimetry.* Oxford, UK: Pergamon Press, 1978.

Khan, F. M. *The Physics of Radiation Therapy,* Fourth Edition. Philadelphia: Lippincott Williams & Wilkins, 2009.

7 Radiation Measurement Quantities

7.1 Introduction

It is important to correlate patient treatment outcome with the amount of radiation received; therefore we need to develop quantitative measures of the characteristics of radiation. We want to describe the intensity of radiation, its ability to ionize matter, the energy absorbed, and the biological damage that results. In the earliest days of radiation therapy the concepts and the measuring instruments were inadequate for accurate quantitative work. Over the years a great deal of effort has been made by physicists to develop the conceptual framework and the instrumentation to make highly reliable radiation measurements. In this chapter we will discuss the conceptual framework, and in chapter 8 we will consider instrumentation. We will not discuss quantities of interest for radiation protection here. That topic will be deferred to chapter 17.

7.2 Exposure

Exposure is a measure of the ability of a photon beam to ionize air. The definition of exposure is:

$$X = \frac{Q}{m},$$ (7.1)

where Q is the sum of all electrical charges of one sign on all ions produced **in air** when all electrons liberated by **photons** in a small volume of (dry) air of mass m are completely stopped in air.

In general, it is necessary to find and count all charge liberated as a result of the photon interactions in m **regardless of where that charge ends up.** Electrons liberated by photons will produce ionization tracks (see Figure 7.1). All of this ionization, coming from tracks originating in m, must be counted in the definition of exposure even though many of these ionization tracks will pass out of the volume of mass m. Each energetic electron, set in motion by a photon, can cause tens to hundreds of thousands of ionizations along its track. Recall from Example 6.3 that a single 1 MeV electron can generate about 30,000 ion pairs in air.

Exposure is a measure of the ability of photon radiation to ionize air. Exposure is:

1. Only defined for photons.
2. Only defined for ionization of air.
3. Not useful above ~3 MeV because of conditions necessary for measurement (see discussion of free air ionization chamber in chapter 8).

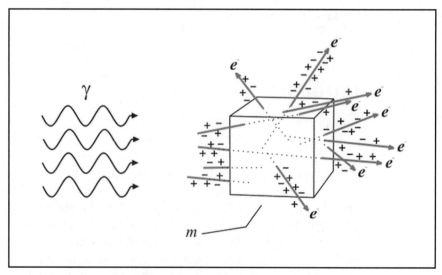

Figure 7.1: Photons irradiate a volume of air mass m. The photons set electrons in motion and the electrons in turn produce further ionization along their tracks. Note that most of the ionization is produced along the tracks of the electrons.

The units of exposure are:

$$[X] = \left[\frac{Q}{m}\right] = \frac{C}{kg}.$$ (7.2)

This is the SI unit of exposure. A more commonly used unit is the roentgen, abbreviated R:

$$1\,R = 2.58 \times 10^{-4}\,\frac{C}{kg}.$$ (7.3)

For some applications, such as radiation protection and imaging, the roentgen is rather large and it is sometimes more convenient to use $mR = 10^{-3}\,R$.

The apparently arbitrary numerical value in equation (7.3) arose from the original definition of the roentgen in terms of antiquated units:

$$X = \frac{Q}{m} = \frac{1 \text{ electrostatic unit (esu)}}{\left(\text{mass of } 1\,cm^3 \text{ air at } 760 \text{ Torr}, 0^\circ C\right)}.$$ (7.4)

The electrostatic unit is an old unit of electrical charge, and 760 Torr of pressure corresponds to the nominal atmospheric pressure at sea level. Under these conditions 1 cm^3 of air has a mass of 0.001293 g. When these units are converted to SI, the result is the numerical value in equation (7.3). An illustration of a calculation involving exposure appears in Example 7.1.

Some representative values of the entrance skin exposure for diagnostic radiographs are:

- 10 mR for a chest x-ray (110 kVp, 3 mAs)
- 300 mR for a lumbar spine exam (70 kVp, 60 mAs)
- 200 mR for a skull film (75 kVp, 50 mAs).

Example 7.1

A volume of 1.0 cm^3 of air is irradiated by x-rays. If the exposure is 1.0 R and if the density of air is 1.20×10^{-3} g/cm^3, what is the ionization charge produced by the x-rays?

The charge produced is given by $Q = X\,m$. Care must be taken to use consistent units: 1.0 R = 2.58×10^{-4} C/kg. The mass of the air is the density times the volume: $m = 1.20 \times 10^{-3}$ g/cm$^3 \times 1.0$ cm^3 = 1.20×10^{-3} g = 1.20×10^{-6} kg.

$Q = 2.58 \times 10^{-4}$ C/kg $\times 1.20 \times 10^{-6}$ kg = 3.3×10^{-10} C = 0.33 nC.

7.3 Charged Particle Equilibrium

The definition of exposure, equation (7.1), requires that all of the charge Q produced by photon interactions in m be measured, regardless of the final location of this charge. Figure 7.1 illustrates that much of this charge may reside outside m. Furthermore, charged particle tracks originating outside m will create ions inside. In general, we are faced with the necessity of locating all electron tracks originating in m and summing all of the charge generated along these tracks. At the same time, we must exclude the charge associated with all tracks originating outside m. This is an almost hopeless task unless a condition called *electronic equilibrium* or *charged particle equilibrium (CPE)* holds.

In a radiation field, if each charged particle of a given type and energy leaving a volume is replaced by a charged particle of the same type and energy entering that volume, then the volume is said to be in charged particle equilibrium. It does not make sense to say that CPE holds unless the volume concerned is clearly specified.

When CPE prevails in a mass m of air, it becomes easy to measure exposure. We do not need to worry about electron tracks leaving the volume because any track that exits is replaced by an identical track entering. For the same reason, we do not need to worry about tracks entering; each one is replaced by an identical track leaving. Under these conditions, we can measure exposure by simply measuring the total charge inside the volume of mass m. This is the importance of CPE. Fortunately, CPE is common. For photon energies above a few MeV however, CPE requires a volume of air that is so large as to be impractical (see chapter 8, section 8.1.1).

7.4 Some Important Radiation Dosimetry Quantities

Fluence is defined as

$$\Phi = \frac{N}{a}, \qquad (7.5)$$

where N is the total number of particles entering a sphere of small cross-sectional area a (see Figure 7.2). The symbol Φ is the capital Greek letter phi. The particles could be photons, electrons, neutrons, etc. The units of fluence can be found from the definition: $[\Phi] = [N/a] = $ m^{-2} or cm^{-2}. The number of particles has no units.

Energy fluence is defined as

$$\Psi = \frac{E_T}{a}, \qquad (7.6)$$

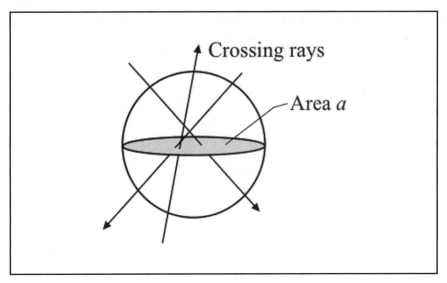

Figure 7.2: Particles entering a sphere of small cross-sectional *a*.

where E_T is the total energy carried by all particles entering a sphere of cross-sectional area *a*. The symbol Ψ is the capital Greek letter psi (pronounced "sigh"). The units of energy fluence are $[\Psi]$ = J/m^2. For a monoenergetic photon beam $E_T = E_\gamma N$ and $\Psi = E_T/a = E_\gamma N/a = E_\gamma \Phi$, where E_γ is the energy of each photon.

The *energy transfer coefficient* (μ_{tr}) is the fraction of the photon energy that is transferred to kinetic energy of charged particles per unit thickness of absorber:

$$\mu_{tr} = \frac{\bar{E}_{tr}}{E_\gamma}\mu, \qquad (7.7)$$

where $\bar{E}_{tr}$ is the average energy *transferred* to kinetic energy of charged particles per photon interaction and μ is the linear attenuation coefficient. For Compton scattering this is the average energy transferred to an electron from a photon of some specified energy. Note that $\mu_{tr} < \mu$ because a photon cannot give up all of its energy to an electron in Compton scattering and therefore $\bar{E}_{tr}/E_\gamma < 1$. The energy absorption coefficient is defined as:

$$\mu_{en} = \frac{\bar{E}_{ab}}{E_\gamma}\mu, \qquad (7.8)$$

where $\bar{E}_{ab}$ is the average energy *absorbed* per interaction from photons.

Electrons can lose energy via two mechanisms: (1) collisions, which lead to ionization and excitation and (2) radiation (bremsstrahlung) that is lost to the local region. Recall that the radiation yield $Y(T_0)$ is the total fraction of the initial kinetic energy T_0 emitted as electromagnetic radiation when a single electron slows down and comes to rest. When electrons are set in motion by photons (even monoenergetic photons), they start off with a variety of values of initial kinetic energy T_0. The average value of $Y(T_0)$, averaged over all values of the starting energy T_0, is given the symbol g. This is the fraction of the initial kinetic energy of *all* the electrons set in motion by photon irradiation that is lost to bremsstrahlung as the electrons are brought to rest in the medium.

There is a relationship between the energy absorption coefficient and the energy transfer coefficient:

$$\mu_{en} = \mu_{tr}(1-g). \tag{7.9}$$

This reflects the fact that some fraction of the transferred energy is radiated. Often g is small and $\mu_{en} \approx \mu_{tr}$. For Co-60 radiation in air, $g = 0.0032$ and for 100 to 135 keV x-rays, $g = 0.0001$.

A very important quantity in radiological physics for indirectly ionizing radiation is *kerma,* which is an acronym for _k_inetic _e_nergy _r_eleased per unit _ma_ss in a medium at a specified point. The definition of kerma is:

$$K = \frac{E_{TR}}{m}, \tag{7.10}$$

where E_{TR} is the sum of all the initial kinetic energies *of all charged particles* (generally electrons for photon irradiation and protons for neutron irradiation) liberated by uncharged ionizing particles in a material of mass m. Note that E_{TR} is not the same as $\bar{E}_{tr}$. The units of kerma are $[K] = [E_{TR}/m] = $ J/kg. In this context, this combination of units has been given a special name: 1 J/kg = 1 gray = 1 Gy. The value of the kerma at a particular location may not be a measure of biological damage there, because it does not necessarily tell how much energy is *absorbed* at that spot. Not all of the energy is retained locally; some is radiated away by bremsstrahlung emission from the charged particles and the charged particles move off to a different locality. The tracks of the charged particles produced may be appreciable in length; therefore energy transferred to charged particles in mass m at a particular location may be absorbed elsewhere.

An alternative but equivalent equation for the kerma, in terms of the energy fluence, is

$$K = \Psi \frac{\bar{\mu}_{tr}}{\rho}, \tag{7.11}$$

where $\bar{\mu}_{tr}$ is the average value of μ_{tr}, averaged over the spectrum of the incoming photons.[1] This equation is equivalent to equation (7.10).

---

[1] This equation is not expected to be obvious.

The kerma can be written as the sum of the collision kerma and the radiative kerma. The collision kerma is energy transferred to charged particles that go on to produce excitations or ionizations. The radiative kerma is the energy transferred to charged particles that ends up being radiated:

$$K = K_c + K_r,$$ (7.12)

where

$$K_c = \Psi \frac{\bar{\mu}_{en}}{\rho} \qquad K_r = \Psi \frac{\bar{\mu}_{en}}{\rho} \frac{g}{1-g}.$$ (7.13)

One of the most important quantities in radiation therapy dosimetry is the *absorbed dose*. It is closely related to biological damage because it is the energy actually absorbed in the medium at a specific location. The definition is:

$$D = \frac{E_{AB}}{m},$$ (7.14)

where E_{AB} is the total energy absorbed from indirectly or directly ionizing radiation inside a mass m of material. The units of dose are J/kg; the same as the units of kerma. The gray (Gy) is the SI unit of dose. An old unit of dose which is still sometimes used is the rad: 1 rad = 100 erg/g. The erg is an antique unit of energy:

100 rads = 1 Gy = 100 cGy
1 rad = 1 cGy.

In the old days, physicians were accustomed to writing radiation dose prescriptions in rads. When told that they needed to adopt proper SI units, many of them simply wrote down the same numerical value for the dose and instead of following this with the unit "rad" wrote "cGy." It is important to understand that the dose may vary from point to point in a medium. A radiation therapy prescription must not only specify the dose to be delivered, but also precisely where that dose is to be delivered.

There is a relationship between dose and collision kerma. Recall that the collision kerma is the energy transferred to charged particles per unit mass that ultimately is absorbed via collisions, as opposed to bremsstrahlung. After the energy is transferred to the charged particles, they move off to another location where they deposit this energy; that is, the energy is absorbed. If CPE prevails in a given region, then for every charged particle that carries its energy out of the region another identical particle will enter. In this case the dose is equal to the collision kerma:

$$D \overset{\text{CPE}}{=} K_c.$$ (7.15)

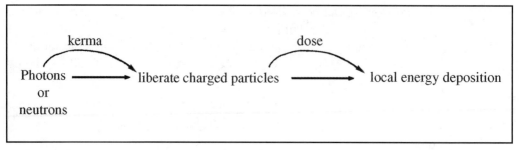

Figure 7.3: Illustration of the relationships in absorption of energy from indirectly ionizing radiation.

As described at the beginning of chapter 6, absorption of energy from indirectly ionizing radiation (photons or neutrons) is a two-step process. The first step involves liberation of charged particles. This is related to kerma. The second step involves the absorption of the energy of the charged particles. This is related to dose. These relationships are illustrated in Figure 7.3. Example 7.2 illustrates some of the concepts of this chapter and the preceding chapter.

Example 7.2

A beam of 10 MeV photons interacts with water. In some small volume of the water at a particular location the photon fluence is 3.86×10^{14} m^{-2} and $\mu/\rho = 0.0222$ cm^2/g, $\mu_{tr}/\rho = 0.0162$ cm^2/g and $\mu_{en}/\rho = 0.0157$ cm^2/g.

a.   What is the energy fluence in units of J/m^2?

The energy fluence for a monoenergetic photon beam is $\Psi = E\, \Phi$ where $E = 10^7$ eV $\times 1.6 \times 10^{-19}$ J/eV $= 1.6 \times 10^{-12}$ J; therefore $\Psi = 1.65 \times 10^{-12}$ J $\times 3.86 \times 10^{14}$ m^{-2} $= 6.37 \times 10^2$ J/m^2.

b.   What is the average energy transferred to an electron by a 10 MeV photon?

From equation (7.7),

$$\bar{E}_{tr} = E_\gamma \frac{\mu_{tr}}{\mu} = E_\gamma \frac{\mu_{tr}/\rho}{\mu/\rho} = 10 \text{ MeV} \frac{0.0162 \text{ cm}^2/g}{0.0222 \text{ cm}^2/g} = 7.3 \text{ MeV}.$$

c.   What is the average energy absorbed by the water per photon interaction?

From equation (7.8),

$$\bar{E}_{ab} = E_\gamma \frac{\mu_{en}}{\mu} = E_\gamma \frac{\mu_{en}/\rho}{\mu/\rho} = 10 \text{ MeV} \frac{0.0157 \text{ cm}^2/g}{0.0222 \text{ cm}^2/g} = 7.1 \text{ MeV}.$$

Example 7.2 (continued)

d. Why is there a difference between the answer to part b and part c and where does the missing energy go?

Not all of the energy that is transferred to electrons is absorbed. Some of the transferred energy is radiated as bremsstrahlung:

$$\bar{E}_{tr} - \bar{E}_{ab} = 7.3 \text{ MeV} - 7.1 \text{ MeV} = 0.2 \text{ MeV}.$$

e. What is the value of g?

From equation (7.9),

$$1 - g = \frac{\mu_{en}}{\mu_{tr}} = \frac{\mu_{en}/\rho}{\mu_{tr}/\rho} = \frac{0.0157 \text{ cm}^2/g}{0.0222 \text{ cm}^2/g} = 0.969,$$

and therefore $g = 0.031$. Notice that the energy lost to bremsstrahlung divided by the average energy transferred is $0.2/7.3 = 0.03 = g$.

f. What is the value of the collision kerma expressed in Gy?

The collision kerma can be calculated using equation (7.13). A consistent set of units must be used and therefore, if Ψ is in units of J/m^2, then μ_{en}/ρ must be expressed in units of m^2/kg. The conversion can be done as follows:

$$1 \frac{\text{cm}^2}{g} = 1 \frac{\text{cm}^2}{g} \times \frac{10^3 g}{kg} \times \left(\frac{1 \text{ m}}{10^2 \text{ cm}} \right)^2 = 10^{-1} \frac{m^2}{kg},$$

so that $\mu_{en}/\rho = 1.57 \times 10^{-3}$ m^2/kg and $K_c = \Psi \, (\mu_{en}/\rho) = 6.37 \times 10^2$ J/m$^2 \times 1.57 \times 10^{-3}$ m^2/kg = 1.00 J/kg = 1.00 Gy.

g. If there is CPE in the given volume, what is the absorbed dose within this volume?

For CPE the absorbed dose is equal to the collision kerma and therefore $D = 1.00$ Gy.

7.5 Dose Buildup and Skin Sparing

In the early days of radiation therapy, only low-energy superficial beams were available. For superficial x-ray beams, the dose delivered to a patient was limited by skin tolerance. Above a certain dose (which may be suboptimal for tumor eradication), adverse skin reactions require discontinuation of radiation treatment. For megavoltage (MV) x-ray beams, the relative dose to the skin is low. This is called *skin sparing* and it is one of the major advantages of MV beams. The other advantage is penetration, as MV beams can penetrate much more deeply than lower-energy beams. Skin sparing is illustrated in Figure 7.4, which shows the dose as a function of depth for a MV x-ray beam. The dose initially rises with increasing depth, reaches a maximum value, and then declines as the depth increases further. The depth at which the dose is a maximum is called "d-max" and will be denoted as d_m in this book. The region over which the dose rises from the skin surface to its maximum value is called the *build-up region*.

At first glance, the build-up phenomenon is rather surprising. For an external beam of photon radiation incident upon matter, the fluence has its maximum value at the surface and it declines with increasing depth of penetration. We might therefore naively expect the dose to be a maximum at the surface and to decline with increasing depth. The attenuation of the photon fluence is only half the story however. We must remember that the absorption of energy by indirectly ionizing photons is a two-step process and that it is the electrons set in motion by the photons that deliver the dose. We must consider the second step to understand buildup.

Why does skin sparing occur for high-energy beams? First consider the hypothetical situation in which there is no attenuation of incoming photons. Examine Figure 7.5, which shows photons incident upon a rectangular block of material. The block has been divided into equal-size

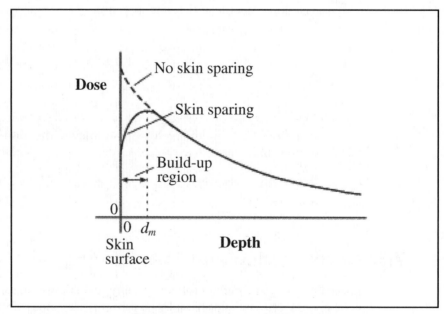

Figure 7.4: A graph of dose vs. depth for a MV photon beam (solid curve). The surface dose is relatively low. With increasing depth the dose rises to a maximum value and then declines. The depth of the maximum dose is called "d-max", denoted in this book as d_m. The phenomenon of relatively low surface dose is referred to as "skin sparing."

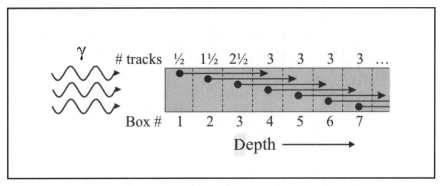

Figure 7.5: Photons are incident upon a rectangular block of material. Electrons are set in motion by photon interactions. The electrons are shown as dots with arrows. It is assumed that one electron is set into motion in each box and that each electron has a range of 3 box lengths. This ignores photon attenuation. The number of electron tracks in each box is listed at the top.

boxes at different depths. As the photons move into the material, they set electrons into motion. For this hypothetical situation the photons are not attenuated as they move deeper into the block. Let us further assume that one electron is set into motion in the first box. Since we have assumed the photons are not attenuated, then one electron will be set into motion in each box, regardless of how deep the box is. Dose is deposited along the electron tracks. We shall assume that the dose in each box is proportional to the number of electron tracks traversing the box. Let us suppose that the electron range is 3 box lengths.

Let us now examine a graph (Figure 7.6) of the number of tracks in each box (call it "Dose") versus the box number (call it "Depth"). The dose rises with increasing depth and reaches a maximum in box 4. Notice that d_m occurs approximately at a depth that corresponds to the electron range (about 3 box lengths). Also note that beyond d_m we have CPE. In box 1 we have one electron leaving and none entering: definitely not CPE. In box 2 we have one electron that enters, but it also leaves; we also have another electron that is generated in the box and leaves. Therefore we have one electron entering and two electrons leaving. We therefore do not have CPE in box 2. In box 3 we have two electrons entering and three leaving. In box 4 we have three electrons entering and three leaving, and thus we have CPE in this box. From here on, each box will be in CPE.

We have assumed that the same number of electrons is set in motion in each box, that is, we have ignored photon attenuation. If we now include attenuation, how do we expect Figure 7.6 to change? The number of electrons set in motion in successive boxes will gradually decrease. There will still be a build-up region; but as we go deeper, the number of electrons set in motion will dwindle and therefore the curve in Figure 7.6 will turn over and begin to decline as the number of tracks becomes fewer and fewer. Figure 7.6 will then begin to look like Figure 7.4.

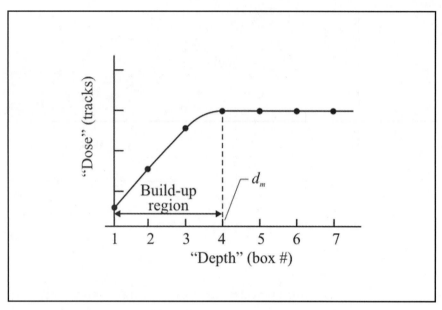

Figure 7.6: The dose distribution resulting from the conditions illustrated in Figure 7.5.

The value of d_m is approximately equal to the range of the electrons set in motion by the photons. There is no discernible buildup for low-energy photons (such as diagnostic or superficial energy) because d_m is very small due to the small range of the electrons set in motion. For Co-60 radiation, which has a mean photon energy of 1.25 MeV, d_m is approximately 0.5 cm. Nominal values of d_m for MV photon beams are listed in chapter 10.

If you think about the previous discussion, you may wonder why there is any surface dose at all. You might expect it to be zero because at the surface no electrons have been set in motion. Yet we see from Figure 7.4 that it is not zero. Our discussion has been oversimplified. Surface dose results from two factors: backscattered electrons and a phenomenon we have not previously considered, electron contamination of the photon beam. As electrons move through the medium, they can be scattered through large angles and some electrons can be scattered back toward, and reach, the surface. These electrons will contribute to dose at the surface. In addition, photon beams have some electrons that "contaminate" them. These electrons are unavoidably produced in the head of the treatment machine as photons scatter off the high-density metal components in the head. Also, some electrons will be produced by interaction of the photons in the air between the source and the patient. This electron contamination will also produce dose at the surface. Generally, an attempt is made to keep this contamination to a minimum. The introduction of beam modifiers such as blocks, wedges, and compensators increases this contamination. We will discuss this further in chapter 14.

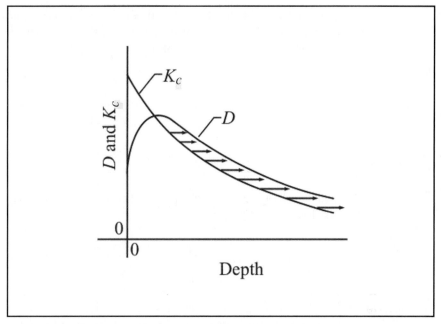

Figure 7.7: The relationship between collision kerma and dose. The dose is characteristic of the collision kerma "upstream."

In a real radiation beam there is no strict CPE at depth because of photon attenuation. Referring again to Figure 7.5, the number of electrons set in motion in each box will decline with depth and therefore we will never have strict CPE, as we did for the case in which there was no attenuation. The energy transferred (per unit mass) to electrons is the collision kerma (we can ignore the small component of energy transfer that leads to later bremsstrahlung emission). We expect the collision kerma to decline steadily with depth due to photon attenuation. This is illustrated in Figure 7.7. The energy transferred to charged particles is absorbed "downstream" (at greater depth). For this reason, the dose at a specific depth is characteristic of the value of the collision kerma "upstream," as portrayed in Figure 7.7, and when true CPE prevails the dose will be equal to the collision kerma.

7.6 Absorbed Dose to Air

We can relate the absorbed dose deposited in air to exposure. We will assume charged particle equilibrium. Recall that the mean energy to produce an ion pair in air is almost constant for all electron energies:

$$\overline{W}_{air} = 33.97 \text{ eV/ion-pair} \quad \text{or} \quad \frac{\overline{W}_{air}}{e} = 33.97 \text{ J/C.} \qquad (7.16)$$

The energy absorbed by the air is $E_{AB} = Q\overline{W}_{air}/e$, where Q is the ionization charge resulting from photon interactions in mass m. If we divide both sides of this equation by the mass:

$$\frac{E_{AB}}{m} = \frac{Q}{m}\frac{\overline{W}_{air}}{e},$$

(7.17)

$$D_{air} = X\frac{\overline{W}_{air}}{e} = \left(K_c\right)_{air}.$$

The quantity $(K_c)_{air}$ is referred to as the *air kerma*. If we express X in roentgens and D_{air} in cGy:

$$D_{air}\left(\text{cGy}\right) = 0.876X\left(\text{R}\right).$$

(7.18)

We will put this result to good use in the next section.

7.7 Dose in a Medium Calculated from Exposure

We are more interested in calculating the dose in a medium such as tissue (or water) rather than the dose in air. However, it is far easier to measure the exposure in air (using a small cavity ionization chamber) than it is to measure the dose in a medium. Let us suppose that we would like to calculate or measure the dose in a medium at a particular location. Let us further suppose that we carve a small cavity out of the medium; that is, we replace the medium at the point of interest by a small air cavity (see Figure 7.8).

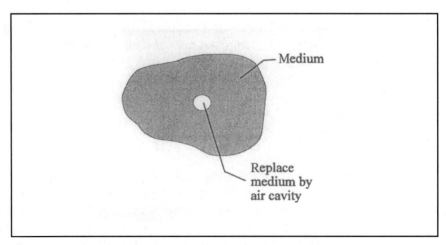

Figure 7.8: The dose in a medium can be calculated by first imagining that we carve a small cavity out of the medium and evaluate the exposure in the air cavity.

We will assume CPE in the air cavity. Now let us imagine that we calculate or measure the exposure in the air cavity. From the value of the exposure it is possible to calculate the dose in the medium. We will first state the result and then derive it. The dose in the medium (in units of cGy) is given by:

$$D_{med}\left(cGy\right) = f_{med} \cdot X\left(R\right) \cdot A, \tag{7.19}$$

where,

f_{med} = roentgen to rad conversion ratio; depends on medium and beam energy,

$X(R)$ = exposure, measured in roentgens, when medium is replaced by an air cavity,

A = fractional attenuation of photons due to the presence of the medium (not to be confused with activity).

Derivation: Assume CPE.

$$D_{air} = \left(K_c\right)_{air} = \Psi_a \left(\frac{\bar{\mu}_{en}}{\rho}\right)_{air}$$

$$D_{med} = \left(K_c\right)_m = \Psi_m \left(\frac{\bar{\mu}_{en}}{\rho}\right)_m$$

We imagine that the medium is replaced by an air cavity for the purpose of determining D_{air}.

$$\frac{D_{med}}{D_{air}} = \frac{\left(\mu_{en}/\rho\right)_m}{\left(\mu_{en}/\rho\right)_a} \left(\frac{\Psi_m}{\Psi_a}\right)$$

Transmission ratio Call it A

$$D_{med} = D_{air} \frac{\left(\mu_{en}/\rho\right)_m}{\left(\mu_{en}/\rho\right)_a} \cdot \frac{\Psi_m}{\Psi_a}$$

$$= X \frac{\overline{W}_{air}}{e} \frac{\left(\mu_{en}/\rho\right)_m}{\left(\mu_{en}/\rho\right)_a} \cdot \frac{\Psi_m}{\Psi_a}$$

$$D_{med}(cGy) = 0.876 \frac{\left(\mu_{en}/\rho\right)_m}{\left(\mu_{en}/\rho\right)_a} \cdot A \cdot X$$

$$\underbrace{\qquad\qquad}_{f_{med}}$$

$$D_{med}(cGy) = f_{med} \cdot X \cdot A$$

Equation (7.19) is only useful in so far as the exposure can easily be measured. As we shall discuss in chapter 8, section 8.3, the exposure is not easily measured for MV beams; therefore equation (7.19) is of use only for Co-60 and lower-energy beams.

The quantity f_{med} is called the f factor or the "roentgens to rads" conversion ratio. The value of this quantity depends on the photon energy as well as the medium. For air $f = 0.876$ and $A = 1$ [see equation (7.18)]. Figure 7.9 shows the f_{med} as a function of photon energy for muscle, water, and bone.

An interesting aspect of Figure 7.9 is that at low energies, the photoelectric effect is especially important as far as dose to bone is concerned. Recall that $\tau/\rho \sim (Z/E_\gamma)^3$. At 100 keV, $f_{bone}/f_{muscle} = 1.8$. For the *same* exposure (in the imaginary cavity) the dose absorbed by bone will be 80% higher than the dose absorbed by muscle. This has implications for treatment with superficial x-rays. Any bone underlying skin treated with superficial x-rays may receive a substantially higher dose than surrounding soft tissue. This is somewhat complicated by the fact that the value of A in equation (7.19) is likely to be lower for bone because bone attenuates more than soft tissue. At high energies, where the Compton effect dominates, the electron density of bone is somewhat smaller than water. At 1 MeV, $f_{bone}/f_{muscle} = 0.94$.

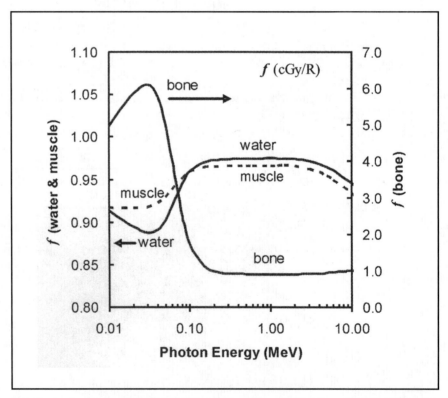

Figure 7.9: The f factor for water, muscle (ICRU 44) and dense bone (ICRU 44) as a function of photon energy. Note that the values for bone must be read from the right-hand vertical scale and the other values are read from the left-hand scale. Bone has a significantly higher f value than water or muscle at energies below about 100 keV. (Mass-energy absorption coefficient data from NIST)

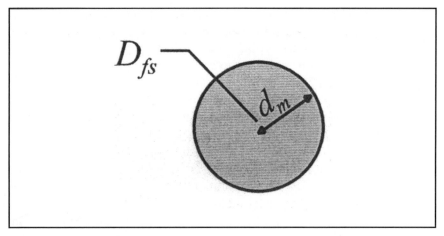

Figure 7.10: Dose in free space refers to the dose at the center of an equilibrium-sized sphere of material that is isolated in "free space."

7.8 Dose in Free Space

The dose in free space D_{fs} is the dose delivered to the center of a sphere of a medium (usually water or tissue) that is just large enough to have CPE at its center (Figure 7.10). The sphere is surrounded only by air (in free space). This is sometimes referred to as the "dose in air," a misleading term as it suggests that it is the dose delivered to air. The sphere should be no larger than the minimum diameter necessary to assure CPE at its center. If the sphere is any larger, it will introduce extra photon attenuation. For Co-60 radiation and a medium composed of water, the sphere would be 0.5 cm in radius—just large enough to guarantee CPE at the center but no larger. For low-energy photon beams (Co-60 and lower) equation (7.19) can be used to calculate D_{fs} (for monoenergetic radiation):

$$D_{fs} = f_{med} X\, A_{eq},\qquad(7.20)$$

where A_{eq} accounts for absorption and scatter in the sphere. The value of A_{eq} is 0.989 for Co-60 radiation. The quantity dose in free space will be used later in connection with external beam dosimetry.

7.9 An Example of Photon Interactions: History of a 5.0 MeV Photon in Water

As an illustration of the ideas discussed in this chapter and in chapter 6, we consider the fate of a 5 MeV photon impinging on a tank of water. This energy is approximately the average energy of a photon in a 15 MV linear accelerator beam (see chapter 9). We assume that the water is sufficiently deep and broad that the photon expends all of its energy in the water without passing through and out of the water. The average distance that a photon will travel in a medium is called the *mean free path*. We expect that the mean free path is inversely related to the linear attenuation coefficient μ. It turns out that the mean free path is equal to $1/\mu$. For a 5 MeV photon in water, $\mu = 0.0303$ cm^{-1} and the mean free path is therefore $1/0.0303 = 33$ cm. Our photon travels an average of 33 cm before interacting.[2] Note that if this photon enters a patient, it might pass through with no interaction at all. There are a number of possible ways in which the photon can, in principle, interact with the electrons and nuclei in the water. Photon interactions with electrons include coherent scattering, photoelectric effect and Compton scattering. Interactions with nuclei include pair production and photonuclear reactions.

A 5.0 MeV photon has the necessary 1.02 MeV threshold energy to produce an electron-positron pair. A 5.0 MeV photon has an 8.5% chance of pair production and a 91.5% chance of interacting via Compton scattering. The likelihood of a photoelectric or coherent interaction is essentially zero at this energy for water. Let us assume, for now, that the first interaction is Compton scattering. The minimum possible energy transfer in a Compton interaction is essentially zero; the maximum for a 5.0 MeV photon is 4.8 MeV, which occurs when the photon is scattered at 180° (the photon cannot give up all of its energy in a single interaction and conserve momentum). A 4.8 MeV electron will travel about 2.5 cm, which is roughly d_m for a 15 MV beam. The average energy transferred to an electron is $\bar{E}_{tr} = 3.14$ MeV. This leaves $5.00 - 3.14 = 1.86$ MeV for the average scattered photon. Under these circumstances the scattering angle of the photon is [see equation (6.3)] 34°. High-energy photons have a tendency to be scattered in the forward direction (through small angles). The scattered electron emerges at a 17° angle. The electron will travel 1.5 cm (approximately $E/2$) and on average it will lose about 1% of its energy to bremsstrahlung emission. The scattered photon will travel a mean distance of about 19 cm before it scatters again. The probability that this photon will interact via pair production is now lower than before—it is about 0.8% and the photoelectric effect remains negligible. Compton scattering transfers an average energy of 0.97 MeV to the scattered electron leaving $1.86 - 0.97 = 0.89$ MeV for the photon. The photon scatters at 45°. The scattered photon will travel a mean distance of 13 cm before interacting again. This time, the probability of pair production is zero because the photon energy is now below the threshold energy necessary to create a pair. Photoelectric interactions will not become of importance until the photon energy is below 100 keV.

Table 7.1 shows successive average Compton scattering events listing the energy of the incident photon, the energy of the scattered pho-

---

[2]This would appear to imply that a significant fraction of the photons travel through a typical patient without interacting. For 5 MeV photons and $x = 30$, $I = I_0 e^{-\mu x} = 0.40\,I_0$ and therefore 40% of the radiation passes through without interacting.

Table 7.1: History of a 5.0 MeV Photon in Water

Interaction no.	Incoming energy (MeV)	Mean free path (cm)	Outgoing energy (MeV)	Scattering angle (°)	Recoil electron energy (MeV)
1	5.000	33.0	1.860	34	3.140
2	1.860	19.4	0.889	46	0.971
3	0.889	13.3	0.512	55	0.377
4	0.512	10.4	0.335	62	0.177
5	0.335	8.7	0.239	67	0.096
6	0.239	7.7	0.181	72	0.058
7	0.181	7.0	0.144	74	0.037
8	0.144	6.5	0.118	77	0.026
9	0.118	6.1	0.100	79	0.019
10	0.100	5.9	0.086	80	0.014
11	0.086	5.6	0.075	81	0.011
12	0.075	5.3	0.067	82	0.008
13	0.067	5.1	0.060	83	0.007
14	0.060	4.9	0.054	83	0.006
15	0.054	4.6	0.050	84	0.005
16	0.050	4.4	0.046	84	0.004
17	0.046	4.1	0.042	85	0.003
18	0.042	3.9	0.039	85	0.003
19	0.039	3.7	0.037	86	0.003
20	0.037	3.4	0.034	86	0.002
21	0.034	3.1	0.032	87	0.002
22	0.032	2.9	0.030	87	0.002
23	0.030	2.8	0.029	86	0.002
24	0.029	2.5	0.027	87	0.000

ton, the angle of scatter, and the energy imparted to the recoil electron. The values in the table are based on the assumption that the photon always travels the mean distance and that the energy transfer to the electron is the average value. The photon will continue to scatter via the Compton effect until its energy becomes low enough that there is an appreciable probability of absorption by the photoelectric effect. For water, the probability of a photoelectric interaction becomes 50%, just below 30 keV. For this reason, we have stopped the table when the outgoing photon energy is 27 keV. The photon will be absorbed and a photoelectron of approximate energy 27 keV will emerge. The table shows that the photon will scatter about 25 times before it is absorbed in a photoelectric interaction. Each of the electrons set in motion by Compton scattering will produce a track of ionization (and hence energy deposition). There is a chance that each of these electrons will produce a delta ray or emit bremsstrahlung radiation, both of which will carry energy away from the track.

The initial 5.0 MeV photon has an 8% chance of producing an electron-positron pair. Let us now consider the possibility that the initial reaction event is pair production. The kinetic energies of the electron and positron will be on average $(5.00 - 1.02)/2 = 1.99$ MeV. The 1.02 MeV is the energy necessary to create the pair. The positron will annihilate with another electron in the water and two 511 keV annihilation photons will be produced traveling in opposite directions. The subsequent fate of these two photons can be followed by consulting Table 7.1 and starting at step 4 of the table where the incoming photon has an energy of 0.512 MeV. These photons will travel an average distance of 10.4 cm before scattering from an electron.

7.10   Monte Carlo Calculations

The interaction of radiation with matter is devilishly complex. The best way to calculate the consequences of the irradiation of matter is to simulate the interactions by following individual particles as they interact. This process is far too laborious to be done by hand and therefore digital computer programs are used. Many of these programs were developed at national laboratories as part of high-energy physics or nuclear weapons research. One of the goals of radiation therapy physics is to compute the energy deposition of radiation in matter. The Monte Carlo method is the "gold standard" for evaluating the detailed consequences of the interaction of radiation with matter. It is the most accurate method of accomplishing this *if implemented properly*. The incident radiation can be photons, electrons, neutrons, or protons. We will be primarily concerned with photons here. Monte Carlo calculations use the basic physics of radiation interactions (see chapter 6).

Incident particles are sent in one at a time and their detailed history is followed. This is called a *particle history*. The computer must keep track of the primary (incident) particle and all other particles created by or set in motion by the incident particle. The secondary particles must also be followed, and they in turn may create or set in motion additional particles. At every step there is a range of possible interactions that can occur. These occur with probabilities that can be calculated from the fundamental physics. These probabilities depend on the type of particle, its energy, and the medium in which it finds itself. The properties of the medium (density and composition) may vary from place to place. At each step, a list of all particles must be kept in memory, along with their energies and directions of motion. The particles are followed and their energy deposition is recorded until they have lost all but an insignificant fraction of their original energy. A large number of histories (perhaps millions to hundreds of millions) must be calculated before a meaningful average emerges (see Figure 7.11).

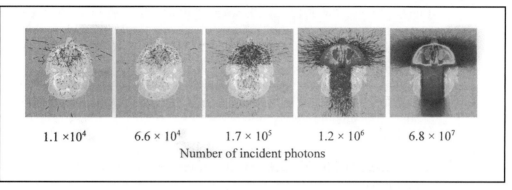

1.1 ×10⁴   6.6 × 10⁴   1.7 × 10⁵   1.2 × 10⁶   6.8 × 10⁷

Number of incident photons

Figure 7.11: Monte Carlo calculation of the dose distribution from a 6 MV anterior and two lateral opposed beams using Peregrine software. The number of particle histories is written under each frame. A large number of particle histories is necessary for an accurate dose calculation. (Courtesy of Lawrence Livermore National Laboratory) See COLOR PLATE 1.

In our discussion of the fate of a 5 MeV photon in water we have chosen average values at every step. In a Monte Carlo calculation all possible events must be taken into account, although each possibility must be constrained by the *probability* of that event. As an example, when the 5.0 MeV photon first interacts with water, there is an 8.5% chance that the interaction will be pair production and a 91.5% chance that it will be Compton scattering. We need a roulette wheel in which the ball will turn up in a bin labeled Compton scattering 91.5% of the time and pair production 8.5% of the time. Monte Carlo computer programs are written to simulate this. The name Monte Carlo is taken from the city in Monaco, which is famous for its gambling casino.

As you might imagine, Monte Carlo calculations are very computationally intensive. These calculations require large amounts of computer time. It is for this reason that they have only recently begun to be used for routine patient dose calculations. Commercially available software packages that are used to calculate the dose distribution in patients are called *treatment planning systems.* Most of these do not use Monte Carlo dose calculation algorithms. The algorithms that are used are much faster and they are reasonably accurate under most circumstances. The current techniques are not highly accurate, however, in or near inhomogeneities, particularly at boundaries, because of a lack of CPE there. Some significant discrepancies between the dose calculated by Monte Carlo techniques and simpler methods have been pointed out in the literature.

A number of Monte Carlo software packages (many of these are in the public domain) are in use for research calculations in radiation therapy: EGS4 (*e*lectron *g*amma *s*hower) for photons and electrons, MCNP (*M*onte *C*arlo *n* *p*article), which can be used for neutrons also, Peregrine (developed at Lawrence Livermore National Laboratory), BEAM (used to model radiotherapy accelerators). Commercial treatment planning systems are just beginning to incorporate Monte Carlo algorithms in their software for dose calculations of photon and electron beams. As computer hardware becomes faster, it seems likely that Monte Carlo dose calculations will become the clinical standard. It is difficult to envision any possible improvement in dose calculation beyond this—the dose calculation problem will be solved once and for all. Monte Carlo calculations can be used for brachytherapy as well as for external beam dose calculations.

7.11 Microscopic Biological Damage

A detailed discussion of the biological effect of radiation on cells is beyond the scope of this book. A very brief overview, however, may assist the reader in making the bridge between this book and radiobiology texts and to appreciate the importance and context of some of the concepts introduced here. The reader is referred to the excellent book by Hall and the section on radiobiology in Johns and Cunningham. This discussion is adapted from those texts. A discussion of the biological effects of low doses of radiation within the context of radiation protection can be found in chapter 17, section 17.3.

High-energy charged particles produce ionization of the atoms in the material through which they pass. The ionization is in the form of tracks through the medium (see Figure 6.7). The charged particles can be the primary radiation, as for an electron or proton beam, or secondary charged particles set in motion by photons or neutrons. Most of the energy absorbed by ionizing radiation is ultimately converted into heat, causing no significant biological effect. Some of the energy however causes molecular bonds to be broken, which can result in biological damage. Biological damage to cells is thought to be caused principally by damage to DNA. If the damage is severe, it may interfere with normal cellular function, in particular the ability to reproduce normally. There are two broad mechanisms by which this damage can occur. The radiation can directly break molecular bonds in the DNA helix. This is called the *direct mechanism*.[3] The direct mechanism is of particular importance for high-LET radiation (such as produced by neutrons or alpha particles), since this is associated with very dense ionization tracks. The *indirect mechanism* of radiation damage is caused by reactive chemical species formed by the interaction of radiation with water. Cells are 70% to 80% water. The radiation products formed in water can attack DNA molecules, causing molecular bonds to break. In particular, *free radicals* formed as a result of the ionization of water are especially damaging. Free radicals are neutral atoms or molecules that

---

[3] Do not confuse this with the term *directly ionizing radiation*.

have an unpaired electron and are thus highly reactive. One of the most damaging of these is the hydroxyl radical, usually denoted OH•. Radicals can diffuse far enough through the intracellular medium to reach DNA molecules. Both the indirect and the direct mechanism operate simultaneously. The indirect mechanism is of particular importance for low-LET radiation (x-ray and electron beams). The tracks from this type of radiation are not as dense and therefore not as likely to cause direct damage to DNA.

The absorbed dose by itself does not "tell the whole story" with respect to biological damage. Biological damage depends on the LET of the radiation. High-LET radiation can be more damaging per unit dose than low-LET radiation. The reader may wish to refer to chapter 17 for a discussion of radiation weighting factors (w_R) that are used in the context of radiation protection.

Chapter Summary

- **Exposure:** Exposure is a measure of the ability of photon radiation to ionize air. $X = Q/m$, where Q is the sum of all electrical charges of one sign on all ions produced **in air** when all electrons liberated by **photons** in a small volume of (dry) air of mass m are completely stopped in air. In general, it is necessary to find and count all charge liberated as a result of the photon interactions in m **regardless of where that charge ends up.** Exposure is: (1) only defined for photons; (2) only defined for ionization of air; (3) not useful above ~3 MeV because of conditions necessary for measurement. The SI unit of exposure is C/kg. The old "pre SI" unit is the roentgen (R); 1 R = 2.58×10^{-4} C/kg. This unit is sometimes rather large and it is then more convenient to use mR = 10^{-3} R.

- **Charged Particle Equilibrium (CPE):** In a radiation field, if each charged particle of a given type and energy leaving a volume is replaced by a charged particle of the same type and energy entering that volume, then the volume is said to be in charged particle equilibrium. When CPE prevails in a mass m of air, it becomes easy to measure exposure. Simply measure the total charge in the mass m.

- **Fluence:** $\Phi = N/a$, where N is the total number of particles entering a sphere of small cross-sectional area a. Units are cm^{-2} or m^{-2}.

- **Kerma:** $\underline{K}$inetic $\underline{e}$nergy $\underline{r}$eleased per unit $\underline{ma}$ss in a medium at a specified point. $K = E_{TR}/m$, where E_{TR} is the sum of all the initial kinetic energies of all charged particles liberated by uncharged ionizing particles in a material of mass m. The units of kerma are J/kg = gray = Gy. Kerma may not be a measure of biological damage because it does not necessarily tell how much energy is absorbed locally.

- **Absorbed Dose:** $D = E_{AB}/m$, where E_{AB} is the total energy absorbed from ionizing radiation inside a mass m of material. The units of dose are the same as the units of kerma. The gray (Gy) is the SI unit of dose. An old unit of dose which is still sometimes used is the rad.

$$100 \text{ rads} = 1 \text{ Gy} = 100 \text{ cGy}$$
$$1 \text{ rad} = 1 \text{ cGy}$$

The dose is equal to the collision kerma when CPE holds (i.e., $D \overset{CPE}{=} K_c$).

- **Absorption of energy from indirectly ionizing radiation** (photons or neutrons) is a two-step process.

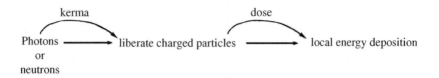

- **Buildup and Skin Sparing:** For megavoltage photon irradiation the relative dose to the skin is low. The dose builds up to a maximum value at a depth denoted d_m and then declines with increasing depth. The depth d_m is approximately equal to the maximum range of the electrons set in motion by the photons. At the

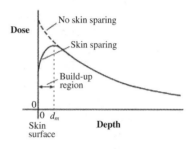

depth of d_m and beyond there is approximate CPE. There is no discernible buildup for low-energy photons because d_m is very small. For Co-60 radiation, which has a mean photon energy of 1.25 MeV, d_m is approximately 0.5 cm.

- **Dose to Air:** The dose absorbed by air can be related to the exposure: D_{air} (cGy) $= 0.876\ X$(R). Air kerma is equal to the dose absorbed by air in CPE.

- **Dose to a Medium:** The dose absorbed by a medium can be related to the exposure in a small air test cavity carved out of the medium. The dose is given by D_{med} (cGy) $= f_{med} \cdot X$(R) $\cdot A$, where $f_{med} =$ roentgen to rad conversion ratio, which depends on the medium and beam energy; X(R) = exposure, measured in roentgens, if medium replaced by air cavity; and A = fractional attenuation of photons due to presence of medium. At low energies, the photoelectric effect is important. At 100 keV, $f_{bone}/f_{muscle} = 1.5$. At high energies where the Compton effect dominates, the electron density of bone is somewhat smaller than the electron density of water. At 1 MeV, $f_{bone}/f_{muscle} = 0.96$.

- **Dose in Free Space:** The dose in free space D_{fs} is the dose delivered to the center of a sphere of a medium just large enough to be in charged particle equilibrium that is surrounded only by air (in free space). For Co-60 radiation and a medium composed of water, the sphere would be 0.5 cm in radius—just large enough to guarantee CPE at the center.

Problems

1. A volume of 0.60 cm^3 of air in CPE is irradiated producing an ionization charge of 20.0 nC. What is the exposure in roentgens (R)? The density of the air is 1.20×10^{-3} g/cm^3.

2. If 100 g of a material uniformly absorbs 10 J of energy from radiation, what is the absorbed dose received by the material?

3. A 10 g mass of tissue is uniformly irradiated and receives 1 cGy of absorbed dose. What is the dose received by 5 g of this same tissue?

4. The fluence of Co-60 radiation at a point in a water phantom is 1.69×10^{16} m^{-2}. Co-60 radiation can be considered monoenergetic, with an energy of 1.25 MeV. For Co-60 in water: μ_{tr}/ρ = 0.0298 cm^2/g, μ/ρ = 0.0641 cm^2/g, μ_{en}/ρ = 0.0296 cm^2/g, Y(0.6 MeV) = 2.16×10^{-3},
   a. What is the energy fluence expressed in units of J/m^2?
   b. On average, how much kinetic energy is transferred to an electron when a photon interacts with it? Express the answer in units of MeV.
   c. How much energy is lost to bremsstrahlung by an electron of this energy as it slows down?
   d. Calculate the collision kerma in units of Gy.
   e. If CPE holds, what is the absorbed dose?
   f. Suppose that a small volume of the water is replaced by compact bone (μ_{en}/ρ = 0.0283 cm^2/g). Assuming that the energy fluence remains the same, what dose will be delivered to the bone?

5. For high-energy photon beams incident upon a medium, why doesn't the dose have its maximum value at the surface? After all, the photons are steadily attenuated as the depth increases. What determines where the dose reaches its maximum value?

6. Why is the absorbed dose lower in bone than in soft tissue when subjected to equal exposure of Co-60 radiation?

7. In section 7.5 we discussed skin sparing and buildup. A simple model was introduced to explain this phenomenon. In this simple model there was no attenuation of photons. We can extend this model by introducing photon attenuation. With photon attenuation, fewer and fewer electrons will be set in motion per block as the depth increases. In the figure below, 100 electrons are set in motion in the first box, 80 in the second, 64 in the third, etc. It is again assumed that the range of the electrons is 3 box lengths.

Complete the table shown below, indicating the number of electron tracks in each box. Three table entries have already been made to serve as an example. The number of tracks in the first box is $\frac{1}{2} \times 100 = 50$, in the second box there are $100 + \frac{1}{2} \times 80 = 140$ tracks, etc. Once the table is complete, plot the points on the accompanying graph and draw a smooth curve through them. You may wish to make a photocopy of the graph.

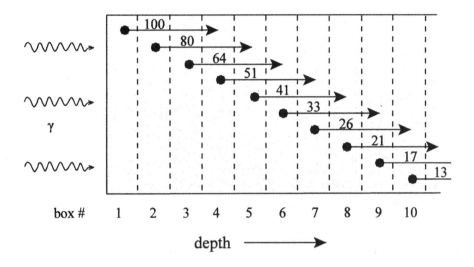

box #	number of electron tracks
1	50
2	140
3	
4	
5	175
6	
7	
8	
9	
10	

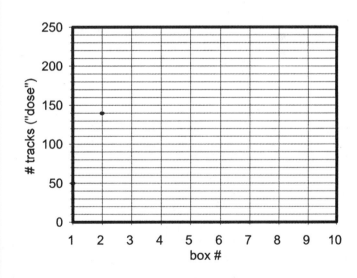

8. Using the values in step 4 of Table 7.1, verify that a 0.512 MeV photon scattering through an angle of 62° has a final energy of 0.335 MeV (as listed in step 4).

9. Add the energies of all of the recoil electrons in Table 7.1. Does the sum have approximately the expected value? Why?

Bibliography

Attix, F. H. *Introduction to Radiological Physics and Radiation Dosimetry.* New York: Wiley InterScience, 1986.

Hall, E. J. *Radiobiology for the Radiologist,* Fifth Edition. Philadelphia: Lippincott Williams and Wilkins, 2000.

International Commission on Radiation Units and Measurements (ICRU) Report No. 44. *Tissue Substitutes in Radiation Dosimetry and Measurement.* Bethedsa, MD: ICRU, 1989.

Johns, H. E., and J. R. Cunningham. *The Physics of Radiology,* Fourth Edition. Springfield, IL: Charles C Thomas, 1983.

Khan, F. M. *The Physics of Radiation Therapy,* Fourth Edition. Philadelphia: Lippincott Williams & Wilkins, 2009.

8 Radiation Detection and Measurement

8.1 Introduction

In the last chapter we discussed the concepts and defined quantities that can be used for radiation measurement—quantities such as exposure, absorbed dose, and dose in free space. In this chapter we will discuss the instruments that can be used to detect and or measure radiation. In chapter 11 we will discuss how measurements of radiation beams, made with instruments discussed in this chapter, can be used to calibrate these beams in terms of absorbed dose in water.

Radiation measurement instruments can be categorized in terms of the type of radiation measurement they are designed for and the type of medium used for detection or measurement. In radiation therapy there are four main applications of radiation instruments: (1) radiation machine calibration, (2) survey work, (3) personnel monitoring, and (4) in vivo patient measurements. Radiation machine calibration involves very accurate measurement of the amount of radiation emitted by a radiation-producing device (e.g., a linear accelerator) that is used for therapeutic treatment. Calibration instruments need to be very accurate, but they do not need to be very sensitive because the level of radiation is high.

Survey meters are used to detect and provide a rough measure of radiation levels in the environment. These meters are used for detecting and locating radiation contamination. Survey meters need to be very sensitive but do not need to be highly accurate. Both calibration instruments and survey instruments need to provide measurements of instantaneous radiation levels. Personnel monitoring devices are used to track the amount of radiation that individual radiation workers receive. These devices need to be sensitive because they are required to measure small amounts of radiation and they need to measure cumulative radiation exposure. In vivo radiation detectors are used to monitor the amount of radiation that patients receive during treatment.

There are three major categories of radiation detectors classified according to the phase of the medium used for detection: gas, liquid, and solid. It is to be emphasized that the medium used for detection may not be the same as the medium in which the radiation is measured. For example, a gas ionization detector may be placed in a solid medium to measure the radiation in the solid. All of the various types of gas detectors are based on the ability of radiation to produce ionization in the gas. The solid and liquid detectors employ a variety of mechanisms to detect and measure radiation. The major types of radiation detection and measurement instruments are:

1. Gas Ionization Detectors
   a. Ionization chambers (used for beam calibration and survey meters).
   b. Proportional counters (used for survey meters).
   c. Geiger-Müller (GM) counters (used for survey meters).
2. Solid-State Detectors
   a. Thermoluminescent dosimeters (TLDs) (personnel monitoring, in vivo dosimetry).
   b. Film (measurement of distribution of dose and for personnel monitoring).
   c. Diodes (in vivo dosimetry, beam measurements).
   d. MOSFETs (metal oxide semiconductor-field effect transistors) (in vivo dosimetry).
   e. Polymer gel (measurement of 3-D distribution of dose).
   f. Scintillation (survey meters).
3. Liquid Dosimeters
   a. Calorimeters (used in standards laboratories, direct measurement of dose).
   b. Chemical (aqueous solution, direct measurement of dose).

The design of an individual radiation measurement instrument depends on the intended application and on the medium used for radiation detection. Each of these detector types will be discussed in this chapter, but first we must digress to consider the medium in which measurements are made.

8.2 Phantoms

It is often necessary to make detailed measurements or to conduct experiments that cannot be performed in a patient. In this case, radiation measurements must be made in an object constructed of a material that is a substitute for the patient. Such an object is referred to as a *phantom*. The chief characteristics of phantoms are their shape and their composition. The phantom material is designed to mimic the patient with respect to radiation scattering and absorption. Note that this depends on the type of radiation to be used.

There are two types of phantoms: geometrical and anthropomorphic. A geometrical phantom is in the form of some simple geometrical shape and makes little attempt to imitate the shape of a patient. Common shapes are cubes, rectangular slabs, cylinders, etc. An anthropomorphic phantom is designed to duplicate the shape of the (average) patient and perhaps even the distribution of materials within the patient.

The term "tissue equivalent" is loosely defined as meaning that the material has the same or very similar radiation properties (scattering and absorption) as tissue with respect to a defined type of radiation (e.g., megavoltage photons, megavoltage electrons, neutrons, etc.). Water is considered to be the best substitute for soft tissue for most types of radiation. Important properties of a phantom material include the elemental composition and the electron density. Compounds or mixtures are often described in terms of the effective atomic number. This is a single value of the atomic number that will correctly describe the absorption properties of x-rays over a reasonably wide range in energy. When the Compton effect dominates, the mass attenuation coefficient depends only on the electron density (electrons per gram), which is independent of Z (for materials with little or no hydrogen content). When the photoelectric effect dominates, the attenuation coefficient is highly sensitive to the value of Z. The effective value of Z is 7.8 for air and 7.5 for water. The value of τ/ρ (photoelectric mass attenuation coefficient) at 20 keV is 0.544 cm^2/g for water and 0.536 cm^2/g for air. One would expect the value of τ/ρ to be slightly higher for air, based on the effective values of Z cited above. The fact that it is not just shows the approximate nature of the effective Z value. The compound lithium fluoride (LiF) is widely used for TLDs. The effective Z for LiF is 8.3 and its electron density is 0.833 times that of water. At an energy of 1 MeV, the Compton mass attenuation coefficient $\tau/\rho = 5.89 \times 10^{-2}$ cm^2/g for LiF and $7.10^{-2} \times 10$ cm^2/g for water. The ratio of these two mass attenuation coefficients is just about the value expected, based on the ratio of the electron density of LiF to that of water.

Geometrical phantoms are usually homogeneous. They are often made of solid materials such as plastics like polystyrene (relative electron density 0.969), acrylic [also known as Lucite™, Plexiglas™, PMMA (polymethyl methacrylate), Perspex™; relative electron density 0.972]. Solids are convenient. They can be set up quickly and do not require that the detector be waterproof. Epoxy resin phantom materials are sometimes referred to as "solid water" (which means ice to most people) or "virtual water." Slabs of this material are typically 30×30 cm^2 in cross section and come in varying thicknesses (see Figure 8.1). Slabs are available which are machined to accept various types of ion chambers. By using different combinations of plates, various ion chamber depths are possible.

Water phantoms are commonly used for radiation therapy dosimetry purposes, especially for radiation calibration and beam measurements. Water is considered the best substitute for tissue for megavoltage beams. A water phantom is essentially a large "fish" tank, which can be filled with water. Computerized scanning water phantoms will be discussed in detail in chapter 9.

Anthropomorphic phantoms are designed to imitate the shape of patients. An example is the "RANDO®" phantom (see Figure 8.2) which is constructed from a tissue-equivalent resin (density 0.985 gm/cm^3) molded around a natural skeleton. This phantom has natural air spaces (pharynges, larynx, trachea, stem bronchi, etc.), which are taken from impressions of a cadaver. RANDO has realistic lungs with a density of 0.32 g/cm^3. "He" can be purchased sectioned into 2.5 cm thick axial

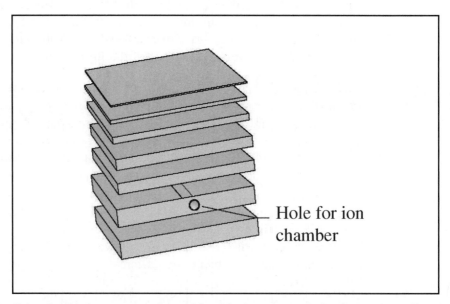

Hole for ion chamber

Figure 8.1: Slabs of solid phantom material, which might be composed of polystyrene, acrylic, or "virtual water."

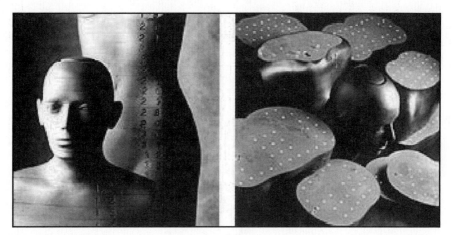

Figure 8.2: RANDO® phantom is an anthropomorphic phantom that is sectioned into slices 2.5 cm thick. Some of the individual slices are shown on the right. Each slice contains an array of plugs that may be removed and replaced by TLD capsules. (Courtesy of The Phantom Laboratory, Salem, NY)

slices. Within each slice there are plugs arranged in a 3×3 cm^2 grid which may be removed and replaced by TLDs.

8.3 Gas Ionization Detectors

All gas ionization chambers rely on the ability of radiation to ionize a gas, producing pairs of ions (see Figure 8.3). In the absence of radiation no current will flow in the circuit shown in Figure 8.3 because charge is unable to flow across the gap between the electrodes. When charged particles pass through the detector, they produce ion tracks consisting of pairs of oppositely charged ions. The ions will be attracted toward the electrode that is oppositely charged. A small electrical current is produced from the collection of these ion pairs. Gas ionization detectors have low efficiency compared to solid-state detectors. This means that the amount of current or total charge registered by the ammeter is relatively small in comparison to that measured from solid-state detectors for a fixed amount of radiation. The density of the ion tracks is much lower in a gas because of its low mass density and low Z value.

8.3.1 Ionization Chambers

In an ionization chamber the charge is collected by the electrodes. If the chamber is irradiated with photons and if the collecting volume is in CPE and if the mass of the gas irradiated can be accurately determined, then the exposure can be determined directly, as we will show.

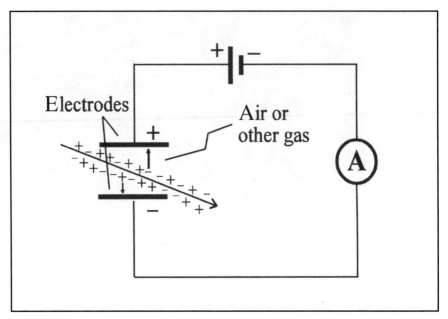

Figure 8.3: A prototypical gas ionization chamber. When radiation passes through the gas between the charged electrodes, it produces ion pairs, which are attracted to the plates having charge of opposite sign. As the charge is collected, it will register as a current on the ammeter.

Ionization chambers have a "flat" energy response for photons above 100 keV. This means that the charge collected depends only on the exposure and not on the energy of the photons. If the charge produced by the ionizing radiation is Q, then Q/X is independent of energy above about 100 keV (refer to Figure 8.14).

An ionization chamber can be used to detect the ionization produced by the passage of charged particles as well as photons. In fact, an ionization chamber cannot distinguish between them.

Free-Air Ionization Chamber

Free-air ionization chambers are used for exposure measurement in national standards laboratories such as the National Institute of Standards and Technology (NIST). These instruments are impractical for field use. NIST sets U.S. national standards for radiation quantities and measurements. NIST can be described as a Primary Standards Laboratory.

Figure 8.4 shows a diagram of a free-air ionization chamber. The x-rays enter the chamber from the left. Ions are produced all along the volume occupied by the beam. Each photon produces one (or at most a few) ionizations, but an electron set in motion by a photon may produce

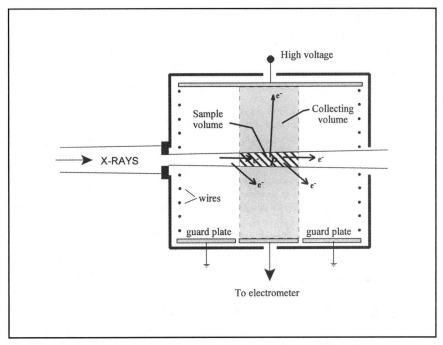

Figure 8.4: A side view of a free-air ionization chamber. The charge is collected from the volume labeled "collecting volume." The exposure is to be measured for the volume labeled "sample volume." Some of the charge produced in the sample volume may leave the collecting volume. Provided every charge that leaves the collecting volume is replaced by one entering (CPE in the collecting volume), then the charge produced in the sample volume will be the same as that collected from the collecting volume. In this way all the charge collected may be assumed to have originated by photon interactions in the sample volume. The wires and the guard plates are used to make the electric field very uniform so that charge will only be collected from the well-defined region labeled collecting volume. (Adapted from Fig. 12.1, p. 293 in Attix, F. H. *Introduction to Radiological Physics and Radiation Dosimetry.* 1986. Copyright Wiley-VCH Verlag GmbH & Co., KGaA. Reprinted with permission.)

tens of thousands of ionizations by the time it comes to rest. The electrons produced by the photons move through the air creating tracks of ionization. The point P in the middle of the volume labeled "Sample volume" is the place at which we wish to measure the exposure. We shall assume that the photon beam is not significantly attenuated along the length of the beam within the sample volume.

In this case, the exposure will be uniform throughout the sample volume. To measure the exposure, we must collect and measure all of the charge produced as a result of photon interactions in the sample volume. The large, shaded volume shown in Figure 8.4 is called the *collecting volume*. The *sample volume* is the cross-hatched region contained within this larger volume. Charge is collected from throughout the entire collecting volume by the electrode at the bottom of the figure.

Some of the electrons produced in the sample volume by photon inter-actions escape from the collecting volume. The full ionization produced by escaping electrons as they come to rest will not be collected. If, how-ever, each one of these escaping electrons is replaced by another elec-tron with the same energy entering the collecting volume, then there will be no net gain or loss of charge in the collecting volume. The col-lecting volume will be in CPE. In this case, the charge collected will be equal to the charge produced (wherever it ends up) by photon interac-tions in the sample volume. The distance from the sample volume to the boundary of the chamber must be greater than the maximum electron range in air. If this were not the case, then an electron could travel up and through the top plate and be lost to the collecting volume. This electron would not be replaced by an incoming electron. As long as the plates are far enough apart, all charge produced in the shaded sample volume will be collected. The exposure can be calculated directly from the equation $X = Q/m$, where Q is the charge collected and m is the mass of the air in the sample volume.

Free-air ionization chambers are practical in the range 10 to 300 keV. Above this photon energy the range of maximum energy electrons becomes large and the chamber must therefore be made quite big. Above about 3 MeV (at best) the plate separation must be impractically large. The maximum range of electrons produced by 3 MeV photons in air is about 10 meters. For this reason, exposure measurements above this energy are impractical. In radiation therapy, many of our beams have energies higher than this and therefore the quantity "exposure" is of limited usefulness.

A free-air ionization chamber is an *absolute dosimeter* for exposure measurements. A free-air ionization chamber can measure exposure (but not dose) without comparison or calibration against another radiation measurement device. An absolute dosimeter is a radiation measurement instrument that does not need to be compared or calibrated against any other radiation measurement device.

Cavity Ionization Chambers

Imagine an air cavity of mass m. This air cavity shall be surrounded by a large air "shell" (see Figure 8.5). The entire cavity plus shell is to be irradiated by photons. We want CPE in the air cavity. The air shell must be thick enough so that the air cavity is *not* in the build-up region of the air shell. If the air shell is too thin, then more electrons will leave the air cavity than will enter it. If the source of the photons were too close to the air cavity, then there might not be CPE in the air cavity. To achieve CPE, the thickness of the air shell must be larger than the maximum range of electrons set in motion by the photon beam. This is just like the

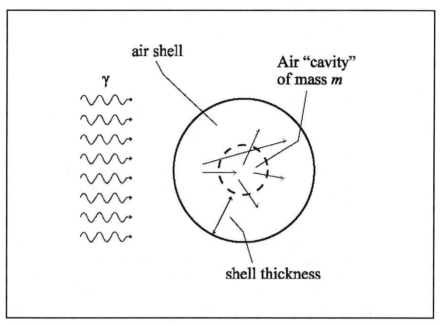

Figure 8.5: An air cavity with a "shell" of air surrounding it which is sufficiently thick to provide charged particle equilibrium inside the air cavity.

free-air ionization chamber. Under these circumstances the exposure in the cavity is given by:

$$X_{cavity} = \frac{Q}{m},\qquad(8.1)$$

where Q is the charge collected from the air cavity.

The same goal can be accomplished in a more practical way by replacing the air shell by a solid material that has an effective atomic number Z as close as possible to air. Air has an effective Z value of about 7.8. The thickness of this solid wall must be large enough to provide CPE in the central air cavity—which is to say that the wall thickness must be greater than the maximum range of electrons set in motion in the wall by the incoming photons. We can think of this wall as "solid air" (see Figure 8.6). As typical solids have a density about 1000 times the density of air, it becomes practical to build such a device that can be used as a field measurement instrument. The wall or shell thickness need be only 1/1000 of the thickness of the air shell in Figure 8.5. We would like the wall to be thick enough to provide CPE but not so thick as to significantly attenuate the incoming photon radiation. At low energy (e.g., diagnostic or superficial) a thin chamber wall is adequate to provide CPE and to minimize attenuation. At higher energies a thicker

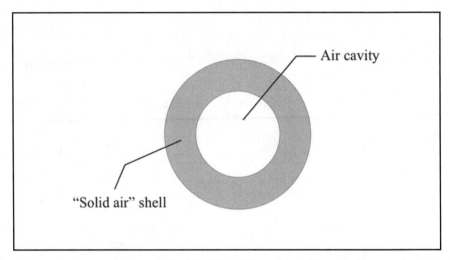

Figure 8.6: An air cavity surrounded by a shell of "solid air." The solid shell is made from an air-equivalent material that is thick enough to provide charged particle equilibrium inside the air cavity. This is the basis for the cavity ionization chamber.

wall may be necessary. Some ion chambers are provided with a "build-up cap," which can be added for high-energy radiation. Special build-up caps are available for Co-60 radiation (average energy 1.25 MeV). The thickness of the cap plus the thickness of the chamber wall is about 5 mm, which corresponds to the value of d_m for Co-60 radiation. When the cap is added, the cap plus wall will provide CPE.

Cavity ion chambers are generally calibrated against a standard such as a free-air ionization chamber. We will discuss chamber calibration in chapter 11.

In addition to being compact, a cavity ion chamber has the added advantage that it can be used to measure other types of radiation, such as electrons. For photon measurements in air, the ionization produced in the cavity originates from electrons that are produced in the build-up cap and the wall of the chamber by photon interactions there. These secondary electrons traverse the cavity, leaving a trail of ionization. If the ion chamber is placed in a medium other than air, such as a water phantom or a solid phantom (see Figure 8.1), the build-up cap is removed and the secondary electrons are generated in the medium by photon interactions in the medium.

For primary electron beam measurements, a thin wall is desirable because the irradiating particles themselves produce the ionization directly as they pass through the cavity. A thick wall would disturb the fluence of these particles. For electron beam measurements, the build-up cap should be removed from the chamber.

Small cavity ion chambers can be used to make measurements in regions where the dose is changing rapidly with position. Such chambers have a high spatial resolution. Since the amount of gas inside such a chamber is small, it will suffer from low sensitivity. The amount of charge produced ($Q = m\,X$) inside the cavity for a given amount of radiation will be small because the mass of gas inside the cavity is small. For large cavity ion chambers, spatial resolution is sacrificed to obtain high sensitivity.

There are three major types of cavity ion chambers:

1. **Thimble chambers.** These are chambers that are cylindrically shaped, somewhat loosely like a sewing thimble. Examples are Farmer chambers, mini-chambers, diagnostic energy chambers, survey meter chambers, etc. (see Figure 8.7).
2. **Flat-cavity chambers.** These are sometimes described as pancake, pillbox, or plane-parallel chambers. These chambers are shaped somewhat like a pillbox. Examples are the plane-parallel chambers

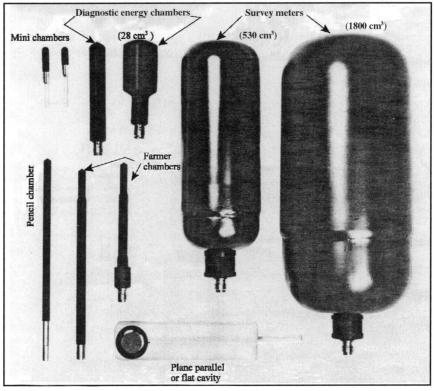

Figure 8.7: Various types of ionization chambers. The large chambers are used in survey meters, the large collecting volume assuring high sensitivity. The diagnostic chambers are of intermediate volume and can be used to measure exposure and beam HVL. Mini chambers are used for therapy beam scanning to determine beam profiles and percent depth dose curves. Farmer chambers are used for therapy beam calibration. The pencil chamber is used for computed tomography (CT) dose measurements. The plane parallel chamber is used for electron beam measurements. (Courtesy of Capintec Inc., Ramsey, NJ)

used in radiation therapy for electron beam measurements, the monitor chambers in the head of a linac, extrapolation chambers, etc. (see Figure 8.7; refer to Figures 8.12 and 8.13).

3. **Well-ionization chambers.** These chambers are used in nuclear medicine for radioactive source strength assay and in therapy for brachytherapy source calibration (see Figure 8.8).

Thimble Chambers

A thimble ionization chamber resembles a sewing thimble (see Figure 8.9). Chamber collecting volumes are 0.1 to 1.0 cm^3 for therapy applications and up to 2000 cm^3 for survey meters. The inside of the thimble wall serves as one of the electrodes. If the wall is made of a nonconducting material, then it is coated with a conducting substance such as Aquadag™ (sometimes called "dag"). Aquadag is a colloidal graphite dispersion in isopropyl alcohol that is coated on the inside of the chamber. In plain English, this is an electrically conducting paint.

A voltage, called the *bias,* is placed between the inner thimble wall and the central electrode. The central electrode is sometimes called the collecting electrode. If the central electrode is made positive, then any negative charge produced in the cavity by the passage of ionizing radi-

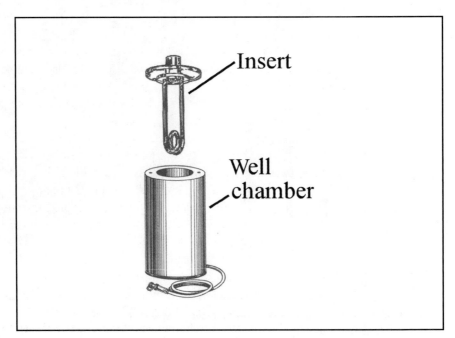

Figure 8.8: A well ionization chamber shown with an insert. Well chambers are used for brachytherapy radioisotope source calibration. A well chamber like this can be used to determine the activity of sources prior to implantation in a patient. The cable is attached to an electrometer. The sources are put into the insert and then the insert is lowered into the well. (Courtesy of Sun Nuclear, Melbourne, FL)

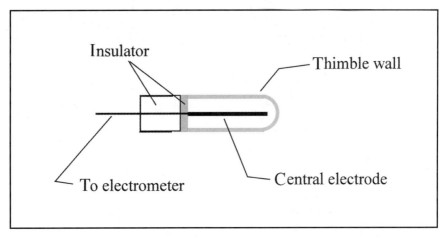

Figure 8.9: A thimble ionization chamber. The inner thimble wall is coated with a conducting material and a bias voltage is placed between the inner thimble wall and the central electrode. Charge is collected at the central (collecting) electrode which then flows out to the electrometer.

ation will be attracted to it. It will then flow out through the wire attached to the central electrode and be counted by the electrometer. In principle, a chamber such as this could be used for direct measurement of exposure (i.e., $X = Q/m$), but it is more accurate to calibrate the chamber. Radiation therapy clinics send their ionization chambers to Secondary Standards Laboratories, which are accredited by the American Association of Physicists in Medicine (AAPM) among others. The instruments used by these laboratories are calibrated by NIST. These secondary laboratories are called Accredited Dosimetry Calibration Laboratories (ADCLs). There are four ADCLs in North America. The calibration process is described in chapter 11.

It is recommended that ion chambers used for external beam radiation therapy be calibrated every 2 years. Ion chambers used for Co-60 teletherapy beam calibration are required by the U.S. Nuclear Regulatory Commission (NRC) to be calibrated every 2 years.

A Farmer chamber is a particular type of thimble ionization chamber that is commonly used for external beam calibration (see Figure 8.10). The chamber is named after its inventor and was first developed in 1956. The collecting volume of a Farmer chamber is approximately 0.6 cm^3. External beam photon calibrations are made almost exclusively with a Farmer chamber. Common materials used for the wall are AE plastic (which is tissue equivalent), acrylic (also called Lucite, Plexiglas, or PMMA) or graphite. Designs vary slightly from manufacturer to manufacturer (see Figure 8.11). The cost of a Farmer chamber is about $2000.

Farmer chambers are often used in a water tank for beam calibration purposes. The most recent beam calibration protocol (AAPM TG-51) requires beam calibration in water as opposed to a solid material such as

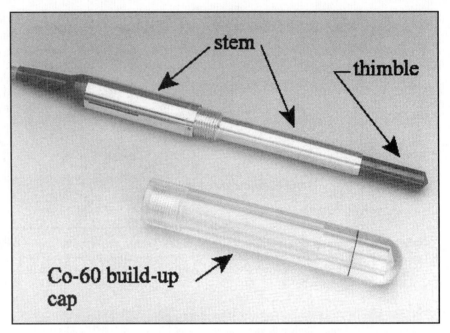

Figure 8.10: A Farmer ionization chamber shown alongside its Co-60 build-up cap. The collecting volume is inside the thimble. (Courtesy of PTW-New York, Hicksville, NY)

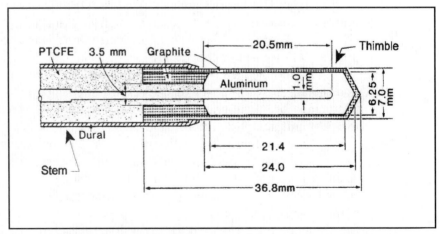

Figure 8.11: The internal structure of a typical Farmer ionization chamber. The collecting volume is approximately 0.6 cm³. The central or collecting electrode is cylindrical with a diameter of 1.0 mm and is made of aluminum. The thimble wall is made of graphite. The PTFCE material is an insulator. (Reprinted from *The Physics of Radiation Therapy,* Third Edition, by F.M. Khan, Fig. 6.10, p. 88, © 2003, with permission from Lippincott Williams & Wilkins.)

polystyrene. Under these circumstances the build-up cap is removed and the chamber must be made waterproof. Some newer Farmer chambers are inherently waterproof. Those that are not can be placed in a specially fitted rubber sleeve, although a 1 mm thick acrylic plastic cap that fits snugly over the thimble is recommended. A rubber sleeve attaches to this cap (with a grommet) to protect the stem and cable from water.

Plane-Parallel Ion Chambers (Flat Cavity)

A Farmer chamber has a diameter that is too large for measurements in regions where dose is changing rapidly with depth, such as in the build-up region or in electron beams. The large inner cavity can disturb low energy electron beams and therefore provide inaccurate readings. To solve this problem, plane-parallel ion chambers are used. These have two thin, closely spaced, parallel collecting plates or electrodes (see Figures 8.12 and 8.13). Such chambers are sometimes called pancake chambers. One of the electrodes is a thin window through which the radiation enters the chamber. The entrance window is made of a foil or plastic membrane, which is 0.01 mm to 0.03 mm thick. For this reason, one should never touch the unprotected entrance window of a plane-parallel chamber. Therapy plane-parallel ion chambers typically have a

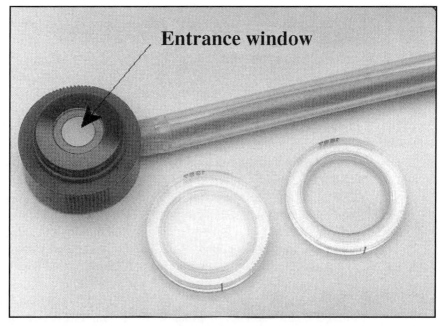

Figure 8.12: A plane parallel Markus chamber commonly used for electron measurements. The spacing between the electrodes is 2 mm. The entrance window is only 0.03 mm thick. A waterproofing cap is shown at bottom left. (Courtesy of PTW-New York, Hicksville, NY)

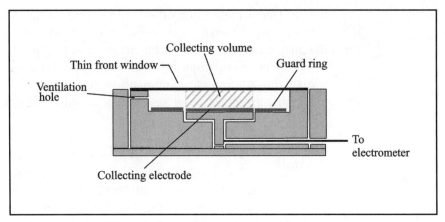

Figure 8.13: Cross section of a plane parallel ionization chamber for use in radiation therapy. (Adapted from *The Physics of Radiotherapy X-Rays from Linear Accelerators* by P. Metcalfe, T. Kron, and P. Hoban, figure 3.21, p. 128, © 1997, with permission.)

2 mm spacing between electrodes (collecting electrode and entrance window) and a collecting diameter of 5 mm. This provides high spatial resolution in the direction parallel to the radiation beam.

8.3.2   Survey Meter Ion Chambers

A survey meter is a sensitive instrument designed to detect the presence of radiation (usually photons) and to provide a rough measure of the radiation rate (often in units of mR/h). Radiation survey meters are portable, hand-held battery-operated radiation detectors. There are many different types of survey meters. One type of survey meter contains a large volume ion chamber. A collecting volume of 500 cm^3 is typical. Compare this volume to the 0.6 cm^3 of a Farmer chamber. The much larger volume makes the chamber a very sensitive survey instrument. An example of this is the type of survey meter that is called a "Cutie Pie."

Ionization chambers have a relatively flat energy response over a wide range of energies (see Figure 8.14).

An example of a survey meter ion chamber is the Victoreen 450P, which has an operating range of 0 to 5 R/h. The chamber volume is 300 cm^3 and is filled with a pressurized gas at 6 times normal atmospheric pressure. This increases the amount of gas inside the chamber. For a given exposure the charge produced will be 6 times larger than for a nonpressurized chamber. The chamber walls are made of a conductive plastic with a wall thickness of 200 mg/cm^2. The bias potential is 90 volts and is derived from two 9-volt transistor batteries.

Ionization chamber survey meters are somewhat slow in responding to changes in radiation levels. Detectors based on GM tubes are better

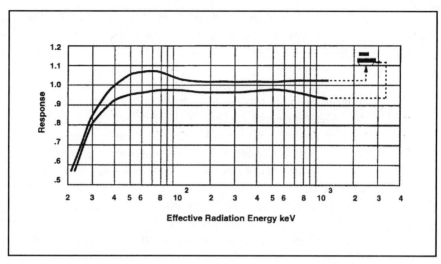

Figure 8.14: Energy response of an ionization survey meter (Victoreen 450P). This is how the reading varies for a fixed exposure rate as the energy of the radiation is changed. The energy response is slightly different depending on whether the radiation enters the meter from the bottom or side. The energy response is flat for energies above about 10^2 keV. The flat energy response makes this an accurate instrument over a wide range in radiation energy. (Courtesy of Fluke Biomedical, Everett, WA).

for finding lost radioactive sources or detecting contamination because they are very sensitive and respond quickly. Ionization survey meters tend to be more accurate in their readings for a large variety of isotopes because of their flat energy response.

8.3.3 Charge Collection and Measurement

The charge collected by a therapy ionization chamber is measured by an electrometer (see Figure 2.3). A modern electrometer performs two functions:

1. It provides a bias voltage between the electrodes of the chamber. A typical bias voltage is ±300 volts for a chamber used for therapy beam measurements.
2. It measures the charge collected. The amount of charge collected by a therapy ion chamber is typically on the order of nC (i.e., 10^{-9} C). This is a very tiny amount of charge. The electrometer is connected to the ion chamber by a cable that has three concentric conductors. This cable is called *triaxial* cable.

Beam calibration protocols require a measurement of the radiation-induced charge to an accuracy of a few percent. Due to this stringent requirement, a number of small corrections must be made to the electrometer reading to determine the actual charge appearing in the ion chamber collecting volume as a result of an irradiation. For survey meter measurements with an ion chamber such corrections are unnecessary. The actual reading of the electrometer is called the "raw" reading and is designated M_{raw}. This reading must be mathematically corrected for a number of small effects so that it corresponds to the true ionization charge produced inside the ion chamber by the radiation.

Measurements made with a calibrated ion chamber are only as good as the electrometer that is used to measure the charge collected. The electrometer may not accurately measure the charge that flows into it. As an example, when the electrometer reads 1.000 nC, perhaps the charge actually collected is 1.003 nC. In this case, we can correct the electrometer reading by multiplying by an electrometer correction factor P_{elec} = 1.003 Coulomb per Reading (C/Rdg). The value of P_{elec} can be provided by an ADCL and an electrometer should be calibrated every 2 years. If an electrometer and an ion chamber will always be used together, they can be calibrated as a set. The cost of electrometer calibration is approximately $100 (in year 2008).

The number of ions generated by a fixed amount of radiation will depend on the mass of the air inside the ion chamber. The greater the mass of the air, the more ions produced. If the air pressure should increase, the mass of the air in the chamber will rise even though the volume of air remains fixed.[1] If the temperature should increase the mass of the air will decline. Ion chamber calibration is referenced to a temperature of 22 °C (295 K) and an air pressure of 760 mm-Hg.[2] This pressure is the nominal atmospheric pressure at sea level. If the temperature and pressure do not have these standard values, then a correction must be made by multiplying by a correction factor. The temperature and pressure correction factor is given by the equation:

$$P_{TP} = \frac{273+T}{295} \times \frac{760}{p}, \tag{8.2}$$

where T is the temperature in Celsius and p is the pressure in units of mm-Hg. Note that $273 + T$ is the temperature in units of Kelvin. Equation (8.2) is based on the ideal gas equation $pV = nRT$. The temperature and pressure correction can be the single largest correction to the raw electrometer reading. It can easily be 4% or 5% at moderate elevations and even higher than this in mountainous regions where the atmospheric pressure is always low.

Note:

a. P_{TP} = 1 for T = 22 °C and p = 760 mm-Hg as expected.

b. As the pressure increases, the mass inside the chamber rises; therefore the amount of ionization goes up and the electro-

---

[1] Ion chambers used for beam calibration are unsealed, i.e., they are not "airtight." The technical term for this is "atmospheric communication."

[2] This is not the SI unit for pressure; nevertheless, it is so commonly used that we will stick to it.

meter reading increases. In this case, P_{TP} must go *down* to compensate [see equation (8.2)].

c. As the temperature goes up, the mass inside the chamber goes down and therefore P_{TP} must go *up* to compensate [see equation (8.2)].

It is necessary for radiation therapy departments to possess a barometer and a thermometer for the purpose of determining P_{TP}.

During routine measurements the collecting electrode of the ion chamber has a certain polarity, either positive or negative. If the polarity is reversed, the magnitude of the electrometer reading may change. The multiplicative term P_{pol} corrects for this. This correction is generally less than 2% (i.e., $0.98 \leq P_{pol} \leq 1.02$). It is evaluated by making measurements at one polarity and then reversing the polarity and repeating the measurements. Although we will not describe the details here, it is relatively simple to calculate this correction factor.

Not all the charge produced by radiation inside an ion chamber is collected. Ionizing radiation produces ions of opposite sign. These ions move under the action of the electric field inside the ionization chamber. The positive ions migrate toward the cathode and the negative ions toward the anode. When the ions are collected at an electrode, they produce a signal, which is measured by the electrometer. During the time that it takes the ions to move to the electrodes, some small number of positive and negative ions will meet and recombine and therefore some charge will be lost to collection. The larger the number of ions per unit volume, the more likely this process is to occur; and therefore the effect is most pronounced in radiation beams of high intensity or dose rate where the ionization density is high. The lower the voltage between the electrodes, the longer it takes for the ions to be collected and the more opportunity there is for recombination.

If the charge collected is denoted as Q' and the charge produced by the radiation (before recombination) as Q, the ion collection efficiency can be defined as[3]

$$f = \frac{Q'}{Q} = \frac{\text{charge collected}}{\text{charge deposited}}. \tag{8.3}$$

This number is always less than or equal to 1.00. The amount of recombination depends on the bias voltage between the electrodes in the ion chamber. A larger bias voltage produces a stronger electric field, causing the ions to migrate more rapidly to the electrodes. This allows less time for the ions to find one another and thus reduces the likelihood of recombination. At low bias, recombination may be significant (see Figure 8.15).

---

[3] Do not confuse the ion collection efficiency with the f_{med} introduced in chapter 7. It is standard notation (perhaps unfortunate) that both these quantities have the symbol f.

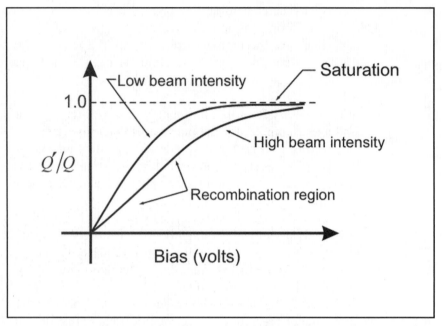

Figure 8.15: The charge collected divided by the charge produced in an ion chamber as a function of the applied bias voltage. At low bias voltage much of the charge is lost to recombination before it can be collected. As the bias is increased less and less recombination occurs until almost all the charge is collected. When the beam intensity is higher the density of ions is higher, recombination is more apt to occur and a higher bias voltage is required to reach saturation.

At high bias almost all the charge produced in the chamber may be collected. This is called *saturation*.

The electrometer reading must be corrected for recombination. The correction to the electrometer reading is the reciprocal of the collection efficiency, namely:

$$P_{ion} = \frac{1}{f}. \tag{8.4}$$

Note that P_{ion} is always greater than or equal to 1.00. The P_{ion} correction is typically less than about 2%; that is, $P_{ion} \lesssim 1.02$. The value of P_{ion} is determined by making measurements at a bias voltage of 300 volts and then again at 150 volts and comparing the measurements. From these measurements it is possible to estimate the value of P_{ion}, although we will not discuss the details here. Ionization chambers used for therapy beam measurements typically operate at a bias of ±300 volts. With this bias voltage, recombination effects are small, generally less than 1% to 2%. Why not just increase the bias further to eliminate recombination as much as possible? If the bias is set too large, gas multiplication will begin to occur and the chamber no longer acts like an ion chamber. We will discuss gas multiplication in section 8.3.4.

After all of the corrections discussed above are evaluated, the charge M produced inside the ionization chamber by ionizing radiation can be related to the value M_{raw} read from the electrometer display as follows:

$$M = P_{ion}P_{TP}P_{elec}P_{pol}M_{raw}. \tag{8.5}$$

An illustration of the application of equation (8.5) is given in Example 8.1.

Example 8.1

A series of ion chamber measurements are made for identical irradiations with a bias voltage of –300 volts. The air temperature is 20 °C and the atmospheric pressure is 730 mm-Hg. For the bias voltage given and for the beam dose rate, the ion collection efficiency is $f = 0.982$. The electrometer in use has a value of $P_{elec} = 1.005$ nC/Rdg. The polarity correction is negligible, i.e., $P_{pol} = 1.000$. The average raw electrometer reading is $M_{raw} = 18.314$ nC.

a. Find the value of the temperature/pressure correction.

$$P_{TP} = \frac{273+T}{295} \times \frac{760}{p}$$

$$= \frac{273+20}{295} \times \frac{760}{730} = 1.034$$

b. What is the value of P_{ion}?

$$P_{ion} = \frac{1}{f} = \frac{1}{0.982} = 1.018$$

c. What is the value of the actual average charge produced by the radiation in the ion chamber?

$$M = P_{ion}P_{TP}P_{elec}P_{pol}M_{raw}$$
$$= 1.018 \times 1.034 \times 1.005 \times 1.000 \times 18.314 \text{ nC} = 19.374 \text{ nC}$$

8.3.4 Proportional Counters

Proportional counters operate at a higher bias voltage than ion chambers. As the bias voltage is increased, ions liberated by radiation are accelerated toward the collecting electrode. If the bias voltage is sufficiently high, the accelerated ions may themselves produce new ionization. This process is called *gas multiplication*. The *gas amplification factor* is the amount by which the original ionization charge is increased by gas multiplication. Gas amplification factors can be as high as 10^6. The amount of charge produced by the passage of radiation through the proportional counter is equal to the original charge produced by the radiation multiplied by the gas amplification factor. Thus the total charge collected is proportional to the original charge produced by the radiation and hence the name *proportional counter*. This allows for the possibility of determining the type of radiation or particle. Since gas multiplication is desired in these counters, the gas that is chosen to fill the sealed chamber is selected for maximum acceleration of free electrons. Common gases are xenon and argon. Proportional counters are not widely used in radiation therapy.

8.3.5 Geiger-Müller (GM) Counter

The GM counter is the radiation detector that most people have heard of—the one seen in B grade science fiction movies from the 1950s. A Geiger counter consists of a tube, which is the actual detector, connected to a counter or rate meter (see Figure 8.16). The counter or rate meter is sometimes sold separately from the tube. A Geiger-Müller tube

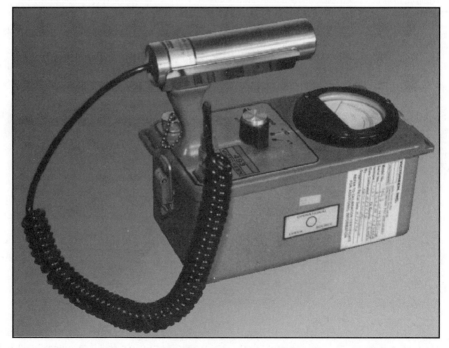

Figure 8.16: A classic GM tube and rate meter. The tube can be removed from its holder at the top. (Courtesy of Fluke Biomedical, Everett, WA)

is used for survey meters. They are very sensitive (for gas detectors), but they are not very accurate. They are designed for maximum gas amplification. They are very good for locating lost radioactive sources or finding radioactive contamination.

The counter sometimes has a loudspeaker that can produce audio clicks corresponding to every count. This feature can be useful when one cannot observe the meter continuously, but it can be unnerving to those who are not familiar with normal levels of operation. The rate meter usually reads in mR/h, μSv/h (see chapter 17) or counts per minute (cpm). It is typical to have a range from 0.01 mR/h up to 1 R/h. Meters have multiple scales: X1 (times 1), X10 (times 10), and X100. The response time can be adjusted: "slow" or "fast." The needle (or the digital readout) can fluctuate rapidly as the counter registers individual counts, particularly at low radiation levels. It is useful under these circumstances to set the response time to "slow." This provides a sort of running average over several seconds. Fast mode is desired when searching for contamination or a lost radioactive source. Some rate meters have an integration mode in which the cumulative number of counts over some time period or the total exposure can be measured.

A GM tube consists of a cylindrical tube filled with an inert gas such as neon and with a co-axial wire running along the central axis of the tube (see Figure 8.17). For detection of beta particles, a thin entrance window is needed so that betas can get inside. A GM tube is operated at higher voltages than a proportional counter (about 900 volts is typical for the type of GM tubes used in radiation therapy).

The passage of a single charged particle can cause a pulse. Of course, many photons can pass through the wall and the gas without interacting and setting a charged particle in motion. When a charged particle traverses the interior of the tube, the high voltage causes avalanche ionization leading to a large pulse of current. All pulses have the same amplitude and therefore no energy discrimination is possible.

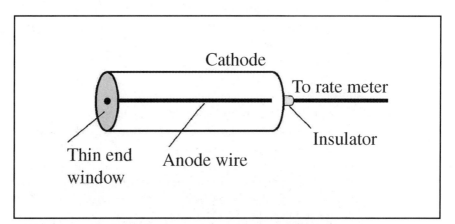

Figure 8.17: A thin end window GM tube. The anode runs coaxially down the tube and the cathode is the outer shell of the tube.

A single ionization event can cause a multiple, pulsating series of discharges that will register as spurious counts. The multiple pulsing is caused by ultraviolet (UV) emission from positive ion collisions with the walls of the detector. The UV interacts with the gas in the detector to produce additional ions. Prevention of such spurious counts is called *quenching*. There are two methods of quenching. The first uses the addition of a quenching gas such as a halogen gas (e.g., Cl_2), which absorbs UV photons without becoming ionized. The second method is to electronically reduce the anode voltage until all positive ions are collected.

When avalanche ionization occurs, a sheath of positive ions forms around the anode, shielding the electric field inside it. The ions must migrate to the cathode before the electric field can build up again for a subsequent avalanche. This leads to a minimum time between detectable pulses called the "resolving time."[4] This time scale is on the order of 100 microseconds. During this period the counter is insensitive to ionizing events. It is possible, in principle, that in a high-intensity radiation field a GM counter can become saturated and read anomalously low. Saturation may occur at an exposure rate of 1000 mR/hour or perhaps even lower. Meters are usually designed to peg at full scale under these circumstances. The user must be aware that it is possible in a very high radiation area that a GM rate meter may read low. GM counters are not recommended for radiation surveys of linear accelerators because linac beams are pulsed.[5] The pulses are brief and are therefore of high intensity.

The energy dependence of a GM detector can be ±30% over the range from 50 keV to 5 MeV. A GM detector should be used for the type and energy of radiation for which it was calibrated.

Advantages

- Very sensitive for a gas detector because of avalanche discharge. The passage of a single ionizing particle can trigger a discharge. They are mostly used as a survey meter and they are very good for locating radioactive contamination or finding lost radioactive sources.

Disadvantages

- There is no energy discrimination.
- Due to the large resolving time it is only possible to measure low count rates.
- Because they register counts, and due to their energy dependence, they are not very accurate for quantitative work.

---

[4] This is sometimes called the "dead time," but that is not strictly correct.
[5] Except perhaps for finding hot spots; see chapter 17, section 17.8.5.

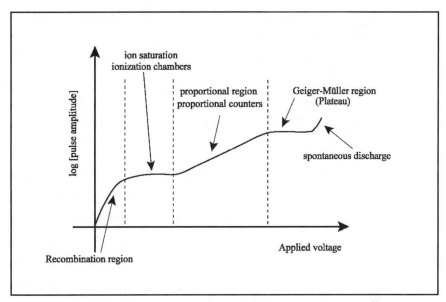

Figure 8.18: This graph summarizes the behavior of gas ionization detectors. At low applied voltage there is a great deal of recombination. At higher voltages saturation is reached. It is in this region that ionization chambers are operated. As the voltage increases further, ion multiplication occurs and the signal becomes proportional to the original charge produced by the radiation. This is the regime of the proportional counter. At still higher voltages avalanche ionization occurs and we reach the conditions under which a GM tube is operated. If the bias is increased further, spontaneous discharge (a spark) occurs. This diagram should not be taken too literally. There is no single instrument that can operate in all these regimes. Each regime requires individual design considerations.

Figure 8.18 provides a useful summary of some of the properties of gas ionization detectors.

8.4 Solid-State Detectors

8.4.1 Thermoluminescent Dosimeters

Thermoluminescent dosimeters (TLDs) are used for in vivo dose verification (e.g., skin dose), phantom measurements, and for personnel radiation monitoring. Ring badges are frequently worn by radiation workers who handle radioactive sources. The ring badges monitor the dose to the workers' hands. These ring badges commonly contain TLDs (see chapter 17).

A wide variety of materials exhibit thermoluminescence. For radiation dosimetry purposes TLD materials are crystals with impurities that are "sensitive" to radiation. When TLDs are irradiated, a small fraction of the absorbed dose is stored in the crystal structure (lattice). When TLDs are then heated, some of the stored energy is released in the form of light. Furthermore, the amount of light energy released increases with increasing absorbed dose in the material. This explains the name *thermoluminescence.*

After TLDs are "read" by heating, it is sometimes necessary to "anneal" them by subjecting them to special heat treatment to "bake" out any residual signal and to condition their sensitivity. TLD material comes in a variety of physical forms: chips, rods, powder, etc. TLD "microrods" are common (see Figure 8.19). These are rods with dimensions 1 mm × 1 mm × 5 to 6 mm. They cost about \$1 to \$2 per rod. The most frequently used TLD material in radiation dosimetry is lithium fluoride (LiF). The effective Z of LiF is 8.2, which is similar to tissue and to air.

The efficiency of TLD material can be defined as:

$$\text{Efficiency} = \frac{\text{TL light energy/mass}}{\text{Absorbed dose}}. \qquad (8.6)$$

The efficiency for LiF is only 0.039%, very tiny!

TLDs are heated during the read process. As the temperature of the TLD increases, the brightness of the thermoluminescence increases until it reaches some maximum value at a temperature called T_{max}, then the brightness begins to decline (see Figure 8.20). Some TLD materials have multiple peaks.

A TLD reader heats the TLD and measures the light emitted during heating (see Figure 8.21). A photomultiplier tube (PMT) detects the light and converts it into an electrical signal. The PMT has a high voltage across it. This is typically in the range of 750 to 900 volts. The circuitry inside the reader must sum the total light output. The result of the reading is displayed in terms of total charge output from the PMT in units of either μC or nC. The highest temperature that the TLD reaches is generally around 300 °C. The TLD reading is directly proportional to the dose for relatively low doses. The TLD material is said to be "linear" at low doses, meaning that twice the dose will result in twice the reading. LiF TLD material is linear up to a dose of about 300 to 400 cGy.

TLDs must be calibrated by exposing them to a known dose and then measuring the response with a TLD reader (usually in μC or nC) (see Figure 8.21). This provides a calibration constant in units of cGy/μC or cGy/nC.

The usual procedure for in vivo dose measurement is to take several TLDs, called standards, and expose them to a known dose that is close to the dose one expects to measure (if that is known). This procedure provides a calibration factor. Several more TLDs, called unknowns, are then used by attaching them to the patient during treatment. The standards and the unknowns should be drawn from the same group or manufacturers "lot." The sensitivity of TLDs may vary from lot to lot. The TLDs are read and the calibration factor from the standards is used to estimate the dose received by the patient. The unknowns are simply placed on the skin if it is desired to determine the skin or entrance dose. If the dose at d_m is desired, then the TLDs will be placed on the patient's

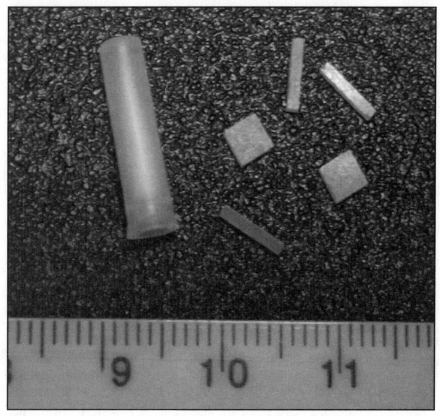

Figure 8.19: Various forms of TLDs: rods, chips, and a capsule containing TLD powder. The scale is in centimeters.

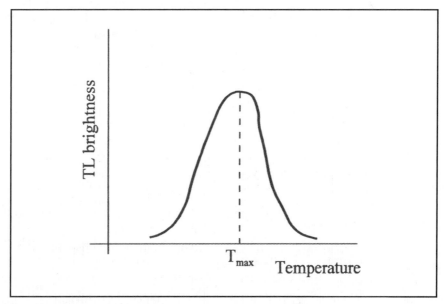

Figure 8.20: TLD "glow" curve shows the brightness of the sample as a function of the temperature. The maximum occurs at a temperature T_{max}. Many TLD materials have multiple glow peak curves. The details of the glow peak and the value of T_{max} depend on the heating rate.

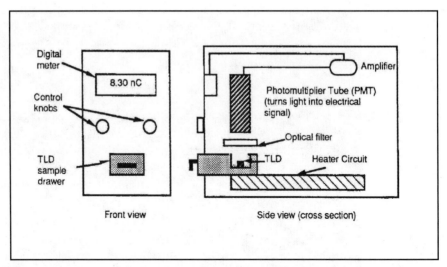

Figure 8.21: A TLD reader. The sample is placed in the drawer on a tray which can be heated. The tray is sometimes called a *planchet*. The drawer is closed and the TLD is heated. The light from thermoluminescence passes through an optical filter and into the photomultiplier tube (PMT). The optical filter absorbs infrared light emitted by the heated planchet and prevents this from reaching the PMT. The PMT converts the light into an electrical current. The charge produced by the PMT is summed and then displayed on the front panel of the reader. (Adapted from *Applied Physics for Radiation Oncology* by R. Stanton and D. Stinson, Fig. 6.10, p. 71. © 2009. Reprinted with permission.)

skin and covered by a tissue-equivalent material of the necessary thickness. This material is sometimes referred to as *bolus*. An example of the measurement process is shown in Example 8.2.

The advantages of TLDs are their small size, reusability, wide dose range (10^{-3} cGy to 10^3 cGy) and their near tissue equivalence (for LiF). They do not need attached wires like diodes or MOSFETs. The disadvantages are that the reading is not instantaneous. They have to be exposed and then taken to the reader. Another disadvantage is the possible loss of a reading. They can only be read once and thus there is no permanent

Example 8.2

A patient's skin dose is to be measured by using TLDs. Six TLDs are removed from a packet. Three of these are used as "standards" and are exposed to a known dose of 100 cGy. Three unknowns are placed on the patient's skin. The average reading of the standards is 64.8 nC and the average reading of the unknowns is 83.2 nC. What skin dose did the patient receive?

The calibration factor of these TLDs is 100 cGy/64.8 nC = 1.54 cGy/nC. The patient dose is 83.2 nC × 1.54 cGy/nC = 128 cGy.

record in the sense that they cannot be read again later. For in vivo dosimetry the use of TLDs is declining in favor of diodes and MOSFETs.

8.4.2 Film

The degree to which film is blackened is related to the dose received by the film. Radiographic film consists of an emulsion 10 to 25 μm thick of microscopic "grains" of silver bromide (AgBr) coated on either one or both sides of a plastic film "base" (see section 4.4). When radiation strikes the grains, they become susceptible to chemical change. They form a so-called "latent image." The development process leaves small grains of metallic silver. The silver in the unexposed areas is washed away and the portion exposed to radiation appears dark. A negative image of the radiation field is the result.

A measure of film blackening is provided by the degree to which the light is attenuated in passing through the developed film. A measure of light attenuation by film is called *optical density.* The optical density is defined in terms of the light intensity incident on the film, I_0, and the intensity of the transmitted light I_t (see Figure 8.22):

$$OD = \log_{10}\left(\frac{I_0}{I_t}\right). \tag{8.7}$$

The percentage of *transmitted light* is $I_t/I_0 \times 100\%$ (note that I_t is in the numerator). Another example of the use of equation (8.7) is given in Example 8.3. As an example, if 10% of the light is transmitted, then $I_0/I_t = 10$ and $OD = \log_{10}10 = 1.0$. The usable range of OD extends up to $OD \cong 2.0$, which corresponds to 1% light transmission. Above this optical density the film is very black and little useful information can be obtained. Optical densities are additive. The optical density of two films together is the sum of the individual optical densities.

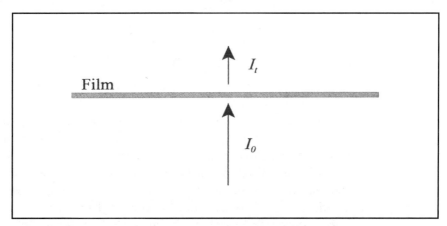

Figure 8.22: Light with intensity I_0 is incident upon a piece of film. The intensity of the transmitted light is I_t.

Example 8.3

What percentage of incident light is transmitted through a film that has an optical density of 2.5? The percentage of transmitted light is $(I_t/I_0) \times 100\%$.

$$\log\left(\frac{I_0}{I_t}\right) = 2.5$$

$$\left(\frac{I_0}{I_t}\right) = 10^{2.5} = 316$$

$$\left(\frac{I_t}{I_0}\right) \times 100\% = 0.32\%$$

Optical density is measured with a device called a densitometer. Figure 8.23 shows a manual densitometer. This device is used to make manual measurements of the OD at various points on a film. A film digitizer (Figure 8.24) measures light transmission over the entire surface of the film. A film digitizer is like a scanner that is used to scan images into a computer, except in this case it is the transmitted and not the reflected light that is measured. The transmission data are fed into a computer producing an image of the film. Software is available which will convert the transmission measurements to optical density. If a calibration curve of the type shown in Figure 8.25 is available for the particular film scanned, then software can be used to construct maps of the dose distribution (isodose curves) over the entire film plane.

Even film that has not been exposed to radiation will, when developed, attenuate some light because of the plastic film base and because some Ag grains are developed even in the absence of radiation exposure. The former is called "base" and the latter is called "fog." A typical optical density for base plus fog is OD $\cong 0.2$. The *net optical density* is defined as the total optical density minus the optical density of base + fog:

$$\text{Net optical density} = OD - OD_{base+fog}. \tag{8.8}$$

Figure 8.25 shows the relationship between net optical density and dose for Kodak XV film and 10 MV x-rays. This graph provides a density-to-dose calibration and it is sometimes erroneously called an "H&D" curve.[6] For low doses the relationship between the net *OD* and dose is linear. As the dose increases, the curve starts to turn over and become non-linear; that is, twice the dose does not result in twice the optical density. As the dose becomes even larger, the film begins to saturate;

---

[6] A true H&D curve is a plot of OD versus log exposure.

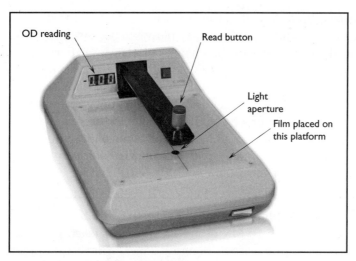

Figure 8.23: A manual densitometer for measuring the optical density (OD) of film. The film is placed on the platform and the arm is pressed down. Light emerging through the aperture passes through the film and the OD is read from the digital display. (Courtesy of X-Rite Incorporated, Grand Rapids, MI)

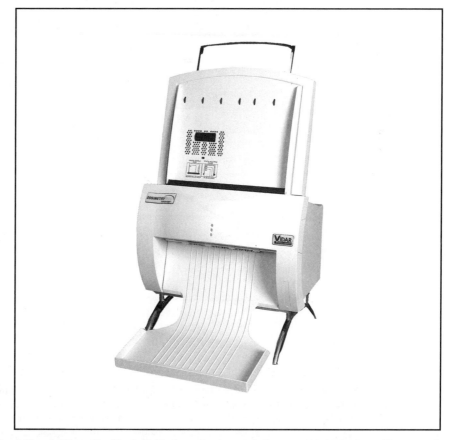

Figure 8.24: A film digitizer. The film is fed in from the top and comes out at the bottom. (Photograph of the Dosimetry PRO® Advantage Film Digitizer courtesy of VIDAR Systems Corporation, Herndon, VA)

that is, there is little or no increase in *OD* as the dose increases. This region is useless for dosimetry purposes because the *OD* is almost completely insensitive to the changes in the dose. For radiation dosimetry purposes it is preferable to work on the linear portion of the curve. This curve provides calibration. One must calibrate film for each radiation type and energy, for each film type (including even the particular batch of film), and for processor conditions, which may vary over time. The use of the calibration curve in Figure 8.25 is demonstrated in Example 8.4.

Example 8.4

Kodak XV film is used to measure the dose in a plastic phantom at a depth d_m for a 10 MV beam. The film was taken from the same lot as that used to construct Figure 8.25. All films were processed at the same time, including a film that had not been exposed to any radiation. The unirradiated film has an optical density of 0.22. The film with the unknown dose has an OD of 1.40. What dose did this film receive?

The net OD of the unknown is 1.40 – 0.22 = 1.18. Consulting Figure 8.25 we see that the film received a dose of approximately 50 cGy.

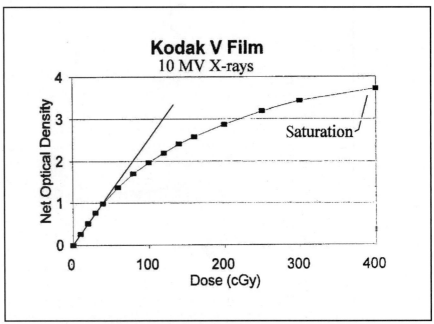

Figure 8.25: The relationship between net optical density and dose for Kodak XV film exposed to 10 MV x-rays. For low doses the relationship is linear. A line has been drawn through the low dose data to illustrate this. For higher doses the relationship becomes non-linear. At the highest doses the curve flattens out because all of the available Ag grains are developed and no more remain, regardless of how high the dose becomes. This phenomenon is called saturation. For dosimetry purposes it is best to work on the linear portion of the curve. This type of film requires a dose of roughly 50 cGy to produce a net OD of 1.0.

An advantage of film is that it has high spatial resolution and it can be used to obtain a detailed "map" or "picture" of a dose distribution. Film can be saved and read again later. It forms a permanent record. It is also widely commercially available and it is relatively inexpensive. The disadvantages of film are that it has to be developed and that it has a strong energy dependence for photons, it is not tissue equivalent, and it is sensitive to light. Film is much more sensitive to low-energy photons than high-energy photons. The AgBr emulsion has a high effective Z and its sensitivity is highly energy dependent, particularly below about 300 keV where photoelectric interactions begin to become important. Recall that $\tau/\rho \sim (Z/E_\gamma)^3$ for the photoelectric effect. Film can be 10 to 50 times more sensitive at low energies!

A new type of film was introduced for radiation dosimetry called *radiochromic film*. A trade name is GafChromic film. This film has the advantage that it is not based on a silver halide but rather a radiation sensitive "monomer." It is roughly equally sensitive to radiation of all energies. The unexposed film is colorless and it turns various shades of blue upon exposure to radiation. It is insensitive to ambient room light and it is self-developing—no processing is required. A disadvantage is that it is very insensitive; it requires a dose of 1000 to 5000 cGy to achieve a reasonable OD. It is also very expensive. The use of film for personnel monitoring of radiation exposure will be discussed in chapter 17.

8.4.3 Diodes

Diodes are small solid-state devices that are used in electronics to convert alternating current to direct current (AC to DC). When these devices are irradiated, they produce a small current even in the absence of an externally supplied bias voltage. Because they are solid detectors, they are very sensitive and they give a real-time readout (see Figures 8.26 and 8.27). These properties make them useful for patient dosimetry. They are also used for depth dose scans and for beam profile measurements (see chapter 9). They are not suitable for beam calibration, but they can be used as a daily check device to monitor linac beam output constancy.

For patient dosimetry, diodes can be used to measure the dose at a depth of d_m. They are placed on the patient's skin. They can be purchased with the appropriate buildup already on them for various energy beams. Diodes with buildup on them cannot be used to measure skin dose. For tissue-equivalent material the build-up thickness is several centimeters for high-energy x-ray beams (see Figure 8.27). This would make the diode detector impractically large. Therefore a high-density non–tissue-equivalent material is used, usually some type of metal. This can lead to anomalous behavior under some circumstances.

The diode is attached via a cable to an electrometer, which measures the total charge flowing out of the diode as a result of irradiation (see Figure 8.26). Diodes used for radiation therapy are unbiased; that is,

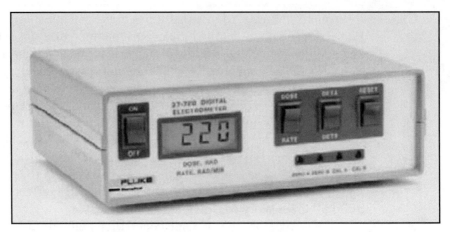

Figure 8.26: A direct reading dedicated electrometer used for diode dose measurements. (Courtesy of Fluke Biomedical, Everett, WA)

there is no voltage placed across them. The electrometer used is usually dedicated (used only for this purpose) and its sensitivity is adjusted so that the dose can be read directly. The adjustment of the sensitivity is part of the calibration process. The diode is exposed to a known dose of radiation and then the electrometer is adjusted to read the known dose. Calibration must be performed periodically since the sensitivity drifts with time and with cumulative radiation exposure. The diode response varies with energy and to a small extent with field size.

Diodes are rugged, reliable, and they give an instant reading. Many clinics routinely monitor patient treatment with in vivo diode dosimetry. Diodes complement portal images (see chapter 19). A portal image tells where the radiation is going but not how much is going there, whereas a diode can. Further discussion of in vivo dosimetry can be found in chapter 18, section 18.3.4.

8.4.4 MOSFETs

MOSFET stands for metal oxide semiconductor-field effect transistor. A MOSFET is a special type of transistor that is sensitive to radiation. A "threshold voltage shift" is measured (in units of mV) which is proportional to the radiation dose. Standard sensitivity MOSFETs have a calibration factor of about 1 mV/cGy, whereas high sensitivity detectors have a calibration factor of 9 mV/cGy. High-sensitivity MOSFETs are well suited for measuring low doses, such as under a block or outside the radiation field. Diodes are not well suited for this.

MOSFETs are small and lightweight (see Figure 8.28). They are easily placed on a patient's skin. They provide an immediate dose read-

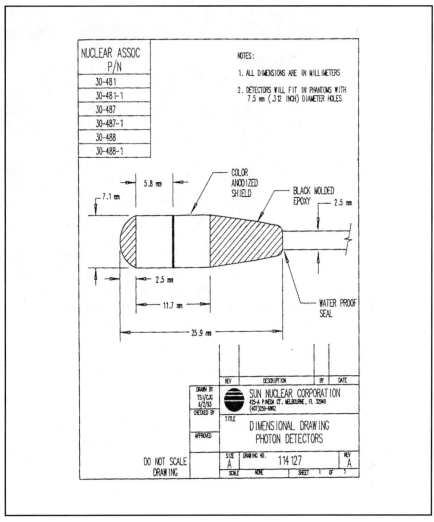

Figure 8.27: Schematic of a diode detector used for patient dosimetry. The diode is placed on the patient's skin and measures the dose at depth d_m. (Courtesy of Sun Nuclear, Melbourne, FL)

ing and they can be reused. The MOSFETs are connected to a reader, which in turn sends a signal to a computer. MOSFETs are read in terms of a "threshold voltage shift" in millivolts (mV). Computer software is used to acquire readings, apply calibration factors, and store readings. One commercially available system allows up to five MOSFETs to be connected to the reader. In this case, one can gather dose measurements at five points. MOSFETs are sold without buildup. For measurements at d_m buildup must be placed over the MOSFET. The detectors have a limited life of about 20,000 mV. For a standard sensitivity MOSFET this corresponds to about 20,000 cGy. This is significantly shorter than the lifetime of a diode.

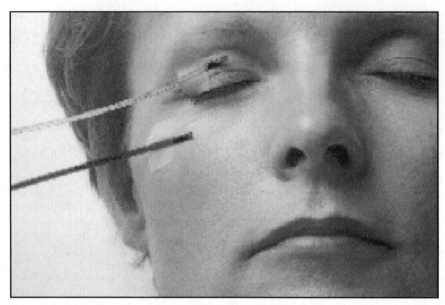

Figure 8.28: MOSFETs applied to a patient's skin. The MOSFET is contained in the dark area at the end of the electrical lead. (Courtesy of Best Medical Canada, www.TeamBest.com)

8.4.5 Polymer Gels

Polymer gels are tissue equivalent gelatin-based materials that can fill containers in the form of spheres or other convenient shapes and be used to assess the full 3-D dose distribution in a phantom. This is a unique capability. Such phantoms can be used to validate radiosurgery dose distributions. Radiation causes polymer chains to form in the tissue-equivalent gel. One frequently mentioned type of polymer gel is called *BANG gel*. Magnetic resonance imaging can be used to measure the 3-D dose distribution in the sample. Calibration data are obtained by irradiating test tubes filled with gel to known doses. Techniques have also been developed to measure the dose distribution using relatively inexpensive CT-like laser scanners. There are commercial firms that will ship a phantom containing a polymer gel to customers. The customer irradiates the phantom and then returns it to the commercial firm for dosimetric evaluation.

8.5 Liquid Dosimeters

8.5.1 Calorimeters

One of the few methods for direct measurement of absorbed dose involves the use of a calorimeter. A *calorimeter* is an insulated container that is used to measure small amounts of heat energy. A calorimeter can function as an absolute dosimeter for the measurement of absorbed dose. Recall that a free-air ionization chamber is an absolute dosimeter for the measurement of *exposure*. Dosimetry calorimeters are generally only found in standards laboratories such as NIST.

Let us assume that all of the energy absorbed in a material by radiation appears ultimately as heat. We either account for, or neglect, any energy stored internally in the material. An example of radiation energy stored in a material is given by thermoluminescence. A thermometer inserted into the calorimeter measures the rise in temperature of an irradiated sample due to the absorption of radiation energy. If the change in temperature of an isolated sample of mass m and specific heat c is ΔT, then the corresponding amount of heat energy is $\Delta Q = m \, c \, \Delta T$. The specific heat of water is 4.186×10^3 J/(kg °C). The absorbed dose $D = E_{AB}/m$ and if $E_{AB} = \Delta Q$, then $D = c \, \Delta T$. An absorbed dose of 1 Gy will raise the temperature of water by only 2.5×10^{-4} °C! Such a small temperature change is difficult to measure.

A calorimeter can be used to calibrate an ion chamber. The calorimeter is used to measure the dose delivered by a radiation beam. The ion chamber is then placed in that radiation beam and the same dose is delivered. The amount of charge collected in the ion chamber is measured. These measurements can be used to provide a calibration of the ion chamber in terms of the known dose measured using the calorimeter.

8.5.2 Chemical Dosimetry

Radiation can induce chemical changes. Chemical dosimetry is generally based on metallic ions in an aqueous solution. Since the concentration of the chemical is very low, these solutions are water equivalent. The most common type is the Fricke dosimeter. This is based on an acidic aqueous solution of ferrous sulfate. Irradiation changes the oxidation state of the iron from +2 to +3, thus producing ferric sulfate from ferrous sulfate. The production of ferric sulfate results in a change in color of the solution. This can be measured with a spectrophotometer.

The amount of ferric sulfate produced can be quantified by the yield or so-called G factor. The G factor is the number of moles of ferric sulfate produced per joule of absorbed energy. A typical G value is 1 µmol/J. The absorption of 1 Gy dose therefore requires the detection of 1 µmol in 1 kg of solution, which may contain 10^{10} µmol. This requires a parts per billion detection. For this reason, chemical dosimetry is not very sensitive and cannot be used to measure small doses. Chemical dosimetry can be used to determine the average dose in an irradiated volume of complex shape. The solution is placed in a container of the desired shape. For example, it can be placed in a Petrie dish for the purpose of evaluating the dose delivered for a radiobiological cell experiment. A lack of stability of the solution has inhibited commercial development of chemical dosimeters. Chemical dosimetry is not usually found in radiation therapy clinics.

Chapter Summary

- There are three major categories of radiation detectors:
  1. **Gas Ionization Detectors** (radiation produces ionization in the gas, collect ion pairs, poor efficiency compared to solid)
     a. Ionization chambers (used for beam calibration and survey meters).
     b. Proportional counters (used for survey meters).
     c. Geiger-Müller (GM) counters (used for survey meters).
  2. **Solid-State Detectors**
     a. Thermoluminescent dosimeters (TLDs) (personnel monitoring, in vivo dosimetry).
     b. Film (measure distribution of dose and for personnel monitoring).
     c. Diodes (in vivo dosimetry, beam measurements).
     d. MOSFETs (in vivo dosimetry).
     e. Polymer gel (measure 3-D distribution of dose).
     f. Scintillation (survey meters).
  3. **Liquid Detectors**
     a. Calorimeters (used in standards laboratories, direct measurement of dose).
     b. Chemical (aqueous solution, direct measurement of dose).

- **Phantoms:** Classified by shape and composition.
  —Shape: Geometrical or anthropomorphic.
  —Composition: Elemental and electron density.
  —Tissue equivalence: Same properties as tissue with respect to radiation absorption and scattering; depends on type and energy of radiation.
  —Effective atomic number: Equivalent atomic number of a compound or mixture that describes radiation absorption and scattering over a range in energy (depends on type of radiation).

- **Survey Meters:** Portable radiation detection devices that are designed to detect the presence of radiation and to make a rough measurement of the radiation level, often in terms of mR/h.

- **Gas Ionization Detectors**
  —Cavity Ionization Chambers
  These are characterized by their shape, collecting volume, and the thickness and composition of their walls. These instruments are used for a wide variety of applications. The larger the volume the more sensitive the instrument but the poorer the spatial resolution. Large volume ion chambers are used for survey meters.

- *Thimble chambers:* Shaped like a thimble; examples are Farmer chamber, mini-chambers for beam scanning, survey meter chambers. Therapy chambers range in collecting volume from about 0.1 cm^3 to 1.0 cm^3. A bias voltage of about 300 V is applied between the inner wall and the central collecting electrode. Ion chambers used for beam calibration should be calibrated by an Accredited Dosimetry Calibration Lab (ADCL) every 2 years. Ion chambers used for Co-60 teletherapy beam calibration are **required** by the U.S. Nuclear Regulatory Commission (NRC) to be calibrated every 2 years.

  External beam calibration is carried out with a Farmer chamber: a thimble chamber with a collecting volume of approximately 0.6 cm^3. When measurements are made in air, a water-equivalent build-up cap is used. The build-up cap ensures CPE inside the chamber; the electrons crossing the interior of the chamber will have properties characteristic of the electrons generated in water. In this way the dose in free space can be measured. The build-up cap also serves to protect the thin chamber wall. The build up cap that comes with a Farmer chamber is designed for Co-60 and therefore has a thickness equivalent to 0.5 cm of water. A Farmer chamber can also be placed directly in a water tank (it may be necessary to cover it with a waterproof protective sleeve first). In this case, the build-up cap is removed and the electrons crossing

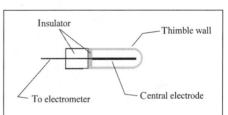

A thimble ionization chamber. The inner thimble wall is coated with a conducting material and a bias voltage is placed between the inner wall and the central electrode. Charge is collected at the central electrode, which then flows out to the electrometer.

  the interior of the chamber are generated in the water. In this way the absorbed dose delivered by a radiation beam can be measured in a water "phantom."

- *Flat-cavity chambers* (also called pancake or plane-parallel): Shaped like a pancake, used for electron beam measurements or measurements in the x-ray build-up region. The electrodes are shaped like parallel plates. One of the electrodes is a thin window through which the radiation enters the chamber. The entrance window is made of a foil or plastic membrane that is 0.01 to 0.03 mm thick. For therapy applications the spacing between the electrodes is typically 2 mm.

- *Well chambers:* Used for assaying radioactive sources in nuclear medicine and for brachytherapy.
- *Electrometer:* Connected to the ion chamber with triaxial cable.
  1. Provides bias voltage across electrodes of ion chamber (usually ±300 volts).
  2. Measures the charge collected from ion chamber, usually on the order of nC.
  3. Calibrated by ADCL: Supply correction factor P_{elec}, *True charge = Reading* $\times P_{elec}$.

  Ionization chamber survey meters have a slow response compared to GM but may have a more accurate reading; no dependence on radiation energy; relatively flat energy response above about 100 keV.
- *Recombination:* Ions may recombine as they drift to the collecting electrode; more likely to occur when the ionization density is high (high radiation level) and the collecting bias is low. The ion collection efficiency is defined as $f = Q'/Q \leq 1$, where Q' is the charge collected and Q is the charge produced by the radiation. Saturation occurs when almost all of the charge is collected.

- **Corrections to Ion Chamber Readings** (necessary only for accurate beam calibration):

$$M = P_{ion}P_{TP}P_{elec}P_{pol}M_{raw}.$$

1. Temperature and pressure

$$P_{TP} = \frac{273+T}{295} \times \frac{760}{p}$$

where T is the temperature in Celsius and p is the atmospheric pressure in mm-Hg.
2. Recombination: $P_{ion} = 1/f$.
3. Electrometer correction: P_{elec}.
4. Polarization: P_{pol}.
   - *Gas multiplication:* When the bias voltage is high, ions liberated by radiation are accelerated toward the collecting electrode; they in turn produce new ions—get pulse, individual count. This occurs in proportional counters and in GM tubes.
   - *Proportional counters:* Gas amplification up to 10^6; signal is proportional to original charge produced by radiation.

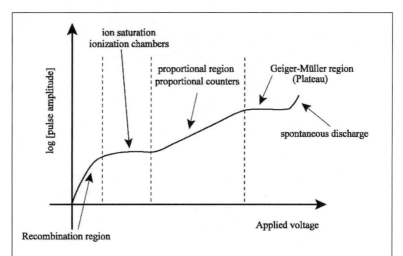

This graph summarizes the behavior of gas ionization detectors. At low applied voltage, there is a great deal of recombination. At higher voltages, saturation is reached. It is in this region that ionization chambers are operated. As the voltage increases, further ion multiplication occurs and the signal becomes proportional to the original charge produced by the radiation. This is the regime of the proportional counter. At still higher voltages, avalanche ionization occurs and we reach the conditions under which a GM tube is operated. If the bias is increased further, spontaneous discharge (a spark) occurs. This diagram should not be taken too literally. There is no single instrument that can operate in all these regimes. Each regime requires individual design considerations.

- *GM Counter designed for maximum gas amplification.* Operates at higher voltages than proportional counter (about 900 volts). High voltage causes avalanche ionization, which leads to a large pulse of current. All pulses have the same amplitude; no energy discrimination is possible. Very good for locating radioactive contamination or finding lost radioactive sources. May not be as accurate as ion chamber survey meter because of strong energy dependence. A quenching gas (e.g., halogen) is necessary to prevent multiple pulsing. Insensitive during "dead time"; can potentially read low in high radiation field.

- **Thermoluminescent dosimeters (TLDs)** are solid-state dosimeters used for in vivo dose verification (e.g., skin dose) and for personnel radiation monitoring. When TLDs are irradiated, a small fraction of the absorbed dose is stored in the crystal structure (lattice). When TLDs are then heated, some of the stored energy is released in the form of light. The most commonly used TLD material in radiation dosimetry is lithium fluoride (LiF). The effective Z of LiF is 8.2, which is similar to tissue and to air. A TLD reader heats the TLD and measures the light emitted during heating. As the temperature of the TLD increases, the brightness of the thermoluminescence increases until it reaches some maximum value at a temperature called T_{max}; then the brightness begins to decline (see glow curve in Figure 8.20). Some TLD materials have multiple peaks. A photomultiplier tube (PMT) detects the light and converts it into an electrical signal. The result of the reading is displayed in terms of total charge output from the PMT in units of either μC or nC. TLDs must be calibrated by exposing them to a known dose and then measuring the response with a TLD reader. This provides a calibration constant in units of cGy/μC or cGy/nC. The advantages of TLDs are their small size, no need for wires, reusability, wide dose range, and their near tissue-equivalence (for LiF). The disadvantages are that the reading is not instantaneous; they have to be exposed and then taken to the reader. Another disadvantage is the possible loss of a reading; they can only be read once and thus there is no permanent record.

- **Film:** The degree to which film is blackened is related to the dose received by the film.
  —*Optical Density:* A measure of film blackening

$$OD = \log_{10}\left(\frac{I_0}{I_t}\right).$$

  where I_0 is the incident intensity and I_t is the transmitted intensity. The percentage of transmitted light is I_t/I_0. The usable range of OD extends up to $OD \cong 2.0$.
  —*Base+Fog:* the optical density of a piece of film that has not been exposed to any radiation. A typical value of base + fog is $OD \cong 0.2$.

  An advantage of film is that it has high spatial resolution and it can be used to obtain a detailed "map" or "picture" of a dose distribution. Film can be saved and read again later. It forms a permanent record. It is also widely commercially available and it is relatively inexpensive. Disadvantages of film are that it has to be developed and that it has a strong energy dependence, it is not tissue equivalent, and it is sensitive to light. Film is much more sensitive to low-energy photons than high-energy photons.

- **Diodes:** Small solid-state devices that produce a small current when irradiated even in the absence of external bias. They are very sensitive and give a real-time readout. Frequently used for patient dosimetry. Can be used to measure the dose at d_m when diode has buildup on it. To keep size reasonable, build-up material is high density, non–tissue equivalent. Diode is attached to a dedicated electrometer that measures the total charge flowing out. Diode/electrometer combination is calibrated to read directly in terms of dose.

- **MOSFETs:** Small, solid-state transistors. Threshold voltage shift (in mV) is proportional to radiation dose; used for patient dosimetry; lifetime of about 200 Gy or less.

- **Polymer Gels:** Gelatin-base materials that have the unique capability of measuring 3-D dose distributions. Read by either MRI or optical CT.

- **Calorimeter:** An insulated container that can be used to measure the small temperature rise associated with absorbed dose. An absolute dosimeter for dose.

- **Chemical Dosimetry:** Based on metallic ions in an aqueous solution; tissue-equivalent; requires large doses; measure dose in liquid of complex shape; requires spectrophotometer to measure change in optical properties of solution.

Problems

1. The value of the Compton mass attenuation coefficient $\sigma/\rho = 2.78 \times 10^{-2}$ cm^2/g for water at 5 MeV. The relative electron density of polystyrene is 0.969 compared to water. What is the approximate value of σ/ρ for polystyrene at 5 MeV?

2. What quantity does an ionization chamber (connected to an electrometer) actually measure?

3. A 0.6 cm^3 Farmer chamber receives a 1 R exposure. The air inside the chamber is at 22 °C and 760 mm-Hg pressure. Calculate the charge produced inside the chamber if the cavity is in CPE. The density of air is 1.21×10^{-3} g/cm^3 at 22 °C and 1 atmosphere of pressure. Express your answer in nC.

4. A typical plane-parallel therapy ion chamber has an entrance window diameter of 5 mm and a plate spacing of 2 mm. If a plane-parallel chamber and a Farmer chamber are subjected to the same irradiation, what will the ratio of their charge readings be (assume no recombination)?

5. The bias potential (voltage between the electrodes) for an ion chamber placed in a radiation field is accidentally changed from 300 volts to 100 volts. What effect will this have on the electrometer reading and why?

6. Why must the value of P_{ion} always be greater than or equal to 1.00. Why can't it be less than 1.00?

7. If the ionization produced inside an ion chamber is 20.0 nC and if 19.2 nC are actually collected, what is the collection efficiency f?

8. Beam calibration measurements using a Farmer chamber result in an average raw electrometer reading of 17.036 nC. The temperature is 19.2 °C and the atmospheric pressure is 729 mm-Hg. The electrometer has a value of $P_{elec} = 1.005$, recently obtained from an ADCL. The ion collection efficiency is $f = 0.997$. The value of the polarity correction is found to be $P_{pol} = 1.001$. Find the true charge produced inside the ion chamber under standard conditions of temperature and pressure.

9. What are quenching gases? What gases are used for this purpose?

10. What is "base" and what is "fog" for photographic film? What is a typical value of the optical density of base + fog?

11. Calculate the optical density of a piece of film that transmits 2% of the light incident upon it.

12. An optical density of 3 corresponds to what percentage of transmitted light?

13. Two radiographic films, each having an OD of 1.2, are placed on top of one another. What is the optical density of the combination? What percentage of incident light is transmitted by the combination?

14. List some of the advantages and disadvantages of the use of photographic film as a dosimeter.

15. Sketch a calibration curve for radiographic film, carefully label the axes, and explain the major features of the curve.

16. List some of the advantages and disadvantages of the use of TLDs for patient dosimetry.

17. A patient's skin dose is to be measured by using TLDs. Six TLDs are removed from a packet. Three of these are used as "standards" and are exposed to a known dose of 100 cGy. Three unknowns are placed on the patient's skin. The average reading of the standards is 84.6 nC and the average reading of the unknowns is 64.3 nC. What skin dose did the patient receive?

18. A 30 mg capsule of LiF TLD powder receives a dose of 1 Gy. How much energy (in joules) is stored for later release as thermoluminescence?

19. What are the applications of diodes in radiation therapy?

20. A sample of water in a calorimeter is irradiated to a uniform dose of 7000 cGy. Assuming that there is no heat loss from the water, calculate the change in the temperature of the water.

21. If your department has a manual densitometer (most do), perform the following exercise. With no film inserted, does the optical density read zero? If not, it should be zeroed—ask for help from a staff member. Select a film and choose a region of moderate optical density. Measure the optical density. Select a second film and choose a region on it and measure the optical density. Place the two films on top of one another at the point of measurement and measure the optical density of the combination. Is the optical

density of the two films together equal to the sum of the individual optical densities? Specify the manufacturer and model of the densitometer used.

22. If your department has an HDR unit, perform a radiation survey of the unit. Ask for help from a therapist or physicist. Use a survey meter. Do a battery test and test the meter with the check source.

Date of survey: _____

Meter manufacturer and model number: _____

Last calibration date: _____

Check source isotope and nominal activity: _____

HDR isotope and activity on this date: _____

Background reading: _____ _____
                                                                            Units

Maximum reading at 1 m from afterloader: _____ _____
                                                                            Units

Maximum reading at surface of afterloader: _____ _____
                                                                            Units

Location of maximum reading at surface: _____

Bibliography

Attix, F. H. *Introduction to Radiological Physics and Radiation Dosimetry.* New York: Wiley InterScience, 1986.

Cember, H. *Introduction to Health Physics,* Third Edition. New York: McGraw-Hill Medical, 1996.

Cherry, S. R., J. Sorenson, and M. Phelps. *Physics in Nuclear Medicine,* Third Edition. Philadelphia: W. B. Saunders, 2003.

Ibbott, G. S. "Detectors for 2D or 3D Dosimetry Measurements" in *General Practice of Radiation Oncology Physics in the 21st Century.* A. S. Shiu and D. E. Mellenberg (eds.). AAPM Medical Physics Monograph No. 26. Madison, WI: Medical Physics Publishing, pp. 329–356, 2000.

Johns, H. E., and J. R. Cunningham. *The Physics of Radiology,* Fourth Edition. Springfield, IL: Charles C Thomas, 1983.

Khan, F. M. *The Physics of Radiation Therapy,* Fourth Edition. Philadelphia: Lippincott Williams & Wilkins, 2009.

Knoll, G. F. *Radiation Detection and Measurement,* Third Edition. New York: John Wiley & Sons, 2000.

Metcalfe, P., T. Kron, and P. Hoban. *The Physics of Radiotherapy X-Rays and Electrons.* Madison, WI: Medical Physics Publishing, 2007.

Shapiro, J. *Radiation Protection: A Guide for Scientists, Regulators and Physicians,* Fourth Edition. Cambridge, MA: Harvard University Press, 2002.

Stanton, R., and D. Stinson. *Applied Physics for Radiation Oncology, Revised Edition.* Madison, WI: Medical Physics Publishing, 2009.

Van Dyk, J. (ed.). *The Modern Technology of Radiation Oncology.* Madison, WI: Medical Physics Publishing, 1999.

Williams, J. R., and D. I. Thwaites (eds.). *Radiotherapy Physics: In Practice,* Second Edition. New York: Oxford University Press USA, 2000.

9 External Beam Radiation Therapy Units

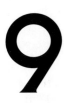

9.1 Introduction
9.2 Medical Electron Linear Accelerators
9.3 Cobalt-60 Teletherapy Units
9.4 Photon Beam Characteristics
The Invention of the Cavity Magnetron
Chapter Summary
Problems
Bibliography

9.1 Introduction

Throughout the history of radiation therapy a variety of machines have been used to produce beams of radiation. Radiation therapy delivered with an external beam is sometimes referred to as *teletherapy*. There are two major classes of external beam treatment units: those that use radioactive isotopes and those machines called accelerators, which employ electric fields to accelerate charged particles. We will confine our discussion here to megavoltage (MV) beams and therefore we will not discuss superficial or orthovoltage x-ray units in this chapter (see chapter 4). Isotope machines have used cesium-137 (Cs-137) and cobalt-60 (Co-60). Cesium is not used any more. Co-60 units have almost completely disappeared, at least in the United States. Co-60 radiation has a relatively low penetrating power and a large penumbra (see section 9.5). In addition, there are stiff regulatory requirements and fees to contend with. Specialized external beam units such as robotic linacs, tomotherapy units, and gamma stereotactic units are discussed in chapter 20. Quality assurance tests for linear accelerators are discussed in chapter 18.

There are two main types of accelerators those that accelerate charged particles in a straight line, called *linear accelerators* (see Figure 9.1), and those that accelerate them in a circular or approximately circular fashion. There are a variety of circular machines: microtrons, cyclotrons, synchrotrons, and betatrons. Circular accelerators for radiation therapy are found in only a handful of centers. Cyclotrons and synchrotrons are discussed in chapter 20 in the context of proton therapy.

An electron linear accelerator (sometimes called a *linac*) accelerates electrons along the length of an evacuated tube (called a *waveguide*) to almost the speed of light. As an example of this, if the electrons are accelerated through the equivalent of 20 million volts (20 MV), at the end of the tube they will travel at a speed that is within 0.03% of the speed of light! The electrons are accelerated by microwaves that travel down the tube. Microwaves are electromagnetic waves, and it is the electric field associated with these waves that accelerates the electrons (see section 2.4).

The electron beam can be used directly to treat patients or it can be aimed at a metallic "target" (see Figure 9.2). The target absorbs the energy of the electrons and converts some of it to very energetic, highly penetrating x-rays via the bremsstrahlung process discussed in chapter 5. The radiation passes through field-defining jaws in the "collimator" which determine the cross-sectional size of the beam (see Figure 9.2). Modern linacs allow selection between two photon beam energies and five or six electron beam energies.

The major components of the treatment machine are the gantry, the gantry stand, the treatment couch, and the treatment console. The console is outside the treatment room and is used to control the machine during the time that the beam is on. The gantry and the couch can move in numerous directions, allowing radiation beams to enter a patient from almost any angle (see Figure 9.1). The gantry can rotate around the patient. The rotation axes of the gantry, the collimator (same as beam central axis), and the couch meet at a common point in space called the *isocenter*.

Digital position indicators (Figure 9.1) show the gantry and collimator angle as well as the collimator jaw settings. The round board on which these numbers are displayed is sometimes called the "pizza" board.

The source-to-axis distance, or SAD, is the distance from the source of radiation to the isocenter. In all modern linacs this distance is 100 cm. In some older linear accelerators, notably the Clinac 4 (Varian Medical Systems, Palo Alto, CA), and in many Co-60 units, the SAD is 80 cm. The SAD of a particular linac always remains the same; it is not adjustable.

The couch top has a portion that has thin Mylar® (a type of plastic) covering a web of nylon or a carbon fiber mesh for patient support. This mesh is sometimes referred to as the "tennis racket" because of its

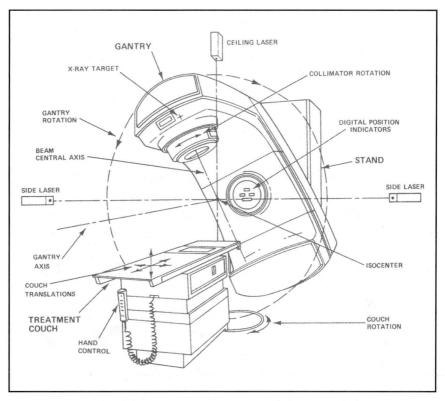

Figure 9.1: The major parts of a medical linear accelerator are the gantry, the gantry stand, and the couch. This diagram illustrates the large variety of mechanical motions possible. Motion is controlled by use of the hand control, which is sometimes called a pendant. The radiation beam is directed along the beam central axis. The gantry can rotate around an axis (labeled gantry axis) that extends out of the page, thus allowing rotation around the patient on the couch. The collimator can rotate around the beam central axis. The treatment couch or table can move up or down, in or out toward the gantry (longitudinal motion) or from side to side (lateral motion). The couch can also rotate around a vertical axis. The axes of rotation of the couch, the gantry, and the beam central axis meet at a point in space called the isocenter. Lasers are used for patient positioning. (Reprinted from Karzmark, C. J., and R. Morton, *A Primer on the Theory and Operation of Linear Accelerators in Radiation Therapy,* Fig. 2. © 1989, with permission.)

resemblance to the same. When the gantry head is underneath the table, it is possible to treat through the Mylar portion of the table.

There is extensive safety circuitry to insure that a linac is not run in a dangerous configuration. If the status of the linac is not safe for the machine settings, then an "interlock" will prevent the beam from turning on.

Figure 9.3 shows a so-called SAD patient treatment. The isocenter is positioned at or near the center of the patient's tumor. With this arrangement the beam is always pointed directly at the tumor for all gantry angles. For a given gantry angle, the distance from the radiation source to the patient skin surface is called the source-to-surface distance, or SSD. The SSD will change when the gantry is rotated to a new angle.

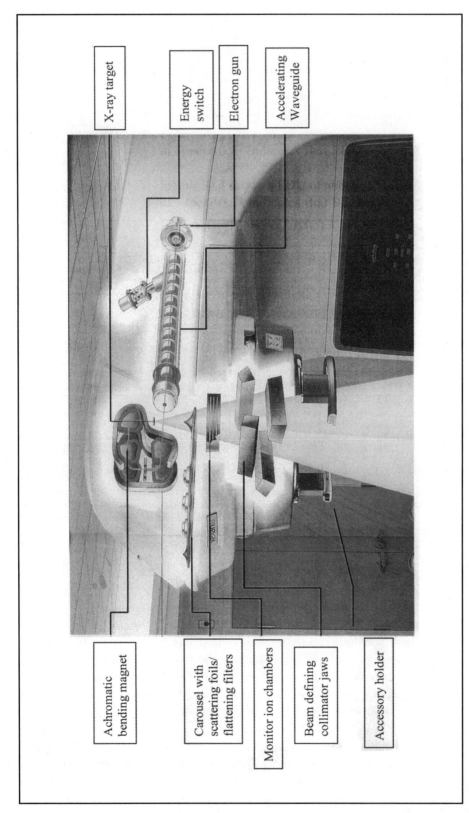

Figure 9.2: The waveguide and the treatment head of a modern dual photon energy linear accelerator. Electrons injected by the electron gun are accelerated down the waveguide. An electromagnet at the end of the waveguide deflects the electron beam downward so that it strikes the x-ray target. The collimator jaws define the cross-sectional size of the beam. Beam "modifiers" can be inserted into the accessory holder. Lead plates that are used to shield against stray "leakage" radiation are not shown. (Copyright © 2010, Varian Medical Systems, Inc. All rights reserved.)

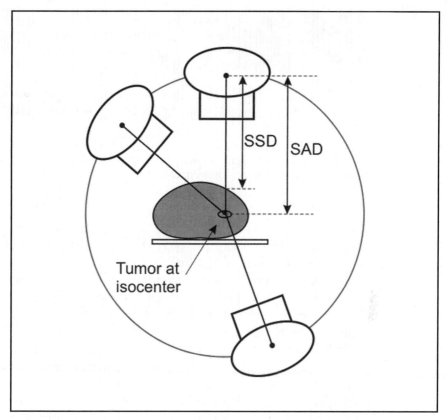

Figure 9.3: Gantry rotation around the patient. Patients are often positioned so that the isocenter is at or near the center of the volume to be treated. This is called an SAD treatment. As the gantry rotates, the beam always points at the isocenter. It is possible to treat through the table. The SSD is the distance from the source to the patient surface. The SSD changes with changing gantry angle.

9.2 Medical Electron Linear Accelerators

Medical electron linear accelerators were first introduced in Britain in the 1950s. They were introduced into the United States in the 1960s and widespread use began in the 1970s. They have almost completely replaced every other type of external beam treatment machine. There are now only three manufacturers of medical electron linear accelerators: Varian, Siemens, and Elekta (formerly Philips). (See Figure 9.4.)

To obtain the benefits of deeply penetrating radiation and skin sparing, megavoltage photons are required. Such photons can be produced by accelerating electrons to high energy and directing them against a metallic target. As the electrons lose energy in the target, they produce x-rays (as well as heat) via the bremsstrahlung mechanism. For some types of therapeutic treatment it is desirable to use the high-energy electron beam directly. In this case, the metal target is removed and the electron beam is allowed to enter the patient.

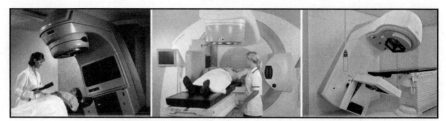

Figure 9.4: Varian, Elekta, and Siemens linear accelerators (from left to right). Notice that the Elekta machine does not have a gantry stand. (Left: Copyright © 2010, Varian Medical Systems, Inc. All rights reserved; middle: courtesy of Elekta, Norcross, GA; right: courtesy of Siemens Medical Solutions USA, Inc., Concord, CA)

When electrons are accelerated through a potential difference V they acquire a kinetic energy $T = Q\,V$ (this was discussed in chapter 2). If electrons are accelerated through a potential difference of 1 million volts, they will acquire a kinetic energy of 1 MeV. As an electron penetrates the x-ray target, it undergoes bremsstrahlung interactions in which photons are radiated. The electrons lose an amount of energy equal to the energy of the photon produced. Generally, an electron will only lose a fraction of its kinetic energy in any single interaction. The photons that emerge from the target will therefore have a range of energies from close to zero up to a maximum value that is equal to the initial kinetic energy of the electron. As an example, if the electrons are accelerated to an energy of 6 MeV, the *maximum* photon energy produced in the target will be 6 MeV. The photons will have a broad range of energies from 0 to 6 MeV. It is therefore not correct to refer to the emerging x-ray beam as a 6 MeV beam. In fact the average energy of the photons in such a beam is approximately 6/3 MeV = 2 MeV. The nomenclature that is used to refer to such a beam is based on the fact that the electrons were effectively accelerated through a potential difference of 6 million volts or 6 MV. The proper way to refer to the "quality" or energy of this x-ray beam is to describe it as a 6 MV beam. The average energy of the photons in a linear accelerator beam in MeV is (very roughly) numerically equal to MV/3. The electron beam itself is nearly monoenergetic with an energy of 6 MeV. It is therefore correct to refer to the electron beam as a 6 MeV beam.

Common x-ray beam energies for medical linear accelerators range from 4 MV to 18 MV. Most linacs have dual photon energies; 6 MV and 15 MV or 6 MV and 18 MV are common. Three photon energies are possible on traveling wave linacs. Linacs also have multiple electron energies ranging from as low as 4 MeV up to 22 MeV. A modern dual-energy linac costs between $1.5 and $3.0 million depending on options. These options include a multileaf collimator (MLC), an electronic portal imaging device (EPID). and a cone beam kVp imager. These options will be discussed in later chapters.

You may wonder: why not just make an x-ray tube and place millions of volts across the electrodes (Figure 9.5)? It is difficult to produce such high voltages directly. An attempt to do so will result in arcing (sparks). It can be done up to a point, but it is unwieldy and expensive. Therefore, other more indirect methods are used. These indirect methods were developed after World War II for research in high-energy elementary particle physics and later adapted to medical use.

The accelerator waveguide is a highly evacuated copper "pipe" in which electrons are accelerated. They are one of the most expensive components of a linear accelerator. Replacement cost is in excess of $100,000. There are two major types of accelerating waveguides: (1) traveling wave and (2) standing wave. Both of these designs use electromagnetic waves to accelerate electrons. These waves are in the microwave region of the spectrum, $\nu \approx 3000$ MHz (S-band radar) for conventional medical linacs ($\lambda = 10$ cm in free space). In both designs, electrons are accelerated in bunches and therefore the radiation output is pulsed. The pipe must be under high vacuum so that the electrons do not collide with air molecules and lose energy.

In a traveling wave linac, the electrons "surf" on a traveling electromagnetic wave (see Figure 9.6). There is a problem with this however: the electrons must travel at the same speed as the electromagnetic wave to "surf" along. In free space, electromagnetic waves travel at speed c; electrons are prohibited from traveling at this speed by the special theory of relativity. To avoid this problem, the electromagnetic wave is sent down a "disk loaded" copper tube or pipe called a *waveguide* (see Figure 9.7). Electrons travel in bunches down the waveguide; disks in

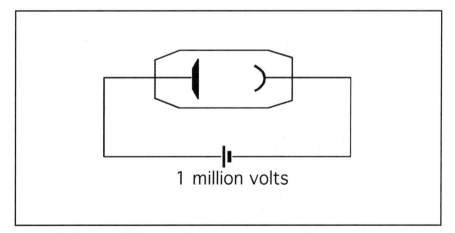

1 million volts

Figure 9.5: An x-ray tube with a potential difference of 1 million volts between the anode and the cathode. This method of producing high-energy x-rays is not practical for reasons explained in the text.

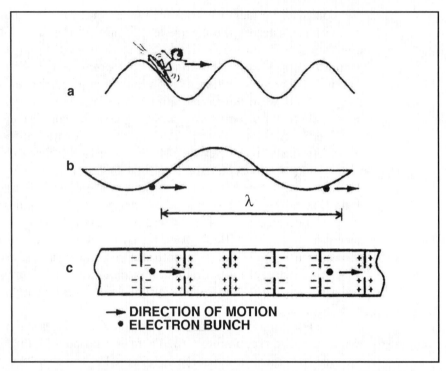

Figure 9.6: Traveling wave acceleration. In (a) a surfer is pushed along by a wave. In a similar way, electron bunches (b) are pushed along by an electromagnetic wave in a traveling wave accelerator waveguide. A snapshot of a waveguide is shown in (c) illustrating the charge distribution inside the waveguide at that instant which accelerates the electron bunches shown toward the right. (Reprinted from Karzmark, C. J., and R. Morton, *A Primer on the Theory and Operation of Linear Accelerators in Radiation Therapy,* Fig. 28. © 1989, with permission.)

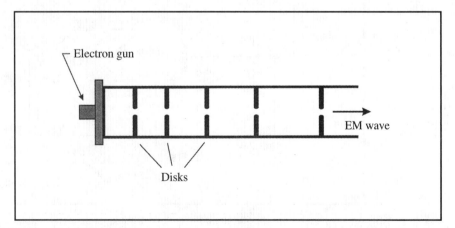

Figure 9.7: An accelerating waveguide for a linear accelerator. The waveguide is disk loaded to slow down the microwave electromagnetic waves so that bunches of electrons may "surf" on these waves down the guide from left to right.

the guide slow down the electromagnetic wave. Toward the end of the waveguide, the disks are spaced farther and farther apart and they have larger openings. The effect of this is to increase the speed of the electromagnetic traveling wave. If this is done in just the right way, the electron bunches will be able to continue to surf on the wave as they speed up and, in this manner, they will gain energy.

The other major type of linear accelerator is the standing wave linac. You can produce standing waves on a string by tying it to a nail on a wall, pulling the string taut, and then plucking it. Such waves are produced in the strings of musical instruments. A standing wave is formed when a traveling wave moving down the string arrives at the wall and is then reflected back. This leads to two traveling waves moving in opposite directions. The two traveling waves add to produce a standing wave. Standing waves are illustrated in Figure 9.8.

How can a standing wave accelerate electrons? The electrons cannot surf along the wave. The acceleration process is illustrated in Figure 9.9, which shows snapshots of a standing wave at three instants in time. This figure shows a graph of the electric field as a function of position at the three instants in time. The electric field is proportional to the height of the graph above the horizontal axis. If the force on electron bunches due to this electric field always acts in the same direction, then the electrons will gain kinetic energy as they move down the waveguide. In the first instant shown, let us suppose that the force on the electron bunch is toward the right. In the middle instant, the electric field has momentarily become zero. There is no force on the electron bunch, but it will

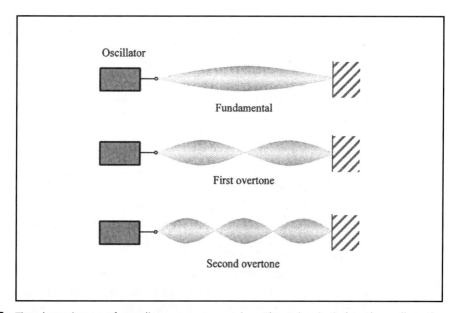

Figure 9.8: Time-lapse image of standing waves on a string. The string is tied to the wall on the right. The "fundamental" is shown at the top. Increasing the frequency of the oscillator produces successive overtones.

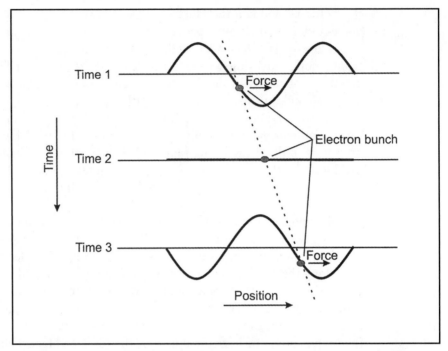

Figure 9.9: An electron bunch undergoing acceleration by a standing wave in a waveguide. This shows three different instants in time starting at the top. At Time 2 the electric field is momentarily zero; it then reverses at the bottom. The height of the wave represents the strength of the electric field. As the electric field oscillates in strength, the electron bunch will experience a force that is constantly toward the right.

continue to move toward the right owing to its velocity in that direction. In the third frame the electric field has returned, and in the meantime the electrons have moved to a new position; however the electrons are in the same relative position with respect to the wave as they were in the first instant and therefore they again experience a force toward the right. If the electron bunch can maintain its *relative* position with respect to the standing wave, it will always be accelerated forward.

In a standing wave accelerator, the microwave power is introduced through the side of the waveguide (see Figure 9.10). Standing wave linacs require a device called a *circulator,* which prevents microwaves from reflecting back into the klystron (discussed later in this chapter). Traveling wave linacs require a "terminating" or "dummy" load to absorb the backward-reflected wave to prevent a standing wave from forming. In a standing wave linac, every other waveguide cavity can be moved off to the side, as shown in Figure 9.10. This is called *side cavity coupling.* It reduces the length of the waveguide by almost a factor of 2, a big advantage. The electrons gain roughly 2 MeV energy per cavity.

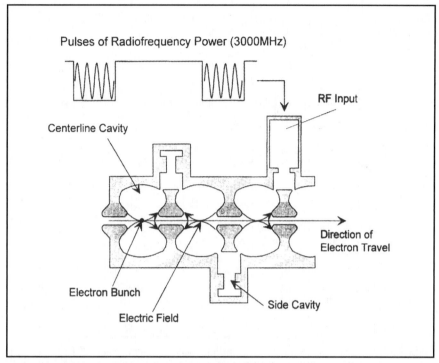

Figure 9.10: A cross-sectional view of a side-coupled standing wave accelerating waveguide. The length of the waveguide is reduced by a factor of 2 by introducing side cavities. The microwave radiofrequency (RF) power is fed into the waveguide through the RF input. Is the electric field in the correct direction? (Courtesy of Siemens Medical Solutions USA, Inc., Concord, CA)

Among the three major manufacturers, Varian and Siemens machines are standing wave linacs; Elekta uses a traveling wave.

The orientation of the accelerating waveguide in a standing wave linac depends on the design energy. This is illustrated in Figure 9.11. For low single-energy linacs, in the range 4 to 6 MV, the waveguide is short enough (perhaps 30 cm) so that it can be oriented vertically. For intermediate energy, in the range 6 to 25 MV, the waveguide is too long to orient vertically. Instead, the waveguide is oriented horizontally and a "bending magnet" is employed to "bend" or deflect the electron beam in a downward direction toward the patient. In the highest energy standing wave waveguides (25 to 35 MeV) or in traveling wave waveguides, the guide may need to be oblique. A dual-energy traveling wave waveguide is about 2.5 m in length. Dual-energy standing wave waveguides are approximately 1.3 m in length. A long waveguide could be oriented vertically, but this would require both a tall ceiling and a pit in the floor so that the gantry could rotate underneath the patient couch.

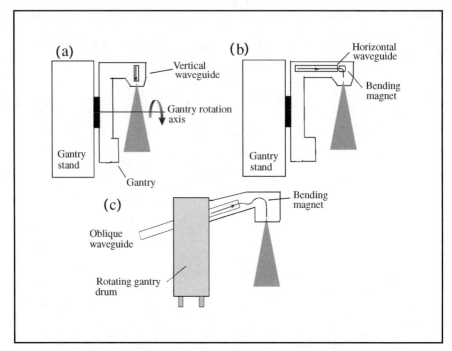

Figure 9.11: Orientation of the accelerating waveguide in linacs of different types. In low single-energy machines (4–6 MV), the waveguide is short enough that it can be mounted vertically as in (a). In higher-energy machines, the waveguide is too long to be mounted vertically and instead is mounted horizontally. This requires a bending magnet to redirect the beam down toward the patient. The addition of the bending magnet makes the linac considerably more complex. Most modern, dual-energy linacs are oriented as in (b). Traveling wave linacs and the highest energy standing wave linacs require an oblique waveguide as in (c).

9.2.1 Source of Microwave Power

Linear accelerators require high-power microwaves to accelerate electrons down the waveguide. There are two different devices that can supply the necessary power: magnetrons and klystrons.

A magnetron generates high-power microwaves (see Figure 9.12). You may even own one without realizing it. A magnetron supplies the microwaves for your microwave oven. Your home oven operates at a frequency of 2450 MHz and is capable of producing about 1 kW of power. By comparison, the magnetron in a linac produces pulses of microwaves with a frequency of approximately 3000 MHz and peak power of about 2.5 to 5.0 MW. This is why a magnetron for a linac costs about $30,000. The magnetron was invented during World War II and it is widely used for radar applications (see the box at the end of this chapter entitled "The Invention of the Cavity Magnetron"). The lifetime of a magnetron is about 2000 hours of operation (perhaps 2 to 4 years).

In a magnetron, electrons move past a cavity (see Figure 9.13) that has a resonant or natural frequency in the microwave part of the

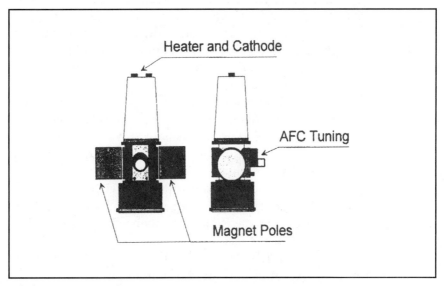

Figure 9.12: A drawing showing two views of the external appearance of a magnetron. The magnets supply the magnetic field in which the electrons spiral. The AFC (automatic frequency control) plunger continually adjusts the frequency of the microwaves to maintain optimum accelerating conditions for the waveguide. (Courtesy of Siemens Medical Solutions USA, Inc., Concord, CA)

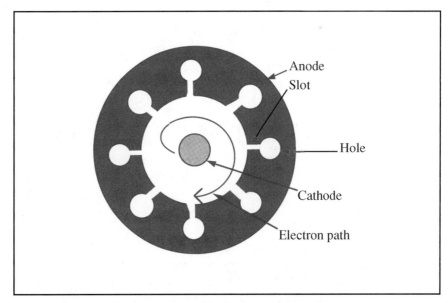

Figure 9.13: A cross section through a magnetron illustrating the principle of operation. Electrons emitted by the cathode spiral toward the anode in a magnetic field that is perpendicular to the page. As the electrons pass the cavities consisting of the holes and the slots, they induce oscillations at microwave frequencies. This is analogous to the sound waves that are produced by blowing air across the top of a soda bottle. (Adapted from Stanton, R., and D. Stinson, *Applied Physics for Radiation Oncology, Revised Edition,* Fig. 9.6, p. 110, © 2009, with permission.)

spectrum. The electrons induce electromagnetic oscillations in the cavity. This is somewhat like blowing air over the top of a soda bottle to produce a loud sound. If conditions are right, the airflow over the top of the bottle induces oscillations of the air inside the bottle, producing a loud sound.

While a magnetron generates high-power microwaves, a klystron amplifies them. Today, klystrons are capable of producing higher power levels than magnetrons: up to about 8 MW peak power. Magnetrons are used in low-energy standing wave linacs and in traveling wave linacs. Klystrons are used in standing wave linacs with energies above about 12 MV. Linear accelerators with klystrons (see Figure 9.14) require a low-energy source of microwaves called an "RF driver." The output pulse power from the RF driver only needs to be about 100 W. Klystrons are bulkier than magnetrons and they sit inside a tank of insulating oil (see Figure 9.15). This precludes gantry mounting and therefore the microwave power must be transmitted farther to reach the accelerating waveguide. Klystrons are sometimes mounted in separate cabinets. The

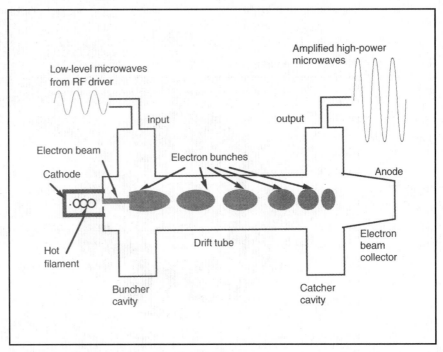

Figure 9.14: The operation of a klystron. Electrons are injected by the cathode into the drift tube and they are accelerated toward the anode at the other end. Low-energy microwaves from the RF driver cause the electrons to break up into bunches. The electron bunches move past the catcher cavity and induce high-power microwave oscillations. (Reprinted from Stanton, R., and D. Stinson, *Applied Physics for Radiation Oncology, Revised Edition,* Fig. 9.7, p. 110, © 2009, with permission.)

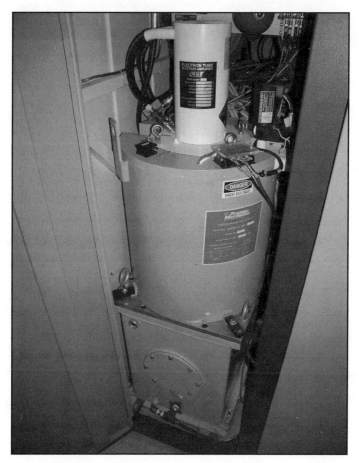

Figure 9.15: A klystron inside the gantry stand of a high-energy standing wave linac. The tank of insulating oil can be seen at the bottom.

microwaves are sent via a transmission waveguide to the gantry stand. A klystron costs about $70,000, considerably more than a magnetron. The operating lifetime of a klystron is about 4 to 7 years.

Let us now consider the entire operation of a linear accelerator as a system. This is illustrated in the block diagram of Figure 9.16. Microwave power is supplied to the accelerating waveguide in short (5 μs) pulses. A power supply furnishes high power DC to the modulator. The modulator contains the so-called "pulse forming network" (pfn). The high-power pulses are delivered simultaneously to the klystron (or magnetron) and the electron gun. The pulses are triggered by a vacuum tube called a *thyratron* that acts as a switch and is capable of handling the high currents. The electron gun injects a pulse of electrons into the accelerating waveguide. The

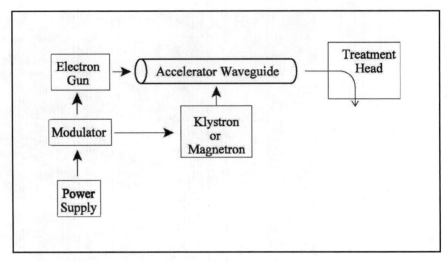

Figure 9.16: A block diagram showing the major components of a linear accelerator.

electrons are accelerated down the waveguide and emerge as a narrow beam about 3 mm in diameter.

In standing wave linacs, the photon beam energy can be changed with the use of an energy switch (see Figure 9.2). The switch essentially shuts off part of the waveguide so that electrons are not accelerated in that part of the guide. For the high-energy photon beam, the entire guide is used to accelerate electrons. In a traveling wave linac, the radiofrequency (RF) power delivered to the guide is changed to change the beam energy.

9.2.2 The Treatment Head

Inside the cover of the treatment head of a linear accelerator is a thick shell of shielding material (not shown in Figure 9.2) so that radiation cannot escape the head (head leakage). We only want radiation to emerge from the machine as part of the useful beam. Radiation escaping from the head contributes dose to the entire body of the patient, and it requires thicker walls to shield personnel outside the room. Head leakage will be discussed further in chapter 17 on radiation protection. There are seven major components inside the head (the first five of these are shown in Figure 9.17 and the last two in Figure 9.20):

    (1) x-ray target; used for photon beams only
    (2) scattering foils; used for electron beams only
    (3) flattening filter; used in x-ray mode only
    (4) monitor ion chambers
    (5) fixed (primary) and movable (adjustable) collimators
    (6) light localizing system (or field defining light)
    (7) optical distance indicator (ODI) or rangefinder.

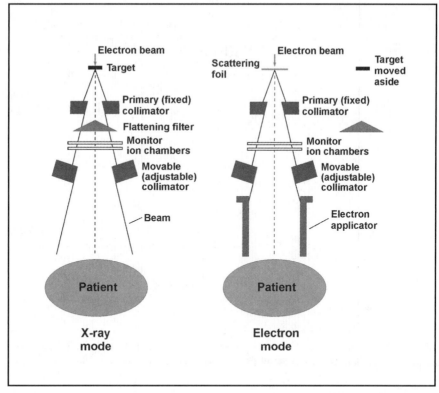

Figure 9.17: Schematic diagram of the components of a linear accelerator treatment head. The two major modes of operation are illustrated; x-ray mode on the left and electron mode on the right. In x-ray mode, a metallic target is placed in the electron beam. In electron mode, the target and flattening filter are moved aside and a scattering foil is placed in the beam to spread out the narrow incident electron beam.

X-Ray Mode

In X-ray mode a target is placed in front of the narrow electron beam. The electrons enter the target and their energy is converted via the bremsstrahlung mechanism into x-rays. Linear accelerators use transmission targets, unlike a diagnostic or superficial therapy x-ray tube (see Figure 9.18). The target is often made out of a high-Z material and it must be water-cooled; otherwise it would quickly melt. Bremsstrahlung x-ray production is strongly peaked in the forward direction at high energies (see Figure 5.11). As a result of this, the radiation intensity emitted by the target is not uniform across the beam. To make the radiation field have uniform intensity, a flattening filter is placed in the beam, which is thicker in the middle (and thus attenuates more) than at the edges. If the flattening filter is designed correctly, the radiation field will be of uniform intensity across the beam (see section 9.4 for a discussion of beam flatness). Flattening filters are made of a high-Z material. If the flattening filter is not precisely positioned, the beam will not be flat or symmetric (see section 9.4).

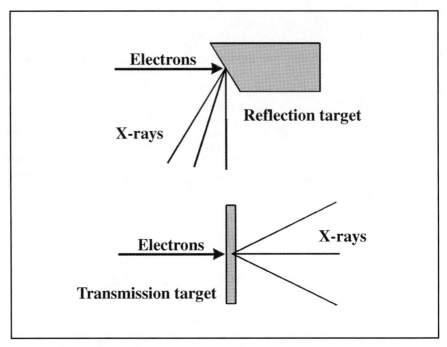

Figure 9.18: Linear accelerators use a transmission target rather than a reflection target like those used for low-energy x-ray production.

The dose delivered to a given location in a patient by a treatment machine depends on: the depth in the patient, the beam energy, the collimator jaw setting, the distance of the patient from the source of radiation, etc. It is therefore not possible to set a treatment machine directly for dose. For a Co-60 unit the beam "time on" is set. A different arrangement is called for in the case of a linac. The intensity of a linac beam may fluctuate slightly from moment to moment and therefore we cannot set the beam time on for a linac. Instead we set *monitor units,* or *MU*. The number of monitor units is a measure of the cumulative amount of radiation passing through the head of the linac. It is part of the treatment planning process to determine, for a particular patient, the relationship between the time on (for a Co-60 unit) or the MU (for a linac) and the desired dose to be given to the patient.

The monitor ion chambers shown in Figure 9.17 and Figure 9.2 serve three purposes. They provide feedback to enable the accelerator to maintain a constant dose rate. Typical "dose" rates range between 200 and 600 MU/min. On some linacs the dose rate can be selected. The ion chambers also track the total or integrated dose; that is, the total MU delivered. This is related to the total amount of radiation passing through them. There are two sets of ion chambers that monitor this. The second is a backup. The output from the backup is sometimes referred to as MU2, and the primary is MU1. A safety interlock will shut off the beam if MU2 exceeds MU1 by a certain amount (typically 10%). If MU1 and

MU2 both fail to shut off the beam, then a backup timer will do so. This timer will shut off the machine after a certain period of time. If there is a power failure, a backup counter keeps track of the number of MU actually delivered. The third purpose that the ion chambers serve is to monitor beam flatness and symmetry (see section 9.4). If the beam flatness or symmetry departs from expectation by more than a specified amount, then an interlock shuts off the beam. Some monitor chambers are unsealed. In this case, transducers in the treatment head must measure the atmospheric pressure and the ambient temperature and apply a correction to the output from the chamber (see section 8.3.3). Sealed chambers require no correction. If a sealed chamber should develop a leak however, the output from the linac may become erratic.

The movable or secondary collimator jaws produce rectangular field sizes ranging from 0×0 cm^2 to 40×40 cm^2 defined at the SAD (usually 100 cm). These jaws are usually made of tungsten. Modern linacs have asymmetric jaw capability (see Figures 9.17 and 9.19). The amount of radiation transmitted through these jaws is typically 0.5% or less.

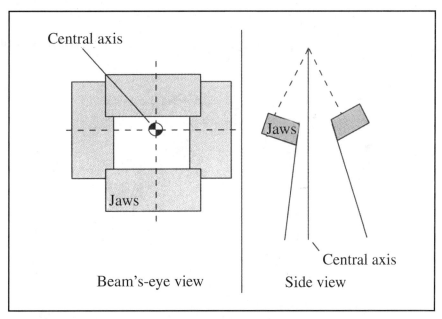

Figure 9.19: A "beam's-eye" view and a side view of a radiation field established by dual asymmetric jaws. Each of the four field edges is defined by movable jaws that can move independently of each another.

The light localizing system (also called the "field defining light," see Figure 9.20) projects a light field down onto the patient that is congruent with the radiation field. The total path length for the light field is the same as for the radiation field and therefore the divergence is also the same. The light localizing system shows where the radiation is going to go. The light localizing system must be checked periodically to ensure that the light field is congruent with the radiation field (see chapter 18 for further discussion). If the light field and radiation field are not congruent, the tilt of the reflecting mirror (not labeled in Figure 9.20) can be adjusted to shift the light field, or the light source can be moved to change the size of the light field. Figure 9.20 also shows the optical distance indicator (ODI), which is sometimes called the "range finder." The ODI projects a scale down onto the patient surface, which indicates the value of the SSD.

In chapter 13 we will discuss multileaf collimators (MLCs). An MLC is used to shape the beam cross section so that it corresponds to the projected view of the target to be treated. In chapter 19 we shall

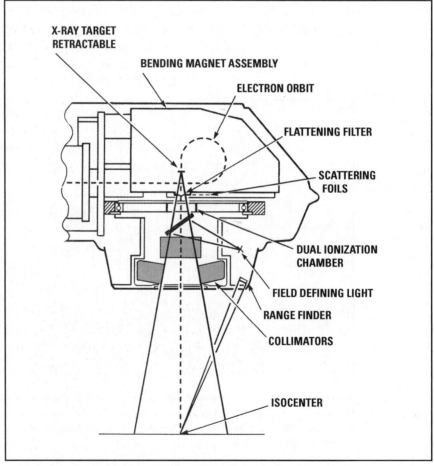

Figure 9.20: The head of a linear accelerator showing the field-defining light. The light source is off to the side of the beam and projects up to a mirror that reflects it downward. The total light path length is the same as for the radiation, and therefore the divergence is the same. The optical distance indicator (ODI) or range finder is also shown. The ODI projects a scale downward onto the surface below. The projected scale indicates the distance of the surface from the source of the radiation. This is called the source-to-surface distance (SSD). (Adapted from Karzmark, C. J., and R. Morton, *A Primer on the Theory and Operation of Linear Accelerators in Radiation Therapy,* Fig. 38. © 1989, with permission.)

discuss electronic portal imaging devices (EPIDs), which are used to verify targeting of the radiation beam.

Electron Therapy Mode

When a linac is run in electron therapy mode, the target and the flattening filter must be moved out of the way (see Figure 9.17). The flattening filter is sometimes moved with the use of a carousel or "Lazy Susan" type of arrangement (see Figure 9.2). The "raw" electron beam cannot be used to treat a patient because it is a very narrow beam of only about 3 mm in diameter.[1] The use of a scattering foil (or multiple foils) is the most common method of spreading the beam. A scattering foil is a thin foil made of a high Z material (copper or lead) that easily scatters electrons. This spreads out the beam. The foil should be just thick enough to spread out the beam but not so thick as to cause significant bremsstrahlung production, which would contaminate the electron beam with x-rays (see chapter 15 on electron beams).

Electrons are easily scattered even by air. To prevent the electrons from straying outside the desired field, the electron beam must be collimated all the way down to the skin surface or as closely as possible. This is accomplished with the use of an electron applicator (sometimes called an "electron cone," see Figures 9.17 and 9.21). Without the applicator, electrons would scatter out of the beam and the beam would not

---

[1] The raw electron beam would tend to drill holes in patients.

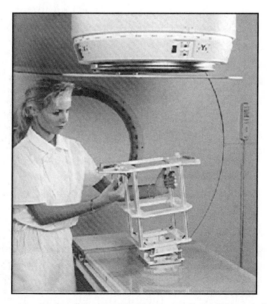

Figure 9.21: A therapist prepares to attach an electron applicator to the collimator of a linac. (Courtesy of Elekta, Norcross, GA)

be flat (see section 9.4) An interlock prevents the linac from running in electron mode unless an applicator is inserted in the collimator by the operator. Applicators come in a variety of field sizes: 10×10 cm^2, 15×15 cm^2 (14×14 cm^2 for Elekta), 20×20 cm^2 and 25×25 cm^2 are common. Smaller cones having a circular aperture of about 5 cm diameter are also common. When an electron cone is inserted, the adjustable collimator jaws must be set to a specific field size that is larger than the cone aperture. This field size may depend on the electron beam energy. For some linacs the jaws are automatically set to the correct value; in older linacs, the jaws must be set manually. An interlock prevents operation with an incorrect setting. If the jaws were set incorrectly, the radiation output would be incorrect and the radiation beam might not be flat.

When the linac is in x-ray mode, the electron beam current inside the waveguide is up to 1000 times higher than when the linac is running in electron mode. If the linac is run in a configuration in which the beam current is this high but there is no target or flattening filter in the beam, then the rate of beam delivery will be several hundred thousand MU per minute. This may be fatal to the patient (see chapter 18, section 18.7 on radiation therapy accidents). A dose rate interlock prevents this.

Bending Magnets

The bending electromagnet in a linac must change the direction of the electron beam from horizontal to vertical (see Figure 2.11). The bending magnet is made from coils of wire, which must be supplied with a high current to produce the magnetic field necessary to deflect the electron beam. Some linacs use an "achromatic" bending magnet that deflects the electron beam through 270° rather than 90° (see Figures 9.2 and 9.22). When the electrons enter the region between the bending magnet poles, they have a small spread in energy. If a 90° bending magnet were used, the paths of electrons with slightly different energies would diverge. A 270° bending magnet causes all the electrons with various energies to converge at the focal spot. This is the arrangement employed in Varian and Siemens linacs; Elekta machines use a more elaborate "slalom" design. When the selection of the beam energy is changed, the bending magnet current must change—this takes a short while.

9.2.3   Linear Accelerator Auxiliary Subsystems

Linear accelerators are complex machines with a variety of subsystems necessary to make all of the major components operate. They have a vacuum system, a water-cooling system, a dielectric gas system, and some have a compressed air system.

The klystron, the electron gun, and the accelerating waveguide need to operate under a high vacuum. The high vacuum serves two purposes.

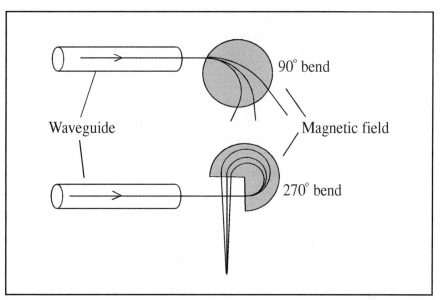

Figure 9.22: The magnetic field is confined to the shaded area. Electrons emerge from the accelerating waveguide with a slight distribution in energy. If a 90° bending magnet is used, the electrons will be spread out by the magnetic field. The path of more energetic electrons will bend less than those with lower energy. By using a 270° bending magnet, all the electrons can be made to come together at the target. An actual achromatic bending magnet system is somewhat more complicated than this. Elekta linacs use a slalom bending magnet system that is different from the design shown here.

It prevents arcing and it prevents collisions between the accelerated electrons and air molecules, which would scatter and decelerate the electrons. A special type of vacuum pump called a "vacuum ion pump" or "vacion pump" is used to provide the necessary high vacuum.

Linacs are not usually completely powered down at the end of a treatment day. Instead, they are put into "standby" mode. In standby mode some of the subsystems, such as the vacuum system, continue to operate. If a linac were to lose part of its vacuum, it might take an excessively long time to reestablish a sufficient vacuum to produce a beam.

Circulating cooling water is necessary for two purposes. The first of these is the obvious one: to carry excess heat away from critical components such as the accelerator waveguide, the microwave power source, the x-ray target, and the bending electromagnet. High-energy microwaves heat the accelerating waveguide. The target is heated by the electron beam, which strikes it. The bending magnet is heated by the high electrical currents that travel through the wire coils. The second function of the cooling system is to keep the accelerating waveguide at a nearly constant temperature (usually 40±5 °C). This is necessary because the propagation properties of microwaves in the accelerating waveguide are exquisitely sensitive to the dimensions of the copper waveguide, and these dimensions are affected by the temperature of the metal.

The water-cooling system employs a heat exchanger. The water that is used internally to cool the parts of the linac directly is in a closed-loop system. The external cooling water is either brought in directly from the municipal water supply or from a device that first cools it called a "chiller." The temperature and the flow rate of the external cooling water must meet certain requirements in order to provide adequate cooling. The internal water enters the heat exchanger, which has a radiator-like structure (designed for maximum heat exchange) immersed in a tank of external cooling water to allow for maximum heat exchange with the hot internal water. The internal cooling water is distilled water. The water level should be checked daily, and distilled water should be added when necessary. There is a demineralizing cartridge in the system to absorb minerals picked up by the internal cooling water. This cartridge needs to be changed from time to time.

Some linacs require a supply of compressed air. Most hospitals have a hospitalwide system of compressed air, and if not, a small compressor can be used. Compressed air is sometimes used to move the target out of the beam (the default position is target in), to operate the energy switch, and to operate the locking pin on the carrousel. A pressure of 45 to 50 psi (pounds per square inch) is common.

Transmission waveguides carry the microwaves from their source (magnetron or klystron) to the accelerating waveguide. These are usually large copper "pipes" of rectangular cross section. The electric field strengths associated with the microwaves are very high and they would cause arcing in air at normal atmospheric pressure. This is the reason that you are warned against putting any metallic objects in your microwave oven because dramatic arcing can occur. To prevent arcing, the transmission waveguide is filled with a pressurized non-conducting (dielectric) gas. The gas used for this purpose is sulfur hexafluoride (SF_6). A nonconducting window (ceramic or quartz) is used where the transmission waveguide joins the accelerating waveguide. This window permits microwave passage but does not allow the SF_6 to enter the accelerating waveguide. There is usually a tank of SF_6 inside the gantry stand with a regulator. As the SF_6 slowly leaks out of the transmission waveguide, it can be replenished from the tank (the required pressure is 25 to 32 psi, or about 2 atmospheres for Varian machines and 0.8 atmosphere for Elekta).

9.2.4 Interlocks and Safety Systems

Medical linear accelerators have an interlock system that prevents or terminates operation under unsafe conditions. Interlocks are intended to safeguard the staff, the patient, and the machine from potential harm. Safety interlocks are designed to protect patients and staff from mechanical, electrical and radiation hazards. Interlock conditions appear on the machine console.

Machine interlocks are designed to protect the machine from operation under conditions which may cause it damage. After the machine is turned on, it must be warmed up before it can produce a beam. The cathodes of the thyratron and the klystron (or magnetron) require a heating period of 5 to 15 min to come up to operating temperature. Operation under cold conditions could cause very expensive damage to one of these components. This is why linacs have a warmup timer and cannot be run until warmup is complete. Any attempt to bypass this is asking for costly trouble. There are interlocks for the vacuum system, cooling water flow and temperature, bending magnet current, and SF_6 pressure. There are limit switches that prevent mechanical movement beyond the design limits. These apply to collimator rotation, gantry rotation, and couch vertical motion.

The door interlock is designed to safeguard the staff. If the door to the treatment room is not closed, the beam cannot be turned on. If the beam is on and the door is opened, the beam will be automatically shut off. The door interlock is usually set up as a double interlock: two separate and independent switches must be closed for the beam to come on and to remain on.

There are a variety of safety systems and interlocks to protect patients from harm and to ensure that they receive the intended treatment. In the United States many states require an audiovisual system. A closed-circuit TV system is used so that the patient can be viewed at all times. There is also a two-way intercom system. There are emergency off buttons on the console and the treatment couch, and there may be others that are wall mounted. During beam operation, the monitor chambers check beam flatness and symmetry and inspect the dose rate. If the dose rate becomes excessive, the beam will turn off. A collision avoidance system is necessary to prevent contact between the patient and the linac head. Some linacs employ a mechanical touch guard system on the treatment head (see the ring near the top of Figure 9.21). If the head of the gantry should touch the patient, switches are activated which stop all motion. Other linacs use a laser or optical system. Electron cones also have a collision detection system built into the bottom end. This is necessary because the bottom of the cone is designed to be close to the patient. Any undue pressure on the bottom of the electron applicator causes an interlock, preventing any further motion.

There are a number of interlocks to help ensure that a patient receives the intended treatment. Beam modifying devices such as cast blocks, compensators, and wedges must be explicitly chosen when programming the treatment console. Each of these devices is coded. When these devices are inserted into the accessory holder, the machine "knows" which one is inserted. If the beam modifier chosen at the console differs from that actually inserted into the machine, an interlock will appear until the discrepancy is resolved. There are limits on the field size for many wedges. When a particular wedge is inserted into the collimator, the machine will trigger an interlock if the field size is too large for that particular wedge. There are also interlocks for electron applicators. The machine will not produce an electron beam unless an electron applicator is inserted. Electron applicators are also coded. The size of the electron applicator must be entered at the console and it must match the applicator actually mounted. The collimator jaws must be set to the correct opening for the applicator mounted and for the electron energy set.

9.2.5 Patient Support Assembly

The patient support assembly, sometimes called the "pedestal," is a fancy name for the patient couch. Important considerations for couch design are safety, accuracy, and rigidity. The couch support is offset from the isocenter so that the end of the couch can extend out over the isocenter, permitting the gantry to rotate underneath it (see Figure 9.1). The couch can move vertically, laterally (from side to side), and longitudinally (in and out). In addition, the couch can rotate about a vertical axis through the isocenter (see Figure 9.1). This is sometimes referred to as a pedestal rotation or "couch kick." Couch movement controls are found on both sides of the couch and on a pendant. Couch motion requires that a "deadman" switch be depressed while activating motion. Emergency off buttons are also located on the couch and the pendant. Couches will also operate in a free-float mode in which the operator can freely move the couch in both a lateral and a longitudinal direction to position a patient or phantom.

The couch top is constructed from carbon fiber and is light, flat, and rigid for setup reproducibility. One portion of the couch top consists of a mesh with a clear plastic placed over it. This allows for maximum radiation transmission for treatment through the couch top. A portion of the couch may have a dense spine or metal side rails. Caution must be used to ensure that radiation beams are not obstructed by these obstacles. The patient load limit ranges from 200 to 250 kg (441 to 551 lb).

9.3 Cobalt-60 Teletherapy Units

Cobalt-60 external beam treatment units were introduced in the early 1950s. These were the first practical megavoltage therapy units. They enjoyed widespread use for many years. Modern megavoltage radiotherapy was developed based on these units. They are simple and highly reliable, much more so than modern linear accelerators. They are now rare in the United States for a number of reasons. They have a larger geometric penumbra (see section 9.4) and a lower beam energy than a

linear accelerator; therefore they do not have the penetrating power of a
linac beam. They cannot produce electron beams. The dose rates for
linacs (up to 600 cGy/min in free space at 100 cm from the source) are
generally higher than for Co-60 units. Gamma stereotactic units utiliz-
ing Co-60 for the treatment of the brain continue in worldwide use.
These specialized units will be described in chapter 20.

The Co-60 is produced in a nuclear reactor via the reaction:
$^{59}_{27}\text{Co} + ^{1}_{0}\text{n} \rightarrow ^{60}_{27}\text{Co} + \gamma$. The half-life is 5.26 years. The activity declines
by approximately 1% per month. The dose rate used to calculate beam
on time for patients should be updated once per month.

 Rule of thumb: The dose rate of a Co-60 machine declines by
approximately 1% per month. (Use with caution!)

This rule of thumb must be used with caution! It can only be applied
over a period of a few months at best. As an illustration, it is clearly not
true that the dose rate delivered by a Co-60 unit declines by 50% in 50
months. When in doubt, perform a full radioactive decay calculation as
discussed in chapter 3.

The decay diagram for Co-60 is shown in Figure 9.23. The mechanism is beta decay. The daughter nucleus is left in an excited state. Two
gamma rays are emitted which are closely spaced in energy. These
gamma rays are the therapeutic radiation and their average energy is
1.25 MeV.

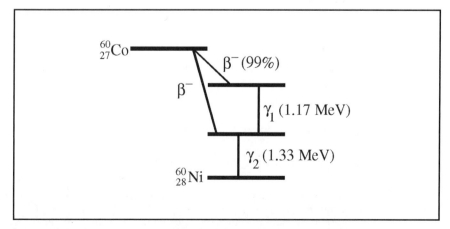

Figure 9.23: Decay diagram for Co-60. The primary β⁻ (labeled 99%) has maximum beta energy of
0.32 MeV. These betas do not escape from the source. There are two closely spaced gammas,
which are emitted. The average energy of these gammas is 1.25 MeV.

The Co-60 is packed in a doubly encapsulated stainless steel cylinder. It is in the form of a solid cylinder, pellets, or disks. Regulatory agencies are now favoring a single, solid cylinder rather than pellets because of the danger that pellets could be dispersed, forming a radiation safety hazard. The encapsulating cylinder is welded closed. There should be no leakage of material from the cylinder. The cylinders range between 1 to 2 cm in diameter. As a result of the large source size, Co-60 units have a larger geometric penumbra than a linac (see section 9.4). A new source may have an activity as high as 10^4 Ci, very high indeed! The dose rate in free space is nominally 240 cGy/min at a distance of 80 cm from such a source.

A diagram of a Co-60 unit is shown in Figure 9.24. The design shares much in common with a linear accelerator.

The SAD of most existing Co-60 units is 80 cm, although newer units are available with SAD = 100 cm, like most linacs.

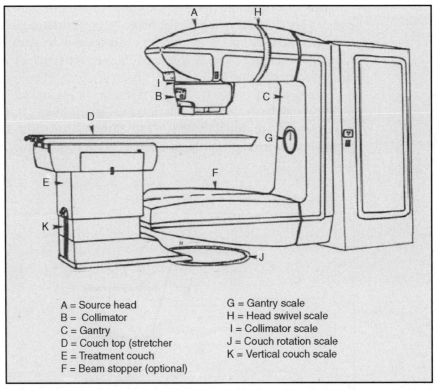

A = Source head
B = Collimator
C = Gantry
D = Couch top (stretcher
E = Treatment couch
F = Beam stopper (optional)

G = Gantry scale
H = Head swivel scale
I = Collimator scale
J = Couch rotation scale
K = Vertical couch scale

Figure 9.24: A typical Co-60 machine and treatment couch. Mechanical movement is very similar to a linear accelerator. This particular unit has a beam stopper (labeled F). A beam stopper is an option available for linacs or Co-60 units. The beam stopper prevents the primary beam from striking any of the walls of the treatment room. This reduces the amount of shielding necessary in the walls. (Reprinted from Bentel, G. C. *Radiation Therapy Planning*, Fig. 2.7, p. 32. © 1992 with permission from MacMillan McGraw-Hill.)

When the beam is off, the source is stored in a shielded part of the head of the treatment unit (see Figure 9.25). There is a mechanism that moves the source into position to turn the beam "on." This mechanism must be designed in such a way that the source will automatically retract if there is a power interruption.

For Co-60 units (and superficial and orthovoltage x-ray units) the dose to be delivered is determined by the setting of a timer. The setting of the timer may not correspond exactly to the effective "on" time of the source. The reason for this is that it takes a certain amount of time for the source to move into position when the beam is turned on and it takes a certain amount of time for the source to be retracted at the end of the treatment (see Figure 9.26).

The timer error is the time that must be added to the timer setting to get the effective time on for the beam. Note that the timer error can be a negative number. The timer error can be calculated by measuring the exposure using an ion chamber for a timer setting of t and then again for a timer setting of $2t$. The time t is typically 1.00 min. Let us denote the timer error as Δ, the actual exposure rate as $\dot{X}$, the measured exposure for timer setting t as X_t, and the measured exposure for timer setting $2t$ as X_{2t}. The timer error and the actual exposure rate are to be determined

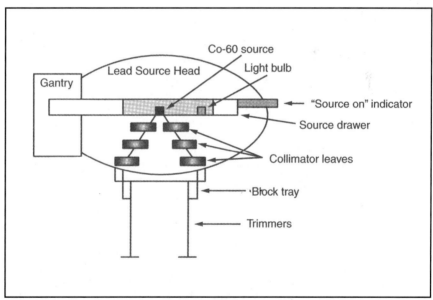

Figure 9.25: This is a simplified schematic cross-sectional view of the head of a Co-60 unit. The source slides back and forth on a "drawer"; it is shown in the "beam on" position. The source slides toward the left into a shielded region when the beam turns off. When the beam is off, the light source occupies the position where the source sits when the beam is on. An indicator rod protrudes from the head of the unit when the beam is on. (Reprinted from Stanton, R., and D. Stinson, *Applied Physics for Radiation Oncology, Revised Edition*, Fig. 10.2, p. 131. © 2009, with permission.)

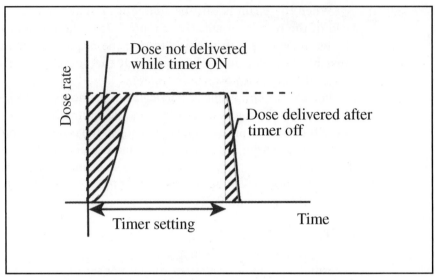

Figure 9.26: The dose rate as a function of time for a Co-60 unit. When the timer turns on, it takes a short while for the source to become fully exposed. During this period there is some dose that is not delivered even though the timer is on. This is shown as the shaded area on the left. When the timer turns off, it takes a short period of time for the beam to turn off because the source has to move back into the shielded position. There is dose delivered during this time even though the timer is off. This is represented by the shaded region on the right. If the shaded areas on the right and on the left were equal, there would be no timer error. In general, they are not equal.

from the measurements. The measured exposure is simply the actual exposure rate multiplied by the effective beam on time and therefore:

$$X_t = \dot{X}(t+\Delta) \quad \text{and} \quad X_{2t} = \dot{X}(2t+\Delta). \tag{9.1}$$

Equations (9.1) are a system of two equations in two unknowns. We wish to solve this system for the unknown Δ (try it). The solution for Δ is:

$$\Delta = \left(\frac{2X_t - X_{2t}}{X_{2t} - X_t}\right)t. \tag{9.2}$$

The timer error is typically on the order of 0.01 minute. The timer error must be subtracted from the time calculated for the desired dose if it is significant. The timer error should be measured once per month. In the United States, the U.S. Nuclear Regulatory Commission *requires* that the timer error be measured once per month. Under normal circumstances the timer error should not change significantly from month to month. If there is a significant change, it may indicate that the source is about to become "stuck" in the open or beam on position. This is an emergency situation.

9.4 Photon Beam Characteristics

A radiation beam spreads or diverges with increasing distance from the source. The width of the beam becomes larger. The field size displayed at the linac console is the length and width of the beam cross section, as measured at the isocenter. We will denote this field size as f. Closer to the source the field size will be smaller, and further from the source it will be larger.

Figure 9.27 shows the geometry of a diverging radiation beam. It is useful to be able to calculate the field size at any distance r other than $r = $ SAD. We will denote this quantity as f_r. In Figure 9.27, triangle ADE is similar to triangle ABC and therefore $f_r/f = r/$SAD and hence:

$$f_r = f \times \frac{r}{\text{SAD}}. \tag{9.3}$$

Although Figure 9.27 shows the case in which $r > $ SAD, equation (9.3) is also applicable when $r < $ SAD.

The properties of radiation therapy beams are measured using a scanning water phantom. This is a tank of water (like a large fish tank, see Figures 9.28 and 9.29), which can be up to 60 cm × 60 cm × 50 cm deep. A radiation detector mounted on a carriage moves through the water. The radiation detector is driven by stepper motors that are computer controlled, and it can be positioned very precisely. The radiation detector is usually an ion chamber, but a diode can be used in some circumstances. The signal from the radiation detector is fed into an electrometer, which is connected to a computer. As shown in Figure 9.28 the computer can drive the detector up and down, from side to side

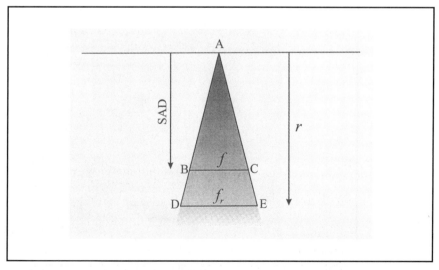

Figure 9.27: A radiation beam diverges with increasing distance from the source. The numerical field size displayed on a linac console is the field size measured at a distance equal to the SAD of the unit.

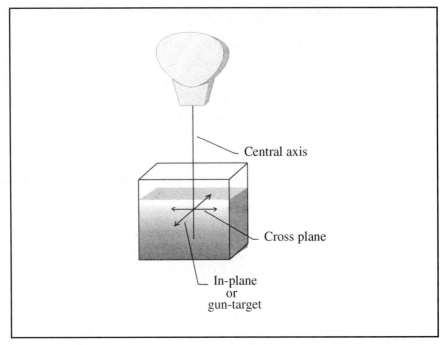

Figure 9.28: A computerized water phantom beam scanner can scan either vertically (along the central axis), in the cross-plane direction (right to left in the plane of this page), or in the in-plane direction (in and out of this page).

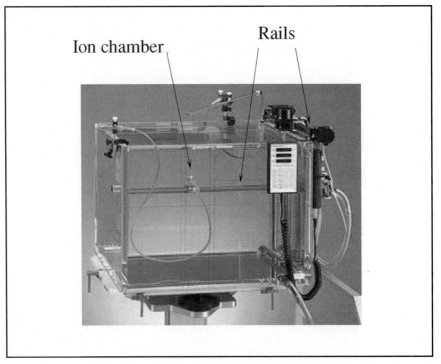

Figure 9.29: A computerized scanning water phantom consists of a tank about $60 \times 60 \times 50$ cm^3, which can be filled with water. A radiation detector in the tank can be moved in any direction: up/down, left/right, or in/out. (Courtesy of PTW-New York, Hicksville, NY)

(called cross plane, transverse plane, or AB plane) and in and out (called in-plane, gun-target, or radial plane). For the in-plane direction, the gun side is the side toward the electron gun and the target side is the side toward the target. The computer records the output from the detector and graphically displays the signal as a function of detector position. When the detector scans a photon beam vertically, the resulting graph is called a *depth dose curve* (see Figure 7.4). The detector can be set at various depths to scan either in the cross plane or in-plane direction. The resulting graphs are called *beam profiles*.

A typical beam profile is shown in Figure 9.30 for an 18 MV 20 cm × 20 cm (jaw setting) beam measured at a depth of 10 cm in the cross-plane direction. The dose at the central axis is set to 100%. Earlier we defined the field size as the width of the beam cross section. A more precise definition is that the field size is the distance between the 50% levels as illustrated in Figure 9.30.

It is desirable to have the intensity of the beam uniform over the irradiated area and to drop abruptly to zero at the edges of the irradiated area as shown in Figure 9.31. The graph of the beam intensity in Figure 9.31 is completely flat over the central portion of the beam. Real radiation beams deviate from this ideal. At the beam edges the profile is rounded

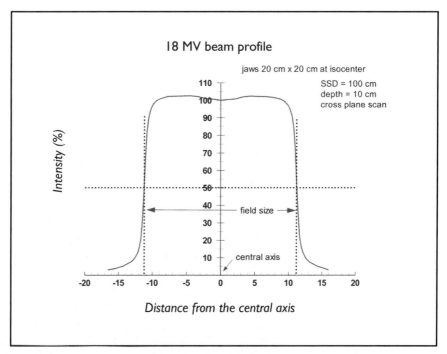

Figure 9.30: A beam profile measured with an ion chamber in a water phantom. This profile was measured by moving the ion chamber in the cross-plane direction at a depth of 10 cm. The intensity at the central axis is set to 100%. The field size is defined as the distance between the 50% intensity points. In this instance, the ion chamber is at a distance of 110 cm (100 cm SSD plus 10 cm deep) and the field size at this distance is expected to be 20 cm × (110/100) = 22 cm [see equation (9.3)]. The measured field size corresponds closely to this.

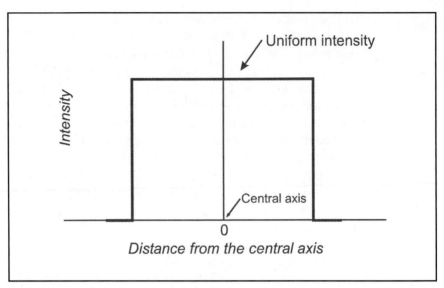

Figure 9.31: An ideal beam profile would be of uniform intensity inside the field and zero intensity outside the field. In the real world, such radiation beams are not possible because of the non-zero source size and scattering in the medium. Both of these effects lead to a penumbra region.

(see Figure 9.30). It is not realistic to expect beams to be flat near the beam edge, and therefore the degree of flatness is evaluated over the inner 80% of the beam. The field size of the beam in Figure 9.30 is 22 cm; 80% of this is 17.6 cm. This beam profile is shown again in Figure 9.32. A measure of beam flatness is defined as:

$$F = \frac{M-m}{M+m} \times 100\%, \qquad (9.4)$$

where M is the maximum intensity value and m is the minimum value measured over the inner 80% of the field.[2] The flatness depends on the depth at which the profile is scanned. The flatness is usually specified at 10 cm deep and sometimes also at d_m. The flatness also depends on the field size, so this too must be specified. The flatness may differ for cross-plane and in-plane profiles. Therefore it should be evaluated for both. For beam flatness measured at a depth of 10 cm, the tolerance is usually 3% when the flatness is as defined in equation (9.4).

Examining Figure 9.32 we see that $M = 103$ and $m = 100$. Substituting these values into equation (9.7) we find that $F = 1.5\%$. This is well within the 3% tolerance. If the flatness does not meet tolerance, it may mean that the axis of the beam is not centered on the flattening filter. In this case, the beam must either be "steered" electronically or the flattening filter must be shifted.

---

[2] Beware: there are many definitions of flatness and symmetry.

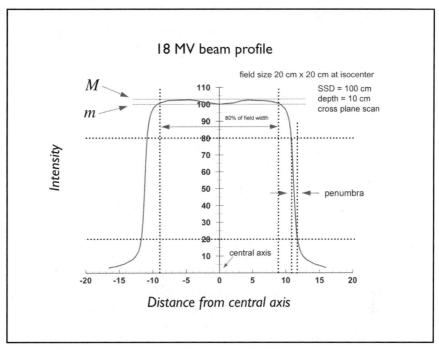

Figure 9.32: Penumbra and flatness for an 18 MV cross-plane beam profile with field size set to 20 × 20 cm² (at isocenter) and a depth of 10 cm. The field size at 10 cm deep is 22 cm. A common definition of the penumbra is that it is the distance between the 80% and 20% intensity levels (the intensity is set to 100% at the central axis). The penumbra is approximately 1.0 cm. Flatness is evaluated over the central 80% of the field which is 0.80 × 22 cm = 17.6 cm in this case. M is the maximum intensity value over this range and m is the minimum.

Another measure of beam shape is beam symmetry about the central axis. There are many different ways to define this. One definition is that the area under the curve on either side of the central axis should be the same within some tolerance.

The penumbra is the region at the edge of the beam over which the beam intensity drops sharply (see Figure 9.32). Whenever a source of light or radiation is not a point source (and of course a point source is an idealization, see section 5.5.1), the source of radiation will not cast a sharp shadow of an object. In the case of visible light, the gray area between the illuminated region and the dark shadow is called the *penumbra*. For a radiation beam the penumbra is the region at the edge of the beam over which the dose rate drops sharply. It is caused by three factors:

(1) non-point source: geometric penumbra
(2) transmission penumbra: collimator jaws or blocks
(3) scattering of photons and secondary electrons: scattered photons and secondary electrons "smear" the edge of the beam.

We will discuss each of these contributions below.

The physical penumbra is the measured penumbra. It encompasses all possible causes, geometric penumbra, scattering, etc. Unfortunately there is no universally agreed upon quantitative definition of penumbra. A common definition is that it is the lateral distance between the 80% and 20% intensity levels measured at a depth of 10 cm and at either the SAD (usually 100 cm) or for SSD = 100 cm, for a field size of 10×10 cm^2. An example is the specification used by Varian Corporation for their Clinac accelerators. They define the physical penumbra as the distance between the 20% and 80% level for a 10×10 cm^2 field at a depth of 10 cm in water (water surface at 100 cm SSD) along the major axes (in-plane and cross plane). This is illustrated in Figure 9.32 (although the jaws are set to 20×20 cm^2 in this figure). The Varian specification is that the physical penumbra shall be less than or equal to 0.9 cm.

Geometric penumbra results from the fact that sources of radiation are not point objects. This can be demonstrated with a flashlight. In a darkened room, project the shadow of your hand onto a wall. If the flashlight is held close to the hand blocking the light, you will see a gray area surrounding the dark shadow of your hand. The gray area is the penumbra. A radiation beam defined by collimator jaws also exhibits a penumbra as shown in Figure 9.33.

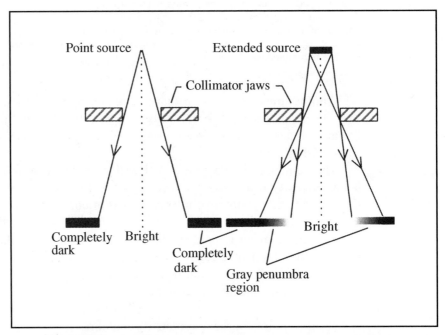

Figure 9.33: Two sources of collimated radiation: a point source on the left and an extended source on the right. The point source casts a very sharp shadow of the collimator jaws. The extended source does not cast a sharp shadow. There is a gray area between the "bright" central region and the region that is completely dark. The gray region is called the *penumbra region.*

It is possible to derive a quantitative relationship for the size of the geometric penumbra. The size of the penumbra depends on the source size, the distance to the collimator (sometimes called the "diaphragm"), and the total distance from the source. The beam may be defined by hand blocks, cast blocks, or an MLC rather than the jaws (see chapter 13).

We will refer to Figure 9.34 for the derivation. The symbols in the diagram have the following meaning:

SSD = source-to-surface distance, where the surface is the surface of the patient or phantom.

SDD = source-to-diaphragm distance. This is the distance to the bottom of the jaws (in the case of blocked fields, this is the distance to the bottom of the block or MLC).

s = the source diameter.

d = depth below the surface.

P = width of geometric penumbra.

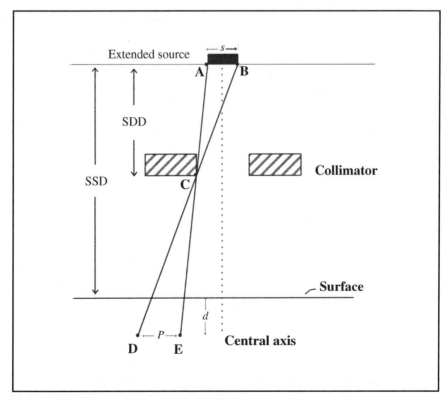

Figure 9.34: Geometry for calculation of geometric penumbra. An extended source of size s produces a geometric penumbra of width P.

Note that triangle ABC is similar to triangle DEC and therefore:

$$\frac{P}{s} = \frac{\text{SSD} + d - \text{SDD}}{\text{SDD}}. \tag{9.5}$$

Notice that SSD + d − SDD is simply the distance from the bottom of the collimator jaw to the position at which the penumbra is measured. Equation (9.5) can be rearranged slightly to yield:

$$P = s\frac{\text{SSD} - \text{SDD} + d}{\text{SDD}}. \tag{9.6}$$

The x-ray source diameter for a linear accelerator may only be 3 to 5 mm (although the flattening filter may effectively enlarge this), whereas a Co-60 source may be up to 2 cm in size. The consequence of this is that the geometric penumbra of a linac is less than for a Co-60 unit because the Co-60 source is considerably larger.

It is useful to understand the systematic changes in the geometric penumbra. When the SSD or depth goes up, the penumbra goes up. When the SDD goes up, the penumbra goes down. You may wish to check this with a flashlight by projecting the shadow of your hand on a wall in a darkened room. In this case, the SDD is the distance from the flashlight bulb to your hand.

Another cause of physical penumbra is transmission penumbra. This is produced when the beam cuts through the edge of a square collimator jaw as shown in Figure 9.35. This can be eliminated by angling the face of the jaws as shown on the right in Figure 9.35. Linear accelerators have such "focused" jaws. The jaws are designed so that they remain focused even when the opening (field size) changes.

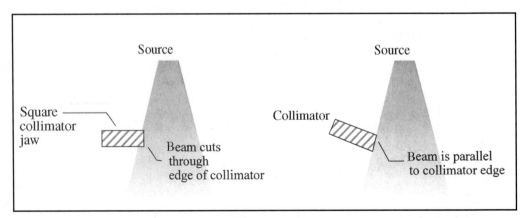

Figure 9.35: On the left, the beam cuts through the edge of the square collimator jaw. Where the beam cuts through the edge, it will be partially transmitted. The partial transmission will result in a penumbra region, even for a point source of radiation. In the diagram on the right, the edge of the collimator jaw has been shaped so that it is parallel to the beam edge. This type of collimator is called a *focused collimator* and it reduces the transmission penumbra.

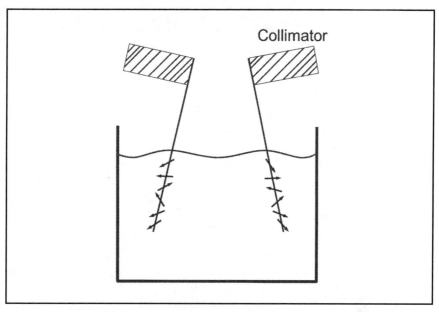

Figure 9.36: Scattered photons and the electron tracks at the edge of a radiation beam "smear" out the dose, even if the edge of the beam is very sharply defined by the collimator.

The third source of physical penumbra results from an unavoidable characteristic of radiation: scattering. This is illustrated in Figure 9.36. Photon scattering and the tracks of secondary electrons smear out the beam edge no matter how sharply it is initially defined.

The Invention of the Cavity Magnetron

Before the invention of the cavity magnetron, radar was unreliable and limited to short range. The shortcomings of early radar were due to the fact that it was not possible to generate microwaves of sufficiently high power and short wavelength to have the needed range and spatial resolution. The cavity magnetron was invented by physicists Randall and Boot at the University of Birmingham, England in early 1940. It was one of the single most important technical developments of World War II. Even early models produced hundreds of times more microwave power output than any other type of microwave-generating device. As the physicist Luis Alvarez commented in the 1980s "If automobiles had been similarly improved, modern cars would cost about a dollar and go a thousand miles on a gallon of gas." Furthermore, the magnetron is a compact device that can be mounted inside airplanes.

The devotees of radar have made a compelling argument that it played a decisive role in WWII. It has been argued that it played a more important role than the atomic bomb, although certainly less dramatic. Admirers of radar like to say that radar ended the war and that the atomic bomb finished it. The invention of the cavity magnetron gave the Allies a distinct advantage, not only for detecting airplanes at long distance, but also for detecting German U-boats. Toward the end of the war a U boat could hardly surface without being pounced upon by Allied aircraft with on-board radar.

At first there was no clear or detailed theoretical understanding of the mechanism of operation of the magnetron. When the device arrived in the United States, a prominent group of theoretical physicists gathered around to look at it. "It's simple," the physicist I.I. Rabi declared. "It's just kind of a whistle." "Okay, Rabi," said E.U. Condon, "How does a whistle work?"

The klystron was developed prior to the invention of the cavity magnetron by brothers Sigurd and Russell Varian at Stanford University. Initially, it was unable to produce the high power output that the cavity magnetron was capable of. Today klystrons are capable of higher power output than magnetrons. Magnetrons are now widely used in police radar and in microwave ovens.

Reading

The Invention that Changed the World by Robert Buderi. New York: Simon and Schuster, 1996.
Winning the Radar War by Jack Nissen. New York: St. Martin's Press, 1987.

Chapter Summary

- There are two main types of external beam treatment units: isotope machines and accelerators.

- Isotope machines use radioisotope Co-60.

- Accelerators use electric fields to accelerate charged particles; linear accelerators (linacs); circular accelerators: microtrons, cyclotrons, synchrotrons, betatrons, etc.

- Linacs accelerate electrons down an evacuated tube (waveguide) to almost the speed of light. The electrons can be used to treat directly or they can be directed onto a metallic target and produce x-rays.

- Isocenter of a linac is the (ideal) point in space where the gantry rotation axis, collimator rotation axis and couch rotation axis meet. The location of this point is fixed.

- **Source-to-axis distance (SAD):** Distance from radiation source to isocenter (usually 100 cm).

- **Source-to-surface distance (SSD):** Distance from the radiation source to the surface of the patient. This distance will generally vary with gantry angle.

- **Linear accelerators:** Photon beam energy stated in terms of MV not MeV; energies range from 4 MV to 25 MV; cannot set beam time on but rather monitor units (MU): MU1 primary setting, MU2 is backup.

- **Accelerating waveguide:** Essentially a pipe under high vacuum; electrons are accelerated down waveguide by 3000 MHz microwaves (S band radar). Two major types: standing wave (Varian, Siemens) and traveling wave (Elekta). In low-energy machines (4 to 6 MV) waveguide can be mounted vertically. In higher-energy machines waveguide is mounted either horizontally or obliquely; therefore a bending magnet is required.

- **Source of microwave power:** (1) magnetron: generates high-power microwaves, which are fed into waveguide; (2) klystron amplifies low-energy microwaves supplied by "RF driver." Klystron can produce higher power than magnetron; generally used in high-energy machines.

- **Electron gun:** Injects pulses of electrons into waveguide.

- **Modulator:** Supplies high-power pulses to the klystron (or magnetron) and to electron gun; pulses are triggered by a vacuum tube called a thyratron that acts like a switch.

- **Treatment head:**
  (1) X-ray target: Used for photon beams only, electron beam strikes target, x-rays produced, transmission target.
  (2) Scattering foils: Used for electron beams only, spreads beam out, makes beam "flat."
  (3) Flattening filter: Used in x-ray mode only, flattens beam.
  (4) Ion chambers: Determine MU1 and MU2; beam symmetry and flatness monitored.
  (5) Fixed (primary) and movable (adjustable jaws) collimators: often independent (asymmetric) jaws, usually up to 40 cm × 40 cm field size. Most linacs have multileaf collimator (MLC) for field shaping.
  (6) Light localizing system (or field defining light).
  (7) Optical distance indicator (ODI) or rangefinder.

- **Co-60 units:** $T_{1/2}$ = 5.26 years, average beam energy 1.25 MeV (not MV!); activity declines roughly 1% per month (Beware: this rule of thumb can only be used over short time intervals!) Source strength up to 10^4 Ci, distance from source-to-axis (SAD) (isocenter) of most Co-60 units is 80 cm.

- **Timer error:** For Co-60, superficial units, time set at console may not be precisely the same as the time source is exposed. Subtract timer error from the time calculated in order to obtain the correct time to set on the timer. Timer error can be positive or negative—typical magnitude is 0.01 min for a Co-60 unit. Must be measured once per month for a Co-60 unit per NRC regulations.

- **Field size:** Distance between 50% levels (central axis 100%).

- **Penumbra:** Region at edge of radiation beam over which dose drops sharply. No universal quantitative definition. One definition: Lateral distance between the 80% and 20% level measured at a depth of 10 cm with SSD = 100 cm and field size 10×10 cm^2. For this definition, penumbra ≤ 0.9 cm (Varian). Caused by: (1) non-point source (called geometric penumbra); (2) transmission through collimator jaws or blocks, and (3) scattering of photons and electrons in the medium.

- **Geometric penumbra** $P = s \dfrac{\text{SSD} - \text{SDD} + d}{\text{SDD}}$, where s is the source size,

  SSD is the source-to-surface distance, SDD is the source-to-diaphragm distance (distance to distal end of jaws or cast block), and d is the depth in the patient. Typical values of the source size are 1 to 2 cm for Co-60 sources and several millimeters for the x-ray source spot size of a linear accelerator. Systematic behavior: $P \uparrow$ when SSD $\uparrow$ or $d \uparrow$; $P \downarrow$ when SDD $\uparrow$.

- **Beam flatness:** Usually evaluated at 10 cm depth, must be flat to ±3% or less, measured over central 80% of the beam.

- **Beam symmetry:** Many ways to define, e.g., area under the beam profile on either side of central axis should be the same to within some tolerance.

Problems

1. Define the term isocenter and source to axis distance (SAD).

2. An electromagnetic wave has a frequency of 3000 MHz.
   (a) Calculate the wavelength in free space. Express your answer in cm.
   (b) If each cavity in an accelerator waveguide is 1/4 of this wavelength long, then how long is each cavity in cm?
   (c) If the energy gain is 2 MeV per cavity and the maximum electron energy is 20 MeV, how long is this waveguide?

3. Explain the major differences between traveling wave and standing wave linacs.

4. (a) How do the features of klystrons and magnetrons differ?
   (b) Why are klystrons used in some accelerators and magnetrons in others?

5. Calculate the geometric penumbra for a Co-60 unit with a source size of 2.0 cm at a total distance of 80 cm (SSD + d). Assume a source to diaphragm distance of 60 cm (in this case, the distance to the block tray). Express the answer in units of mm.

6. Repeat the calculation of problem 5 for a 4 MV linac at a distance of 100 cm and a source-to-diaphragm distance of 60 cm. Assume the source size is 3 mm. Express the answer in units of mm.

7. Why might it be important to measure the timer error of a Co-60 unit on a regular basis?

8. An 18 MeV electron beam strikes the target in a linear accelerator. What is the maximum energy, average energy, and minimum energy of the photons produced.

9. Why don't we have to worry about timer error for linear accelerators?

10. For a Co-60 unit, the measured exposure is 200.0 R for a timer setting of 1.00 minute. For a timer setting of 2.00 minutes, the measured exposure is 401.8 R.
    (a) Calculate the timer error.
    (b) What is the exposure rate in units of R/min?

11. For the beam profile shown: measure (a) the field size and (b) the flatness. Does the beam meet typical specifications for flatness? You will need to use a ruler and to make careful measurements.

18 MV beam profile

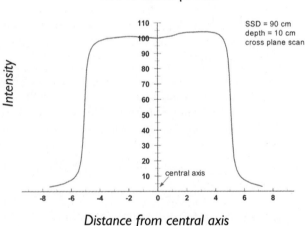

Distance from central axis

12. The bottom of the lower jaws on a linac (see Figure 9.2) is at a distance of 44 cm from the source and the bottom of the upper jaws is at 36 cm. Assuming a source size of 3 mm, compute the geometric penumbra for both sets of jaws at the isocenter (100 cm).

13. It is incorrect to apply the rule of thumb in section 9.3 over a period of more than a few months. If you were to use it over a period of 5.25 years, what relative activity would remain after this time interval? What is the true relative activity after this time interval?

14. If you have access to a linac, ask a medical physicist to give you a tour. You should look at the console, the information displayed on the console and how to program the console for simple beam delivery, the backup MU counter and the door interlock. Inside the room, locate the emergency off switches; observe gantry and collimator rotation and the pendant used to control these functions. Observe couch movements (lateral, longitudinal, vertical, and rotation). Observe operation of the light field and the ODI. Rotate the gantry to 180°. Use a flashlight to look into the head of the machine. Identify the upper and lower jaws and the MLC. Examine an electron applicator and see how it is attached to the collimator. Check the collision avoidance on the applicator. For a Varian or Siemens machine, examine a wedge and see how wedges are mounted on the collimator. Examine the magnetron or the klystron (and the RF driver if present) and the thyratron if accessible. Look at the heat exchanger, water level indicator, the water temperature gauge, and the demineralizing cartridge; the SF_6 supply and gauge.

Bibliography

Bentel, G. C. *Radiation Therapy Planning*. New York: Macmillan, 1995.

Greene, D., and P. C. Williams. *Linear Accelerators for Radiation Therapy*. Bristol, PA: Taylor & Francis, 1997.

Karzmark, C. J., and R. Morton. *A Primer on the Theory and Operation of Linear Accelerators in Radiation Therapy*. Madison, WI: Medical Physics Publishing, 1989.

Karzmark, C. J., C. S. Nunan, and E. Tanabe. *Medical Electron Accelerators*. New York: McGraw-Hill, 1993.

Khan, F. M. *The Physics of Radiation Therapy,* Third Edition. Philadelphia: Lippincott Williams & Wilkins, 2009.

Metcalfe, P., T. Kron, and P. Hoban. *The Physics of Radiotherapy X-Rays and Electrons*. Madison, WI: Medical Physics Publishing, 2007.

Scharf, W. H. *Biomedical Particle Accelerators*. Woodbury, NY: American Institute of Physics, 1997.

Stanton, R., and D. Stinson. *Applied Physics for Radiation Oncology, Revised Edition*. Madison, WI: Medical Physics Publishing, 2009.

Van Dyk, J. (ed.). *The Modern Technology of Radiation Oncology*. Madison, WI: Medical Physics Publishing, 1999.

Williams, J. R., and D. I. Thwaites (eds.). *Radiotherapy Physics: In Practice,* Second Edition. New York: Oxford University Press USA, 2000.

10 Central Axis Dose Distribution

10.1 Introduction

Given the nature of a particular x-ray radiation beam, we need to be able to describe and predict the dose distribution in patients that results from the application of that beam. This task will occupy us over the next several chapters. It is important to always keep in mind that dose can vary from point to point in three dimensions. It is not very informative to say that a patient receives, for example, 5000 cGy. At what anatomical location is this dose absorbed and what is the distribution of dose throughout the rest of the patient's body? The dose distribution depends on characteristics of the beam and characteristics of the patient. In general, the dose distribution in a patient depends on: beam energy, depth, field size, beam modifiers (e.g., wedges), distance from the source of radiation, patient skin contour, tissue inhomogeneities (such as lung, bone, and air cavities), etc. Portions of the beam are usually blocked to shape the beam cross section so that it corresponds to the shape of the target. Furthermore, most patients are treated with multiple beams. In general, dose calculation presents a very complex physical problem. In this chapter we shall concentrate on a description of the relative dose distribution in one dimension—along the central axis. We will gradually add complexity as we proceed.

At the beginning of this chapter we confine ourselves to a discussion of beams with a square cross section. Toward the end of the chapter we will consider beams that are rectangular in cross section. In a later chapter we will handle beams that are arbitrarily shaped and we will consider points that are off the central axis. We will then treat the case in which the surface of the phantom is not flat, or in which the surface is not perpendicular to the beam central axis. We will consider what happens when the phantom is not infinite in depth or lateral extent. We will also consider the effects of inhomogeneities in the phantom, such as those presented by air cavities or lung tissue.

The dose at some given fixed point in a patient or in a phantom can be written as the sum of two contributions: primary radiation and scatter radiation:

$$\text{Dose}_{total} = D_{primary} + D_{scatter}. \tag{10.1}$$

The primary dose contribution is from radiation that comes directly from the source without having been scattered (see Figure 10.1).[1] The

---

[1] We know from the discussion in chapter 6 that the deposition of energy by photons is actually a two-step process. The photon first transfers its energy to electrons in the medium and it is the electrons that deposit dose along their track length. The primary component of dose is that component deposited by electrons set in motion by photons that have not been scattered.

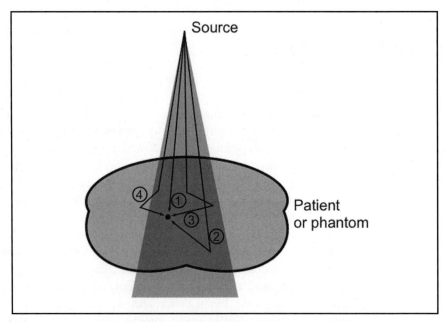

Figure 10.1: Examples of the different types of contribution to absorbed dose at point P. Number ① shows the primary component, which travels directly to P without scattering with intervening matter. Number ② shows a photon that scattered once and which subsequently deposits its remaining energy at point P. Numbers ③ and ④ show multiply-scattered photons. The scatter contribution to the dose increases as the volume of material irradiated increases.

primary contribution to the absorbed dose is relatively easy to calculate. It also generally (but not always) contributes most of the dose. The scatter component of dose is from photons that deposit energy after having undergone one or more scattering events. Photons that have scattered only once are the predominant component of scatter dose, although multiple scattering is not negligible. The scatter contribution increases as the volume of material irradiated increases. For this reason the scatter contribution rises with increasing field size. It is quite difficult to directly compute the scatter contribution to the dose. One method of doing this is the Monte Carlo method discussed earlier in chapter 7, section 7.10.

The scatter component can contribute significantly to the total dose. As an example, for a 4 MV beam at a depth of 3.0 cm along the central axis and for a field size of 10×10 cm^2:

$$\frac{D_{scatter}}{D_{primary}} \approx 0.10, \tag{10.2}$$

or about 10%. We cannot ignore the scatter contribution if we wish to compute dose to an accuracy of a few percent.

Consider an observation point on the central axis. The scatter component of the dose rises with increasing field size. This is because more matter is irradiated as the field size increases, and therefore more radiation can be scattered toward the observation point. When the field size becomes very large, radiation scattered far from the central axis will be attenuated before it can reach the central axis. In this case a further increase in field size will result in a negligible increase in the dose.

In discussing relative dose distribution, our approach is to start with simple conditions and to gradually add complexity. We begin by considering the dose distribution along the central axis of a beam of square cross section that is incident at right angles to a flat infinite (this means infinite in the lateral directions and infinitely deep), homogeneous phantom (see Figure 10.2). We can consider the material to be water and we will assume that tissue is equivalent to water. The distance from the source to a point of interest X is designated r. This distance is sometimes called the "source-to-point distance." The source-to-axis distance (SAD) is fixed and is 100 cm for most linear accelerators (linacs). The source-to-surface distance (SSD) is the distance from the source to the surface of the phantom. The depth of the point of interest below the surface is denoted d and the depth of maximum dose is d_m. A radiation beam of square cross section has a field size designated by f, the length of a side of the square. For a 10×10 cm^2 field, $f = 10$ cm. The field size depends on the distance from the source because of beam divergence (see section 9.4). Therefore it is important to clearly understand the distance from the source at which the field size is specified. The field size displayed on the treatment machine console and on the gantry digital display is the field size at the isocenter, which is usually 100 cm from the source.

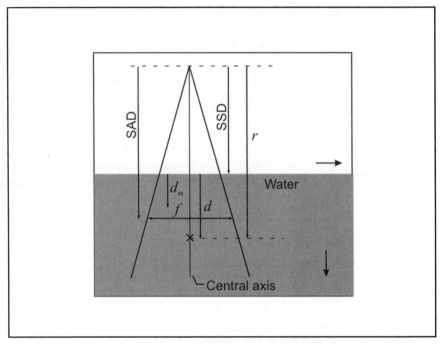

Figure 10.2: An x-ray beam entering a water phantom that is infinitely deep and infinite in lateral extent. The field size set, f, (e.g., 10 × 10 cm²) is defined at the SAD of the treatment unit. The quantity d_m is the depth of maximum dose.

The dose at depth d on the central axis at a distance r from the source and for a set field size f (see Figure 10.2) is denoted $D_d (r, f)$. Under these simple conditions the dose on the central axis depends on: depth, beam energy (quality), SSD, and field size.

There are four widely used quantities that describe dose as a function of depth and field size:

1. Percent depth dose: PDD.
2. Tissue-air ratio: TAR.
3. Tissue-phantom ratio: TPR.
4. Tissue-maximum ratio: TMR.

We will discuss each of these quantities in turn below.

10.2 Percent Depth Dose (PDD)

Recall from the discussion in chapter 7, section 7.5 that absorbed dose rises with depth from the surface and reaches its maximum value at a depth "d-max" (d_m) and then declines as the depth increases. Nominal

Table 10.1: Nominal Values of d_m

Beam quality	Co-60	4 MV	6 MV	10 MV	15 MV	18 MV
d_m (cm)	0.5	1.2	1.5	2.5	3.0	3.3

(Values are taken from *British Journal of Radiology (BJR) Supplement 25,* Central Axis Depth Dose Data for Use in Radiotherapy. London: British Institute of Radiology, 1996.)

values of d_m are listed in Table 10.1. The values in your clinic may be somewhat different from these, depending on the spectrum of your beams. We shall assume that d_m is independent of SSD and field size for now.[2]

The percent depth dose (PDD) at a depth d, for a field size f and at a source-to-surface distance (SSD) is defined as:

$$\text{PDD}(d, f, \text{SSD}) = \frac{D_d(\text{SSD}+d, f)}{D_{d_m}(\text{SSD}+d_m, f)} \times 100\%, \qquad (10.3)$$

where D_d is the dose at depth d (at a distance of SSD + d from the source of radiation) and D_{d_m} is the dose at depth d_m. It is important to note that the field size f is as *measured at the surface* of the patient or phantom. By definition PDD = 100% at $d = d_m$. The depth dose, DD(d, f, SSD), is equal to PDD/100%; that is, it is the decimal equivalent of the percent depth dose. If PDD = 65%, then DD = 0.65. Tables of generic PDD for a variety of beam energies are given in appendix B. PDD tables are usually tabulated only for a standard SSD (almost always SSD = 100 cm). If the SSD is not the standard value, then the numbers in the table cannot be directly used. See Examples 10.1 and 10.2.

Example 10.1

A patient is to be treated with a dose of 150 cGy delivered to a depth of 7 cm on the central axis using a 10×10 cm^2 field size at SSD = 100 cm. If PDD(7, 10, 100) = 74.5%, what dose is delivered to d_m?

$$\text{DD} = 0.745 = \frac{D_d}{D_{d_m}} \Rightarrow D_{d_m} = \frac{D_d}{0.745} = \frac{150}{0.745}$$

$$D_{d_m} = 201 \text{ cGy}$$

---

[2] Although, see section 10.3 in which there is a discussion of the weak dependence of d_m on field size and SSD.

Example 10.2

For a field size $f = 10$ cm, estimate the PDD at a depth of 10 cm for a 4 MV beam and a 15 MV beam from Figure 10.3. Also, look up the PDD in appendix B.

  4 MV: Figure 10.3 shows a PDD of about 63%. The table for 4 MV in appendix B indicates that PDD = 62.1%.

15 MV: Figure 10.3 shows a PDD of about 77%. The table for 15 MV in appendix B indicates that PDD = 76.5%.

Figure 10.3 shows a graph of PDD versus depth for a variety of commonly available beam energies at SSD = 100 cm and a field size of 10×10 cm^2. For clinical application, PDD data should be measured for each individual treatment unit. Two linacs with stated beam energies of 6 MV, for example, may have somewhat different PDD data.

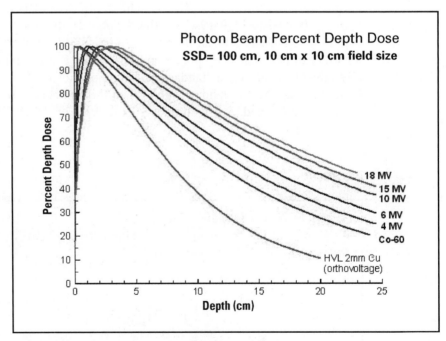

Figure 10.3: Percent depth dose curves for SSD = 100 cm, field size 10×10 cm^2 and for a variety of beam energies. The higher the energy, the more penetrating the radiation. For $d > d_m$ the PDD is higher for higher energies. For $d < d_m$ the PDD is generally *lower* for higher energy beams, although this depends on the degree of electron contamination. Higher energy beams generally have a lower surface dose and thus enhanced skin sparing. [The data for Co-60 and half-value layer (HVL) 2 mm Cu are taken from *British Journal of Radiology (BJR) Supplement 25,* Central Axis Depth Dose Data for Use in Radiotherapy. London: British Institute of Radiology, 1996.]

PDD data are measured using a scanning water phantom (see chapter 9). An ionization chamber is placed in the water phantom and positioned on the central axis at depth d, and the charge collected by the ionization chamber, $M_{raw}(d)$, is measured for a fixed number of monitor units (MU). The ionization chamber is then moved to depth d_m and $M_{raw}(d_m)$ is measured for the same number of monitor units. The dose at depth d is proportional to $M_{raw}(d)$, and for photons (but not for electrons) the proportionality constant is independent of depth; therefore PDD$(d, f, \text{SSD}) = [M_{raw}(d)/M_{raw}(d_m)] \times 100\%$. A real water phantom is not infinitely wide or infinitely deep; however, if there is a sufficient amount of water, it may not matter. As an example, suppose that we wish to measure the PDD up to a depth of 30 cm for an 18 MV, 40×40 cm^2 beam using a water phantom that is 60 cm wide by 60 cm long by 50 cm deep. In this case there will be approximately 10 cm of water between the beam edges and the tank walls, and up to 20 cm of water below the deepest depth of measurement. Experience has shown that approximately 5 cm of water surrounding the beam and below the depth of maximum measurement provides almost as much scatter as an infinite amount of water. In other words, making the water phantom bigger in this case would make a negligible difference to the measured values of the PDD.

It is important to understand how the PDD depends on depth, beam energy, field size, and SSD. This discussion will be confined to depths greater than the depth of maximum dose. As the beam energy rises, the beam becomes more penetrating and the PDD goes up.

The decrease in the PDD with increasing depth is due to two factors: the inverse square factor, which is independent of the material present, and attenuation due to the matter.

The PDD rises with increasing field size. It is not totally obvious that this should be so. Recall that both primary and scattered photons contribute to the dose. For larger field sizes more of the medium is irradiated and thus there will be more scattered photons reaching the central axis. In the definition of PDD [equation (10.3)], therefore, both D_d and D_{d_m} will increase. It is not evident which will increase more rapidly. It turns out that D_d rises faster than D_{d_m} and therefore PDD goes up as the field size increases. This is a less pronounced effect with higher energy beams than for lower energy beams.

The PDD increases with increasing SSD, all other variables held constant *including depth and field size* at the surface.[3] Both D_d and D_{d_m} decrease as the SSD increases. The question is, which decreases the fastest? Let us compare the PDD for two different values of the

---

[3] If the SSD increases, then the jaws must be adjusted (closed slightly) to keep the field size at the surface the same.

SSD, namely SSD_1 and SSD_2. The ratio of these two PDDs is called the Mayneord F factor or Mayneord correction:

$$\frac{PDD(d, f, SSD_2)}{PDD(d, f, SSD_1)} = F$$

$$F = \left(\frac{SSD_2 + d_m}{SSD_1 + d_m} \cdot \frac{SSD_1 + d}{SSD_2 + d} \right)^2.$$

(10.4)

It can be shown that (don't you hate it when they say this?) $F > 1$ for $SSD_2 > SSD_1$, that is

$$PDD(d, f, SSD_2) > PDD(d, f, SSD_1) \quad \text{when } SSD_2 > SSD_1 \quad (10.5)$$

Example 10.3

A patient is treated with a Co-60 beam at $SSD_2 = 100$ cm. The standard $SSD_1 = 80$ cm. If PDD(10, 10, 80) = 55.6%, what is PDD(10, 10, 100)?

$$\frac{PDD(10, 10, 100)}{PDD(10, 10, 80)} = F = \left(\frac{SSD_2 + d_m}{SSD_1 + d_m} \cdot \frac{SSD_1 + d}{SSD_2 + d} \right)^2$$

$$F = \left(\frac{100 + 0.5}{80 + 0.5} \cdot \frac{80 + 10}{100 + 10} \right)^2 = 1.043,$$

therefore, PDD(10, 10, 100) = 58.0%. Notice that the PDD has indeed increased with increasing SSD, but that the change has been small.

It is not difficult to derive the expression for the Mayneord factor. As we shall see, it is simply a consequence of the inverse square law.

We will make two assumptions:

1. The attenuation of the radiation *by the material* it traverses in reaching a depth d does not change as the SSD changes. Regardless of the SSD, the amount of material that the beam has to traverse in reaching depth d remains the same.
2. The scattered radiation contribution is independent of SSD. This assumption is not quite correct because the volume of irradiated material changes slightly as the SSD changes (carefully examine Figure 10.4).

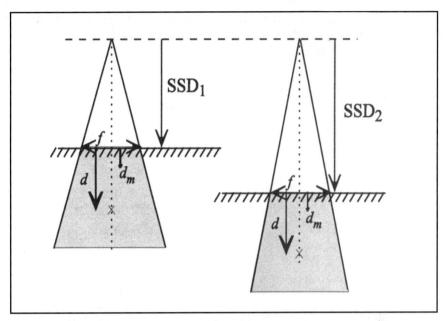

Figure 10.4: PDD rises with increasing SSD. Note that the field size at the surface is held constant. The volume of material irradiated is shaded and is slightly different in the two cases.

The dose at any distance from a source is inversely proportional to the square of the distance from the source:

$$D_d\left(\text{SSD}+d,f\right)\propto\frac{1}{\left(\text{SSD}+d\right)^2}, \qquad D_{d_m}\left(\text{SSD}+d_m,f\right)\propto\frac{1}{\left(\text{SSD}+d_m\right)^2}, \quad (10.6)$$

where the symbol $\propto$ means "proportional to." We now derive the expression for F as follows:

$$\frac{\text{PDD}\left(d,f,\text{SSD}_2\right)}{\text{PDD}\left(d,f,\text{SSD}_1\right)}=\frac{D_d\left(\text{SSD}_2+d,f\right)}{D_{d_m}\left(\text{SSD}_2+d_m,f\right)}\times\frac{D_{d_m}\left(\text{SSD}_1+d_m,f\right)}{D_d\left(\text{SSD}_1+d,f\right)}$$

$$=\left(\frac{\text{SSD}_2+d_m}{\text{SSD}_2+d}\right)^2\left(\frac{\text{SSD}_1+d}{\text{SSD}_1+d_m}\right)^2 \qquad (10.7)$$

$$=\left(\frac{\text{SSD}_2+d_m}{\text{SSD}_1+d_m}\cdot\frac{\text{SSD}_1+d}{\text{SSD}_2+d}\right)^2$$

$$=F.$$

We can give an explanation for the increase in PDD with SSD in words as follows. The PDD at a fixed depth and field size increases with increasing SSD because inverse square *variations over a fixed distance interval* are smaller at large total distance than at small distance. You may need to read the last sentence several times before it makes sense.

The Mayneord correction is only approximate because of assumption 2 listed above. The larger the change in the SSD, the more unreliable it becomes.

The ratio of the dose at different depths can be found by using PDDs. Suppose we wish to know D_{d_2} (SSD+d_2, f), given the value of D_{d_1} (SSD+d_1, f). We can accomplish this as follows.

$$D_{d_2}\left(\text{SSD}+d_2,f\right)=\frac{D_{d_m}\left(\text{SSD}+d_m,f\right)\times\text{PDD}\left(d_2,f,\text{SSD}\right)}{100\%}$$

and   (10.8)

$$D_{d_1}\left(\text{SSD}+d_1,f\right)=\frac{D_{d_m}\left(\text{SSD}+d_m,f\right)\times\text{PDD}\left(d_1,f,\text{SSD}\right)}{100\%},$$

therefore:

$$\frac{D_{d_2}\left(\text{SSD}+d_2,f\right)}{D_{d_1}\left(\text{SSD}+d_1,f\right)}=\frac{\text{PDD}\left(d_2,f,\text{SSD}\right)}{\text{PDD}\left(d_1,f,\text{SSD}\right)}.$$ (10.9)

The dose at depth d_m divides out and the ratio of the doses is simply given by the ratio of the PDD. If D_{d_1} (SSD+d_1, f) is known, then D_{d_2} (SSD+d_2, f) can be easily found using equation (10.9). This relationship is only useful if the value of the SSD is the standard value (i.e., SSD = SAD, usually 100 cm), otherwise a Mayneord factor is necessary to convert to the standard tabulated values of PDD. See Example 10.4.

Example 10.4

A dose of 100 cGy is delivered to a depth of 10 cm on the central axis of a 15×15 cm^2 beam. Given that PDD(5, 15, 100) = 84.2% and that PDD(10, 15, 100) = 64.2%, what dose is delivered at 100 cm SSD to a point on the central axis at a depth of 5.0 cm?

$$\frac{D_{d_2}\left(\text{SSD}+d_2,f\right)}{D_{d_1}\left(\text{SSD}+d_1,f\right)}=\frac{\text{PDD}\left(d_2,f,\text{SSD}\right)}{\text{PDD}\left(d_1,f,\text{SSD}\right)}$$

$$\frac{D_5}{D_{10}}=\frac{84.2\%}{64.2\%}=1.31$$

$$D_5=1.31D_{10}=131 \text{ cGy}$$

10.3 Dependence of d_m on Field Size and SSD

We have not addressed this so far, but d_m depends weakly on field size (and perhaps on SSD), particularly for higher energy beams. For large

Table 10.2: Partial PDD Table for a 15 MV Beam

Depth	Field Size (cm)							
(cm)	4	6	8	12	16	20	24	30
1.8	92.9	93.5	94.1	96.0	97.5	98.7	99.7	100.8
2.0	95.9	96.3	96.7	98.1	99.2	100.0	100.7	101.4
2.2	96.7	97.1	97.4	98.5	99.4	100.0	100.5	101.1
2.4	97.6	97.8	98.1	98.9	99.5	100.0	100.4	100.9
2.6	98.4	98.6	98.7	99.3	99.7	100.0	100.3	100.6
2.8	99.2	99.3	99.4	99.6	99.9	100.0	100.1	100.3
3.0	100.0	100.0	100.0	100.0	100.0	100.0	100.0	100.0
3.2	99.6	99.6	99.6	99.5	99.5	99.4	99.4	99.4

field sizes d_m may become smaller; that is, the location at which the dose is maximum moves toward the surface. This is probably a result of increased electron contamination that occurs when the collimator is open wider. This poses a problem for PDD [and tissue-maximum ratio (TMR)] measurements—what value of d_m should be used for calculation of these quantities? The consensus of opinion seems to be that the largest value of d_m should be used; this is the value of d_m for the *smallest* field size. We shall denote this value of d_m as d_0 in this book. Note that this means that some values of the PDD may be greater than 100%! This is okay provided that one is consistent in the use of the PDD values.

Data are given in Table 10.2 for an actual 15 MV linac beam. For $f = 4$ cm, $d_m = 3.0$ cm, whereas for $f = 30$ cm, $d_m = 2.0$ cm. In this dataset the PDDs have been set equal to 100% at a depth of $d_0 = 3.0$ cm for all field sizes.

At very large SSD the value of d_m can decrease due to electron contamination generated by the photon beam as it traverses the intervening air. This may be of importance for total body irradiation, which is often delivered at an SSD of several meters.

We now modify our definition of PDD slightly to take account of the fact that d_m can vary somewhat with field size:

$$\text{PDD}(d,f,\text{SSD}) = \frac{D_d(\text{SSD}+d,f)}{D_{d_0}(\text{SSD}+d_0,f)} \times 100\%. \qquad (10.10)$$

PDD(d_0, f, SSD) = 100% for all field sizes.

10.4 Tissue-Air Ratio (TAR)

The PDD is a very convenient quantity for treatments when the SSD equals the SAD of the treatment unit (usually 100 cm for linacs). This is the situation for single beam treatments in which the SSD is set to the SAD of the treatment unit. PDD is very inconvenient for treatments which are isocentric [i.e., the isocenter of the treatment machine is located inside the patient (see Figure 9.3)]. Such treatments usually involve multiple beams. This is sometimes referred to as an "SAD treatment." For SAD treatments the skin is at a different distance for each gantry angle. In this case PDD is very inconvenient because of the need for a Mayneord correction.

The tissue-air ratio (TAR) is more convenient for SAD treatments because it is independent of SSD. The TAR is defined as:

$$\text{TAR}(d,f) = \frac{D_d(r,f)}{D_{fs}(r,f)}, \tag{10.11}$$

where D_d is the dose on the central axis at depth d for field size f and D_{fs} is the dose in free space at the same distance from the source (see Figure 10.5). Note the field size f is measured at depth d, unlike for PDD where the field size is measured at the surface.

The TAR is a ratio of doses that are both measured at the same distance from the source.[4] For this reason TAR is independent (approximately) of distance from the source. The TAR increases with increasing beam energy because higher energy radiation is more penetrating. TAR decreases with increasing depth because of attenuation. As the field size increases (with depth held constant), the value of D_d rises because of the increased scatter contribution. D_{fs} however does not change. The net result is that TAR rises as the field size becomes larger.

---

[4]The scatter contribution may change slightly when the distance from the source is changed.

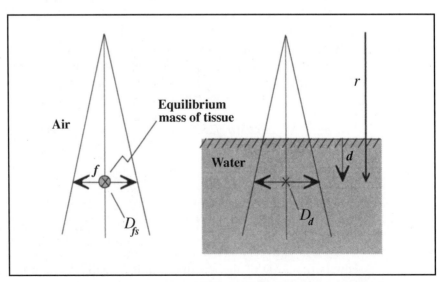

Figure 10.5: This diagram illustrates the definition of TAR. Note that the field size is defined at depth d unlike PDD where the field size is defined at the surface.

10.5 Backscatter and Peak Scatter Factors

Imagine making a measurement of the dose in free space delivered by a treatment beam. This could be done by using an ionization chamber with sufficient buildup on it as shown in Figure 10.6. Then move the ionization chamber and place it in a semi-infinite phantom at depth d_0, keeping it at the same distance from the source. The primary radiation contribution to the dose measured by the ionization chamber will remain the same because the radiation traverses the same amount of material to reach the measurement point. The scatter contribution to the dose will rise however, because much more material is irradiated.

The peak scatter factor (PSF) tells us the enhancement in dose in going from "free space" to "in phantom." The definition of the PSF is

$$\text{PSF}\left(f\right) = \frac{D_{d_0}\left(r,f\right)}{D_{fs}\left(r,f\right)}. \tag{10.12}$$

You can see from the definition of PSF that it is simply the TAR at depth d_0:

$$\text{PSF}\left(f\right) = \text{TAR}\left(d_0, f_{d_0}\right), \tag{10.13}$$

where f_{d_0} is the field size at depth d_0. The value of the PSF must always be greater than 1.000. For megavoltage beams, values of PSF range between 1.06 and 1.09 for a 10×10 cm^2 field. For a 10×10 cm^2 Co-60 beam the PSF = 1.065.

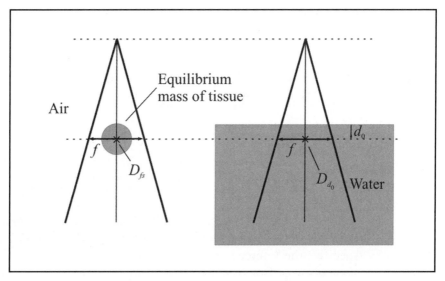

Figure 10.6: Illustration of the meaning of PSF. The PSF is the enhancement factor in the dose that occurs when going from "in free space" to inside a full scattering medium.

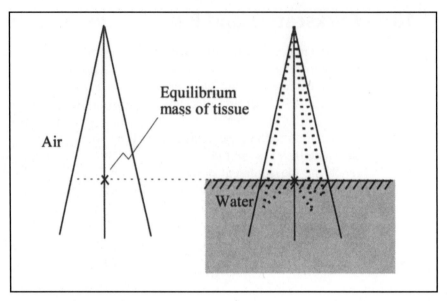

Figure 10.7: Illustration of the backscatter factor (BSF) for low-energy radiation in which d_0 is essentially zero. There is an enhancement in dose over that measured in free space because photons (and electrons set in motion by the photons), which interact at depth, can be scattered back toward the surface.

For low-energy x-rays (diagnostic/superficial) d_0 is essentially zero. In this case the peak scatter factor is usually referred to as the backscatter factor (BSF) (see Figure 10.7). The enhancement in dose under these circumstances is due to backscatter of photons (or of the electrons set in motion by the photons). The value of the BSF can be as large as 1.5 for large fields at orthovoltage energies. This is a 50% enhancement in dose over that measured in free space.

10.6 Tissue-Phantom Ratio (TPR) and Tissue-Maximum Ratio (TMR)

The tissue-phantom ratio (TPR) is defined as:

$$\text{TPR}(d,f) = \frac{D_d(r,f)}{D_{d_r}(r,f)}, \qquad (10.14)$$

where D_d is the dose measured at depth d (and field size f) and D_{d_r} is the dose at some specified reference depth d_r on the central axis. The user specifies the reference depth. Both of these doses are measured at the *same* distance from the source (see Figure 10.8).

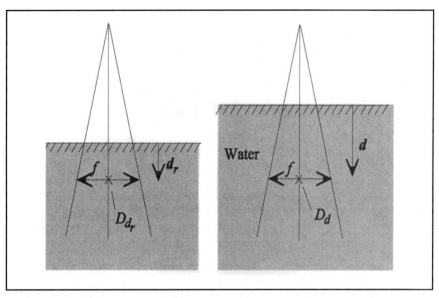

Figure 10.8: Quantities used in the definition of the tissue-phantom ratio (TPR). Both doses are measured at the same distance from the source.

No air measurements are required (as with TAR) and no buildup caps are necessary.

The TPR is independent of SSD (provided that the scatter component does not depend on beam divergence) because both doses are measured at the same distance from the source.

The tissue-maximum ratio (TMR) is a special case of the TPR in which $d_r = d_0$:

$$\text{TMR}\left(d,f\right) = \frac{D_d\left(r,f\right)}{D_{d_0}\left(r,f\right)}. \tag{10.15}$$

Most clinics use TMR for MU calculations. Compare the definition of TMR with the definition of PDD [equation (10.10)]. For the PDD the quantities in the numerator and the denominator of equation (10.7) are measured at different distances, so that PDD combines both the inverse square effect and attenuation by matter. TMR is a measure of attenuation by matter *only,* because the quantities in both the numerator and the denominator in equation (10.15) are measured at the *same* distance from the source of radiation. An application of TMR is illustrated in Example 10.5.

There is a relationship between TMR and TAR:

$$\text{TMR}\left(d,f\right) = \frac{\text{TAR}\left(d,f\right)}{\text{PSF}\left(f\right)}. \tag{10.16}$$

We now derive this result:

$$D_d = D_{fs} \times \text{TAR}$$

$$D_{d_0} = D_{fs} \times \text{PSF}$$

$$\text{TMR} = \frac{D_d}{D_{d_0}} = \frac{D_{fs} \times \text{TAR}}{D_{fs} \times \text{PSF}} = \frac{\text{TAR}}{\text{PSF}}. \tag{10.17}$$

Example 10.5

A dosimeter is placed in a water phantom at a depth of 5.0 cm on the central axis of a 10 MV, $10 \times 10 \text{ cm}^2$ radiation beam. The distance from the source to the dosimeter is 100 cm. Irradiation yields a dose reading of 100 cGy. The dosimeter is "zeroed" and additional water is poured into the water phantom tank until the depth of the dosimeter is 10 cm. The dosimeter is irradiated again without changing any linac settings. What is the new dose reading?

$$\text{TMR}(5,10) = \frac{D_5(100,10)}{D_{d_0}(100,10)}$$

$$\text{TMR}(10,10) = \frac{D_{10}(100,10)}{D_{d_0}(100,10)}$$

$$\frac{D_{10}(100,10)}{D_5(100,10)} = \frac{\text{TMR}(10,10)}{\text{TMR}(5,10)} = \frac{0.828}{0.951} = 0.871$$

$$D_{10}(100,10) = D_5(100,10) \times 0.871 = 87.1 \text{ cGy}.$$

The TMR values are obtained from appendix B.

10.7 Equivalent Squares

We now add a complication. Suppose the field aperture is rectangular rather than square. In principle, if we have a rectangular field, we must write the PDD as a function of both the length L and width W of the rectangle: PDD(d, L, W, SSD). It would be prohibitive to have tables of PDD for every combination of L and W. Fortunately, this is not necessary. Any size rectangle can be "converted" into an "equivalent" size square. For any combination of L and W there is a square field size f that has the same PDD, TMR, and TAR (on the central axis) as a function of depth as the rectangular field. It is fortunate that the value of the equivalent square side length is independent of beam energy and depth.

There are two methods of determining the value of the equivalent square length f:

1. Consult a table of equivalent squares such as that which appears in the *British Journal of Radiology Supplement 25* (BJR 25). This is the most accurate method. This table is reproduced in appendix B of this book. (See Example 10.6.)
2. Use the "area over perimeter" rule. This is a simple empirical formula for computing the equivalent side length f.

Example 10.6

> What is the equivalent square field size for a 12 cm × 8 cm field? Consult the table in appendix B. (Answer: 9.6 cm.)

Area Over Perimeter Rule

The area over perimeter rule is an empirical formula that can be used with fairly high accuracy to calculate the size of a square that is equivalent to a rectangle of given L and W.[5] The rule states that the area divided by the perimeter of the equivalent square is equal to the area divided by the perimeter of the rectangle.

$$\left(\frac{A}{P}\right)_{square} = \left(\frac{A}{P}\right)_{rectangle} , \qquad (10.18)$$

where A is the area and P is the perimeter. The side length of the equivalent square is f. The expression for f may be derived from equation (10.18) as follows:

$$\left(\frac{A}{P}\right)_{square} = \left(\frac{A}{P}\right)_{rectangle}$$

$$\frac{f^2}{4f} = \frac{LW}{2(L+W)} \qquad (10.18a)$$

$$\frac{f}{4} = \frac{LW}{2(L+W)}.$$

---

[5] An empirical formula is usually one that is "cooked up" to give the correct numerical values and it is not derived from fundamental physical principles. There is no fundamental physical basis for equating the area divided by the perimeter of the square and rectangle.

Solving for f,

$$f = \frac{2\,LW}{L+W} = 4\left(\frac{A}{P}\right)_{rectangle}.$$ (10.19)

This rule predicts PDDs to an accuracy of approximately 0.5% or better, provided that the length of the rectangle L is less than 20 cm and that L/W is less than 4. Notice that if $L = W$, that $f = L$ as expected. (See Example 10.7.)

Example 10.7

For a T-L spine treatment with an unblocked (open) field the collimator setting is 20 cm by 5 cm. What is the size of the equivalent square?

a. Table lookup (see appendix B): $20 \times 5 \Rightarrow 7.9 \times 7.9$.

b. A/P rule: $f = \dfrac{2\,LW}{L+W} = \dfrac{2 \times 20 \times 5}{20+5} = 8.0.$

Note that the two methods yield almost identical results.

In some circumstances it is useful to have equivalent squares for circular fields. We wish to have a value of the radius R of a circular field that is equivalent to the square field of side length f. A reasonably accurate empirical rule is obtained by setting the *area* of the square field and circular field equal to one another (rather than the area divided by the perimeter as for rectangles):

$$\pi R^2 = f^2 \Rightarrow R = \frac{f}{\sqrt{\pi}}.$$ (10.20)

We will use this result in chapter 13.

10.8 Linear Interpolation

When performing a lookup in a PDD, TAR, or TMR table, it is sometimes necessary to interpolate between values of the field size or the depth. We first consider a specific example and then later we will generalize.

For a 4 MV beam at a depth of 10 cm the PDD is 66.7% for $f = 15$ cm and PDD = 68.2% for $f = 20$ cm. What is the value of the PDD for $f = 19$ cm?

Let us set up a table with all of the data in it.

f	PDD
$15 = x_1$	$66.7 = y_1$
$19 = x$	y
$20 = x_2$	$68.2 = y_2$

The difference between 15 and 20 is 5; 19 is 4/5 of the way between 15 and 20; therefore PDD(10, 19, SSD) = 66.7 + 4/5 (68.2 – 66.7) = 67.9%.

This value of the PDD seems reasonable. Always ask yourself when you get done with a calculation whether your answer makes sense. If it does, it is not guaranteed to be correct, but if it does not, chances are that it is *not* correct.

We can generalize from this example. Given some quantity y which is a function of $x[y = f(x)]$ and known values of (x_1, y_1) and (x_2, y_2), we want the value of y that corresponds to x when x is between x_1 and x_2. Generalizing from the example:

$$y = y_1 + \frac{x - x_1}{x_2 - x_1}(y_2 - y_1). \tag{10.21}$$

Equation (10.21) is simply the equation for the straight line connecting points (x_1, y_1) and (x_2, y_2), hence the name "linear interpolation." This assumes that the graph of $y = f(x)$ is a straight line in the interval between (x_1, y_1) and (x_2, y_2). Even if the graph is not a straight line in this interval however, this will still work reasonably well provided that $x_2 - x_1$ is small. Note that if the value of x is midway between x_1 and x_2, one can simply average the y values.

Example 10.8

a. Estimate the value of the PDD for the field size of Example 10.7 for a 6 MV beam and a depth of 5.0 cm, given that PDD(5, 5, 100) = 84.5% and PDD(5, 10, 100) = 86.3%.

$$PDD = 84.5 + \frac{8-5}{10-5}(86.3 - 84.5) = 85.6\%$$

b. For a 6 MV beam, TAR(10, 10) = 0.841 and TAR(10, 15) = 0.878. Estimate the value of TAR(10, 12).

$$TAR(10,12) = 0.841 + \frac{12-10}{15-10}(0.878 - 0.841) = 0.856$$

Chapter Summary

- The total dose at a point consists of the dose from primary radiation plus the dose from scatter radiation. Scatter component can contribute up to 10% to 15% in regions irradiated by the primary beam.

Table 10.1: Nominal Values of d_m

Beam quality	Co-60	4 MV	6 MV	10 MV	15 MV	18 MV
d_m (cm)	0.5	1.2	1.5	2.5	3.0	3.3

- For PDD, TAR, TPR, and TMR, know the defining equation and be able to draw diagrams (as in Figures 10.5 and 10.8, reproduced below) illustrating measurement. This is very helpful for problem solving.

- Percent depth dose: $\text{PDD}(d,f,\text{SSD}) = \dfrac{D_d(\text{SSD}+d,f)}{D_{d_0}(\text{SSD}+d_0,f)} \times 100\%$, where d is the depth, d_0 is the nominal value of d_m, f is the field size measured at the surface, and SSD is the source-to-surface distance.

- The decrease in PDD with increasing depth is due to two factors: (1) inverse square and (2) attenuation by matter.

- PDD systematic behavior (up arrow indicates increasing, down arrow indicates decreasing): PDD $\uparrow$ as beam energy $\uparrow$, PDD $\uparrow$ as $f\uparrow$, PDD $\uparrow$ as SSD $\uparrow$.

- $\dfrac{\text{PDD}(d,f,\text{SSD}_2)}{\text{PDD}(d,f,\text{SSD}_1)} = F = \left(\dfrac{\text{SSD}_2+d_0}{\text{SSD}_1+d_0} \cdot \dfrac{\text{SSD}_1+d}{\text{SSD}_2+d}\right)^2$ (Mayneord factor)

- PDD is convenient for calculations when SSD = SAD, but inconvenient otherwise (e.g., isocentric treatment: use TAR, TMR).

- Tissue-air ratio: $\text{TAR}(d,f) = \dfrac{D_d(r,f)}{D_{fs}(r,f)}$, where d is the depth and f is the field size defined at depth d (**not** at the surface as for PDD). The TAR is independent of distance as both doses in the definition of the TAR are measured at the same distance from the source. Draw diagrams if necessary when solving problems; it helps!

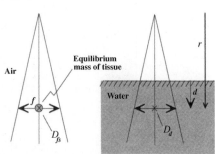

- – TAR systematic behavior: independent of distance from source; TAR ↑ as beam energy ↑; TAR ↓ as d ↑; TAR ↑ as f ↑.

- – Backscatter factor (BSF) or peak scatter factor (PSF): PSF = TAR(d_0, f_{d_0}) describes the enhancement in dose in going from free space to in-phantom. At low energies (diagnostic range) d_0 is close to zero; PSF usually called BSF under these circumstances.

- – Value of BSF can be as high as 1.5 for large field sizes at ortho-voltage energies. For Co-60, 10×10 cm^2 field, PSF = 1.065.

- • Tissue-phantom ratio/tissue-maximum ratio (TPR/TMR):

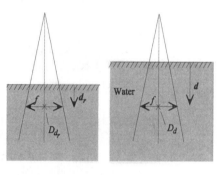

$$\text{TPR}(d,f) = \frac{D_d(r,f)}{D_{d_r}(r,f)},$$

where D_d is the dose at depth d on the central axis and D_{d_r} at some specified reference depth on the central axis. Both doses are measured at the same distance from the source, therefore TPR is independent of distance (and SSD).

TMR = TPR with $d_r = d_0$, i.e., $\text{TMR}(d,f) = \dfrac{D_d}{D_{d_0}}$

- • $\text{TMR}(d,f) = \dfrac{\text{TAR}(d,f)}{\text{PSF}(f)}$

- • PDD combines both the inverse square effect and attenuation by matter. TMR is a measure of attenuation by matter only.

- • Equivalent squares for rectangular fields have the same PDD, TAR, and TPR: empirical rule, area (A) divided by perimeter (P) is the same for the square and rectangle: $f = \dfrac{2\,LW}{L+W} = 4\left(\dfrac{A}{P}\right)$, f is side length of equiv-alent square, L is the length of the rectangle, and W is its width. The equivalent square of a circular field of radius R has side length $f = R\sqrt{\pi}$.

- • Linear interpolation: given two data points (x_1, y_1) and (x_2, y_2), find the value of y corresponding to a value of x between x_1 and x_2 (i.e., $x_1 < x < x_2$):

$$y = y_1 + \frac{x - x_1}{x_2 - x_1}\left(y_2 - y_1\right).$$

Problems

It may be necessary to consult the data in appendices B and C for some of these problems.

1. A dose of 180 cGy is delivered to a depth of 7.0 cm on the central axis with a 6 MV beam having field size 10×10 cm^2 and SSD = 100 cm.
   a. What is the dose deposited at depth d_0 on the central axis?
   b. What is the dose deposited at a depth of 12 cm on the central axis?

2. The SSD of a 6 MV photon beam is increased from 100 cm to 150 cm. By what factor will the PDD increase at a depth of 10 cm when the field size is held fixed at the surface?

3. For the following rectangular fields, determine the equivalent square field size by a table lookup (appendix B) and by calculation. Compare the answers.
   a. 5 cm $\times$ 20 cm
   b. 5 cm $\times$ 30 cm
   c. 5 cm $\times$ 60 cm

4. TMR is defined as D_d/D_{d_0}. DD is defined as D_d/D_{d_0}. Why isn't TMR = DD?

5. What is the value of TMR(d_0, f) for any beam energy? Why?

6. What physical principle accounts for the change in PDD with SSD?

7. Why are TAR and TMR approximately independent of distance from the source of radiation?

8. By definition TMR(d_0, f) = DD(d_0, f, 100) = 1.00. At depth $d > d_0$ is the value of the TMR expected to be larger or smaller than the value of the DD? Explain.

9. Use interpolation to find PDD(10, 8.3, 100) from the 6 MV beam data in appendix C.

10. Calculate TMR(10, 10) for a 6 MV beam given that TAR(10, 10) = 0.841 and PSF(10) = 1.084. Look up the value in appendix C and compare.

11. A patient's spine is treated with a single 6 MV beam at a depth of 5.0 cm, SSD = 100 cm, field size 5 cm × 30 cm. The patient is 20 cm thick.
    a. What is the PDD at the depth of the spine?
    b. What is the ratio of the exit dose at a depth of 20 cm to the dose at the depth of the spine? (Ignore the lack of backscatter at the exit surface.)
    c. The SSD is changed to 130 cm. The jaws are adjusted so that the field size on the skin surface remains 5 cm × 30 cm. What is the new PDD at the depth of the spine?
    d. What is the new ratio of the dose given at a depth of 20 cm to that given at the depth of the spine?

Bibliography

British Journal of Radiology (BJR) Supplement 25. Central Axis Depth Dose Data for Use in Radiotherapy. London: British Institute of Radiology, 1996.

Jani, S. K. *Handbook of Dosimetry Data for Radiotherapy.* Boca Raton, FL: CRC Press, 1993.

Johns, H. E., and J. R. Cunningham. *The Physics of Radiology,* Fourth Edition. Springfield, IL: Charles C Thomas, 1983.

Khan, F. M. *The Physics of Radiation Therapy,* Fourth Edition. Philadelphia: Lippincott Williams & Wilkins, 2009.

Metcalfe, P., T. Kron, and P. Hoban. *The Physics of Radiotherapy X-Rays and Electrons.* Madison, WI: Medical Physics Publishing, 2007.

Stanton, R., and D. Stinson. *Applied Physics for Radiation Oncology, Revised Edition.* Madison, WI: Medical Physics Publishing, 2009.

Williams, J. R., and D. I. Thwaites (eds.). *Radiotherapy Physics: In Practice,* Second Edition. New York: Oxford University Press USA, 2000.

11 Calibration of Megavoltage Photon Beams

In this text we will not discuss calibration of superficial or orthovoltage x-ray units, or electron beams. The reader is advised to consult the bibliography (if necessary) for a discussion of these topics. In the previous chapter we discussed relative dose distributions along the central axis. *Beam calibration* is the process of determining the absolute dose at a particular point on the central axis under carefully specified conditions. The quantities discussed in the previous chapter, such as percent depth dose, may then be used to find the dose at any other point on the central axis.

We do not set a Co-60 unit or linac console for "dose." For a Co-60 unit we set the time on a timer. For a linac we set the number of monitor units (MU) (see chapter 9). The task of beam calibration is to relate machine settings (time or MU) to the dose delivered to a specified point under carefully defined conditions. The actual dose delivered to a specified point in a particular patient depends on numerous factors, which will be discussed in chapters 12 and 13.

The American Association of Physicists in Medicine (AAPM) recommends annual beam calibration. In the United States, Co-60 units are regulated by the U.S. Nuclear Regulatory Commission (NRC) or "Agreement States" (see chapter 17). The NRC *requires* annual beam calibration. Spot checks, also called constancy checks, are performed on a more frequent basis. Beam calibration is one of the most important tasks of the medical physicist. If it is not done correctly, *every* patient will receive an incorrect treatment. Beam calibration should only be performed by, or under the close supervision of, a board certified medical physicist.

Until the year 1999 the standard protocol for the calibration of megavoltage linac beams was prescribed by the AAPM Task Group 21 (TG-21) report in a 1983 publication. This protocol was in almost universal use throughout North America. The TG-21 protocol was superseded in 1999 by the TG-51 protocol. In European countries there are other protocols in use, such as the one published by the IAEA (International Atomic Energy Agency). We will concentrate on the TG-51 protocol here; however, many of the steps described in this chapter are common to all of the protocols.

The International Commission on Radiation Units and Measurements (ICRU) calls for dose delivery accuracy of ±5%. Beam calibration is only one component in the treatment chain. There are many other steps involved in treatment, each of which has an inherent uncertainty. To deliver dose with an accuracy of ±5%, it is necessary to calibrate the beam with considerably better accuracy than this, say 2%. It is this stringent requirement for accuracy that makes beam calibration procedures so complex. Numerous small corrections need to be made to ion chamber readings to achieve the desired accuracy. These were discussed in section 8.3.3.

11.1 Normalization Conditions

To understand beam calibration, it is first necessary to carefully define what it is we are trying to determine. For this purpose we define "normalization conditions." *Normalization conditions* are the conditions under which the dose per monitor unit (or per minute), designated $\dot{D}_0$, is specified for the purpose of dose calculations. All *dosimetry calculations are based on the normalization conditions*. Radiation therapy departments vary in how they specify normalization conditions. It is *extremely* important to understand the normalization conditions in use in a particular clinic before attempting to make any dose calculations, otherwise serious errors may result. The normalization depth is designated d_0 and is usually the nominal value of d_m for that beam energy. In chapter 10 we discussed the fact that d_m may vary with field size. The normalization depth is usually set equal to the largest value of d_m (the value of d_m for the smallest field size).

11.1.1 Normalization Conditions for Co-60

For Co-60 it is common, *but not universal,* to specify the normalization dose rate in water in units of cGy/min, for a field size of 10×10 cm^2 at a distance from the source equal to SAD + d_0, at a depth of d_0, on the central axis and for a particular date. The dose rate will decrease by *approximately* 1% per month due to radioactive decay. It is common to give tables listing the dose rate under the normalization conditions month by month. Most Co-60 units have an SAD of 80 cm and the value of $d_0 = 0.5$ cm; therefore the normalization distance is typically 80.5 cm.

11.1.2 Normalization Conditions for Linear Accelerators

It is common, but not universal, to adjust the linac so that the dose rate of $\dot{D}_0$ is 1.000 cGy/MU delivered to a point in water at a depth of d_0 on the central axis and at a source distance equal to SAD + d_0 for a field size of 10×10 cm^2 (see Figure 11.1). In the notation of the previous chapter $\dot{D}_0 = \dot{D}_{d_0}\left(\text{SAD}+d_0,10\right)$ for this choice of normalization conditions. For most linear accelerators, the SAD = 100 cm. If the linac has more than one photon beam energy, the other beams must be adjusted separately to give

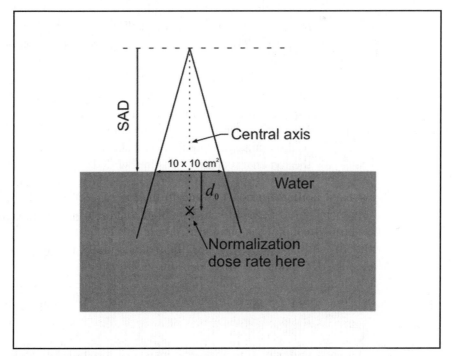

Figure 11.1: Typical normalization conditions for dose specification. The dose per monitor unit (or per minute for Co-60) is specified on the central axis at a source distance of SAD + d_0 and at a depth of d_0 in water for a field size of 10×10 cm^2.

1.000 cGy/MU under the same conditions as above. The value of d_0 will be different for different beam energies.

Note that the dose rate in cGy/MU (cGy/min for Co-60) varies with the field size set. It is a universal convention to calibrate for a 10×10 cm^2 beam. For other field sizes the output is measured relative to 10×10 cm^2. As an example, for a Co-60 unit, the output for a 20×20 cm^2 field is about 5% larger than for a 10×10 cm^2 field. This will be discussed further in chapter 12.

The normalization conditions are *not* necessarily the same as the calibration conditions. Therefore the dose at the normalization point must be calculated from the dose at the calibration point. Calibration conditions are discussed below. The goal of beam calibration is to determine the dose per MU (or per minute for a Co-60 beam) under normalization conditions such as described above.

11.2   Steps in Beam Calibration

We begin with an overview of the entire process of the TG-51 protocol before we launch into details.

Step 1.   Calibration of the ionization chamber and the electrometer at an Accredited Dosimetry Calibration Laboratory (ADCL). Do not confuse calibration of the *ion chamber* with calibration of the *beam*. Once the ion chamber and electrometer are calibrated, they can be used to calibrate any number of beams.

Step 2.   The user determines the beam "quality" by making depth dose measurements.

Step 3.   The ion chamber is placed in the beam under carefully defined conditions, called *calibration conditions*. The ion chamber is exposed to a fixed amount of radiation (time for a Co-60 unit or MU for a linac). The radiation ionizes the air inside the thimble of the ionization chamber. The charge produced is collected from the ion chamber and measured with a calibrated electrometer.

Step 4.   The dose per MU (or per time for Co-60) is calculated using the equations in this chapter for carefully specified conditions, called *normalization conditions,* based on the measured charge collected under calibration conditions.

Step 5.   The linac is adjusted to deliver 1.000 cGy/MU for the normalization conditions.

Step 6.   A system for periodic constancy checks is established, to be performed on a daily basis and, with greater accuracy, on a monthly basis.

The remainder of this chapter consists of a detailed discussion of these steps. We are about to enter the "forest." Do not lose sight of the entire forest while we are examining individual trees.

11.3 Ion Chamber Calibration

Ion chamber calibration is step 1 in section 11.2. Photon beam calibration measurements are made almost exclusively with a Farmer ion chamber. Ion chambers should be calibrated every 2 years. Calibration of ion chambers for radiation therapy applications is performed by secondary (to National Institute for Standards and Technology [NIST]) calibration laboratories called Accredited Dosimetry Calibration Laboratories (ADCLs). The ADCL's instruments are calibrated by NIST. Thus we say that the Farmer chamber calibration is "traceable to NIST." These laboratories are accredited by the American Association of Physicists in Medicine (AAPM). There are three of them in North America.[1] The cost of ion chamber calibration is approximately $700.

The ADCLs provide two types of calibration: in-air and in-water. For calibration in air, the ion chamber is surrounded by air only, with no extraneous material nearby. We will not discuss this type of calibration here. For calibration in water, the ion chamber is placed in a water phantom (tank).

Calibration factors for ion chambers depend on the energy of the beam in which they are calibrated. Linear accelerator beams have a broad spectrum in energy, which is described as the "quality" of the beam. Ideally, a clinic's ion chamber would be calibrated in a beam that has the same quality as the clinic's treatment machine. This is impractical because the calibration laboratories cannot possess every different type of linac. Even beams with the same stated energy in MV sometimes do not have the same energy spectrum. For example, one manufacturer's 6 MV beam may not have the same spectrum as another manufacturer's (see Table 11.1).

One type of beam that is readily available and that has a well-defined spectrum is a Co-60 beam. For this reason, all megavoltage ion chamber calibration is performed in a Co-60 beam. It is then part of the beam calibration process for the user to correct for the beam quality of the users beam. We will discuss how the user can assess the quality of his/her beam later in this chapter.

---

[1]Check out the web site for K&S Associates at http://www.kslab.com/services/calibrations/index.shtml; for the University of Wisconsin at http://uwrcl.medphysics.wisc.edu; for The University of Texas M.D. Anderson Cancer Center at http://rpc.mdanderson.org/adcl/.

Table 11.1: Published Values* of %dd(10) for 6 MV Beams

Linac	%dd(10) (for SSD = 100 cm)
Varian Clinac 2500	66.7
Siemens Mevatron KD	68.2
Elekta (Philips) SL 25	68.1
Mitsubishi EXL-8	67.5

*Data taken from *Handbook of Dosimetry Data* by S. K. Jani.

Ion Chamber Calibration in Water

With the advent of TG-51, ion chambers are to be calibrated at the ADCLs by placing them in a water phantom at a depth of 5.0 cm (see Figure 11.2). The old method of ion chamber calibration is based on an "in-air" measurement in a Co-60 beam. This means that the ion chamber is surrounded by air rather than water. The problem then becomes one of using this ion chamber to determine the dose to water. This makes the old TG-21 protocol very complex. The TG-51 protocol is conceptually much simpler as the ion chamber is calibrated in the same medium (i.e., water) in which we desire to determine the dose.

When the ion chamber is calibrated in water, the build-up cap is removed. If the ion chamber is not already waterproof, it is made waterproof by using a rubber or plastic sheath. The ion chamber is placed in a water tank at a depth of 5.0 cm on the central axis of a $10 \times 10 \text{ cm}^2$ Co-60 beam. The surface of the water is set at a distance of 95 cm from the source (SSD). The total distance from the source to ion chamber is 100 cm (see Figure 11.2).

The absorbed dose calibration factor of the chamber for Co-60 is given by

$$N_{D,w}^{^{60}Co} = \frac{D_w^{^{60}Co}}{M_{raw} \times P_{TP} \times P_{pol} \times P_{ion} \times P_{elec}}, \qquad (11.1)$$

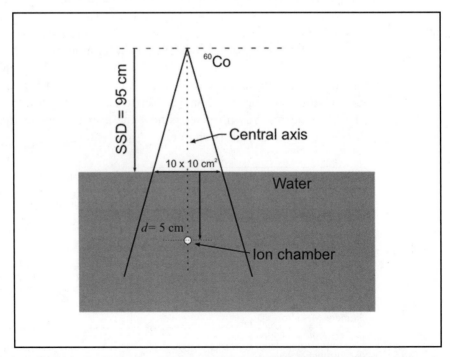

Figure 11.2: Conditions for ion chamber calibration in terms of absorbed dose. Note that these conditions are different than for beam calibration.

where D_w^{60Co} is the known dose delivered to the water at the center of the ion chamber in the absence of the ion chamber and the quantity in the denominator is just the corrected ADCL electrometer reading (see chapter 8). The ADCL measures the value of D_w^{60Co} using its own instruments, which have been calibrated by NIST. The units of the calibration factor are $\left[N_{D,w}^{60Co} \right] = Gy/C$ and a typical value is 5.0×10^7 Gy/C for a Farmer chamber. An ion chamber calibration report is reproduced in Figure 11.3.

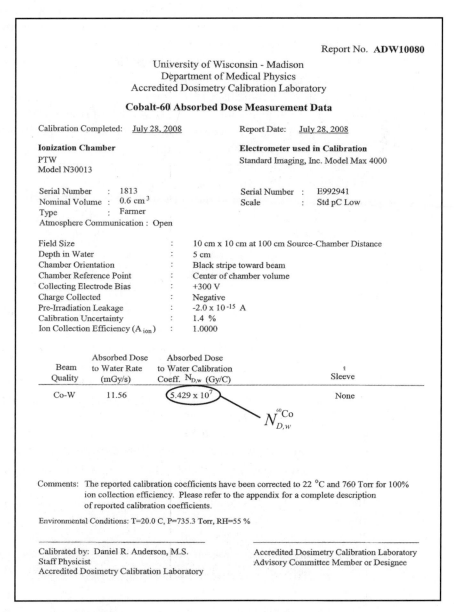

Figure 11.3: An ion chamber calibration report for a Farmer chamber from an Accredited Dosimetry Calibration Laboratory (ADCL). (Courtesy of Larry A. DeWerd, Ph.D., University of Wisconsin, Madison, WI)

11.4 Beam Quality

Determination of beam quality is step 2 listed in section 11.2. The term "beam quality" describes the energy distribution of photons in the beam. The x-ray photons produced by a linear accelerator are not mono-energetic; that is, the photons do not have a single energy. This is in contrast to Co-60 photons which are nearly monoenergetic with average energy of 1.25 MeV. A crude way of describing a beam is in terms of the stated beam energy (sometimes called "nominal accelerating potential"). For example, we may describe a beam as a 6 MV beam. What this generally means is that the electrons emerging from the waveguide have an energy of 6 MeV before striking the x-ray target. The photons exiting the target will have a variety of energies ranging from 0 to 6 MeV. The stated energy is not an adequate description of beam quality for calibration purposes because a 6 MV beam from one manufacturer may have different depth dose values than a 6 MV beam from a different manufacturer. Depth dose is, however, a good beam quality specifier.

TG-51 requires that beam quality be specified by the quantity %dd(10)$_x$, which is the percent depth dose at a depth of 10 cm in water, for a field size of 10×10 cm^2 and an SSD of 100 cm, in the absence of electron contamination. The subscript x in %dd(10)$_x$ indicates that the effect of electron contamination is to be removed from the depth dose. This will be explained shortly. The percent depth dose at a depth of 10 cm is given by,

$$\%\mathrm{dd}(10) = \frac{M_{raw}(10)}{M_{raw}(d_0)} \times 100\%, \tag{11.2}$$

where $M_{raw}(10)$ and $M_{raw}(d_0)$ are the raw electrometer readings at a depth of 10 cm and at a depth of d_0 (for the same number of MUs delivered).[2] Note that there is no subscript x on %dd(10) in equation (11.2). The definition of %dd given in equation (11.2) involves a ratio of raw electrometer readings. If the dose is proportional to M_{raw} and if the proportionality constant is independent of depth, then the definition in chapter 10 is equivalent to the definition given here. This is true for photon beams but *not* electron beams.

Table 11.1 shows that %dd(10) differs for different brands of linacs even though these beams all have the same stated beam quality in MV. Each of these beams has a slightly different energy spectrum even though they are all labeled 6 MV. The use of the quantity MV is inadequate to specify beam quality for the purpose of beam calibration because of the accuracy required.

It is part of the calibration procedure for the user to measure %dd(10)$_x$. In principle, this is straightforward; in practice, there is a complication.

---

[2]In this chapter we will use the TG-51 notation for percent depth dose (%dd). Throughout the rest of the book we will use the notation PDD(d, f, SSD) introduced in chapter 10.

For beams with energy 10 MV and above, there may be a significant amount of electron contamination. Electron contamination results from the interaction of x-rays with the components in the head of the treatment machine. Some of the x-ray photons give up a portion of their energy to electrons (primarily via Compton interactions), which then become a contaminant of the beam (see section 7.5). Some of these electrons may reach a depth of d_0 where they will contribute to the dose. The percent depth dose in the absence of electron contamination, $\%dd(10)_x$, is used in the TG-51 protocol to specify the quality of the beam. If there is significant electron contamination, $M_{raw}(d_0)$ may be larger than it would be otherwise, while the value of $M_{raw}(10)$ will be unaffected because the electrons cannot penetrate this deep. This implies that $\%dd(10)$ will always be less than $\%dd(10)_x$ [see equation (11.2)].

To deal with the problem of electron contamination, the task group calls for the insertion of a lead filter into the beam to stop electrons that are produced in the treatment unit head when the beam energy is 10 MV or above. For energies below 10 MV, electron contamination is negligible and $\%dd(10)_x = \%dd(10)$. One difficulty is that the lead filter will itself introduce electron contamination! The amount of electron contamination introduced by the lead is, however, known and can be removed mathematically from the measured percent depth dose. The lead should be 1 mm thick and it should be placed at a distance of either 30 cm or 50 cm from the water surface. Equations are given in the protocol to convert from the measured percent depth dose, $\%dd(10)_{Pb}$, with the lead in place, to $\%dd(10)_x$, the percent depth dose in the absence of electron contamination. The lead filter is only used for beam quality measurements; it is then removed before making any further measurements. The reader desiring further detail is referred to the TG-51 protocol document (see bibliography).

11.5 The Task Group 51 Dose Equation

The TG-51 protocol is based on the equation

$$D_w^Q = M N_{D,w}^Q, \tag{11.3}$$

where D_w^Q is the absorbed dose to water per monitor unit at the location of the center of the ion chamber in the absence of the ion chamber, M is the charge produced per monitor unit in the sensitive volume of the chamber by the ionizing radiation [equation (8.5)] and $N_{D,w}^Q$ is the absorbed dose calibration factor for beam quality Q. The calibration factor depends on the beam quality and the ion chamber.

The ADCLs provide values of $N_{D,w}^{^{60}Co}$, the Co-60 absorbed dose calibration factor. The user must then determine his/her own beam quality and convert from the Co-60 calibration factor:

Table 11.2: Values of k_Q for a PTW N30001 Farmer Ion Chamber*

%dd(10)$_x$	k_Q	Beam Energy (Approximate)
58	1.000	Co-60
63	0.996	4 MV
66	0.992	6 MV
71	0.984	8 MV
81	0.967	21 MV
93	0.945	>50 MV

*Values taken from TG-51 protocol and *British Journal of Radiology Supplement 25.*

$$N_{D,w}^Q = k_Q N_{D,w}^{^{60}Co}. \tag{11.4}$$

The value of k_Q depends on the ion chamber and the beam quality. For Co-60, $k_Q = 1.000$ by definition. The TG-51 protocol provides tables and charts of values for k_Q. Table 11.2 lists values of k_Q for a commonly used ionization chamber.

The equation for the dose can now be written:

$$D_w^Q = M k_Q N_{D,w}^{^{60}Co}. \tag{11.5}$$

The value of $N_{D,w}^{^{60}Co}$ is obtained from the ADCL for the ion chamber to be used, k_Q converts the calibration factor for Co-60 to the users calibration factor for the users beam and ion chamber (see Table 11.2), and M is the corrected electrometer reading [equation (8.5)].

11.6 Calibration Conditions

Measurements made under beam calibration conditions are listed as step 3 in section 11.2. There is some latitude allowed in the calibration conditions. The depth of the center of the ion chamber must be 10 cm and the field size must be 10×10 cm^2, but the SSD can be either 100 cm or 90 cm. Figure 11.4 shows the calibration conditions for an SSD of 100 cm. Once the dose is determined at the calibration point, the dose at the normalization point must be calculated from it (step 4 of section 11.2). If the normalization conditions are those shown in Figure 11.1 and the calibration conditions are as in Figure 11.4, then the dose at the normalization position can be calculated from the dose at the calibration position by dividing by the percent depth dose, %dd(10). In equation form:

$$\dot{D}_0 = \frac{D_w^Q}{\left[\%dd(10)/100\%\right]}, \tag{11.6}$$

where $\dot{D}_0$ is the dose rate (per MU) at the normalization point at a depth of d_0, D_w^Q is the dose per monitor unit at the calibration point at 10 cm

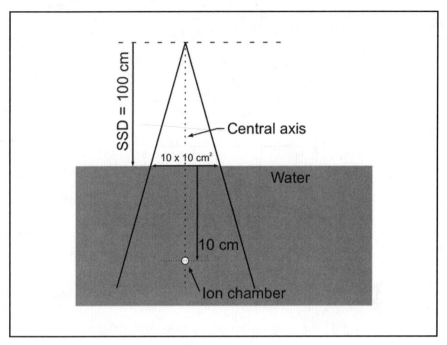

Figure 11.4: One possibility for beam calibration conditions. The ion chamber is placed at a depth of 10 cm and the SSD is 100 cm.

deep, and %dd(10) is the percent depth dose for an SSD = 100 cm, field size 10×10 cm^2 (without any correction for electron contamination).[3] It is presumed that %dd(d_0) = 100%. If the value of $\dot{D}_0$ is not 1.000 cGy/MU, then the physicist can adjust the amplification of the monitor chamber signal so that $\dot{D}_0$ is 1.000 cGy/MU. This is step 5 listed in section 11.2. This completes the TG-51 calibration protocol, but it remains to establish the constancy checks (step 6 of section 11.2).

11.7 An Example of TG-51 Calculations

The TG-51 protocol is to be used to calibrate a 10 MV beam. The Farmer chamber is a PTW N30001 with a value of $N_{D,w}^{^{60}Co} = 5.330 \times 10^7$ Gy/C. The electrometer used with the ion chamber has P_{elec} = 1.003. The calibration conditions are SSD = 100 cm, depth = 10 cm. field size = 10×10 cm^2. The water temperature is T = 21.8 °C and the atmospheric pressure is p = 745 mm-Hg. The normalization conditions are SSD = 100 cm, d_0 = 2.5 cm, field size = 10×10 cm^2. For this beam %dd(10)$_x$ = 74.3% and %dd(10) =73.8%. P_{pol} = 1.000 and P_{ion} = 1.002. For 100 MU delivered, the average (uncorrected) electrometer reading is 13.996 nC.

---

[3] Technically, the denominator of equation (11.6) should be the clinically used depth dose.

1. Find k_Q for this beam.
    Interpolate in Table 11.2.

    Interpolation for k_Q

%dd$(10)_x$	k_Q
71	0.984
74.3	?
81	0.967

    $$k_Q = 0.984 + \frac{0.967 - 0.984}{81 - 71}(74.3 - 71.0) = 0.978$$

2. Find P_{TP}.

    $$P_{TP} = \frac{273 + T}{295} \times \frac{760}{p} = \frac{273 + 21.8}{295} \times \frac{760}{745} = 1.019$$

3. Find M, the charge produced by the radiation per monitor unit.

    $$M = P_{ion} P_{TP} P_{elec} P_{pol} M_{raw} / (100 \text{ MU})$$
    $$= (1.002)(1.019)(1.003)(1.000)(13.996 \text{ nC})/100 = 0.1433 \text{ nC/MU}$$

4. What is the dose per MU delivered to the point of calibration?

    $$D_w^Q = M k_Q N_{D,w}^{^{60}Co} = (0.1433 \times 10^{-9} \text{C/MU})(0.978)(5.330 \times 10^7 \text{Gy/C})$$
    $$= 0.00747 \text{ Gy/MU}$$
    $$= 0.747 \text{ cGy/MU}$$

5. What is the dose per MU for the normalization conditions?

    $$\dot{D}_0 = \frac{D_w^Q}{\left[\%dd(10)/100\%\right]} = \frac{0.747 \text{ cGy/MU}}{(73.8\%/100\%)} = 1.012 \text{ cGy/MU}$$

    and therefore $\dot{D}_0 = 1.012$ cGy/MU. The normal procedure would now be to adjust the sensitivity of the linac monitor ion chambers so that $\dot{D}_0 = 1.000$ cGy/MU.

11.8 Constancy Checks of Beam Calibration

Beam calibration is a laborious and lengthy process. It may take 8 to 12 hours to calibrate both photon beams and all of the electron beams (which we have not discussed here) of a linac. It is recommended that this process be performed annually. It is necessary however to check the "output" more frequently than once per year. There should be some check of the output each day before patient treatment and a more accurate check once per month during the monthly quality assurance tests (see chapter 18 for a detailed discussion of linac QA).

The monthly constancy check is established immediately after calibration. This is step 6 listed in section 11.2, the final step in beam calibration. Generally, this is done by setting up some sort of a convenient solid plastic or tissue-equivalent phantom. The solid phantom is much easier to set up than the water phantom. Often the plastic comes in the form of slabs or sheets that can be stacked upon one another (see Figure 8.1). One of the slabs should have a machined cavity that is designed so that an ion chamber can be inserted into it. The ion chamber does not have to be a Farmer chamber; a plane-parallel chamber can be used for this purpose. An arrangement of the slabs is selected so that the ion chamber is at some specified depth (perhaps d_0). This configuration of ion chamber and plastic slabs is irradiated under some standard conditions (e.g., ion chamber on the central axis at a depth d_0, 10×10 cm^2 field size, SSD = 100 cm) and the electrometer reading is noted. In this way, the beam calibration can be related to the reading of the electrometer using this standard setup (temperature and pressure corrections must be taken into account). This setup is reproduced in subsequent months. Ion chamber measurements in the solid phantom can then be easily used to determine whether the beam calibration has changed. If a significant change has occurred, the physicist can adjust the monitor chamber gain so that the beam calibration is reset to 1.000 cGy/MU under normalization conditions. The whole process of beam calibration and establishment of the monthly and daily checks is repeated yearly as part of the annual QA tests of the linac.

An independent check of beam calibration is essential. If an error is made in the TG-51 calibration, then monthly checks will simply confirm the constancy of the erroneous calibration. The Radiological Physics Center (RPC) in Houston has a mailed dosimetry program.[4] The RPC sends a set of dosimeters that are embedded in plastic blocks, along with detailed instructions on how to irradiate the dosimeters. After irradiation, the dosimeters are mailed back to the RPC where they are read. The RPC then sends a report to the clinic indicating the measured dose delivered to the dosimeters. The accuracy is approximately ±5%. Member institutions of various clinical protocol groups such as the RTOG (Radiation Therapy Oncology Group) are required to participate in the RPC mailed dosimetry program.

---

[4] Web site: http://rpc.mdanderson.org/rpc/index.htm.

Chapter Summary

- Cannot set Co-60 unit or linac for dose, instead set time or MU.

- **Normalization Conditions:** Conditions under which dose/MU (or dose/min for Co-60) is specified for purpose of dose calculations in patients; varies from clinic to clinic; common normalization conditions: physicist adjusts linac to deliver $\dot{D}_0$ = 1.000 cGy/MU on the central axis, SSD = 100 cm, depth = d_0, field size 10 × 10 cm^2. The value of d_0 is commonly set to the nominal (smallest field size) value of d_m.

- **Calibration:** Relate machine settings to the dose delivered to a specific point under carefully defined normalization conditions, accuracy of 1%–2% required.

Calibration Steps: Broad Outline

1. Calibration of ionization chamber and electrometer at an ADCL in a Co-60 beam. Do not confuse calibration of the *ion chamber* with calibration of the *beam*.
2. Place the Farmer ion chamber in the beam under carefully defined conditions, called *calibration conditions*. Expose the ion chamber to a fixed amount of radiation (time for a Co-60 unit or MU for a linac). Charge is collected from the ion chamber and measured with a calibrated electrometer.
3. Calculate the dose per MU (or per time for Co-60) for *normalization conditions* based on the charge collected under calibration conditions.
4. Adjust linac to deliver 1.000 cGy/MU for normalization conditions.

- Establish a system for monthly and daily constancy checks of the beam calibration.

- **TG-51 Calibration**
  The equation for the dose delivered to water per monitor unit, D_w^Q, from a beam quality Q is:

$$D_w^Q = M k_Q N_{D,w}^{^{60}Co},$$

where $N_{D,w}^{^{60}Co}$ is the absorbed dose calibration factor (in water) for the user's ion chamber in a Co-60 beam, k_Q converts the Co-60 absorbed dose calibration factor from Co-60 to the beam quality of the user's beam, and M is the charge produced in the sensitive volume of the ion chamber per monitor unit by the passage of radiation through it.

- **TG-51 Procedure**
  1. Obtain an absorbed dose calibration factor, $N_{D,w}^{^{60}Co}$ in a Co-60 beam, for your Farmer chamber from an ADCL.
  2. Determine the beam quality by measuring the percent depth dose $\%dd(10)_x$ (in the absence of electron contamination) at a depth of 10 cm with an SSD = 100 cm and for a 10×10 cm^2 field size.
     a. If the beam energy is less than 10 MV, $\%dd(10)_x = \%dd(10)$.
     b. If the beam energy is greater then or equal to 10 MV, insert a lead filter and measure $\%dd(10)_{Pb}$. Use the equations given in the protocol to calculate $\%dd(10)_x$.
  3. Find the value of k_Q for your Farmer chamber model using the tables in the protocol and the value of $\%dd(10)_x$ determined above. This permits conversion from a Co-60 beam quality to the users beam quality:

$$N_{D,w}^{Q} = k_Q N_{D,w}^{^{60}Co}.$$

  4. Set the surface of the water phantom to a distance of 100 cm. Position the ion chamber at a depth of 10 cm, set the field size for 10×10 cm^2. Read M_{raw} from the electrometer. Correct the raw reading by using the equation:

$$M = P_{ion} P_{TP} P_{elec} P_{pol} M_{raw}.$$

  5. Calculate the dose per monitor unit to water at the position of the center of the ion chamber using the formula:

$$D_w^{Q} = M k_Q N_{D,w}^{^{60}Co}.$$

  6. Determine the dose per monitor unit for the normalization conditions. For the normalization conditions described in Figure 11.1. this involves a division of D_w^{Q} by $(\%dd(10)/100\%)$.

Problems

1. For the TG-51 protocol, what is the only acceptable medium in which the dose can be measured?

2. Why is the stated beam energy in MV an inadequate measure of beam quality for calibration purposes?

3. What quantity is used to specify beam quality in the TG-51 protocol and how is it measured?

4. Is %dd(10)$_x$ less than or greater than %dd(10)? Explain.

5. What is the value of k_Q for a Co-60 beam and why does it have this value?

The following information is to be used for problems 6 through 14.

A PTW N30001 Farmer ion chamber has a value of $N_{D,w}^{^{60}Co}$ = 5.330×10^7 Gy/C.

The electrometer used with the ion chamber has P_{elec} = 1.003.

The calibration conditions are SSD = 100 cm, depth = 10 cm.

Field size = 10×10 cm^2.

The water temperature is T = 23.5 °C and the atmospheric pressure is p = 730 mm Hg.

For problems 6 through 10, an ion chamber is used to calibrate a 6 MV beam with %dd(10)$_x$ = %dd(10) = 66.4%. The average electrometer reading for SSD = 100 cm, d_0 = 1.5 cm is M_{raw} = 12.218 nC for 100 MU delivered. P_{ion} = 1.002, P_{pol} = 1.000.

---

6. What is the value of the temperature and pressure correction factor?

7. What charge per monitor unit (in units of nC) is produced by the ionizing radiation inside the thimble of the Farmer chamber?

8. What is the value of $N_{D,w}^Q$ for this ion chamber and this beam? Give an answer with an accuracy of at least three significant digits.

9. What is the dose per monitor unit at a depth of 10 cm?

10. What is the dose rate $\dot{D}_0$ in cGy/MU at depth d_0 (SSD = 100 cm) on the central axis for a 10×10 cm^2 field size?

For problems 11 through 14, an 18 MV beam is calibrated with the ion chamber described above and SSD = 100 cm, d_0 = 3.3 cm.

Data for this beam are: $\%dd(10)_x$ = 82.0%, $\%dd(10)$ = 79.4%, P_{pol} = 1.000, P_{ion} = 1.005, the average electrometer reading is M_{raw} = 14.569 nC for 100 MU delivered.

---

11. What is the corrected value of the electrometer reading per monitor unit?

12. What is the value of $N_{D,w}^Q$ for this ion chamber and this beam?

13. What is the dose per monitor unit at a depth of 10 cm?

14. What is the dose rate $\dot{D}_0$ in cGy/MU at depth d_0 (SSD = 100 cm) on the central axis for a 10×10 cm^2 field size?

Bibliography

AAPM TG-21. (1983). "A protocol for the determination of absorbed dose from high-energy photon and electron beams." *Med Phys* 10(6):741–771.

AAPM TG-51. Almond, P. R., P. J. Biggs, B. M. Coursey, W. F. Hanson, M. Saiful Huq, R. Nath, and D. W. O. Rogers. (1999). "AAPM's TG-51 protocol for clinical reference dosimetry of high-energy photon and electron beams." *Med Phys* 26(9): 1847–1970. Also available as AAPM Report No. 67.

British Journal of Radiology (BJR) Supplement 25. Central Axis Depth Dose Data for Use in Radiotherapy. London: British Institute of Radiology, 1996.

Hanson, W. F. "AAPM TG-51 Protocol: The Absorbed Dose Calibration" in *General Practice of Radiation Oncology Physics in the 21st Century*. Proceedings of the AAPM 2000 Summer School. AAPM Medical Physics Monograph No. 26. Madison, WI: Medical Physics Publishing, 2000.

Jani, S. K. *Handbook of Dosimetry Data*. Boca Raton, FL: CRC Press, 1993.

K&S Associates web site at http://www.kslab.com/services/calibrations/index.shtml.

Ma, C.-M., C. W. Coffey, L. A. DeWerd, C. Liu, R. Nath, S. M. Seltzer, and J. P. Seuntjens. (2001). "AAPM protocol for 40–300 kV x-ray beam dosimetry in radiotherapy and radiobiology." *Med Phys* 28(6):868–893. Also available as AAPM Report No. 76.

Rogers, D. W. O. "Fundamentals of Dosimetry Based on Absorbed Dose Standards" in *Teletherapy: Present and Future*. Proceedings of the AAPM 1996 Summer School. Madison, WI: Advanced Medical Publishing, pp. 319–356, 1996.

The University of Texas M.D. Anderson Cancer Center Accredited Dosimetry Calibration Laboratory (ADCL) web site at http://rpc.mdanderson.org/adcl/.

The University of Wisconsin Accredited Dosimetry Calibration Laboratory (ADCL) web site at http://uwrcl.medphysics.wisc.edu.

12 Calculation of Monitor Unit/ Timer Setting for Open Fields

12.1 Introduction

We do not set patient dose directly at the console of a treatment unit. For a Co-60 unit, the dose rate is measured under carefully specified conditions and a timer is set to deliver the proper dose for specific patient treatments. The rate at which dose is delivered by a linear accelerator is not as steady and reliable as the dose rate from a Co-60 unit. For this reason, monitor ion chambers are used in linacs to measure the cumulative amount of radiation passing through them (see chapter 9). This is measured in monitor units (MU). The actual amount of time necessary to deliver a fixed number of MU may vary slightly from one delivery to the next. The number of MU needed for a linac treatment or the timer setting for a Co-60 unit is calculated and set for each individual patient beam. These computations are often referred to as "meter set calculations." For a particular patient, the MU, or time set, depends on the dose to be delivered and the dose rate (either dose per unit time for a Co-60

12-1

unit or dose/MU for a linac) at the location where the dose is to be deposited.

Every radiation therapy patient receives a customized *treatment plan.* The details of the treatment plan depend on the patient's anatomy (size and shape) and on the physician-prescribed amount and distribution of dose. Computerized treatment planning systems are used to calculate the needed MU and the dose distribution throughout the patient. It is important to have some understanding of the principles of MU and dose calculations. Furthermore, in simple cases it may not be necessary to use a computer to calculate MU; a manual calculation may be faster and just as accurate. It is also often the case that MUs for a patient are checked by performing a manual calculation. It is very unlikely for a computer to make arithmetical errors, but an error in the data files used by the computer or in the patient-specific input that was entered into the computer ("garbage in, garbage out") is possible.

In essence, the idea is a simple one. The physician prescribes a specific dose D to a well-defined location in the patient called the *prescription point.* The timer setting for a Co-60 unit is then given by:

$$t = \frac{D}{\dot{D}} - \Delta,\tag{12.1}$$

where $\dot{D}$ is the dose rate (dose/time) at the prescription point and Δ is the timer error for the Co-60 unit (note that the timer error can have a negative value).[1] For a linear accelerator the monitor unit setting, μ, is given by:

$$\mu = \frac{D}{\dot{D}},\tag{12.2}$$

where $\dot{D}$ is now the dose per monitor unit at the prescription location.[2] In equations (12.1) and (12.2) the value of $\dot{D}$ depends on the depth, distance from the source, beam energy, and field size. The problem of determining the meter setting is then a problem of calculating the dose rate $\dot{D}$ at the prescription point in the patient. Regardless of your clinic's system of dosimetry and regardless of the field shape or the presence of beam modifiers, *all meter set calculations are based on either equation (12.1) or (12.2).* As Co-60 units are becoming rare, we will not discuss calculation of the timer setting for these units. The meter set calculation problem is sometimes turned around. Sometimes we know μ and we wish to find D at some specified point other than the prescription point.

---

[1] This assumes that the timer error is as defined in chapter 9, equation (9.2).
[2] It should be clear from the context that μ is not the linear attenuation coefficient.

Within the context of meter set calculations, the term "dose rate" means the dose/MU for a linac and the dose/time for Co-60 machines. For a linac this is not the temporal dose rate (dose/time). The temporal dose rate is the (dose/MU) × (MU/min) = dose/min. The number of MU/min that a linac can deliver depends on the specific model. Common values are 300 to 400 MU/min. Values as high as 600 MU/min are available. The higher the number of MU/min, the more quickly the treatment can be delivered.

In this chapter we shall concern ourselves only with the simplest possible case—the one in which there are no beam modifiers and the cross section of the field is rectangular in shape. Such a field is referred to as an *open field*. For most patient treatments a multileaf collimator or customized blocks are used to shape the radiation field (beam or portal, as it is sometimes called) to make the treatment as conformal as possible. There are other auxiliary devices that are sometimes inserted in the beam to produce a more ideal dose distribution, such as wedges, compensators, beam spoilers, etc. We will consider the complications introduced by these devices in later chapters. For now, we restrict ourselves to calculations of dose delivery at a point on the central axis of the treatment machine.

The SAD for a treatment machine is fixed; it cannot be changed. It is the distance from the source to the axis of rotation of the gantry (see chapter 9). The SSD on the other hand will vary depending on how far the patient is from the source of the radiation. The SAD is 100 cm for all contemporary linear accelerators. Most Co-60 units have an SAD = 80 cm, although some newer Co-60 units have an SAD of 100 cm.

Meter set calculations can be confusing because of the large variety of methods employed at various treatment centers. There are two major systems in use. The first of these is based on dose rate in free space, percent depth dose (PDD), and tissue-to-air ratio (TAR). The second is based on dose rate in phantom, PDD, and tissue-maximum ratio (TMR). The second system seems to have gained favor and is used by most clinics. We will therefore concentrate on the second system. It is the responsibility of the physics staff to establish the method of meter set calculation.

12.2 Normalization Conditions

It is customary to establish certain conditions under which the dose delivered to water (or muscle) per monitor unit (for a linac) or per minute (for a Co-60) unit is specified. The term "output" is often used (BEWARE: this term means different things to different people). It is an unfortunate truth that terminology in radiation oncology dosimetry is far from standardized. The linear accelerator is adjusted by a physicist to deliver a certain dose per monitor unit under carefully specified conditions. These conditions will be referred to as *normalization conditions*. Whenever we go to a clinic that is new to us, we question the staff carefully about the normalization conditions used for their dosimetry system. The method by which meter set calculations are performed depends critically on the normalization conditions and the system of dosimetry in use. Mistakes in dose delivery are easily possible without a clear and precise understanding of these conditions.

The following factors must be clearly stated for the normalization conditions: the distance from the source to the normalization point, the field size (specified at the SAD), and the normalization depth from the phantom surface, referred to as d_0. The depth d_0 is often taken to be d_m. In chapter 10 we saw that the value of d_m may depend on field size. The value of d_0 is taken as the largest value of d_m. As an example, we cite a commonly used normalization configuration. The dose rate is established as 1.000 cGy/MU for a 10×10 cm^2 field size (measured at isocenter) in water at a specified depth d_0 and for an SSD of 100 cm. A survey by Bjärngard et al.[3] has shown that about 75% of institutions specify normalization conditions in this way.

Under normalization conditions, there is a clearly specified value of the dose rate, $\dot{D}_0$, either per minute (Co-60) or per monitor unit (linacs). For Co-60, the dose rate is measured under the specified conditions. This dose rate declines with time because of the radioactive decay of Co-60 and therefore must be updated monthly. For a linac, the dose rate is usually set to a value of 1.000 cGy/MU under the normalization conditions. If physicists measure the dose rate for a linac under the normalization conditions and find that it is not 1.000 cGy/MU, then they can adjust the dose rate by adjusting the sensitivity or gain of the monitor chambers. Note that the beam itself is not adjusted during this procedure, rather it is the sensitivity of the monitor chamber that is changed. This is accomplished by adjusting trimmer potentiometers inside the console cabinet or through software commands. The value of $\dot{D}_0$ is established as part of the beam calibration process described in chapter 11.

Let us define $\dot{D}_d\left(r,f\right)$ as the dose rate at a depth d "in phantom" at a distance r from the source of the radiation and for a field size f (measured at the SAD). The field size f is the field size read on the machine console or gantry display. The notation that we have introduced here is very similar to the notation of chapter 10; we have simply placed dots over the *D's* to indicate *rates*. The normalization dose rate shown in Figure 12.1 can be written as $\dot{D}_0 = \dot{D}_{d_0}\left(\text{SAD}+d_0,10\right)$.

---

[3] Bjärngard, B. E., R. Bar-Deroma, and A. Corrao. (1994). "A survey of methods to calculate monitor settings." *Int J Radiat Oncol Biol Phys* 28(3):749–752.

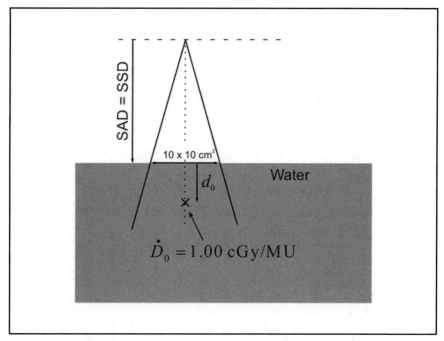

Figure 12.1: Typical normalization conditions for linac dose calculations. The linac is set to deliver 1.000 cGy/MU in phantom (water) at a depth d_0 with the SSD set to the machine SAD (usually 100 cm) and a field size set to 10×10 cm^2.

In Table 12.1 and in appendix C we provide data for a fictitious linac called the "Mevalac." This is a dual-energy machine with photon energies of 6 MV and 18 MV and electron beam energies ranging from 6 to 18 MeV. The values of d_0 for the 6 MV and 18 MV beams are 1.5 cm and 3.0 cm, respectively. The normalization conditions for this machine are the same as those shown in Figure 12.1. The SAD is 100 cm.

12.3 Head Scatter and Phantom Scatter

The dose rate in phantom from a Co-60 unit or a linac at a standard fixed distance depends on the field size setting. The dose rate rises as the field size increases. There are two reasons for this: *head scatter* (sometimes called "collimator scatter") and *phantom scatter*. We will consider the physical cause of each of these contributions in turn below.

For a linear accelerator, head scatter is due to photon scattering in the head of the accelerator, primarily in the flattening filter. If you were to position your eye at the isocenter of a linac and look back up toward the source, you would, if the ion chamber were not in the way, be able to see a portion

Table 12.1: Scatter Correction Factors for the Mevalac (SAD = 100 cm)

$\dot{D}_0$ = 1.000 cGy/MU for f = 10 × 10 cm^2 field at depth d_0, SSD = 100 cm

6 MV: d_0 = 1.5 cm, $\dot{D}_{d_0}$(100,10) = 1.030 cGy/MU

18 MV: d_0 = 3.0 cm, $\dot{D}_{d_0}$(100,10) = 1.061 cGy/MU

Field size (cm)	6 MV			18 MV		
	$S_{c,p}$	S_c	S_p	$S_{c,p}$	S_c	S_p
3	0.919	0.954	0.963	0.881	0.946	0.931
4	0.939	0.963	0.975	0.919	0.956	0.961
5	0.949	0.969	0.979	0.936	0.962	0.973
6	0.964	0.979	0.984	0.955	0.973	0.982
7	0.974	0.985	0.989	0.968	0.980	0.987
8	0.984	0.991	0.993	0.980	0.988	0.992
9	0.992	0.995	0.997	0.990	0.994	0.996
10	1.000	1.000	1.000	1.000	1.000	1.000
11	1.007	1.004	1.003	1.008	1.006	1.002
12	1.014	1.007	1.007	1.016	1.013	1.003
13	1.019	1.010	1.010	1.022	1.016	1.006
14	1.025	1.012	1.012	1.029	1.019	1.009
15	1.030	1.015	1.015	1.035	1.023	1.012
16	1.035	1.018	1.017	1.040	1.026	1.013
17	1.040	1.022	1.018	1.045	1.029	1.015
18	1.045	1.025	1.019	1.049	1.033	1.016
19	1.050	1.029	1.021	1.054	1.036	1.017
20	1.055	1.032	1.022	1.059	1.040	1.018
21	1.058	1.035	1.022	1.062	1.042	1.019
22	1.061	1.037	1.022	1.064	1.044	1.019
23	1.063	1.040	1.023	1.067	1.046	1.020
24	1.066	1.042	1.023	1.069	1.048	1.020
25	1.069	1.045	1.023	1.072	1.050	1.021
30	1.080	1.053	1.026	1.081	1.058	1.021
35	1.084	1.058	1.025	1.084	1.062	1.021
40	1.087	1.061	1.025	1.084	1.066	1.017

of the flattening filter. The larger the jaw opening, the larger the portion of the flattening filter that you could see. By the same token, the larger the collimator opening, the more radiation scattered by the flattening filter that can reach the isocenter and the less that is blocked by the jaws. Therefore as the field size increases, the dose rate rises. Note that this effect is completely independent of whether or not a patient is in the beam.

Recall from chapter 10 that the dose (this also applies to the dose rate) in phantom consists of a primary component and a scatter component. As the field size changes, the primary component changes because of a change in head scatter conditions, as we noted above. The scatter component in the phantom (sometimes called "phantom scatter") also changes because of a change in the volume of matter irradiated. When the field size is increased, a larger amount of material is irradiated and there is an increase in the phantom scatter dose.

Both head scatter and phantom scatter cause the dose rate measured in phantom to increase with an increase in field size. We have seen that the dose rate under normalization conditions is often set to 1.000 cGy/MU for a linac or measured (in cGy/min) for a Co-60 unit. Normalization conditions entail the use of a 10×10 cm^2 field size. The dose rate under normalization conditions is established at the time of beam calibration. The change in the dose rate resulting from a change in field size is evaluated by making relative measurements. As a specific example, let us consider the 6 MV Mevalac beam. Suppose that for a 10×10 cm^2 beam, SSD = 100 cm, an ion chamber is placed at a depth of $d_0 = 1.5$ cm, 100 MU is delivered, and the raw electrometer reading for the irradiation is 19.234 nC. Now the field size is increased to 20×20 cm^2 and the 100 MU irradiation is repeated. The electrometer now reads 20.292 nC. The dose rate for the 20×20 cm^2 field is therefore $20.292/19.234 \times 1.000$ cGy/MU = 1.055 cGy/MU (see Table 12.1). This is how the entries in column 2 of Table 12.1 have been obtained.

These relative measurements are parameterized by the scatter correction factor $S_{c,p}$. This quantity is defined as:

$$S_{c,p}\left(f\right)=\frac{\dot{D}_{d_0}\left(\text{SAD}+d_0,f\right)}{\dot{D}_{d_0}\left(\text{SAD}+d_0,10\right)}. \quad (12.3)$$

Note that $\dot{D}_{d_0}\left(\text{SAD}+d_0,10\right)=\dot{D}_0$ is the normalization dose rate, usually set to 1.000 cGy/MU.

Once we know the normalization dose rate and once we have a table of values for $S_{c,p}(f)$, the dose rate at depth d_0 and distance SAD + d_0 can be calculated for any field size. The subscripts "c" and "p" in $S_{c,p}$ indicate that this factor accounts for both head scatter ("c" for collimator) and phantom scatter ("p" for phantom).

For a rectangular collimator setting, the values of $S_{c,p}(f)$ can be determined from the equivalent square of the rectangle using the area over perimeter rule [equation (10.19)].[4] As an example, for a 10 cm $\times$ 15 cm field, the equivalent square is 12×12 cm^2 and for the 6 MV Mevalac beam, $S_{c,p}(12) = 1.014$, according to Table 12.1.

We shall see later that it is sometimes useful to separate the effects of collimator scatter from the effects of phantom scatter. This is accomplished by assuming that $S_{c,p}(f)$ is the product of a collimator scatter factor $S_c(f)$ and a phantom scatter factor $S_p(f)$:

$$S_{c,p}\left(f\right)=S_c\left(f\right)\times S_p\left(f\right). \quad (12.4)$$

The collimator scatter factor can be measured by placing an ion chamber with a suitable build-up cap in the beam on the central axis at a fixed distance from the source. The ion chamber is to be surrounded

---

[4]It is not at all obvious that this should work for $S_{c,p}$, but it seems to.

only by air to avoid any extraneous scatter contribution. The thickness of the build-up cap should be sufficient to provide approximate charged particle equilibrium for the collecting volume of the ion chamber. Under these circumstances, the raw charge collected from the ion chamber is proportional to the dose rate in free space and therefore:

$$S_c(f) = \frac{\dot{D}_{fs}(r,f)}{\dot{D}_{fs}(r,10)}. \tag{12.5}$$

In making these measurements, the smallest field size used must be large enough so that the ion chamber and build-up cap are completely covered by the radiation beam. The build-up cap can be thought of as a "mini-phantom." As the field size is increased, no additional phantom material will be irradiated and therefore there will be no additional phantom scatter. Any change in $\dot{D}_{fs}$ must originate in the treatment machine. Notice that $S_c(10) = 1.000$, by definition [see equation (12.5)]. The values of $S_p(f)$ can now be found from the measured values of $S_{c,p}(f)$ and $S_c(f)$:

$$S_p(f) = \frac{S_{c,p}(f)}{S_c(f)}. \tag{12.6}$$

Note that $S_p(10) = 1.000$. Values of $S_c(f)$ and $S_p(f)$ can be found in Table 12.1.

12.4 Dose Rate Calculations

When the SSD = SAD (this is referred to as an SSD treatment), the PDD is usually used for meter set calculations. When the prescription point is at the isocenter (SAD treatment), it is most convenient to use either TPR or TMR. It may be that neither SSD = SAD nor the prescription point is at the isocenter. In this instance meter set calculations are usually made by using either tissue-phantom ratio (TPR) or TMR. The different possibilities are discussed in the remainder of this chapter.

12.4.1 Percent Depth Dose Calculations (SSD = SAD)

The method of calculation outlined in this section is useful if the patient skin surface is at a distance equal to the SAD of the unit. This is frequently the case for single beam treatments, such as for supraclavicular fields, spinal fields, etc., because it is convenient to set up the patient this way.

For percent depth dose calculations we use:

$$\mathrm{DD}(d,f,\mathrm{SSD}) = \frac{\dot{D}_d(\mathrm{SAD}+d,f)}{\dot{D}_{d_0}(\mathrm{SAD}+d_0,f)}, \tag{12.7}$$

where the dots over the doses indicate a dose rate (per time for Co-60 or per MU for a linac). Equation (12.7) looks a little bit different from the definition of DD in chapter 10 [see equation (10.10)]. Instead of a ratio of doses, we have a ratio of dose rates. The ratio of doses at two points has the same value as the ratio of dose rates at those points. In this case d_0 is the value of d_m for the smallest field size. Appendix C contains tables of the percent depth dose for the Mevalac.

Rearranging equation (12.7), the dose rate at depth d is then given by:

$$\dot{D}_d\left(\text{SAD}+d,f\right)=\dot{D}_{d_0}\left(\text{SAD}+d_0,f\right)\times\text{DD}\left(d,f,\text{SAD}\right), \qquad (12.8)$$

and from equation (12.3):

$$\dot{D}_{d_0}\left(\text{SAD}+d_0,f\right)=\dot{D}_{d_0}\left(\text{SAD}+d_0,10\right)\times S_{c,p}\left(f\right), \qquad (12.9)$$

therefore

$$\dot{D}_d\left(\text{SAD}+d,f\right)=\dot{D}_{d_0}\left(\text{SAD}+d_0,10\right)\times S_{c,p}\left(f\right)\times\text{DD}\left(d,f,\text{SAD}\right). \qquad (12.10)$$

Note that the value of $\dot{D}_0=\dot{D}_{d_0}\left(\text{SAD}+d_0,10\right)$ is usually 1.000 cGy/MU. The term $S_{c,p}(f)$ in equation (12.10) should technically be replaced with $S_c\left(f\right)\times S_p\left(f_{d_0}\right)$, where f_{d_0} is the field size measured at a depth d_0. If d_0 is the nominal value of d_m, then $S_c\left(f\right)\times S_p\left(f_{d_0}\right)\approx S_{c,p}\left(f\right)$. Equation (12.10) is the equation for the dose rate that is used in MU calculations when SSD = SAD. Note that it is easy to remember equation (12.10) if you can simply remember the definition of depth dose and $S_{c,p}$.

Equation (12.10) looks more daunting than it really is because of the use of functional notation. For example, we write $\dot{D}_{d_0}\left(\text{SAD}+d_0,10\right)$ instead of just $\dot{D}_0$. The latter notation does not tell us *where* $\dot{D}_0$ is to be measured (nor the field size); in this case at a distance of SAD + d_0. We recommend that the beginner write out equation (12.10) with the full functional notation so that the circumstances under which various quantities are specified are clear. Confusion over this issue is a major source of incorrect dose rate calculations. Once the functional dependencies are clear, equation (12.10) can be written more concisely as:

$$\dot{D}_d=\dot{D}_0\times S_{c,p}\times\text{DD}. \qquad (12.11)$$

This is the same as equation (12.10), although it certainly appears much simpler!

The dose rate calculated by using equation (12.10) can be easily understood in terms of steps beginning with the normalization dose. The normalization dose for a 10×10 cm^2 field is first converted to a dose for a field size f by multiplication by $S_{c,p}(f)$. The dose at depth d is then calculated by multiplying by the depth dose.

Example 12.1

A dose of 180 cGy is to be delivered at 10 cm deep on the central axis with a 15×15 cm^2 field size and an SSD = 100 cm. The beam is the 18 MV beam from the Mevalac. How many MU should be delivered? Consult appendix C for PDD data and Table 12.1 (or appendix C) for $S_{c,p}(f)$.

$$\mu = D/\dot{D} \quad \text{and}$$

$$\dot{D}_d(\text{SAD} + d, f) = \dot{D}_0 \times S_{c,p}(f) \times \text{DD}(d, f, \text{SAD})$$

$$= 1.000 \times 1.035 \times 0.788$$

$$= 0.816 \text{ cGy/MU}$$

$$\mu = D/\dot{D}_d = (180 \text{ cGy})/(0.816 \text{ cGy/MU}) = 221 \text{ MU}$$

Congratulations! You have done your first MU calculation. Note that values of μ are usually rounded to the nearest integer.

Example 12.2

A patient is to be treated with a 4 MV beam ($d_0 = 1.2$ cm) at an SSD of 100 cm with a field size of 5 cm $\times$ 20 cm. The prescribed dose is 200 cGy to be delivered to a depth of 5.0 cm on the central axis. Given that $\dot{D}_{d_0}(100,8) = 0.974$ cGy/MU and PDD(5,8,100) = 83.0%, calculate the necessary number of monitor units.

The equivalent square field size of a 5 cm $\times$ 20 cm field is an 8×8 cm^2 field.

$$\dot{D}_d(105,8) = \dot{D}_{d_0}(101.2,8) \times \text{DD}(5,8,100)$$

Note that we do not need the factor $S_{c,p}$ because we are given $\dot{D}_{d_0}(101.2,8)$; it is already built into this.

We are given $\dot{D}_{d_0}(100,8)$ *not* $\dot{D}_{d_0}(101.2,8)$. We must first calculate $\dot{D}_{d_0}(101.2,8)$ using an inverse square correction (ignoring small changes in phantom scatter):

$$\dot{D}_{d_0}(101.2,8) = \dot{D}_{d_0}(100,8) \times (100.0 / 101.2)^2$$

$$= 0.974 \times 0.976$$

$$= 0.951 \text{ cGy/MU}.$$

$$\dot{D}_d(105,8) = 0.951 \times 0.830 = 0.789 \text{ cGy/MU}$$

$$\mu = D/\dot{D}_d = 200 \text{ cGy} / (0.789 \text{ cGy/MU}) = 254 \text{ MU}.$$

12.4.2 Isocentric Calculations

SAD calculations are specifically suited to isocentric treatments. These are treatments in which the isocenter is placed where the prescribed dose is to be delivered. This is usually the method of choice when multiple beams are employed. Once the patient is set up for treatment, it is then simply a matter of rotating the gantry (and if necessary, the collimator and pedestal) of the treatment unit to prepare for the next treatment field. The patient is not moved between treatment fields.

For isocentric treatment the most convenient method of meter set calculation is to use TMR. For TMR meter set calculations at the isocenter, we go back to the definition of TMR [equation (10.15)] just as we did for PDD:

$$\dot{D}_d\left(\text{SAD},f\right)=\dot{D}_{d_0}\left(\text{SAD},f\right)\times\text{TMR}\left(d,f\right), \qquad (12.12)$$

where the reference depth is assumed to be d_0. Equation (12.12) is just a rearrangement of the definition of TMR [equation (10.15)] where we have replaced dose by dose rate. For TMR dose rate calculations you do not need to remember a new equation, just the definition of TMR. Inserting the scatter correction factor into equation (12.12) we obtain:[5]

$$\boxed{\dot{D}_d\left(\text{SAD},f\right)=\dot{D}_{d_0}\left(\text{SAD},10\right)\times S_{c,p}\left(f\right)\times\text{TMR}\left(d,f\right).} \qquad (12.13)$$

Note that $\dot{D}_{d_0}$ is measured at a distance of SAD from the source. The quantity $\dot{D}_{d_0}\left(\text{SAD},f\right)\neq\dot{D}_{d_0}\left(\text{SAD}+d_0,f\right)$ because the latter is measured at a distance of SAD + d_0. We can relate these quantities however by using the inverse square law:

$$\dot{D}_{d_0}\left(\text{SAD},f\right)=\dot{D}_{d_0}\left(\text{SAD}+d_0,f\right)\times\left(\frac{\text{SAD}+d_0}{\text{SAD}}\right)^2. \qquad (12.14)$$

For the 6 MV Mevalac beam, the value of

$$\dot{D}_{d_0}\left(100,10\right)=\dot{D}_{d_0}\left(100+d_0,10\right)\times\left(\frac{100+1.5}{100}\right)^2=1.030\text{ cGy/MU}, \qquad (12.15)$$

and likewise for the 18 MV beam $\dot{D}_{d_0}(100,10)=1.061$ cGy/MU. These values are listed for convenience in Table 12.1.

Examples 12.3 and 12.4 illustrate isocentric monitor unit calculations.

---

[5] This derivation is not rigorous because we ignore small changes in phantom scatter.

Example 12.3

A patient is treated isocentrically on the Mevalac with a 6 MV beam and with a 15×15 cm^2 field. Given that TMR(5, 15) = 0.935, how many MUs should be set to deliver a dose of 180 cGy at a depth of 5.0 cm on the central axis?

$$\dot{D}_d = \dot{D}_{d_0}(100,10) \times S_{c,p}(15) \times \text{TMR}(5,15)$$
$$= 1.030 \times 1.030 \times 0.935$$
$$= 0.992 \text{ cGy/MU}$$

$$\mu = D/\dot{D}_d = 180 \text{ cGy}/(0.992 \text{ cGy/MU}) = 181 \text{ MU}$$

Example 12.4

Determine the number of monitor units necessary to deliver a dose of 200 cGy to a tumor at depth 8 cm on the central axis at the isocenter of a 4 MV linac with SAD = 80 cm. The collimator setting is 6×6 cm^2. The $\dot{D}_{d_0}(80,6) = 0.960$ cGy/MU and TMR(8,6) = 0.787.

$$\dot{D}_d = \dot{D}_{d_0}(\text{SAD},f) \times \text{TMR}(d,f)$$
$$\dot{D}_d = 0.960 \times 0.787$$
$$= 0.756 \text{ cGy/MU}$$

$$\mu = D/\dot{D}_d = 200 \text{ cGy}/(0.756 \text{ cGy/MU}) = 265 \text{ MU}$$

12.4.3 Dose Rate at an Arbitrary Distance

We have seen in chapter 11 that TAR and TMR are independent of distance. This makes these quantities well suited for monitor unit calculations when the prescribed dose is to a point at any arbitrary distance, such as when the SSD is greater than the SAD of the unit (see Figure 12.2). This is sometimes referred to as *treatment at an extended distance*. Recall that TMR is independent of distance [see equation (10.15)] because the dose in the numerator and the dose in the denominator are both measured at the same distance. Let us begin by rewriting the definition of TMR:

$$\text{TMR}(d,f_d) = \frac{\dot{D}_d(r,f_d)}{\dot{D}_{d_0}(r,f_d)}. \tag{12.16}$$

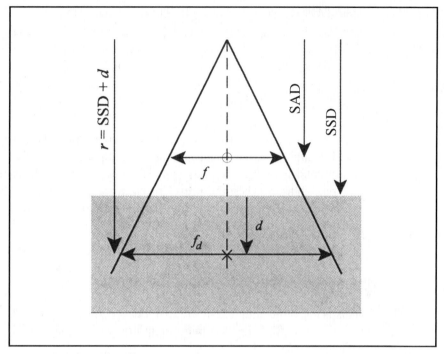

Figure 12.2: Treatment at an extended SSD. The total treatment distance is r = SSD + d. The field size at the treatment distance is $f_d = f \times$ (SSD + d)/SAD.

In this definition we have used dose rates instead of doses, the distance to the point at which the dose is prescribed is an arbitrary distance r and f_d is the field size at depth d. When r = SAD, $f_d = f$. For TMR calculations:

$$\dot{D}_d\left(r,f_d\right)=\dot{D}_{d_0}\left(r,f_d\right)\times\text{TMR}\left(d,f_d\right), \qquad (12.17)$$

where r = (SSD + d) and f_d is the field size at the depth d. We need to find the value of $\dot{D}_{d_0}\left(r,f\right)$. Let us first suppose that the patient surface is at r = 100 cm. We know how to find values of $\dot{D}_{d_0}\left(100+d_0,f\right)$. Now let us suppose that we move the patient further away so that r = SSD + d. At this distance the dose rate at depth d_0 on the central axis will change for two reasons: inverse square changes in the incident radiation fluence and a change in the amount of phantom material irradiated, which will change the phantom scatter factor. We therefore expect that

$$\dot{D}_{d_0}\left(\text{SSD}+d,f_d\right)=\dot{D}_{d_0}\left(100+d_0,f\right)\times\left(\frac{100+d_0}{\text{SSD}+d}\right)^2\times\frac{S_p\left(f_d\right)}{S_p\left(f\right)}. \qquad (12.18)$$

Substituting this result into equation (12.17) we get:

$$\dot{D}_d\left(r,f_d\right)=\dot{D}_{d_0}\left(100+d_0,f\right)\times\left(\frac{100+d_0}{\text{SSD}+d}\right)^2\times\frac{S_p\left(f_d\right)}{S_p\left(f\right)}\times\text{TMR}\left(d,f_d\right). \qquad (12.19)$$

Using equations (12.3) and (12.4) we can write:

$$\dot{D}_d\left(r,f_d\right)=\dot{D}_{d_0}\left(100+d_0,10\right)\times S_c\left(f\right)\times S_p\left(f_d\right)\times\left(\frac{100+d_0}{\text{SSD}+d}\right)^2$$
$$\times\text{TMR}\left(d,f_d\right). \tag{12.20}$$

Notice that when $r = 100$ (i.e., an isocentric treatment) that $f_d = f$, SSD + $d = 100$ and equation (12.20) reduces to equation (12.13) for isocentric treatments. Equation (12.20) is quite general in that it applies to dose rate calculations when the prescription point is at an arbitrary distance.[6]

Once the functional dependencies are clear, equation (12.20) can be written more concisely as:

$$\dot{D}_d=\dot{D}_0\times S_c\times S_p\times\left(\frac{100+d_0}{\text{SSD}+d}\right)^2\times\text{TMR}. \tag{12.21}$$

This is the same equation as (12.20), but it certainly appears much simpler!
Example 12.5 demonstrates an application of equation (12.20).

Example 12.5

A 36 cm long radiation field is necessary to treat the entire spinal column of a patient. The spinal column is at an average of 5.0 cm deep. The patient is treated at an extended SSD of 115 cm. The total distance from the source to the treatment depth is then 120 cm. At a distance of 120 cm, the 30 cm field length diverges to $30\times(120/100)=$ 36 cm. The collimator jaws are set to 30 cm $\times$ 4 cm. The equivalent square field size is $f = 7.06$ cm and $f_d = 7.06\times(120/100)=8.5$ cm. If the 6 MV Mevalac beam is used, calculate the number of monitor units necessary to deliver a dose of 150 cGy. The TMR(5,8.5) = 0.921.

$$\dot{D}_d\left(r,f_d\right)=\dot{D}_{d_0}\left(100+d_0,10\right)\times S_c\left(f\right)\times S_p\left(f_d\right)\times\left(\frac{100+d_0}{\text{SSD}+d}\right)^2\times\text{TMR}\left(d,f_d\right)$$

$$\dot{D}_d\left(120,8.5\right)=\dot{D}_{d_0}\left(100+1.5,10\right)\times S_c\left(7.1\right)\times S_p\left(8.5\right)\times\left(\frac{100+1.5}{115+5}\right)^2\times\text{TMR}\left(5,8.5\right)$$

$$=1.000\times0.986\times0.995\times0.715\times0.921$$

$$=0.646\text{ cGy/MU}$$

and therefore μ = (150 cGy)/(0.646 cGy/MU) = 232 MU.

---

[6]The derivation of eq. (12.20) is not rigorous; we have swept some nuances "under the carpet." The result is, however, generally accepted.

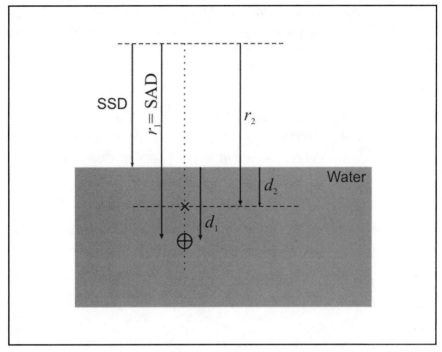

Figure 12.3: The geometry for a calculation of the ratio of the doses at two depths when the SSD is not the standard value.

For an SAD or isocentric treatment, it is useful to be able to calculate the dose at depth d_2 (see Figure 12.3), given the dose at depth d_1.[7] Let us assume that depth d_1 corresponds to the isocenter, then the dose there can be written as $D_{d_1}(\text{SAD}, f)$ and $\text{SSD} = \text{SAD} - d_1$. The distance from the source to depth d_2 is $r_2 = \text{SSD} + d_2$. Then the ratio of the dose at depth d_2 to the dose at depth d_1 is:

$$\frac{D_{d_2}\left(r_2, f_{d_2}\right)}{D_{d_1}\left(r_1, f_{d_1}\right)} = \frac{S_p\left(f_{d_2}\right)}{S_p\left(f_{d_1}\right)} \times \frac{\left(\dfrac{100+d_0}{\text{SSD}+d_2}\right)^2}{\left(\dfrac{100+d_0}{\text{SSD}+d_1}\right)^2} \times \frac{\text{TMR}\left(d_2, f_{d_2}\right)}{\text{TMR}\left(d_1, f_{d_1}\right)}$$

$$= \frac{S_p\left(f_{d_2}\right)}{S_p\left(f_{d_1}\right)} \times \left(\frac{r_1}{r_2}\right)^2 \times \frac{\text{TMR}\left(d_2, f_{d_2}\right)}{\text{TMR}\left(d_1, f_{d_1}\right)}$$

$$\frac{D_{d_2}\left(r_2, f_{d_2}\right)}{D_{d_1}\left(r_1, f_{d_1}\right)} \approx \left(\frac{r_1}{r_2}\right)^2 \times \frac{\text{TMR}\left(d_2, f\right)}{\text{TMR}\left(d_1, f\right)}.$$

(12.22)

---

[7]For an SSD treatment the ratio of dose at different depths is simply given by the ratio of percent depth doses as discussed in chapter 10.

The presence of the ratio $(r_1/r_2)^2$ in equation (12.22) is easily understood when we recall that TMR does not include inverse square attenuation but only attenuation by the intervening matter.

Example 12.6

Refer to Example 12.3. Calculate the dose delivered on the central axis to: (a) a depth of $d_0 = 1.5$ cm and (b) a depth of $d = 10$ cm.

(a) $$\frac{D_{d_2}\left(r_2,f_{d_2}\right)}{D_{d_1}\left(r_1,f_{d_1}\right)} \approx \left(\frac{r_1}{r_2}\right)^2 \times \frac{\text{TMR}\left(d_2,f\right)}{\text{TMR}\left(d_1,f\right)}$$

$d_1 = 5.0$ cm, $d_2 = 1.5$ cm, $r_1 = 100$ cm, $r_2 = 96.5$ cm, TMR(5,15) $= 0.935$, and TMR(1.5,15) $= 1.000$;

therefore $\dfrac{D_{d_2}}{D_{d_1}} \approx \left(\dfrac{100.0}{96.5}\right)^2 \dfrac{1.000}{0.935} = 1.149$ and $D_{d_2} = 207$ cGy.

(b) $d_1 = 5.0$ cm, $d_2 = 10.0$ cm, $r_1 = 100$ cm, $r_2 = 105.0$ cm, TMR(5,15) $= 0.935$ and TMR(10,15) $= 0.811$,

$$\frac{D_{d_2}}{D_{d_1}} \approx \left(\frac{100.0}{105.0}\right)^2 \frac{0.811}{0.935} = 0.787 \text{ and } D_{d_2} = 142 \text{ cGy.}$$

12.4.4   The Equivalence of PDD and TMR Calculations

The percent depth dose and TMR methods described above for MU calculations are equally valid in the sense that in a given situation either one of these can be used; it is just that it is very inconvenient to use PDD when the SSD is not equal to the SAD, and it is inconvenient to use TMR when the SSD is equal to the SAD.

To illustrate the equivalence of the two methods let us repeat Example 12.1 using TMR.

Example 12.7

A dose of 180 cGy is to be delivered at 10 cm deep on the central axis with a 15×15 cm^2 field size and an SSD = 100 cm. The treatment unit is the 18 MV beam from the Mevalac. Calculate the dose rate at the prescription location using TMR data and show that it has the same value as obtained in Example 12.1 using PDD data.

We will compute the dose rate using equation (12.20), which is valid for arbitrary prescription point distance. The value of $r = 110$ cm, $f_d = 15 \times (110/100) = 16.5$ cm, $d_0 = 3.0$ cm and TMR(10,16.5) = 0.897.

$$\dot{D}_d\left(r, f_d\right) = \dot{D}_{d_0}\left(100 + d_0, 10\right) \times S_c\left(f\right) \times S_p\left(f_d\right) \times \left(\frac{100 + d_0}{\text{SSD} + d}\right)^2 \times \text{TMR}\left(d, f_d\right)$$

$$\dot{D}_d\left(110, 16.5\right) = \dot{D}_{d_0}\left(100 + 3.0, 10\right) \times S_c\left(15\right) \times S_p\left(16.5\right) \times \left(\frac{100 + 3.0}{110}\right)^2 \times \text{TMR}\left(5, 16.5\right)$$

$$= 1.000 \times 1.023 \times 1.014 \times 0.877 \times 0.897$$

$$= 0.816 \text{ cGy/MU}$$

This value is the same as the dose rate obtained in Example 12.1. You can see that this method of calculation is much more laborious than the PDD method.

Chapter Summary

- For Co-60 unit, set timer for time: $t = \dfrac{D}{\dot{D}} - \Delta$, where D is the dose

  to be delivered to the prescription point, $\dot{D}$ is the dose rate (dose per *minute,* calculated as shown below) at the prescription point, and Δ is the timer error [as defined in chapter 9, equation (9.1)].

- For linac, set MU, $\mu = \dfrac{D}{\dot{D}}$, where D is the dose to be delivered to the

  prescription point and $\dot{D}$ is the dose rate (dose per MU, calculated as shown below) at the prescription point.

- Meter set calculations depend on normalization conditions in use in the clinic. These are the conditions under which the standard dose rate is specified. Typical normalization conditions are: 1.000 cGy/MU on the central axis in water with SSD = 100 cm, at depth d_0 for a field size of 10×10 cm^2 (as measured at the isocenter). In this case, $\dot{D}_{d_0}(100 + d_0, 10) = 1.000$ cGy/MU.

- Different clinics use different dosimetry systems; some use dose rate in free space and others use dose rate in phantom. Here we use dose rate in phantom.

- Calculation of Dose Rate

  (1) Patient SSD = SAD (usually SSD = 100 cm):

  $$\boxed{\dot{D}_d\left(\mathrm{SAD}+d, f\right) = \dot{D}_{d_0}\left(\mathrm{SAD}+d_0, 10\right) \times S_{c,p}\left(f\right) \times \mathrm{DD}\left(d, f, \mathrm{SAD}\right)}$$

  (12.10)

  (2) Isocentric (to calculate dose at the isocenter):

  $$\boxed{\dot{D}_d\left(\mathrm{SAD}, f\right) = \dot{D}_{d_0}\left(\mathrm{SAD}, 10\right) \times S_{c,p}\left(f\right) \times \mathrm{TMR}\left(d, f\right)} \qquad (12.13)$$

  (3) Arbitrary distance:

  $$\boxed{\dot{D}_d\left(r, f_d\right) = \dot{D}_{d_0}\left(100+d_0, 10\right) \times S_c\left(f\right) \times S_p\left(f_d\right) \times \left(\frac{100+d_0}{\mathrm{SSD}+d}\right)^2 \times \mathrm{TMR}\left(d, f_d\right)}$$

  (12.20)

- All methods are equivalent. In a given situation it is a matter of the input data available and which method is most convenient.

- Extended distance: SSD > SAD: r = SSD + d and the field size at depth d in the patient is

$$f_d = f \times \frac{\mathrm{SSD} + d}{\mathrm{SAD}}.$$

- Ratio of doses at two depths:

$$\frac{D_{d_2}\left(r_2, f_{d_2}\right)}{D_{d_1}\left(r_1, f_{d_1}\right)} \approx \left(\frac{r_1}{r_2}\right)^2 \times \frac{\mathrm{TMR}\left(d_2, f\right)}{\mathrm{TMR}\left(d_1, f\right)}$$

Problems

You may need to consult the data in appendix C to solve some of these problems.

1. For the Mevalac 6 MV beam, 111 MU is delivered.

   (a) Find the dose delivered to a point on the central axis at a depth of 1.5 cm for SSD = 100 cm, f = 10 cm.

   (b) The field size is changed to f = 25 cm. Find the dose at the same point as in part (a).

2. Consult Table 12.1 and verify that $S_{c,p}(20) = S_c(20) \times S_p(20)$ for 18 MV and f = 20 cm.

3. A dose of 200 cGy is to be delivered to a depth of 10 cm SAD using a single 6 MV 10 × 10 cm^2 Mevalac beam. Determine the number of MUs to set.

4. Repeat the MU calculation of Example 12.1 using the 6 MV Mevalac beam instead of the 18 MV beam.

5. A patient is treated with a posterior-anterior (PA) spinal field. The collimator is set to 30 cm × 6 cm. The SSD = 100 cm and the physician wishes to deliver a dose of 150 cGy to a depth of 3.75 cm

on the central axis with the 6 MV beam of the Mevalac. How many MU are necessary to deliver the dose?

6. A patient is to be treated isocentrically with 6 MV photons on the Mevalac with a 6 cm × 20 cm open field to a depth of 3.0 cm. If a dose of 200 cGy is to be delivered to a point at the given depth on the central axis, how many MU should be set on the console?

7. A patient is to be treated on the Mevalac using the 6 MV beam. The treatment is set up with SSD = 100 cm. The collimator setting is 15 cm × 9 cm. Calculate the number of MU necessary to deliver a dose of 100 cGy to a point on the central axis at a depth of 8.0 cm.

8. For problem 4, determine the dose delivered at a depth of $d = 5.0$ cm on the central axis.

9. Repeat the MU calculation of problem 7 using TMR rather than PDD. Do you get the same number of MU?

10. An extended distance is used to treat the entire spinal column of a patient. The spinal column is at an average of 5.0 cm deep. The patient is treated at an extended SSD of 120 cm. The collimator jaws are set to 30 cm × 4 cm. The 6 MV Mevalac beam is used to deliver a dose of 150 cGy. Calculate the number of MU necessary.

11. Refer to Example 12.3. Calculate the dose at a depth of 8.0 cm on the central axis.

Bibliography

Bjärngard, B. E., R. Bar-Deroma, and A. Corrao. (1994). "A survey of methods to calculate monitor settings." *Int J Radiat Oncol Biol Phys* 28(3):749–752.

Khan, F. M. *The Physics of Radiation Therapy,* Fourth Edition. Philadelphia: Lippincott Williams & Wilkins, 2009.

Purdy, J. A., J. F. Williamson, J. W. Wong, and E. E. Klein. "Clinical Photon Beam Dosimetry" in *Advances in Radiation Oncology Physics.* J. A. Purdy (Ed.). AAPM Medical Physics Monograph No. 19. Proceedings of the AAPM 1990 Summer School. Woodbury, NY: American Institute of Physics, 1992.

Stanton, R., and D. Stinson. *Applied Physics for Radiation Oncology, Revised Edition.* Madison, WI: Medical Physics Publishing, 2009.

13   Shaped Fields

13.1   Introduction

To reduce the amount of normal tissue that is exposed to radiation, it is useful to shape the beam aperture so that it conforms closely to the volume containing disease and to block the volume outside this region. Figure 13.1 shows an example of this for a patient with head and neck cancer. The shape of the beam aperture as seen from the point of view of the radiation source is called a "beam's-eye view."

Methods that are used to accomplish field shaping are: asymmetric jaws, hand blocks, cast blocks, and multileaf collimators (MLCs). We will discuss each of these in turn. Following the discussion of the method of field shaping, we turn to the question of MU calculations for shaped fields.

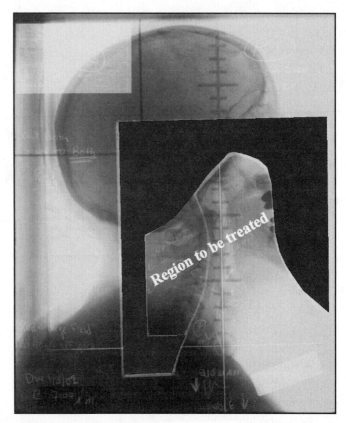

Figure 13.1: A negative of a radiograph of a patient with head and neck cancer taken with a simulator. A radiation oncologist has drawn in the shaped field to be treated. The shaded area is the region to be blocked. The inferior border of the region to be treated will be defined by the collimator jaw. The simulator has wires that project as lines on the radiograph. The location of the wires shows where the collimator jaws will be positioned.

13.2 Field Shaping Methods

13.2.1 Asymmetric Jaws

A linac has two sets of collimator jaws for a total of four jaws (see Figure 13.2 and Figure 13.11). One set defines field length; the other set defines field width. Newer linacs allow each of these jaws to be moved independently of the others, and therefore jaw settings can be asymmetric with respect to the central axis. This can eliminate the need for some types of blocks and it can allow some blocks to be made smaller and lighter. It also allows for easy half-beam blocking, which is useful for tangential breast treatments. In Figure 13.2 the rectangular aperture has dimensions (Y1 + Y2) by (X1 + X2). The transmission through the jaws is less than through blocks, typically 0.5% or less. Therefore the jaws should be used to provide as much of the blocking as possible. In section 13.5 we will discuss MU calculations when asymmetric jaws are used.

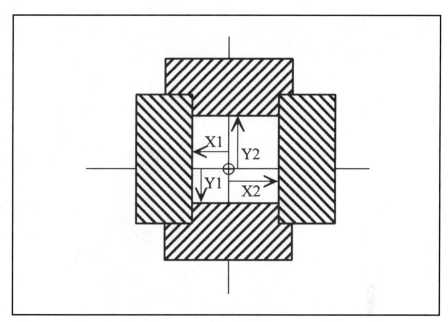

Figure 13.2: Beam's-eye view of the jaws of a linac capable of asymmetric jaw setting. Each jaw can be moved independently of the other. The central axis is denoted by the circle.

13.2.2 Blocks

Hand Blocks

Hand blocks were used in the old days—and they are sometimes still used today on a temporary basis when there is no time to fabricate cast blocks (e.g., for a "sim and treat") and if an MLC is not available. These prefabricated blocks are made of lead or some other high-density material. The blocks are placed on a tray (they can be bolted down) inserted into the accessory holder (see Figure 9.2). The light field is used to position the block over the desired region of the patient's anatomy by looking at the shadow of the block on the patient (see Figure 13.3).

Cast Blocks

Unlike hand blocks, cast blocks are custom-made for each individual patient and are bolted in a fixed position on the block tray. Furthermore cast blocks are "focused" (see Figure 13.4). The blocks are made of a low-melting-temperature metal alloy called "Lipowitz metal." A well-known brand name is Cerrobend®. The density of Lipowitz metal is 9.4 g/cm^3, about 83% of the density of lead. Lipowitz metal is composed of 50% bismuth, 26.7% lead, 13.3% tin, and 10.0% cadmium. Cadmium and lead are toxic heavy metals. Cerrobend melts at 70 °C, quite low compared to the 327 °C melting temperature of lead. It can easily be cast into any shape. Cast blocks are usually designed so that the transmission

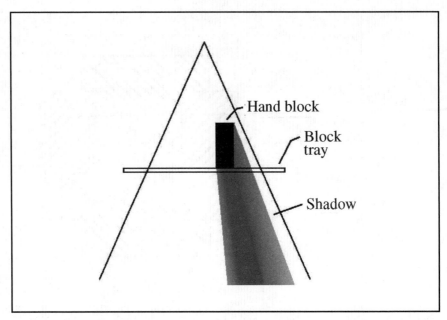

Figure 13.3: Hand blocks are placed on the block tray to "shadow" a portion of the patient's anatomy which is to be spared radiation. The blocks are positioned by hand using the shadow cast by the light field. These blocks are not "focused" and therefore the penumbra around the block will be large.

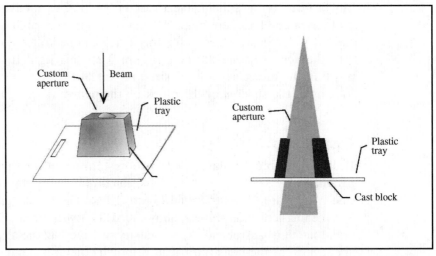

Figure 13.4: On the left is a perspective view of a cast block mounted on a plastic tray. The aperture is custom shaped for the individual patient and the specific beam. The tray slides into the accessory holder on the collimator of the treatment machine (see Figure 9.2). On the right, a cross section through the block shows that the blocks are cut so that they are "focused." This reduces penumbra associated with the block.

through them is 5% or less. How many HVLs does this require? We have learned how to solve problems like this: $(\frac{1}{2})^n = 0.05$, where n is the number of HVLs needed. The solution of this equation is $n = 4.3$. A typical block thickness for Cerrobend is 6 to 8 cm.

The tray attenuates the beam by typically 5% or less. To account for this, we introduce the tray transmission factor (tray factor) TF for block trays. The tray factor ranges between 0.95 and 1.00, depending on beam energy and tray thickness. The tray factors for the Mevalac are 0.956 for the 6 MV beam and 0.970 for the 18 MV beam.

Cast blocks are usually made in a dedicated "mold room." Mold room safety is discussed in chapter 18. Figure 13.5 shows a photograph of a device that is used to construct molds to make cast blocks. A template of the aperture shape is placed on the light table with the position of the intended isocenter located at the center of the table (marked on the table). The template can be a radiographic film such as the one

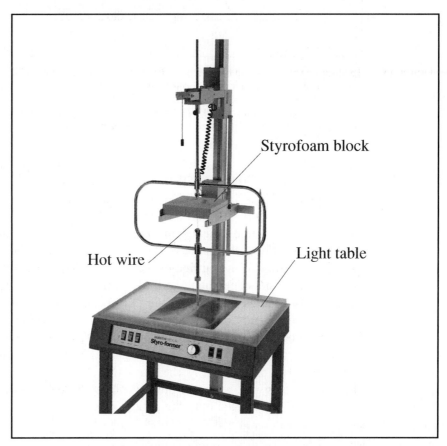

Figure 13.5: A block cutter is used to cut a Styrofoam™ mold, which can then be used to fabricate a cast block. An x-ray film (or DRR) with the field aperture drawn on it is placed on the light table. The Styrofoam block is placed on a ledge. A stylus is used to trace the field aperture. A heated wire connected to the stylus cuts the Styrofoam in the same shape as the aperture. (Courtesy of Best Medical, Springfield, VA, www.TeamBest.com)

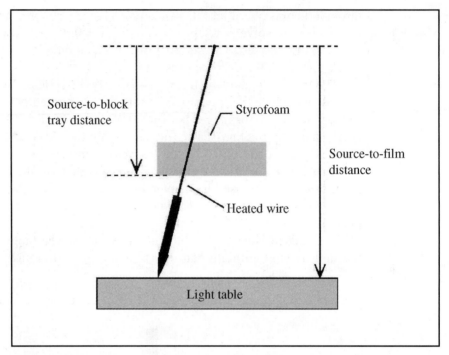

Figure 13.6: The base of the Styrofoam block is placed at the same distance from the wire pivot point as the tray is from the linac radiation source. The assembly is positioned so that the light table is at the same distance as the source-to-film distance. In this way, the aperture will be the correct size and the block will have the same divergence as the radiation beam. (Courtesy of Best Medical, Springfield, VA, www.TeamBest.com)

shown in Figure 13.1 or it can be a computer-generated template (digitally reconstructed radiograph, or DRR) from a treatment planning system. For a radiographic film, the physician actually draws the aperture on the film (using a China Marker™ or wax pencil). When this film is exposed, the distance from the x-ray focal spot to the film is recorded. A Styrofoam™ block is placed on a ledge above the table. A stylus attached to a heated wire is used to trace the outline of the aperture. The heated wire cuts the Styrofoam in the same shape as the outline (see Figure 13.6). The cut Styrofoam serves as a mold. Molten Cerrobend is poured into this mold. After the Cerrobend cools and solidifies, the Styrofoam is broken away. The cast block is then bolted to a tray for insertion into the collimator. The bottom of the Styrofoam block is placed at the same distance from the heated wire pivot point as the block tray is from the x-ray source on the linac. In this way, when the block is placed in the linac beam, the size of the aperture projected onto the patient will be correct.

13.2.3 Multileaf Collimators

A multileaf collimator (MLC) is used for field or portal shaping without the need for custom-made cast blocks. The MLC consists of a series of motorized tungsten leaves (see Figures 13.7 through 13.10). The leaves

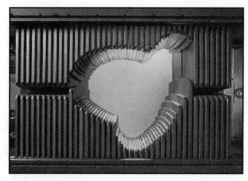

Figure 13.7: A close-up photo of MLC leaves looking up into the collimator head. (Copyright © 2010, Varian Medical Systems, Inc. All rights reserved.). See COLOR PLATE 2.

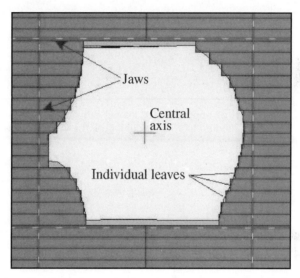

Figure 13.8: An MLC portal outline (beam's-eye view) as shown on a computer display. This MLC is a tertiary system. The position of the secondary jaws is shown. There are locations where the leaves overlap the desired treatment outline and other spots where they underlap. This produces a "scalloped" contour. The leaf width is 1.0 cm projected to isocenter. Varian SHAPER program software. (Copyright © 2010, Varian Medical Systems, Inc. All rights reserved.). See COLOR PLATE 3.

move under computer control. MLC-shaped fields may be able to replace 85% of custom cast blocks. An MLC aperture cannot easily replace an "island block," such as might be used to shield a kidney from radiation delivered to the surrounding abdomen.

MLC beam shapes are described in terms of the coordinates of the leaf ends (see Figures 13.8 and 13.10). Beam shapes can be specified in two ways. If the portal outline is drawn on a radiographic plane film as in Figure 13.1, then this film can be placed on a digitizing tablet and the shape "digitized" into a computer. The second method is to define the beam's-eye portal outline with treatment planning software. In either case, the computer calculates the positions of the leaf ends and stores the data in a file for that patient. The collimator is sometimes rotated to get an optimum fit to the desired beam outline. The file containing the

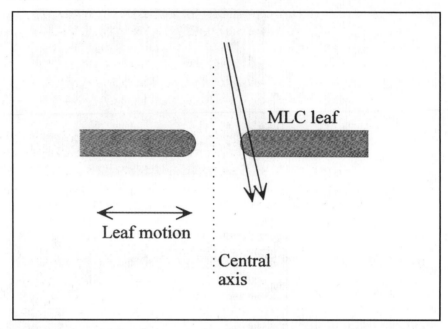

Figure 13.9: A side view of opposing MLC leaves, showing partial transmission through a rounded leaf edge, leading to a larger penumbra than if the leaves were focused.

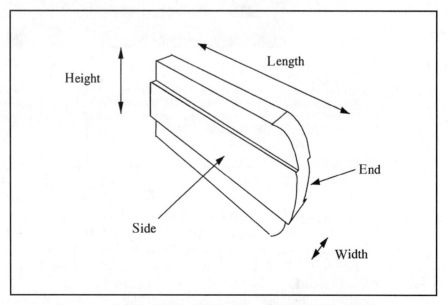

Figure 13.10: A perspective view of an MLC leaf with the nomenclature used to describe the leaves. (Reprinted from AAPM Report No. 72, © 2001, with permission from American Association of Physicists in Medicine (AAPM).)

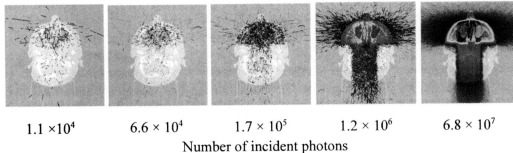

1.1×10^4 6.6×10^4 1.7×10^5 1.2×10^6 6.8×10^7

Number of incident photons

COLOR PLATE 1. Figure 7.11: Monte Carlo calculation of the dose distribution from a 6 MV anterior and two lateral opposed beams using Peregrine software. The number of particle histories is written under each frame. A large number of particle histories is necessary for an accurate dose calculation. (Courtesy of Lawrence Livermore National Laboratory)

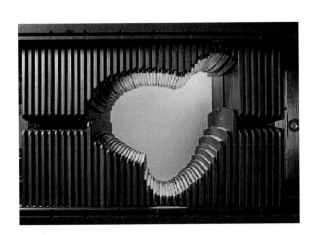

COLOR PLATE 2. Figure 13.7: A close-up photo of MLC leaves looking up into the collimator head. (Copyright © 2010, Varian Medical Systems, Inc. All rights reserved.)

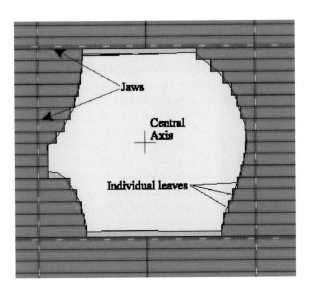

COLOR PLATE 3. Figure 13.8: An MLC portal outline (beam's-eye view) as shown on a computer display. This MLC is a tertiary system. The position of the secondary jaws is shown. There are locations where the leaves overlap the desired treatment outline and other spots where they underlap. This produces a "scalloped" contour. The leaf width is 1.0 cm projected to isocenter. Varian SHAPER program software. (Copyright © 2010, Varian Medical Systems, Inc. All rights reserved.)

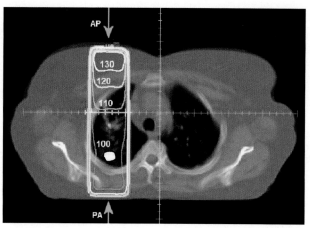

COLOR PLATE 4. Figure 14.14: Two 6 MV parallel-opposed beams are used to treat a posterior lung tumor (white for visualization). The isocenter is at the center of the tumor. Both beams deliver an equal dose to the isocenter (50%). The dose distribution is normalized to 100% at the isocenter. Because the tumor lies so far posterior, the dose to anterior tissue is high. The maximum dose is 139%.

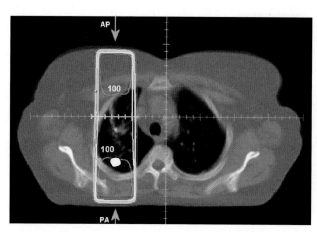

COLOR PLATE 5. Figure 14.15: This is the same as COLOR PLATE 4 except the beams have now been weighted to reduce the excess dose to the anterior tissue. The PA beam has been weighted 65% and the AP beam 35% at the isocenter. This means that 65% of the dose (at isocenter) is delivered by the PA beam and 35% by the AP beam. The high-dose region in the anterior tissue has now been reduced.

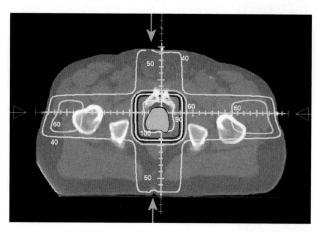

COLOR PLATE 6. Figure 14.25: A four-field box dose distribution resulting from four beams. The beams are all 15 MV equally weighted. The isocenter is at the center of the coordinate system where the dose has been normalized to 100%. The isodoses are displayed in increments of 10% from 100% down to 40%. Each tick mark on the grid represents 1 cm. This is a prostate treatment. The prostate is represented by the uniformly gray structure at the center of the axial slice. The dose is high and uniform where the beams overlap and relatively low elsewhere.

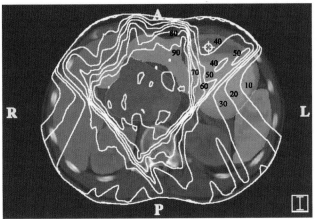

COLOR PLATE 7. Figure 14.29: The dose distribution on an axial CT slice. We are concerned with the dose distribution in the patient's stomach, which is anterior and on the patient's left (your right). The isodose lines are labeled in this region (in percent). In section 14.7, we calculate the "dose area histogram" for the stomach.

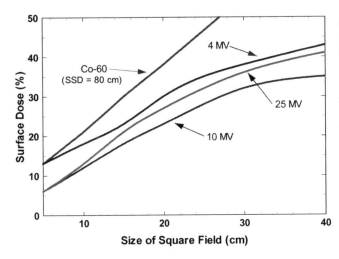

COLOR PLATE 8. Figure 14.40: Surface dose as a function of field size for different energy beams. The SSD = 100 for all beams except Co-60. The 10 MV curve is below the 25 MV curve. (Data taken from Khan, F. M. *The Physics of Radiation Therapy*, Third Edition, 2003.)

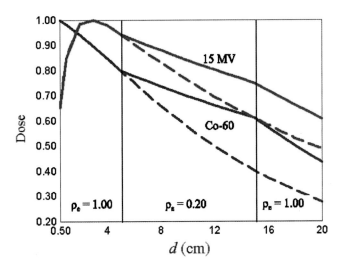

COLOR PLATE 9. Figure 14.48: The depth dose as a function of the geometric depth for a 10×10 cm^2 Co-60 beam and for a 10×10 cm^2 15 MV beam in the presence of an inhomogeneous (solid curves) slab 10 cm thick with a relative electron density of 0.20. The dashed curves are the depth dose values, assuming a homogeneous water phantom. The corrected depth dose is based on equation (14.19). The effect of the inhomogeneity on the Co-60 beam is greater than for the 15 MV beam because the Co-60 beam has a steeper gradient and is therefore affected more by the absence of matter. Nonequilibrium effects are not included in this figure.

COLOR PLATE 10. Figure 16.8: A wide array of applicators are available for brachytherapy. (Courtesy of Nucletron B.V., Veenendaal, The Netherlands)

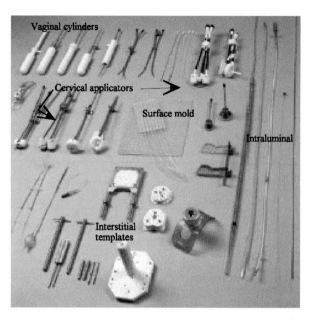

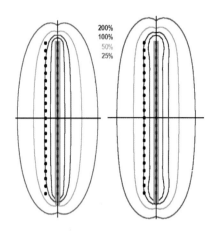

COLOR PLATE 11. Figure 16.14: The dose distribution around a linear array of sources. The vertical shaded tube is a catheter containing the sources. There are 21 sources in each catheter, spaced 0.5 cm apart. The total active source length is therefore 10 cm. Next to each catheter is a series of dots arranged vertically. The dots are at a distance of 1.0 cm from the catheters and serve as reference markers. The dose has been normalized to 100% at a distance of 1.0 cm from the center of the active length of the catheters. The goal is to treat to 100% at all of the marker points. The sources in the catheter on the left all have equal activity. The sources in the catheter on the right do not have equal activity; the activity is higher at the ends than in the middle. Note that the 100% line on the left is "pinched" in near the ends of the catheter, whereas the 100% line on the right uniformly covers the desired treatment length.

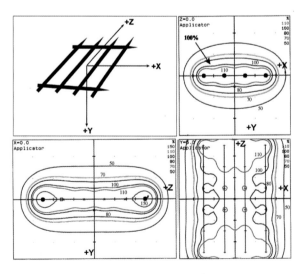

COLOR PLATE 12. Figure 16.17: The interstitial 3×5 cm^2 planar implant discussed in Example 16.6. The interior needles are parallel to the Z axis and the crossing needles are parallel to the X axis. The activity is distributed according to Paterson-Parker rules. The dose distribution is shown in three planes. The distance between tick marks is 1.0 cm. In the $Z = 0$ plane, the 100% isodose line can be seen to be about 1 cm thick in the Y direction and to extend about 0.5 cm beyond the peripheral needles for a total width of about 4 cm. In the $X = 0$ plane, the 100% line is seen to bulge where the crossing needles intersect this plane. The $Y = 5$ plane shows the dose distribution in a plane 5 mm above the plane of the needles. It seems plausible that the dose in this plane is constant over the 3×5 cm^2 area to within $\pm 10\%$.

WIRE DIAMETER
0.59 mm

Ir-192 LINE SOURCE
DIAMETER: 0.34 mm
LENGTH: 5 mm

WIRE: NiTi
SUPERELASTIC ALLOY

COLOR PLATE 13. Figure 16.28: HDR Ir-192 source embedded in wire. (Copyright © 2010, Varian Medical Systems, Inc.)

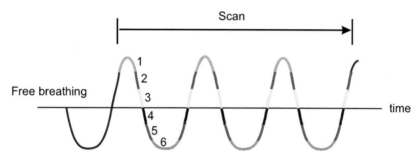

COLOR PLATE 14. Figure 19.20: Retrospective 4D CT. The patient breathes freely while a very low pitch scan is acquired. Every portion of the relevant anatomy is imaged through a minimum of one respiratory cycle. The breathing cycle is divided into phases. In this figure there are a total of six phases. Eight to ten phases are common. All axial images acquired during a particular phase are grouped together into sets.

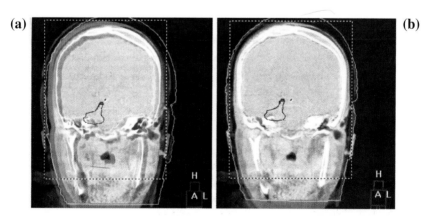

COLOR PLATE 15. Figure 19.33: Cone-beam image-guided radiation therapy. (a) A patient's cranium as imaged with the Elekta XVI (x-ray volume imaging) system shown in Figure 19.32. Contours of a brain tumor (in red) have been imported from the treatment planning CT. This is the view prior to image registration. The planning CT image is in pink and the cone beam CT is in green. There is a clear mismatch between the two image sets. (b) This is the same as (a) except that this is the image after registration. The patient is now positioned very accurately for treatment. (Courtesy of Elekta, Norcross, GA)

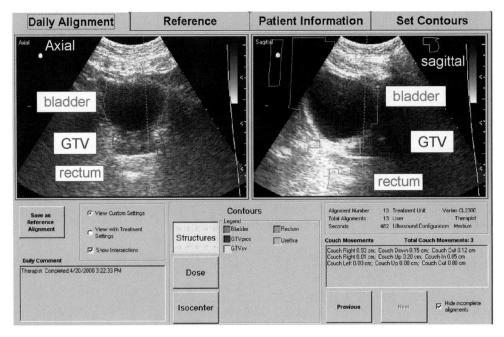

COLOR PLATE 16. Figure 19.35: A screen capture from the NOMOS BAT (B-mode Acquisition and Targeting) ultrasound IGRT system. The image on the left is an axial image. A sagittal image is shown on the right. The operator has superimposed contours of the bladder, GTV, and rectum from the treatment plan. These contours have been aligned with the corresponding structures in the ultrasound images. The shift necessary to bring about this alignment on the computer is then used to calculate how the patient should be moved. This information is shown in the box on the lower right. (Courtesy of Best Medical, Springfield, VA, www.TeamBest.com)

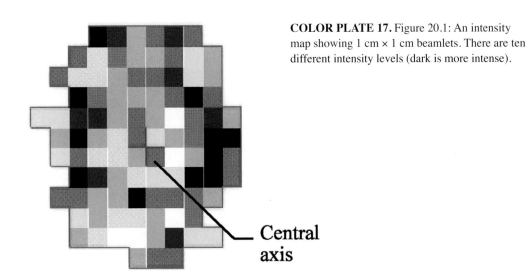

COLOR PLATE 17. Figure 20.1: An intensity map showing 1 cm × 1 cm beamlets. There are ten different intensity levels (dark is more intense).

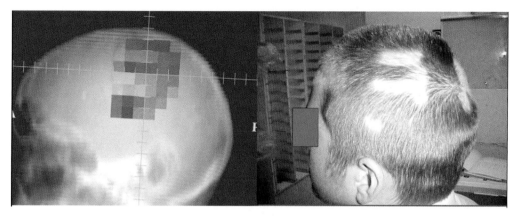

COLOR PLATE 18. Figure 20.2: Intensity map for an IMRT beam superimposed on a patient DRR (left) and reflected in hair loss on the patient's scalp (right).

COLOR PLATE 19.
Figure 20.4: The dose distribution in a geometric phantom illustrates the power of IMRT. The target is the hollow sphere with an organ at risk inside (not shown). Seven gantry angles and five different intensity levels were used. The 100% isodose line wraps tightly around both the inside and outside of the sphere giving outstanding conformity.

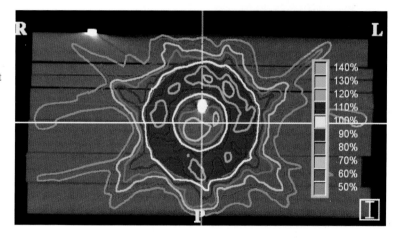

The uniformity of the dose distribution in the target however is relatively poor. The hot spot is 148%. The phantom is a stack of square slabs of virtual water.

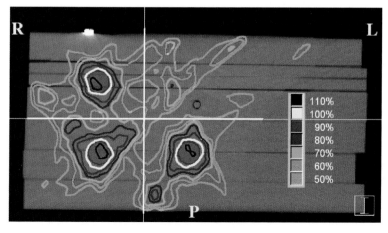

COLOR PLATE 20.
Figure 20.5: The dose distribution in a geometric phantom with three targets. The targets are cylinders with axes perpendicular to the page. The conformality is impressive considering that only a single isocenter was used. Seven gantry angles were used. The maximum dose in the targets is 115%. The intersection of the white lines shows the location of the isocenter.

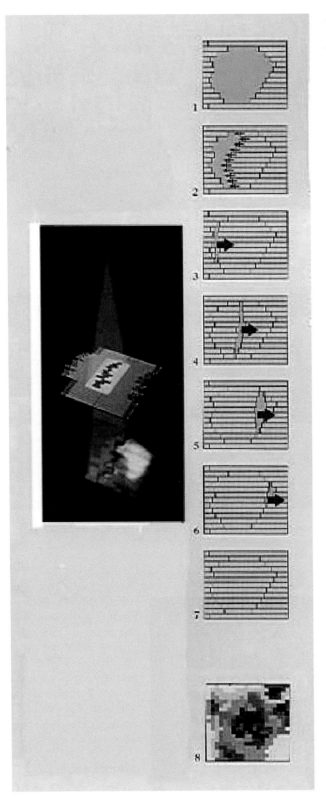

COLOR PLATE 21. Figure 20.8: Illustration of DMLC IMRT delivery. The illustration on the left side of the figure shows the cone beam shaped by the MLC at some instant. The first frame at the top on the right shows an open field used for portal verification. The second frame shows the leaves closing down in preparation for treatment delivery. In frames 3 through 7 the beam is turned on and the "window" is shown sweeping across the field. The dose rate may vary during the sweep. The frame on the bottom right shows the resulting intensity map for this port. (Copyright © 2010, Varian Medical Systems, Inc. All rights reserved.)

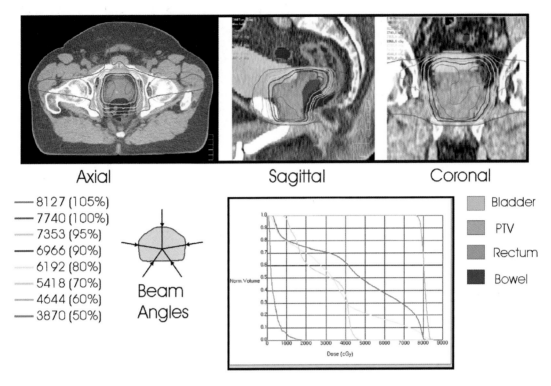

Axial   Sagittal   Coronal

— 8127 (105%)
— 7740 (100%)
— 7353 (95%)
— 6966 (90%)
— 6192 (80%)
— 5418 (70%)
— 4644 (60%)
— 3870 (50%)

Beam Angles

Bladder
PTV
Rectum
Bowel

COLOR PLATE 22. Figure 20.13: Prostate IMRT plan using five 18 MV co-planar beams. The prescription dose is 7740 cGy.

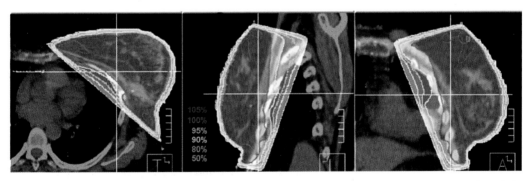

105%
100%
95%
90%
80%
50%

COLOR PLATE 23. Figure 20.14: Breast aperture-based optimized treatment plan. From left to right: axial slice, sagittal slice, and coronal view. The white lines in the axial view show the location of the sagittal and coronal cut planes. The dose distribution is displayed as a "color wash." The red areas have doses between 100% and 105%. The color legend is shown in the middle (sagittal) frame. The beams are two 6 MV tangent beams matched at the posterior border as described in chapter 14, section 14.14. The segments for the lateral beam are shown in COLOR PLATE 24.

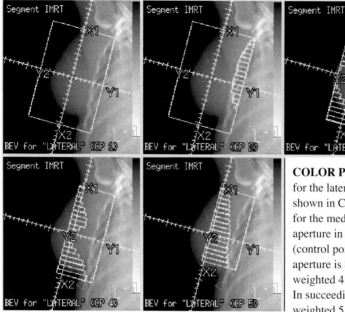

COLOR PLATE 24. Figure 20.15: Apertures for the lateral beam of the dose distribution shown in COLOR PLATE 23. The apertures for the medial beam are similar. The first aperture in the upper left corner is an open field (control point 1: CP1). The weighting of this aperture is 81.3%. In the second aperture (CP2, weighted 4.6%) some of the lung is blocked. In succeeding apertures (CP3, CP4, and CP5, weighted 5.4%, 3.5%, and 5.2%, respectively) anterior portions of the breast, which are thinner, are blocked to suppress hot spots there.

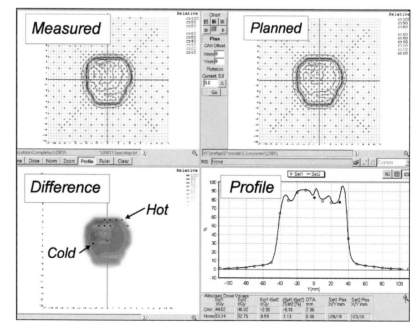

COLOR PLATE 25. Figure 20.17: MapCHECK™ screen showing the comparison between measured IMRT field (AP prostate) labeled "Measured" and the dose distribution calculated by the treatment planning system (labeled "Planned"). The device shown in Figure 20.16 was used to acquire these data. The criteria for acceptance are that the percent difference is 3% or less and the distance to agreement is 3.0 mm or less. The diodes that fail to meet these criteria are shown as "hot" or "cold" dots in the "Difference" window on the lower left. In this example, 96% of the diodes pass and the difference between the measured and calculated dose at the norm point is 1.1%. A profile is shown in the lower right window. This is a profile along the green vertical line shown in the "Difference" window. The solid line is the calculated profile and the dots are the measured values.

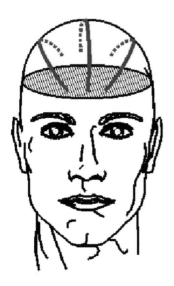

COLOR PLATE 26. Figure 20.23: Dynamic stereotactic radiosurgery treatment technique using a linear accelerator to create multiple non-coplanar arcs. Each arc corresponds to gantry rotation at a separate couch angle. The beam is on while the gantry is rotating. If a jet of red ink were issuing from the collimator, it would trace the patterns shown on the patient's scalp (beam entry trace). Only three arcs are shown for clarity. Typically 4 to 11 arcs are used.

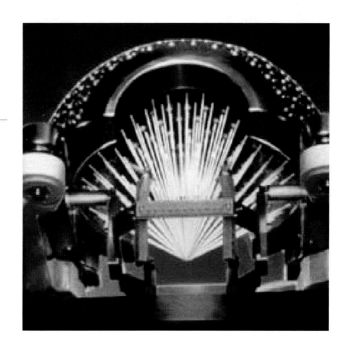

COLOR PLATE 27. Figure 20.27: Light converging on the unit center as it traverses the collimator plugs in a Gamma Knife helmet. The head frame is in the foreground at the bottom. The patient target is positioned at the unit center. (Courtesy of Elekta, Norcross, GA)

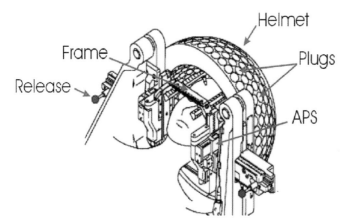

COLOR PLATE 28. Figure 20.28: The Gamma Knife® frame and helmet are attached to the end of the couch. The 201 plugs in the helmet provide final collimation. Four helmets are available with plug aperture diameters of 4, 8, 14, and 18 mm. The automatic positioning system (APS) will move the patient with respect to the unit center. The patient is removed by pulling on the release knob shown. (Courtesy of Elekta, Norcross, GA)

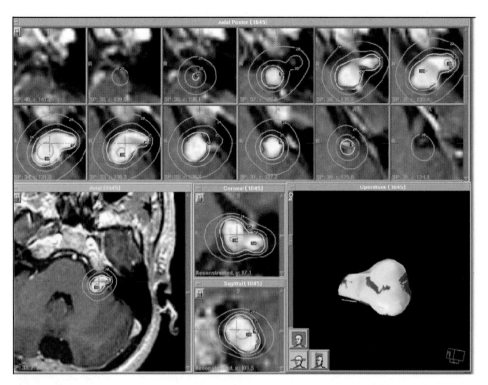

COLOR PLATE 29. Figure 20.30: Gamma Knife treatment plan. The lower left-hand panel shows an axial image zoomed out. The upper panel shows various zoomed axial slices covering the inferior to superior extent of the target. The two middle frames on the bottom show a coronal and sagittal slice. The window on the lower right shows a 3-D rendering. The target contour is red. The yellow contour is the prescription isodose line (50%). The other two isodose lines are 35% and 20%. The 50% prescription isodose surface is highly conformal. (Courtesy of Elekta, Norcross, GA)

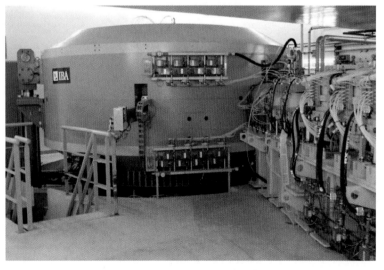

COLOR PLATE 30. Figure 20.37: Photograph of an IBA isochronous cyclotron used for proton radiation therapy. The beam line is visible on the right. (Courtesy of Penn Medicine, Philadelphia, PA, and IBA, Louvain-la-Neuve, Belgium; www.iba-worldwide.com)

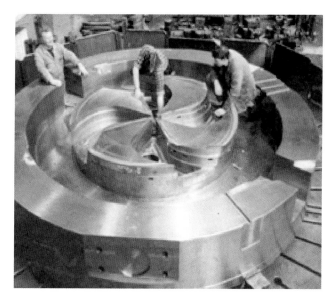

COLOR PLATE 31. Figure 20.38: Magnet yoke for an isochronous cyclotron showing spiral-shaped magnetic pole pieces. (Courtesy of IBA, Louvain-la-Neuve, Belgium; www.iba-worldwide.com)

COLOR PLATE 32. Figure 20.41: A passive scattering system for a proton beam. The first scatterer is a set of movable lead wedges. This creates a Gaussian beam profile. The second scatterer is thicker at the center than at the periphery and functions like a flattening filter. The lead provides the scattering and the polycarbonate is shaped to ensure that the beam energy does not vary laterally. Passage through the second scatterer results in a flattened beam profile and a uniform energy across the beam. The beam then traverses a patient-specific collimator and compensator. The compensator is designed so that the range of the protons corresponds to the location of the distal edge of the target (see also COLOR PLATE 34).

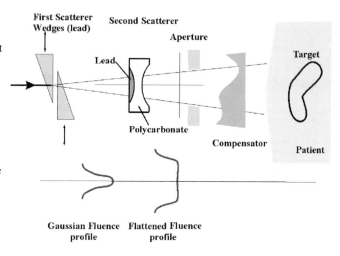

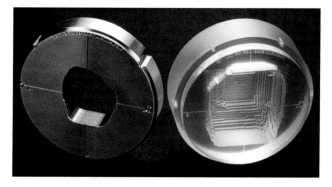

COLOR PLATE 33. Figure 20.42: A patient-specific aperture (left) and range compensator (right) for proton therapy. The aperture shapes the beam laterally and the range compensator shapes the distal edge of the Bragg peak. The aperture is made of brass. These must be stored for a time after use because they become activated. They are then recycled. The compensators are made out of acrylic. (Courtesy of *the.decimal point*; http://www.thedotdecimal.com)

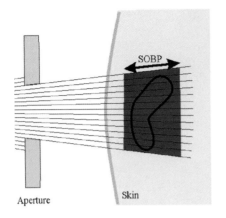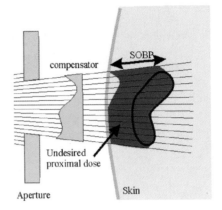

COLOR PLATE 34. Figure 20.43: Customized patient proton treatment with a passive scattering system. The diagram on the left shows the spread-out Bragg Peak (SOBP) prior to the insertion of a compensator. The diagram on the right shows the SOBP after the insertion of a customized compensator. The conformity with the distal edge of the tumor is excellent, but the shift in the SOBP produces unwanted dose proximal to the target.

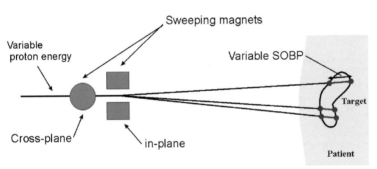

COLOR PLATE 35. Figure 20.44: In proton active scanning, the target is "painted" with a pencil beam steered by a set of orthogonal magnets. The energy of the pencil beam is changed dynamically so that at any given lateral position the distal edge of the SOBP corresponds to the distal boundary of the target.

COLOR PLATE 36. Figure 20.46: Photograph of a proton therapy beam line. Quadrupole magnets in the beam line provide focusing. (Courtesy of Penn Medicine, Philadelphia, PA, and IBA, Louvain-la-Neuve, Belgium; www.iba-worldwide.com)

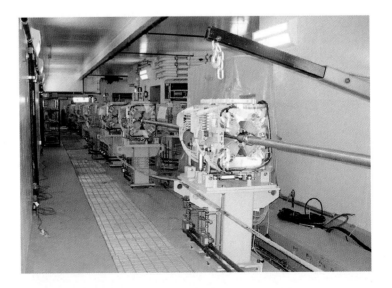

COLOR PLATE 37. Figure 20.47: The gantry of an IBA proton therapy cyclotron. The entire structure rotates on the two rings shown. The beam enters from the right at the center of the gantry structure. To appreciate the scale, notice the man standing in the lower right. (Courtesy of Penn Medicine, Philadelphia, PA, and IBA, Louvain-la-Neuve, Belgium; www.iba-worldwide.com)

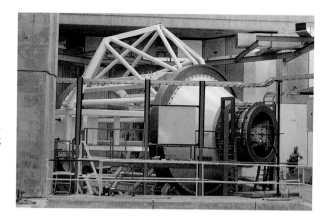

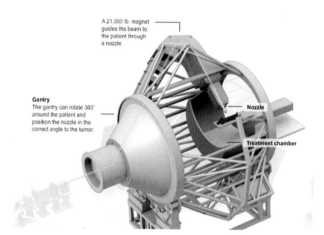

COLOR PLATE 38. Figure 20.48: Diagram showing a drawing of the gantry in the photo in COLOR PLATE 37. This illustrates the path of the beam and shows the treatment chamber with the beam nozzle. (Courtesy of IBA, Louvain-la-Neuve, Belgium; www.iba-worldwide.com)

COLOR PLATE 39. Figure 20.50: The effect of a thin sliver inhomogeneity. In (a) there has been no modification of the compensator to account for the inhomogeneity for proton therapy. As a result, there is a cold spot in the target volume. (b) The compensator has been modified to adjust for the presence of the bone sliver. (c) shows what can happen if there is even a slight misalignment of the compensator. In (d) we see what is called "opened" compensation. The target is fully covered in the event of a small misalignment but the critical structure receives some dose. (Reprinted from Goitein, M., A. J.

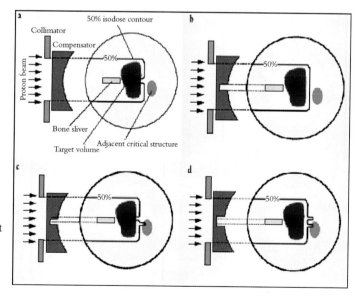

Lomax, and E. S. Pedroni, Fig. 1, p. 46, "Treating Cancer with Protons." *Physics Today* 55(9): 45–50, © 2002 with permission from the American Institute of Physics.)

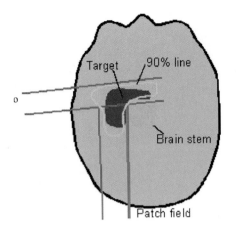

COLOR PLATE 40. Figure 20.52: A proton therapy "patch" field is used in this illustration to fill in coverage of a tumor that wraps around the brain stem. The distal edge of the patch field is adjusted to coincide with the edge of the lateral beam.

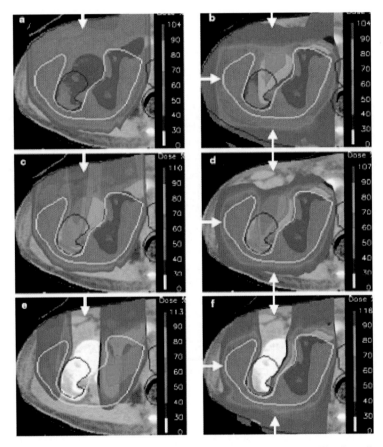

COLOR PLATE 41. Figure 20.53: Treatment of Ewing's sarcoma with protons. The dose distribution is shown by a colorwash (see legend on the right of each frame). The target is the yellow contour. Critical structures are outlined in red. The arrows show beam directions. In (a) a single passively scattered beam is used. Note the good conformity laterally and at the distal edge of the target but not at the proximal target border. In (b) we have a three-field dose distribution from passively scattered beams. (c) shows a single field delivered by an actively scanned beam. (d) shows three fields delivered by actively scanned beams. Each of these fields delivers a near uniform dose. (e) One of the intensity-modulated fields shown in panel (f). Panel (f) shows a three-field optimized IMPT plan. The dose distribution is extraordinarily conformal. (Reprinted from Goitein, M., A. J. Lomax, and E. S. Pedroni, Fig. 4, p. 50, "Treating Cancer with Protons." *Physics Today* 55(9):45–50, © 2002 with permission from the American Institute of Physics.)

leaf positions is loaded into the linac control computer, which will then drive the leaves to the required locations. The position of each leaf must be monitored by the linac to ensure that it is where it is supposed to be.

An MLC offers the following advantages over cast blocks:

(1) Fabrication of cast blocks is a time-consuming, laborious process which requires working with toxic heavy metals. Furthermore, changes to a beam portal can be made rapidly, efficiently, and accurately with an MLC.

(2) The MLC eliminates the need to lift and mount heavy cast blocks on the treatment head. A blocking tray and block can weigh over 25 pounds. Treatment with an MLC is faster because it is not necessary to mount a cast block.

(3) There is no need to store bulky cast blocks.

(4) Transmission is generally lower through MLC leaves than through a cast block. As an example, the transmission through the Varian MLC leaves is approximately 2% (although interleaf transmission is higher).

(5) The use of an MLC makes intensity-modulated radiation therapy (IMRT) possible (see chapter 20).

Depending on the manufacturer, the MLC either replaces one set of jaws or is used as a tertiary field-shaping device, just like a cast block (see Figure 13.11). If the MLC is described as a tertiary field-shaping device, it is below the jaws. The term "tertiary" is used because the field is shaped by: (1) the primary collimator, (2) movable secondary jaws, and finally, by (3) a block or an MLC. A tertiary MLC reduces the available clearance between the head of the linac and the isocenter, decreasing the collision-free zone for patient treatment. The Varian MLC is a tertiary field-shaping device, whereas Elekta uses the MLC to replace the upper jaw and the Siemens MLC replaces the lower jaws. For a tertiary MLC the leaves can be withdrawn entirely and the jaws can be used to define rectangular fields.

The number of leaves ranges from approximately 52 to 120. They are arranged in opposing pairs as shown in Figure 13.9. The leaf width, as projected to the isocenter, ranges from 0.4 cm to 2.0 cm. The most common leaf width is 1.0 cm. Smaller leaf width gives more conformal coverage (less scalloping, see Figure 13.8) but more leaves are required. Some physicians prefer cast blocks for small, highly shaped fields.

Because of limits on the motion of the MLC leaves, the largest useable MLC field may be smaller than the largest field that can be set with the jaws. One manufacturer with a 52-leaf MLC is limited to a 26 cm × 40 cm field. The 26 cm side is in the direction of the leaf width. The ends of the leaves can be rounded, as in Figure 13.9, or they can have a focused shape to reduce penumbra associated with the leaves.

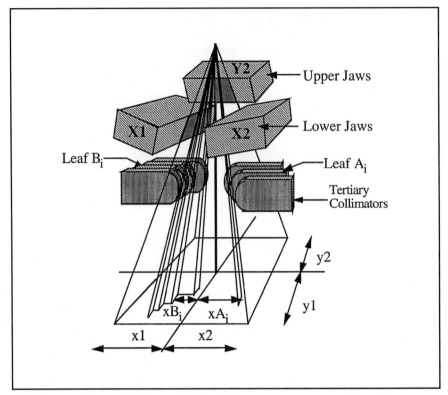

Figure 13.11: An MLC that provides tertiary beam shaping. The primary collimator is not shown. The secondary collimation is provided by the jaws. For clarity, jaw Y1 is not shown. The MLC provides final field shaping. (Reprinted from AAPM Report No. 72, © 2001, with permission from American Association of Physicists in Medicine (AAPM).)

For some field-shaping applications it is necessary for leaves to travel across the midplane. This is sometimes called "overtravel." One manufacturer has an overtravel of 10 cm.

The transmission through a leaf (intraleaf transmission) of a tertiary MLC is approximately 2%, varying somewhat with energy. Transmission between leaves (interleaf transmission) is larger. Interleaf transmission is reduced by introducing steps or a tongue-and-groove arrangement, as shown in Figure 13.12.

13.3 Dose Rate Calculations for Shaped Fields: Symmetric Jaws, Central Axis

Fields that are shaped are sometimes called *blocked* or *irregular* fields because they are not generally rectangular (see Figure 13.13). Fields that are not blocked are sometimes called *open* fields. So far, our dose rate calculations have been restricted to open fields (no field shaping) and to points on the central axis, but, in practice, shaped fields are almost always used. We need to extend our calculation technique to include dose delivered along the central axis for shaped fields and later for dose delivered to points off the central axis.

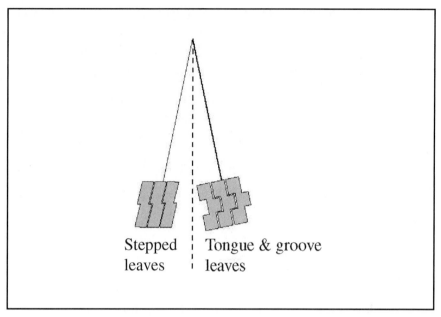

Figure 13.12: Side view of two different types of MLC leaf shapes used to reduce leakage between leaves. In this diagram, leaf motion is perpendicular to the page.

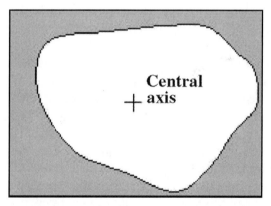

Figure 13.13: Beam's-eye view of a shaped field. The shaded region is blocked. We wish to determine the dose/MU on the central axis at some depth d.

Figure 13.13 is a "beam's-eye view" of a shaped radiation field. Our goal is to determine the dose rate on the central axis at some arbitrary depth for such a field. From the dose rate we can either calculate MU when the dose is specified or we can calculate the dose when the MU are specified. Recall that the absorbed dose at a point consists of a primary component and a scatter component. Provided that the central axis is not blocked, the primary component of the dose is assumed to be unaffected by the blocking. The scatter contribution however will clearly be reduced by the blocking. The amount of reduction in the scatter component will depend on where the field is blocked and on how much of the field is blocked. The scatter contribution also depends on energy and depth. The scatter contribution to the dose is greater for a lower-energy beam than for a high-energy beam. For these reasons, field blocking has the largest effect on the dose rate for highly blocked low-energy beams.

The equations of the previous chapter for dose rate require some modification for shaped fields. We will assume tertiary blocking throughout unless otherwise stated. We assume that tertiary field shaping does not affect collimator scatter and that S_c depends only on jaw setting f. Phantom scatter is affected by the amount of material irradiated. When part of a field is blocked to achieve field shaping, the value of S_p will change. The TAR, TMR, and PDD values will also change when any blocking is introduced to shape a field. To account for these changes, we use an effective or equivalent blocked field size denoted f'_d. This is the side length of the equivalent square of the shaped field at depth d *in the patient.* If f_d is the equivalent square field size of the jaw setting, then for a blocked field $f'_d < f_d$. The correct value of the TMR for a shaped field is TMR(d, f'_d). Equation (12.20) for the dose rate should now be written:

$$\dot{D}_d\left(r, f'_d\right) = \dot{D}_{d_0}\left(100 + d_0, 10\right) \times \left(\frac{100 + d_0}{\mathrm{SSD} + d}\right)^2 \times S_c\left(f\right) \times S_p\left(f'_d\right)$$
$$\times \mathrm{TMR}\left(d, f'_d\right) \times \mathrm{TF}, \qquad (13.1)$$

where $r = \mathrm{SSD} + d$ is the distance from the source to the point of calculation, f is the equivalent square field size for the jaw setting as measured at isocenter, f'_d is the equivalent square field size for the blocked field in the patient at depth d, and TF is the tray transmission factor (use TF = 1.00 for MLC field shaping). Notice that the head scatter factor for tertiary field shaping depends on the collimator jaw setting f and therefore is assumed to be unaffected by the blocking. The TMR depends on the equivalent field size f'_d of the blocked field. This equation is valid for any SSD provided that f'_d is defined at depth d in the patient. Equation (13.1) applies for tertiary blocking such as found on a Varian linac. If the MLC replaces one set of jaws (Elekta and Siemens), then S_c should be calculated for the blocked field size at isocenter.

For percent depth dose calculations the modified version of equation (12.10) is:

$$\dot{D}_d\left(r, f'_d\right) = \dot{D}_{d_0}\left(100 + d_0, 10\right) \times S_c\left(f\right) \times S_p\left(f'_{d_0}\right) \times \mathrm{DD}\left(d, f'_0, 100\right) \times \mathrm{TF}, \quad (13.2)$$

where, f'_0 is the blocked field size at the skin surface. Notice that the field size for the phantom scatter factor is the field size in the patient at depth d_0 and the field size for the DD is the blocked field size at the surface of the patient (f'_0).

The most difficult part of blocked field dose rate calculations is the determination of the value of f'_d, or equivalently, the value of $\mathrm{TMR}(d, f'_d)$ or $\mathrm{DD}(d, f'_0, 100)$. We defer this problem briefly to first consider an example.

Example 13.1

A patient is to be treated with an isocentric blocked field 6 MV Mevalac beam. The prescription calls for a dose from this beam of 90 cGy to mid depth. The patient thickness is 24 cm. The jaw setting is 18.0×18.0 cm^2. The tray factor for the 6 MV beam is 0.956. The side of the equivalent square for the irregular field size is $f'_d = 17$ cm. Calculate the required MU.

$$\dot{D}_d\left(r, f'_d\right) = \dot{D}_{d_0}\left(100 + d_0, 10\right) \times \left(\frac{100 + d_0}{\mathrm{SSD} + d}\right)^2 \times S_c\left(f\right) \times S_p\left(f'_d\right)$$
$$\times \mathrm{TMR}\left(d, f'_d\right) \times \mathrm{TF}$$
$$= 1.000 \times \left(\frac{100 + 1.5}{100}\right)^2 \times S_c\left(18\right) \times S_p\left(17\right) \times \mathrm{TMR}\left(12, 17\right) \times \mathrm{TF}$$
$$= 1.000 \times 1.030 \times 1.026 \times 1.018 \times 0.767 \times 0.956$$
$$= 0.789 \ \mathrm{cGy/MU}$$

$$\mu = \frac{D}{\dot{D}} = \frac{90 \ \mathrm{cGy}}{0.783 \ \mathrm{cGy/MU}} = 115 \ \mathrm{MU}$$

Values of dosimetric quantities for the Mevalac can be found in appendix C.

13.3.1 Approximate Methods for Estimating the Equivalent Square of a Blocked Field

In section 13.3.2 we will discuss a rigorous method for determination of the equivalent square field size of a blocked field. There are at least two methods however that are far easier and are frequently used to estimate the value of the equivalent field size. We emphasize that these methods are approximate only. They are useful for checking MU calculations. More exact methods should be used to calculate MU for patient treatments.

The first of these involves estimating the fraction of the area that is blocked. We start with the equivalent square of the open or unblocked field. The unblocked field is a rectangular field of width W and length L and therefore (at the isocenter) $f = 2LW/(L + W)$. We estimate the fraction of the area that is blocked. We will denote this by the symbol a. The value of a is usually determined by visual inspection. We next subtract the area blocked from the area of the open field: $f_d^2 - a f_d^2 = f_d^2(1-a)$. This is the unblocked area. We then find the side length of the square that has the same area as the unblocked area by taking the square root:

$$f_d' \approx f_d \sqrt{1-a}, \tag{13.3}$$

where the symbol $\approx$ means approximately equal to. There is no physical basis for this method. In fact, strictly speaking, it is incorrect. Nevertheless this method is commonly used and it is often reasonably accurate. It should be used with caution. Clearly equation (13.3) cannot be strictly correct. The dose rate and therefore the size of the equivalent field must depend not only on how much area is blocked but also the *location* of the blocked area. The further away the blocked area from the central axis, the less effect we expect it to have.

Example 13.2

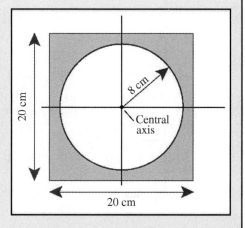

A 20×20 cm^2 square field is blocked as shown in the figure at right. The open portion of the field is a circle with a radius of 8 cm.

(a) Estimate the equivalent square field size using equation (13.3).

The area blocked is equal to $(20)^2 - \pi (8)^2 = 200$ cm^2. The fractional area blocked is therefore $a = 200/400 = 0.5$ and thus $f_d' = 20\sqrt{0.5} = 14.1$ cm.

(b) Calculate the equivalent field size using equation (10.20). The equivalent field size of a circular field is given by
$f_d' = R\sqrt{\pi} = 14.1$ cm.

In this simple case (a circular field centered on the central axis) the estimate from equation (13.3) gives exactly the accepted answer based on equation (10.20).

The second method that is frequently used to estimate the equivalent square of a blocked field we shall call the "guestimate" method. As its name implies, it is based on a judicious estimate.

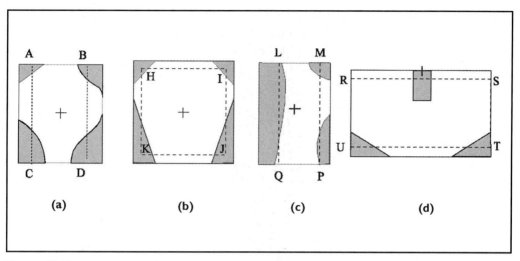

Figure 13.14: Examples of blocked fields and the approximate corresponding rectangular fields. The shaded portion of the field is blocked. Equivalent rectangles are illustrated by the dashed lines. In (a), a lateral pelvis field, the equivalent rectangle is estimated to be ABCD. In (b), an anterior pelvis field, the equivalent rectangle is estimated to be HIJK. In figure (c), an "off cord" head and neck field, the equivalent rectangle is LMPQ. In (d), a field used to treat supraclavicular lymph nodes, the equivalent rectangle is RSTU.

This method is illustrated by the diagrams in Figure 13.14. In these diagrams, it is the shaded area that is blocked. For each field, the jaws are set to define the outer rectangle. The dose rate is to be determined at the center of the field. Our "guestimates" for the equivalent fields are given by the dashed rectangles. One then finds the equivalent square of the dashed rectangle. In summary: Draw an equivalent rectangle centered on the point of interest and then determine the side length of the square that is equivalent to this. It is plain that this method is somewhat subjective and therefore must be used with care.

There are three factors that influence the value of f'_d:

(1) Source distance: the further the point of interest is from the source ($r = $ SSD $+ d$), the more beam divergence and the larger the field [see equation (9.3)].
(2) Blocking: the more blocking, the smaller the value of f'_d.
(3) A portion of the beam is not intercepted by the patient.

The last factor requires some explanation. The shaped beam may not completely intercept tissue. Two examples are shown in Figure 13.15.

Figure 13.15 shows a whole brain irradiation field on the left and a head and neck "off cord" field on the right. In the whole brain field (a), the field is larger than the patient's head and the periphery of the field does not intercept any tissue. In the neck field (b), the anterior portion of the field does not intercept any tissue. Those portions of these shaped

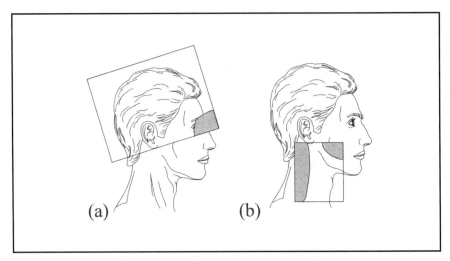

Figure 13.15: Examples of fields that are not completely intercepted by the patient: (a) is a whole brain field and (b) is a lateral "off cord" neck irradiation (see Figure 13.1). A portion of both of these fields intercepts air and those portions do not contribute to the scatter component of the dose.

fields that do not intercept any tissue (sometimes called "flash") cannot contribute to scatter, and therefore those portions of these fields should be considered as blocked for the purpose of calculating f'_d. Example 13.3 shows an application of this concept.

Example 13.3

A shaped lateral whole brain field is shown in the figure at right. This is similar to Figure 13.15(a). The dark shaded region in the lower right is the eye block. A cast block is used for this. The lighter shading represents flash and therefore it does not contribute to the scatter dose. The linac jaws are set to 23 cm by 17 cm. It is desired to deliver a dose of 150 cGy on the central axis (at the location

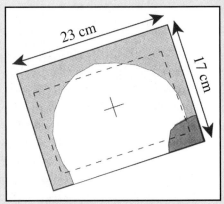

A whole brain field similar to the one shown in Figure 13.15(a).

of the crosshair) to mid depth in the patient's brain using the Mevalac 6 MV beam and an isocentric technique. The thickness of the patient's head (sometimes called the "separation") is 15 cm along the central axis. Estimate the MU required by: (a) estimating the fraction of the area blocked and (b) drawing an equivalent rectangle.

Example 13.3 (continued)

(a) The equivalent square of the open 23 cm × 17 cm field is $f = 19.6$ cm. We estimate that roughly half of the area is blocked and therefore $f'_d = 19.6\sqrt{1-0.50} = 13.9$ cm. The depth $d = 7.5$ cm. The dose rate is given by equation (13.1):

$$\dot{D}_d\left(r, f'_d\right) = \dot{D}_{d_0}\left(100 + d_0, 10\right) \times \left(\frac{100 + d_0}{\text{SSD} + d}\right)^2 \times S_c\left(f\right) \times S_p\left(f'_d\right)$$
$$\times \text{TMR}\left(d, f'_d\right) \times \text{TF}$$
$$= 1.000 \times \left(\frac{100 + 1.5}{100}\right)^2 \times S_c\left(19.6\right) \times S_p\left(13.9\right)$$
$$\times \text{TMR}\left(7.5, 13.9\right) \times 0.956$$
$$= 1.000 \times 1.030 \times 1.031 \times 1.012 \times 0.878 \times 0.956$$
$$= 0.901 \text{ cGy/MU}$$

and therefore $\mu = 150/0.901 = 166$ MU.

(b) The estimated equivalent rectangle is drawn in the figure in this example. The dimensions of this rectangle are 19 cm × 13 cm. The equivalent square is therefore $f'_d = 15.4$ cm. The dose rate is:

$$\dot{D}_d\left(r, f'_d\right) = 1.000 \times \left(\frac{100 + 1.5}{100}\right)^2 \times S_c\left(19.6\right) \times S_p\left(15.4\right)$$
$$\times \text{TMR}\left(7.5, 15.4\right) \times 0.956$$
$$= 1.000 \times 1.030 \times 1.031 \times 1.016 \times 0.881 \times 0.956$$
$$= 0.908 \text{ cGy/MU}$$

and therefore $\mu = 150/0.908 = 165$ MU. The number of MU is almost the same as estimated in part (a). This calculation ignores the three-dimensional nature of the patient's head—it assumes the surface of the patient's head is flat. Treatment planning software is capable of taking this into account.

13.3.2 Clarkson Integration

The methods described in the previous section for estimating the TMR of irregular fields are obviously somewhat crude. More sophisticated and more accurate methods have been developed, and one of these, called *Clarkson integration,* will be discussed here. As usual, it is useful to think in terms of the scatter contribution and the primary contribution to the dose. The primary contribution is not affected by blocking (provided that the point of interest does not lie near or under the block edge). It is helpful to separate the scatter and primary contributions to the dose. If we can calculate the scatter component, which *is* affected by blocking, and then add this to the primary component, we would then have the total dose.

The primary component of the dose at source distance r and depth d is $D_d(r,0)$; that is, it is the dose in the limit of zero field size. The scatter component must therefore be the total dose minus the primary component: $D_d(r, f_d) - D_d(r,0)$. We accomplish the separation of scatter and primary components of dose by introducing the scatter-maximum ratio, SMR:

$$\text{SMR}(d,f_d) = \frac{D_d(r,f_d) - D_d(r,0)}{D_{d_0}(r,0)}. \tag{13.4}$$

The SMR is the scatter component of the dose at depth d divided by the primary dose at the same distance but at depth d_0. We can express equation (13.4) in a more fundamental way by substituting expressions for the doses using equation (13.1) ($f'_d = f_d$, no blocking yet and we use doses instead of dose rates):

$$D_d(r,f_d) = D_{d_0}(100+d_0,10) \times \left(\frac{100+d_0}{r}\right)^2 \times S_c(f) \times S_p(f_d) \times \text{TMR}(d,f_d) \times \text{TF}$$

$$D_d(r,0) = D_{d_0}(100+d_0,10) \times \left(\frac{100+d_0}{r}\right)^2 \times S_c(f) \times S_p(0) \times \text{TMR}(d,0) \times \text{TF}$$

$$D_{d_0}(r,0) = D_{d_0}(100+d_0,10) \times \left(\frac{100+d_0}{r}\right)^2 \times S_c(f) \times S_p(0) \times \text{TMR}(d_0,0) \times \text{TF}.$$

$$\tag{13.5}$$

Substitution of equations (13.5) into equation (13.4) gives (after the dust clears) and realizing that $\text{TMR}(d_0,0) = 1$, by definition

$$\text{SMR}(d,f_d) = \frac{S_p(f_d)}{S_p(0)} \text{TMR}(d,f_d) - \text{TMR}(d,0). \tag{13.6}$$

The values of the SMR can be calculated from the values of $\text{TMR}(d,f_d)$ and $S_p(f_d)$. This does require extrapolation of $\text{TMR}(d,f_d)$ and $S_p(f_d)$ to zero field size to obtain $\text{TMR}(d,0)$ and $S_p(0)$. Values of SMR for the 6 MV Mevalac beam can be found in appendix C. For the 6 MV Mevalac beam $S_p(0) = 0.925$. In the limit of zero field size, the $\text{TMR}(d,0)$ can be written as:

$$\text{TMR}(d,0) = e^{-\mu(d-d_0)}, \tag{13.7}$$

where μ is the linear attenuation coefficient (not to be confused with the number of monitor units). It should not be too surprising that the TMR can be expressed this way for zero field size. Recall that TMR depends only on attenuation by matter and not on distance (inverse square). In the limit of zero field size, we have narrow beam geometry and we expect that the dose should decrease exponentially beyond the build-up region. The dose exhibits a buildup and TMR is related to dose; this is the reason that d_0 appears in equation (13.7). For the Mevalac 6 MV beam, the value of $\mu = 0.0467$ cm^{-1}, obtained from extrapolation of TMR values to zero field size. The average energy of the photons in a 6 MV beam is approximately $6/3 = 2$ MeV. The value of μ for 2 MeV photons in water is 0.0493 cm^{-1}, close to the value obtained by extrapolation of the TMR to zero field size.

Now let us introduce blocking. If an effective or average SMR can be calculated independently for the irregular field, then the TMR for this field can be calculated by rearranging equation (13.6):

$$\text{TMR}\left(d, f_d'\right) = \frac{S_p(0)}{\overline{S}_p}\left[\text{TMR}\left(d, 0\right) + \text{SMR}_{\text{eff}}\right], \tag{13.8}$$

where $\overline{S}_p$ is an effective or average value of S_p and SMR$_{\text{eff}}$ is the average value of the SMR for the blocked field.

We can calculate the effective SMR of an irregular field using the Clarkson integration technique. In Clarkson integration, we use a series of *pie*-shaped segments to build the shape of the irregular field. This is best illustrated by an example. Figure 13.16 shows the beam outline drawn by a physician for the treatment of a patient's right upper lung and mediastinum. Our task is to find the SMR for the shaped field for the Mevalac 6 MV beam at a depth of 12.0 cm on the central axis. The central axis is at the origin in Figure 13.16. We have drawn a few representative pie-shaped segments. The idea is that we use a series of pie-shaped segments of varying radii to approximate the shape of the blocked field. In this example, we will fill the blocked field with 18 of these segments. Each segment is like a portion of a circle (the circle being an entire pie). There is a radius associated with each pie segment. There are 18 of these radii, R_1 through R_{18}, and therefore each segment is $360°/18 = 20°$ in angular extent. We can calculate the SMR of each pie sector because it is 1/18 of a circle. We can then add all of the contributions to obtain the total SMR for the blocked field.

The quantity SMR(12 cm, R_n) is the SMR for *a circle of radius R_n*. Each pie-shaped sector is 1/18 of a circle, therefore:

$$\text{SMR}_{\text{eff}} \approx \frac{1}{18}\text{SMR}\left(12, R_1\right) + \frac{1}{18}\text{SMR}\left(12, R_2\right) + \cdots + \frac{1}{18}\text{SMR}\left(12, R_{18}\right)$$
$$= \frac{1}{18}\left[\text{SMR}\left(12, R_1\right) + \text{SMR}\left(12, R_2\right) + \cdots + \text{SMR}\left(12, R_{18}\right)\right]. \tag{13.9}$$

The value of R_1 is 9.7 cm; to evaluate SMR(12, R_1) we need to consult the table of SMR values for the Mevalac in appendix C. Linear interpolation

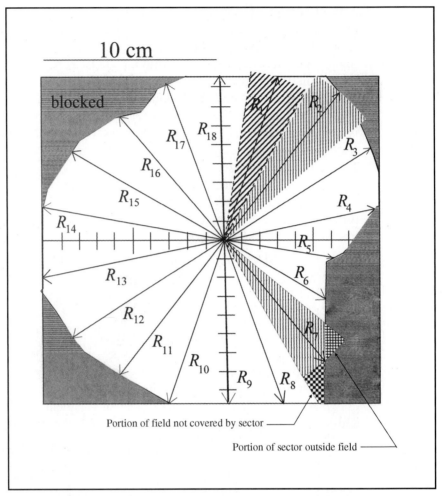

Figure 13.16: Illustration of the Clarkson integration technique used to calculate the TMR for a blocked field. The shape of the irregular field is approximated by filling it with pie-shaped sectors, three of which are shown. The scatter contribution to the dose is determined by adding the contribution of all the sectors.

is necessary. The value of SMR(12,9.7) = 0.231. If all 18 SMRs are evaluated in this way, then the sum is:

$$\text{SMR}_{eff} = \frac{1}{18}\Big[\text{SMR}\big(12, R_1\big) + \text{SMR}\big(12, R_2\big) + \cdots + \text{SMR}\big(12, R_{18}\big)\Big] \quad (13.10)$$
$$= 0.227.$$

The value of TMR(12,0) = $e^{-0.0467(12-1.5)}$ = 0.612 from equation (13.7). For $\bar{S}_p$ we will use the value of S_p for the average radius 9.4 cm. In this case $\bar{S}_p$ = 1.017 and therefore the effective value of the TMR using equation (13.8) is 0.763.

The jaw setting for the field in Figure 13.16 is 19 cm × 18 cm. The equivalent square for the jaws is thus approximately 18.5. It appears as if about 25% of the field is blocked. Using equation (13.3) we find f'_d = 16 and TMR(12,16) = 0.764, almost identical to the value above.

If you examine Figure 13.16 you will notice that the circular sectors do not perfectly fill the field. For example, consider the sector that is associated with R_7. There is a portion of the sector that is outside the field (under the blocked region) and there is a portion of the irregular field that is not included in the sector. This contributes to some error in our calculation. If the areas of these two portions were the same, they would cancel one another.

One way to reduce the error is to make the sectors smaller in angular extent and therefore to use more pieces of "pie" to cover the field. For example, we could use 36 sectors (10° in angular extent) instead of 18. We would expect the result to be more accurate in this case. There is a price to be paid for this however; the amount of computation rises with the number of sectors used.

This technique of dividing up the irregular field into sectors and then adding the scatter contribution from each sector is known as *Clarkson integration*. The reader familiar with calculus will note the similarity of this method to mathematical integration. This technique is readily adaptable to computer implementation. It is the sort of tedious calculation that computers are well suited for. Clarkson integration, or variants thereof, has been widely used by computer treatment planning software for calculating dose rates for irregular fields.

We can calculate the component of the dose that is due to scatter from SMR values. We rewrite equation (13.4) for the SMR as:

$$\text{SMR}\left(d,f\right)=\frac{D_{scatt}}{D_{d_0}\left(100,0\right)}, \tag{13.11}$$

where D_{scatt} is the scatter dose at the isocenter, at depth d and for field size f. Let us solve this equation for the scatter dose and substitute the equation for $D_{d_0}\left(100,0\right)$ [see equation (13.5)]:

$$D_{scatt} = D_{d_0}\left(100+d_0,10\right)\times\left(\frac{100+d_0}{100}\right)^2\times S_c\left(f\right)\times S_p\left(0\right) \tag{13.12}$$
$$\times\,\text{TMR}\left(d_0,0\right)\times\text{TF}\times\text{SMR}\left(d,f\right).$$

We would like to calculate the ratio of the scatter dose to the total dose on the central axis at the isocenter, at depth d for field size f:

$$\frac{\text{Scatter dose}}{\text{Total dose}}=\frac{D_{scatt}}{D_d\left(100,f\right)}. \tag{13.13}$$

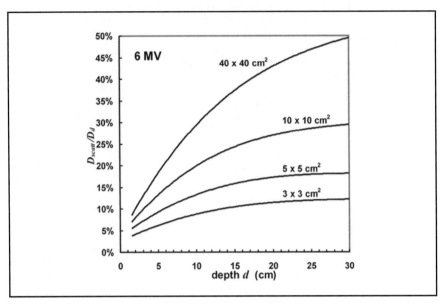

Figure 13.17: Fraction of the total dose due to scatter on the central axis at isocenter for various square fields for a 6 MV beam as a function of depth. The scatter contribution rises with increasing field size and depth.

If we substitute the expression for D_{scatt} [equation (13.12)] and the equation for $D_d(100, f)$ [equation (13.5)], we get

$$\frac{D_{scatt}}{D_d(100, f)} = \frac{S_p(0)}{S_p(f)} \times \frac{\text{TMR}(d, 0)}{\text{TMR}(d, f)} \times \text{SMR}(d, f). \qquad (13.14)$$

A plot of this ratio for the 6 MV Mevalac beam appears in Figure 13.17. As we would expect, the scatter contribution to the total dose rises with increasing field size and depth.

13.4 Dose Rate Calculations for Shaped Fields at Points Away from the Central Axis

Until now, we have only considered the calculation of dose rate at points on the central axis of the beam. Suppose we wish to calculate the dose rate at a point that is not on the central axis. In addition, the distance to the calculation point may be nonstandard (i.e., SSD ≠ 100 cm, r ≠ SAD).

Recall that dose is a combination of primary dose and scatter dose. As we move off the central axis, we do not expect the dose to change dramatically until we approach the edge of the field. We recall from chapter 9 that linac flattening filters are designed to produce reasonably flat beams at least over the inner 80% of the field (see Figure 9.32). Nevertheless, there will be some change in the dose. When we get close to the field edge (into the penumbra), the dose will drop rapidly because of the decrease in the scatter contribution. Dose rate calculations in the

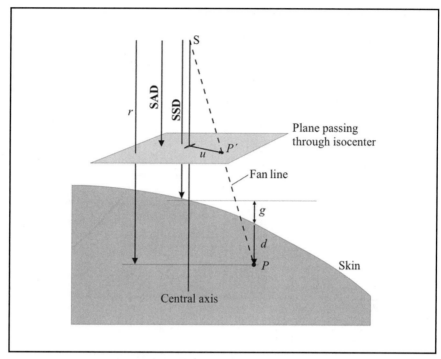

Figure 13.18: Cross-sectional view of the geometry for off-axis dose calculations. If the skin is sloping, there will be an "air gap" g, which may be positive or negative. The off-axis distance u is defined on a plane perpendicular to the central axis at the isocenter.

penumbra are unreliable because of the steep gradients there. MU calculations should therefore not be based on dose rate calculations within about 1.5 cm of any edge of a blocked beam.

Figures 13.18 and 13.19 show two views of an off-axis point. Figure 13.18 shows a side view and Figure 13.19 is a beam's-eye view. We wish to calculate the dose rate at point P in Figure 13.18, which is at depth d. A line drawn from the radiation source (S in Figure 13.18) to point P is called a fan line or ray line. This line crosses the plane through the isocenter at point P' (see Figure 13.19). The point P' is at position (x, y) in the isocenter plane. We will designate the distance from the central axis to the point P' as u. The dose rate at point P will depend on u. To calculate the dose rate at P, we introduce the off-axis ratio OAR(d, u). The OAR depends on the position of point P with respect to the central axis. It is usually assumed for simplicity that the OAR depends only on the distance u of the fan line from the central axis. The distance from the central axis is $u = \sqrt{x^2 + y^2}$. The OAR is the ratio of the open field dose rate at an off-axis point to that for the same field shifted such that the point of calculation lies on the central axis. It is customary to measure the distance off-axis in a plane passing through the isocenter as in Figure 13.18.

In Figure 13.18 the distance from the source to the plane passing through point P and perpendicular to the central axis is r. The SSD is the distance from the source to the point where the central axis meets

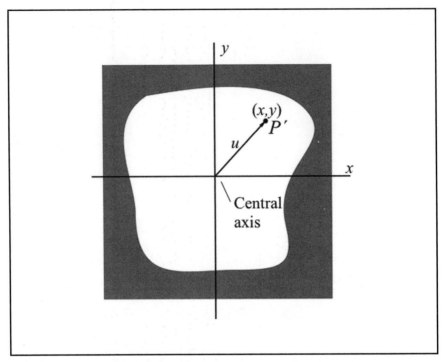

Figure 13.19: Beam's-eye view of a shaped field with an off-axis point P' as seen on the plane through the isocenter. The off-axis point is at a distance u from the central axis. We wish to compute the dose rate at a point along a ray line from the source through P' at a specified depth.

the skin surface. Note that r need not equal SSD or SAD. The skin slopes away from the central axis. The air gap g is the vertical distance between a plane passing through the skin at the central axis and the skin surface vertically above point P. For the case shown in the diagram, the air gap is considered to be a positive quantity. The air gap can be negative—as in the case where the skin slopes up away from the central axis in Figure 13.18. The depth d is the vertical distance of point P below the skin surface.[1] The quantity u (seen in both Figures 13.18 and 13.19) is the distance of the fan line from the central axis as measured in a plane perpendicular to the central axis at the isocenter.

Table 13.1 lists values of the OAR for the 6 MV Mevalac beam; Table 13.2 lists the OAR values for the 18 MV beam. These tables also appear in appendix C. As expected $\text{OAR}(d, 0) = 1.000$. Examination of the tables shows that the OAR can be as large as 7% or more.

Off-axis ratios can be obtained from beam profiles. This can be accomplished by measuring beam profiles as discussed in section 9.4. The reader is warned that there is no standardized nomenclature for the term "off-axis ratio." This term is sometimes used to refer to primary, or

---

[1] You may object that the correct depth to use is the depth measured along the fanline between point P and the surface. We will assume that the difference between these is small. This is reasonable as long as u is small compared to SAD.

Table 13.1: 6 MV Off-Axis Ratios (OARs) for the Mevalac

Depth d (cm)	Distance off axis u (cm)*					
	0	2	4	6	8	10
1.5	1.000	1.011	1.027	1.037	1.053	1.071
5.0	1.000	1.007	1.023	1.030	1.041	1.056
10.0	1.000	1.006	1.016	1.024	1.029	1.036
15.0	1.000	1.008	1.015	1.017	1.019	1.019

*The distance off axis, u, is measured on a plane perpendicular to the central axis at a source distance of 100 cm. These are in-phantom off-axis ratios.

Table 13.2: 18 MV Off-Axis Ratios (OARs) for the Mevalac

Depth d (cm)	Distance off axis u (cm)*					
	0	2	4	6	8	10
3.0	1.000	1.012	1.036	1.042	1.050	1.050
5.0	1.000	1.011	1.030	1.033	1.039	1.038
10.0	1.000	1.011	1.024	1.026	1.029	1.024
20.0	1.000	1.000	1.009	1.003	0.992	0.977

*The distance off axis, u, is measured on a plane perpendicular to the central axis at a source distance of 100 cm. These are in-phantom off-axis ratios.

"in-air" OARs, which are different from the OARs used here based on water phantom measurements.

The dose rate at the off-axis point P is calculated as follows:

$$\dot{D}_d\left(r, f_d'\right) = \dot{D}_{d_0}\left(100 + d_0, 10\right) \times \left(\frac{100 + d_0}{r}\right)^2 \times S_c\left(f\right) \times S_p\left(f_d'\right) \times \text{TMR}\left(d, f_d'\right)$$

$$\times \text{OAR}\left(d, u\right) \times \text{TF}, \tag{13.15}$$

where

r is the distance from the source to point P (see Figure 13.18),

f_d' is the side length of the blocked equivalent square in the patient at depth d,

$\dot{D}_{d_0}\left(100 + d_0, 10\right) = 1.000$ cGy/MU (for the Mevalac normalization),

OAR(d,u) is the off-axis ratio measured at a distance u (on the isocenter plane, see Figure 13.18),

TMR(d, f_d') is the TMR at depth d, and

TF is a tray factor, which is necessary if a cast block is used.

Notice that equation (13.15) reduces to equation (13.1) when $u = 0$.

Example 13.4

A beam's-eye view of a rectangular field is shown in the diagram. A dose of 100 cGy is to be delivered to a depth of 10 cm on the central axis (C) using the 6 MV Mevalac beam. The SSD is 90 cm.

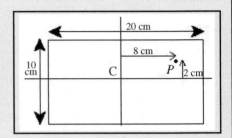

(a) Calculate the number of MU necessary to deliver the prescribed dose.

This is an isocentric treatment since the SSD = 90 cm and the depth is 10 cm. The TMR isocentric method of calculation may be used in this case. The equivalent square field size is $f'_d = 13.3$ cm.

$$\dot{D}_d\left(100,13.3\right)=\dot{D}_{d_0}\left(100,10\right)\times S_{c,p}\left(13.3\right)\times \text{TMR}\left(10,13.3\right)$$
$$=1.030\times1.021\times0.808$$
$$=0.850 \text{ cGy/MU}$$

and therefore $\mu = D/\dot{D} = 100/0.850 = 118$ MU.

(b) We wish to calculate the dose at point P and at depth 10 cm. There is no air gap.

This is simply the dose on the central axis multiplied by the OAR. The distance off axis is $u=\sqrt{8^2+2^2}$ = 8.3 cm and OAR(10,8.3) = 1.030. Therefore D = 103 cGy.

This dose is fairly close to the dose on the central axis—after all the flattening filter is designed for this purpose!

13.5 Dose Rate Calculations with Asymmetric Jaws

An illustration of asymmetric jaws is shown in Figure 13.2. As with all dose rate calculations, we must consider the effects of head scatter and phantom scatter. Phantom scatter is determined by the shape of the aperture. This is taken into account in the TMR and in S_p. As we have discussed, the head scatter is influenced by the jaw settings. We desire to know the value of S_c, but what field size should be used to look up this number? Although the field is rectangular, it is not centered on the central axis (denoted by the circle in Figure 13.2). It is usually *assumed* that the head scatter can be evaluated by calculating the equivalent square of the rectangle even though the central axis is not at the center of this rectangle. In Figure 13.2 the dimensions of the rectangle are (Y1 + Y2) by (X1 + X2). Example 13.5 demonstrates a dose rate calculation with asymmetric jaws.

Example 13.5

The blocked field shown in the diagram to the right is a "supraclav" field for a breast cancer treatment. All dimensions shown in this figure are as seen in a plane through the isocenter. The prescription calls for delivery of a dose of 180 cGy at point P [coordinates (–5.0, 2.5) on the isocenter plane] to a depth of 3.0 cm below the skin surface.

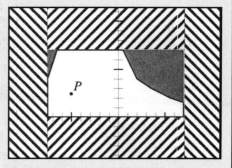

The crosshatch area is blocked by the jaws. The shaded area is blocked by the MLC.

The SSD = 100 cm; the air gap $g = 1.0$ cm. The jaw settings are Y1 = 0.0 cm, Y2 = 7.0 cm, X2 = 7.5 cm, and X1 = 8.0 cm. The field is shaped with the MLC. Using the data for the 6 MV Mevalac beam, calculate the required number of MU.

The jaws are asymmetric. The distance from the source is r = SSD + g + d = 100 + 1 + 3 = 104 cm. The dimensions of the rectangular jaw aperture are (7.0 + 0.0) × (7.5 + 8.0) or 7.0 × 15.5 cm². The equivalent square is $f = 9.6$ cm. It appears as if approximately one-third of the open field area is blocked and therefore $f' = 9.6\sqrt{1-0.33} = 7.9$ cm. This is the blocked field size at a distance of 100 cm from the source. The blocked field size in the patient at a distance of 104 cm is $f'_d = 7.9 \times (104/100) = 8.2$ cm. The off-axis distance is $u = \sqrt{5^2 + 2.5^2} = 5.6$ cm and the OAR (see Table 13.1) is approximately OAR(3.0, 5.6) ≈ 1.017.

(Continued on next page)

Example 13.5 (continued)

Equation (13.15) may be used to calculate the dose rate at point P.

$$\dot{D}_d\left(r,f_d\right)=\dot{D}_{d_0}\left(100+d_0,10\right)\times\left(\frac{100+d_0}{r}\right)^2\times S_c\left(f\right)\times S_p\left(f_d'\right)\times \text{TMR}\left(d,f_d'\right)$$

$$\times \text{OAR}\left(d,u\right)\times \text{TF}$$

$$=1.000\times\left(\frac{100+1.5}{104}\right)^2\times S_c\left(9.6\right)\times S_p\left(8.2\right)\times \text{TMR}\left(3,8.2\right)$$

$$\times \text{OAR}\left(3,5.6\right)\times \text{TF}$$

$$=1.000\times0.952\times0.998\times0.994\times0.977\times1.017\times1.000$$

$$=0.921\,\text{cGy/MU}$$

Therefore $\mu = 180/0.921 = 195$ MU.

13.6 Dose Under a Blocked Region

Even if no primary radiation penetrates a blocked region (and of course some small percentage always does), the blocked region will receive some dose because of scattered radiation, particularly when the region is close to the block edge. At low beam energy, photons undergo Compton scattering at larger angles than at high energy (see Table 7.1 and Figure 6.5) and, hence, the scatter component of the absorbed dose tends to be larger. The most accurate method for determining the dose under a blocked area is to calculate the SMR at the point in question, using Clarkson integration. This is one way that computer treatment planning systems perform these calculations. If the block is rectangular, we can use a trick to estimate the dose under it.

This is best illustrated by an example adapted from the book by Khan.[2] Using the Mevalac 6 MV beam, a dose of 200 cGy is to be delivered to a depth of 10 cm, SSD = 100 cm, at point P in Figure 13.20. The tray factor is 0.956. The transmission through the block itself is 0.05.

(a) Calculate the number of monitor units to deliver the desired dose to point P.

We need to make some assumptions. Ignore (1) any off-axis ratio (assume a flat beam) and (2) contribution from the "other side" (see

---

[2] Khan, F. M. *The Physics of Radiation Therapy,* Third Edition. Philadelphia: Lippincott Williams & Wilkins, 2003.

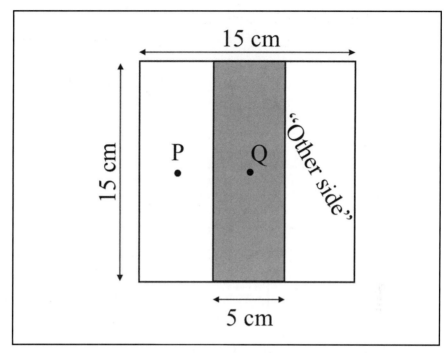

Figure 13.20: A beam portal with central blocking in the shaded area. Given the dose at point *P*, we wish to estimate the dose under the block at point *Q*. All dimensions are as measured at the isocenter.

Figure 13.20). The dimensions of the unblocked area surrounding point *P* are 5 cm × 15 cm. The equivalent square for this rectangle is 7.5 × 7.5 cm^2.

$$\dot{D}(110,7.5) = \dot{D}_{d_0}(100+d_0,10) \times S_c(15) \times S_p(7.5) \times \mathrm{DD}(10,7.5,100) \times \mathrm{TF}$$
$$= 1.000 \times 1.015 \times 0.991 \times 0.662 \times 0.956 \qquad (13.16)$$
$$= 0.637 \text{ cGy/MU}$$

Therefore μ = 200/0.637 = 314 MU.

(b) Estimate the dose under the block at point *Q*.

We will use a trick to estimate this. Examine Figure 13.21. To a first approximation, the *dose* at point *Q* in the *open* (unblocked) field is equal to the dose from the open part of the blocked field plus the dose from the blocked part of the field. In Figure 13.21 we cannot add the full contribution from the narrow open field because the block does transmit some primary dose. To account for this, we multiply the second term by (1 − *T*), where *T* is the transmission through the block. In Figure 13.22 we rearrange the "equation" shown in Figure 13.21.

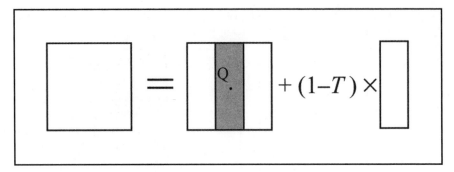

Figure 13.21: A trick used to estimate the dose under a block (shaded area). The block transmission is T.

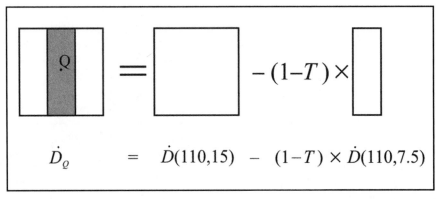

$$\dot{D}_Q \quad = \quad \dot{D}(110,15) \quad - \quad (1-T) \times \dot{D}(110,7.5)$$

Figure 13.22: A rearrangement of the "equation" shown in Figure 13.21. This allows an estimate of the dose at point Q under the block.

The dose rate at point Q can thus be written:

$$\dot{D}_Q = \dot{D}(110,15) - (1-T) \times \dot{D}(110,7.5). \tag{13.17}$$

The dose rate for the 15×15 cm^2 open field is:

$$\dot{D}(110,15) = \dot{D}_{d_0}(100+d_0,10) \times S_{c,p}(15) \times \mathrm{DD}(10,15,100) \times \mathrm{TF}$$
$$= 1.000 \times 1.030 \times 0.700 \times 0.956 \tag{13.18}$$
$$= 0.689 \text{ cGy/MU},$$

and from part (a) $\dot{D}(110,7.5) = 0.637$ cGy/MU; therefore $\dot{D}_Q = 0.084$ cGy/MU. The dose at point Q is therefore $D_Q = \dot{D}_Q \times \mu = 0.084 \times 314 = 26$ cGy.

(c) What is the ratio of the dose under the block at point Q to the dose in the open region at point P?

$$D_Q/D_P = 0.13 = 13\% \tag{13.19}$$

The lesson here is that the dose under a block can be substantially higher than transmission alone would indicate because of scattered radiation. This is particularly true at lower energies where photons are more likely to be scattered through large angles. This is of great importance when blocking critical structures such as the spinal cord.

Chapter Summary

- **Asymmetric jaws** (independent jaws); facilitate half beam blocking (e.g., tangential breast); jaw transmission usually less than 0.5%.

- **Blocks**

  - Hand blocks: when there is no time to fabricate custom cast blocks (e.g., sim & treat).

  - Cast blocks: made of alloy Lipowitz metal (brand name Cerrobend®); 50% bismuth, 26.7% lead, 13.3% tin, 10.0% cadmium (lead, tin, and cadmium are toxic heavy metals); melts at 70 °C; blocks are focused.

  - Typical block thickness of 6 to 8 cm; transmission < 5%.

  - Mounted on plastic tray inserted into collimator head; tray transmission factor (TF) usually ranges from 0.95 to 1.00.

- **Multileaf Collimator (MLC)**

  - Series of thin leaves (e.g., 26 pairs, 40 pairs, 60 pairs) shape field; replace most blocks; many advantages over cast blocks.

  - Either replaces set of jaws or used as tertiary field shaping like block.

  - Leaf width projected to isocenter: 0.4 to 2.0 cm.

  - Some specifications: leaf transmission (2%), largest field size (e.g., 26 cm × 40 cm), leaf shape(focused?), overtravel, interleaf transmission: reduced by tongue and groove, etc.

- **Shaped or blocked fields** are sometimes called irregular fields.

  - Dose rate is reduced by blocking because of a decrease in scatter.

  - Amount of reduction depends on: (1) amount of field blocked and (2) location of blocking.

  - Blocking has greatest effect for large depths and low-energy beams because scatter component is largest under these circumstances.

- **Depth dose calculations** (for SSD = 100 cm calculations):

$$\dot{D}_d\left(r, f_d'\right) = \dot{D}_{d_0}\left(100 + d_0, 10\right) \times S_c\left(f\right) \times S_p\left(f_{d_0}'\right) \times DD\left(d, f_0', 100\right) \times TF. \quad (13.2)$$

- TMR calculations (useful for isocentric calculations but valid for any distance $r = SSD + d$):

$$\dot{D}_d\left(r, f_d'\right) = \dot{D}_{d_0}\left(100 + d_0, 10\right) \times \left(\frac{100 + d_0}{SSD + d}\right)^2 \times S_c\left(f\right) \times S_p\left(f_d'\right) \\ \times TMR\left(d, f_d'\right) \times TF. \quad (13.1)$$

- Approximate methods to find equivalent square of blocked field; f_d'. Any portion of the beam not intercepted by the patient (flash) must be considered blocked. Two methods:

(1) Estimate fraction of area blocked a:

$$f_d' \approx f_d \sqrt{1 - a}.$$

(2) Draw equivalent rectangle, calculate equivalent square.

- **Clarkson integration:** A semi-rigorous method to determine the TMR (or TAR) of a blocked field. Separate the dose into primary and scatter. Calculate the scatter component of the blocked field and add to the primary component to find TMR of blocked field. Accomplish by approximating the field by a series of pie-shaped sectors and adding SMR of all sectors to find effective SMR for blocked field.

- Dose rate at points away from the central axis:

  – Distance from central axis, u, is measured in a plane perpendicular to central axis at the isocenter.

  – OAR(d,u) is the off-axis ratio at depth d and distance off axis u (see appendix C for values).

$$\dot{D}_d\left(r, f_d'\right) = \dot{D}_{d_0}\left(100 + d_0, 10\right) \times \left(\frac{100 + d_0}{r}\right)^2 \times S_c\left(f\right) \times S_p\left(f_d'\right) \times TMR\left(d, f_d'\right) \\ \times OAR\left(d, u\right) \times TF \quad (13.15)$$

- **Dose rate for asymmetric jaws:** Head scatter can be evaluated by calculating the equivalent square of the rectangle formed by the jaws even though the central axis is not at the center of this rectangle.

- **Dose under a blocked region** can be significant because of scatter. Dose will be highest for small block, low-energy. and greater depth.

Problems

Consult appendix C for Mevalac beam data.

1. (a) How does the attenuation of a typical block compare with the intraleaf attenuation of a tertiary MLC?
   (b) What is the typical value of leaf width as projected to isocenter?
   (c) How does leaf design reduce interleaf leakage?

2. A patient is to be treated isocentrically with 6 MV whole brain radiation using a lateral field on the Mevalac. The collimator jaws are set to 20 cm × 26 cm. The blocked equivalent field size is $f_d' =$ 15.8. The dose to be delivered by this beam is 100 cGy on the central axis at a depth of 7.5 cm. The tray factor is 0.956. Use the data in appendix C to calculate the required MU.

3. An "off cord" lateral head and neck field is shown in the figure to the right. The jaw setting is 16 cm × 12 cm. A dose of 90 cGy is to be delivered to a point on the central axis at mid depth (5.0 cm). Calculate the MU required to deliver 90 cGy using an isocentric 6 MV (Mevalac) beam by estimating the area blocked by the MLC and the area to be excluded due to flash.

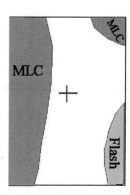

4. Consider a 10 × 10 cm² radiation field.
   (a) Determine the ratio of the scatter contribution to the total dose for the 6 MV Mevalac beam at depths of 5 cm and 10 cm using equation (13.14).
   (b) Check the answer to part (a) by consulting Figure 13.17.

5. For what combination of beam energy and field size is the fraction of the dose due to scatter the greatest?

6. The truly correct method for determining the equivalent square field for a rectangular field is to perform a Clarkson integration for the rectangular field, to find the SMR for that rectangular field, and then to locate in a table the size of the square which has the same SMR. Consider a rectangle of length 20 cm and width 4 cm. For the 6 MV Mevalac beam at a depth of 10 cm, determine the

SMR at the center of the rectangle. Take advantage of the symmetry of the rectangle and perform the Clarkson integration over only one quadrant and then multiply by 4. The diagram below shows *one quadrant* of the rectangle. Six radial spokes have been drawn in for you at 15° intervals.

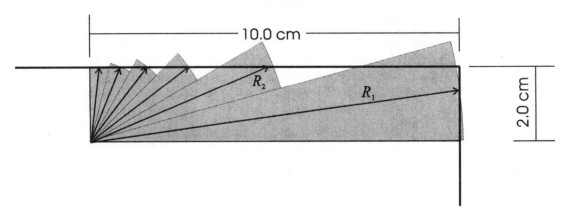

Clarkson integration over one quadrant of a rectangular 20 cm × 4 cm field. Each sector has an angular size of 15°. This diagram is drawn to scale.

(a) Complete the table at the right. Use a ruler to measure the radii and use the SMR data in appendix C. Compute the effective SMR for the entire field (remember to multiply by 4).

(b) Use the effective SMR and the data in appendix C to find the side length of the equivalent square.

(c) Use the area over perimeter rule to determine the equivalent square of the rectangle and compare the result to part (b).

(d) How could the accuracy be improved?

n	R_n (cm)	SMR$(10, R_n)$
1		
2		
3		
4		
5		
6		

7. A 6 MV blocked field is shown in the diagram below. The central
    block is a circle of diameter 6 cm. The open portion of the field is
    a circular annulus with an outer diameter of 12 cm. The jaws are
    set to 13×13 cm^2.
    (a) Using the equivalent square of the circular field for field "a",
        calculate the dose rate at a depth of 5 cm (isocenter) on the
        central axis.
    (b) Using the equivalent square of the circular field for field "b",
        calculate the dose rate at a depth of 5 cm (isocenter) on the
        central axis.
    (c) Calculate the dose rate on the central axis for the blocked field
        on the left in the diagram. Assume a block transmission of 5%.
    (d) If 200 MU are delivered, what is the dose on the central axis at
        a depth of 5 cm?

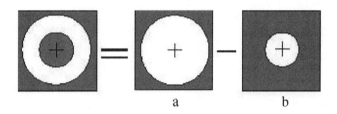

                        a   b

8. A supraclavicular field is shown in the diagram below. This field is
    to be treated with the 6 MV Mevalac beam with SSD = 100 cm to
    the central axis. The jaw settings are X1 = 7, X2 = 10, Y1 = 3.5,
    and Y2 = 2. A dose of 180 cGy is to be delivered to point P at
    coordinates $(x, y) = (4, 2)$ [coordinates refer to the plane perpendic-
    ular to the central axis through the isocenter] and depth 3.0 cm.
    The air gap at this point is +2.0 cm. Calculate the number of MU
    required.

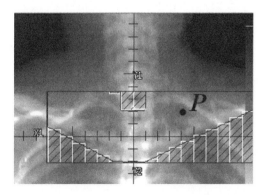

Bibliography

American Association of Physicists in Medicine (AAPM) Report No. 72. *Basic Applications of Multileaf Collimators,* Report of the AAPM Radiation Therapy Committee Task Group No. 50. Madison, WI: Medical Physics Publishing, 2001.

Khan, F. M. *The Physics of Radiation Therapy,* Third Edition. Philadelphia: Lippincott Williams & Wilkins, 2003.

Metcalfe, P., T. Kron, and P. Hoban. *The Physics of Radiotherapy X-Rays and Electrons.* Madison, WI: Medical Physics Publishing, 2007.

Stanton, R., and D. Stinson. *Applied Physics for Radiation Oncology, Revised Edition.* Madison, WI: Medical Physics Publishing, 2009.

Van Dyk, J. (ed.). *The Modern Technology of Radiation Oncology.* Madison, WI: Medical Physics Publishing, 1999.

Williams, J. R., and D. I. Thwaites (eds.). *Radiotherapy Physics: In Practice,* Second Edition. New York: Oxford University Press USA, 2000.

14 Dose Distributions in Two and Three Dimensions

"The answer to any question in radiation therapy physics is: *scatter.*"
—Gary Ezzell, Ph.D.

14.1 Isodose Charts

We have examined the distribution of dose in one dimension (depth) in chapter 10. In chapter 13 we considered points away from the central axis. The goal in this chapter is to examine the distribution of dose in two and three dimensions. We will examine what happens when the beam central axis is not perpendicular to the surface and when the surface is not flat. We will consider the effect of the use of multiple beams. We will look at beam modifiers such as wedges and compensators and learn how to modify dose rate calculations to accommodate the presence of these devices.

The technique that is customarily used to display dose in a plane is to construct isodose charts. Isodose charts are like topographical maps, which have contour lines on them representing altitude. Each contour on a topographical map depicts a curve along which the altitude is constant. Isodose charts display curves along which the dose is a constant. An isodose chart may have as many as 10 or 15 isodose curves on it. Each separate isodose curve corresponds to a different value of the dose. The use of an isodose chart makes it possible to show the spatial distribution of dose in a plane. Isodose curves may be displayed in terms of either absolute dose or percentages. Here we will display them as percentages. It is common to display these charts with increments of 10% in dose. The location where the dose is set to 100% is often called the *normalization point*. If the maximum dose is more than the dose at the normalization point, then there may be isodose curves with values above 100%. If the absolute dose is known at the normalization point, it is easy to determine the dose at any other point.

The simplest example of an isodose chart shows the dose distribution from a single beam of radiation that is perpendicularly incident on a flat phantom surface. An example appears in Figure 14.1.[1] This isodose chart and the others in this chapter were generated with a computerized treatment planning system. It is also possible to generate these charts by measurement using a water phantom scanning system of the type discussed in chapter 9. The isodose curves displayed in Figure 14.1 are percentages. The value of the dose is set to 100% at a depth of d_m (1.2 cm for this 4 MV beam). Figure 14.2 shows the dose distribution from the same beam in a plane perpendicular to the central axis at a depth of d_m. Example 14.1 demonstrates an application of isodose curves.

Figure 14.3 shows the same type of isodose chart except that the beam energy is 15 MV. Note that for both Figures 14.1 and 14.3, the isodose lines are spaced farther apart at depth. Comparing isodose lines between Figures 14.1 and 14.3, we see that the lines are farther apart in

---

[1]Many of the dose distributions displayed in this chapter have been produced by "VRSPlan," which is a modified version of the treatment planning software "GRATIS" written by George Sherouse, Ph.D.

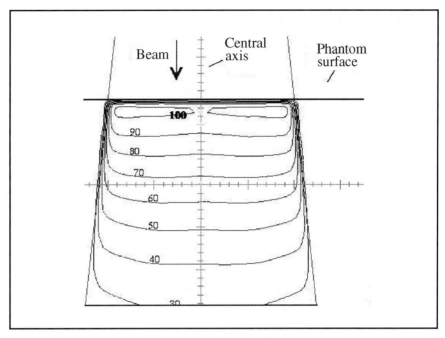

Figure 14.1: The isodose distribution for a 4 MV beam (20×20 cm^2) normalized to 100% at $d_m = 1.2$ cm (SSD = 100) on the central axis. The beam is incident from above. The phantom has a flat surface, which is represented by the horizontal line at the top. The distance between tick marks on the scale is 1.0 cm.

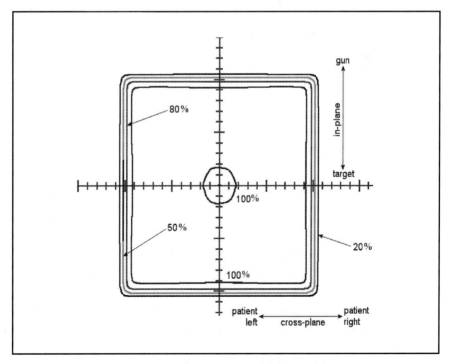

Figure 14.2: Isodose lines for a 4 MV, 20×20 cm^2 beam in a plane perpendicular to the central axis at a depth of $d_m = 1.2$ cm. This is the same beam depicted in Figure 14.1 in a different plane. The central axis extends into this page. The distance between tick marks is 1.0 cm.

Example 14.1

A 4 MV 20 × 20 cm^2 beam (SSD = 100 cm) is used to deliver 90 cGy to a depth of 10 cm on the central axis. Use Figure 14.1 to estimate the dose delivered to a point at a depth of 15 cm and at a perpendicular distance of 7 cm (measured at depth 15 cm) from the central axis.

On the central axis, the depth dose appears to be approximately 67% at a depth of 10 cm. At a depth of 15 cm and at a distance of 7 cm from the central axis (in either direction, the distribution is symmetric), the PDD appears to be 50%. The dose at this point is therefore 50/67 × 90 = 67 cGy.

Figure 14.3 than in Figure 14.1, as we expect, since the 15 MV beam is more penetrating. Notice that the isodose lines curve toward the surface near the edge of the beam. This is because of the decreased scatter contribution near the beam edge. Near the central axis, scatter can come from all sides. Near the beam edge, most of the scatter comes from only one side. It is also true that near the edge of the beam the primary rays have to travel a little farther from the source.

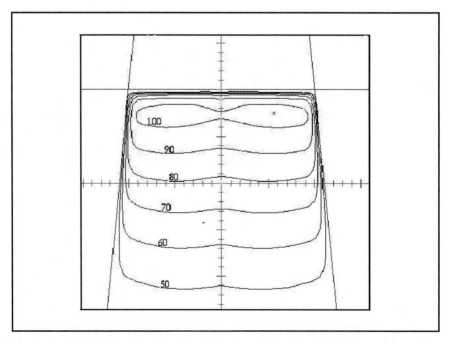

Figure 14.3: The isodose distribution from a 15 MV beam (20 × 20 cm²) normalized to 100% at d_m = 3.0 cm (SSD = 100 cm). The distance between tick marks is 1 cm.

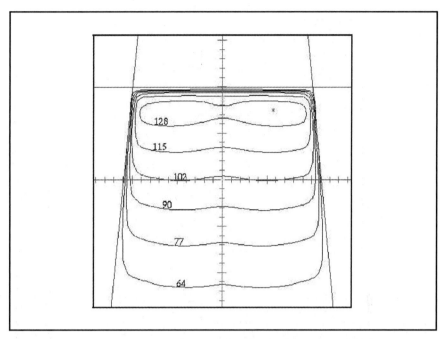

Figure 14.4: The same beam as in Figure 14.3. The normalization has been changed by setting 100% at a depth of 10 cm. Note that the relative dose distribution remains *exactly* the same, only the normalization point has been changed. The isodose curves are the same curves as in Figure 14.2, only the *labels* have been changed.

The characteristics of the isodose distribution depend on beam energy, field size, source size, SSD, source-to-diaphragm distance, etc.

If one were to take PDD values along the central axis from Figure 14.1 or 14.3 and graph these as a function of depth, one would obtain a depth dose curve like those displayed in Figure 10.3. In Figure 14.1 the location of the maximum dose is off the central axis (within the closed loops labeled 100). If one were to draw a horizontal line in Figure 14.1 or 14.2 and make a graph of the percentage along this line as a function of distance from the central axis, one would obtain a beam profile like that shown in Figure 9.30. Do not confuse beam profiles with isodose distributions.

Figure 14.4 shows the dose distribution for the same beam as in Figure 14.3. The normalization has been changed, so that the dose at depth 10 cm on the central axis has been set to 100%. It is a common misconception that a change in normalization changes the relative dose distribution—it doesn't! It only changes the labels that we attach to particular isodose curves. The relative distribution of dose remains the same. The absolute dose however could change drastically. If the prescription calls for 200 cGy to be delivered to the 100% line, then the maximum dose in Figure 14.3 will be 200 cGy, whereas the maximum dose in Figure 14.4 will be 128% of 200 cGy or 256 cGy.

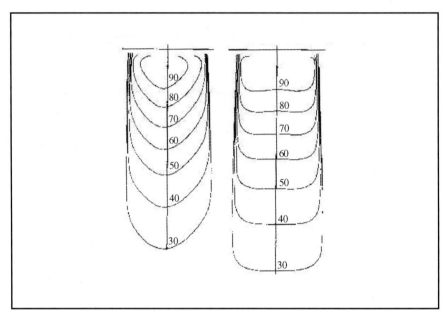

Figure 14.5: 10 MV beam dose distributions. The distribution on the left is without a flattening filter. The flattened beam on the right shows mild "horns" near the surface. (From *Radiation Therapy Physics,* 3rd Edition, W. R. Hendee, G. S. Ibbott, and E. G. Hendee. Fig. 4.11, p. 68. Copyright © 2005 John Wiley & Sons, Inc. Reproduced with permission from John Wiley & Sons, Inc.)

Figure 14.5 shows an isodose chart for a 10 MV beam both with and without a beam flattening filter in place. It is apparent that the dose distribution is highly nonuniform in the direction perpendicular to the central axis in the absence of a flattening filter. This is because bremsstrahlung emission is highly peaked in the forward direction as discussed in section 5.4 in chapter 5 and in chapter 9. For the beam on the right, the dose rises slightly when moving away from the central axis near the surface. This can also be seen in Figures 14.1 and 14.3. The beam is said to exhibit "horns" (examine the 90% isodose curve) near the surface. The beam has been overflattened here. A flattening filter cannot be designed to provide a perfectly flat beam at all depths. Some compromise is necessary. In order to have a beam that is flat at depths that are characteristic of treatment, it may be necessary to accept horns near the surface.

Figure 14.6 shows the effect of source size on the dose distribution. Both beams displayed are 10×10 cm^2 with an SSD of 50 cm (and a source-to-diaphragm distance of 27 cm). Notice the change in the penumbra as the source size increases. This is expected, based on the discussion of geometric penumbra in section 9.4 in chapter 9.

14.2 Skin Contour

In the previous section, we considered dose distributions resulting from a beam that is perpendicularly incident on a flat skin surface. Let us

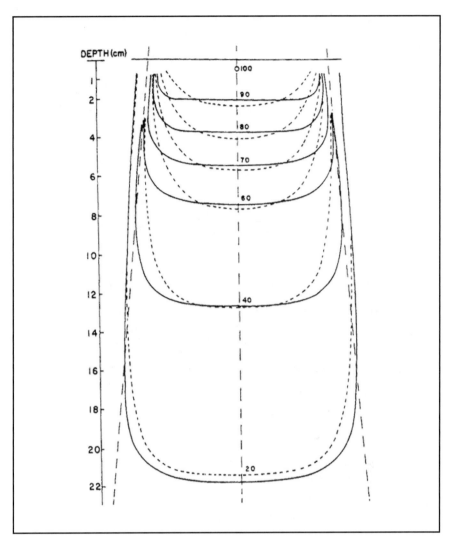

Figure 14.6: The influence of the source size on the dose distribution. Both beams are 10 × 10 cm² with an SSD of 50 cm. The solid curves are for a source with a 1 cm diameter; dashed curves for a source size of 2 cm diameter. (Reprinted from Hendee, W.R. *Medical Radiation Physics,* 1st edition. Chicago, IL: Year Book Medical Publishers, Inc., © 1970 with permission from the author.)

now consider what happens if the skin surface is slanted or curved. Figure 14.7 shows the isodose chart for a surface that is tilted 45° with respect to the horizontal. Note that the isodose curves tend to follow the tilt of the surface, particularly near the surface. Another example is shown in Figure 14.8.

The examples in Figures 14.7 and 14.8 have been generated by a computerized treatment planning system. Useful insight can be obtained however by studying manual methods for skin contour correction. Given an isodose chart like the one in Figure 14.1, there are three methods available for correcting percent depth doses for skin contour: isodose

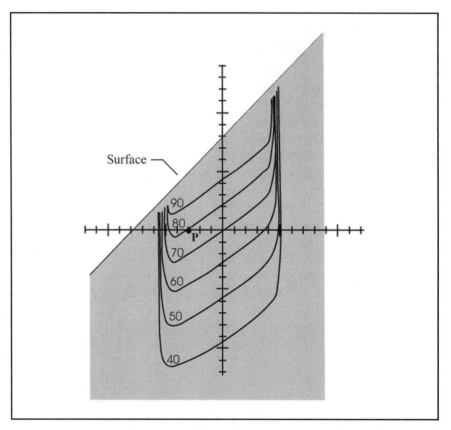

Figure 14.7: The effect of a sloping skin surface on the dose distribution of a 4 MV beam (10×10 cm^2, SSD = 100 cm). The skin slope is 45° with respect to the horizontal. The isodose curves have a tendency to follow the slope of the skin surface. This dose distribution was calculated with treatment planning software.

shift, effective SSD, and ratio of TAR (rTAR). These methods are reliable for angles of incidence up to about 45 degrees[2]. Note that the method discussed in section 13.4 in chapter 13 for calculating the dose rate at off-axis points, including an air gap, remains valid and very general.

14.2.1 Isodose Shift Method

Refer to Figure 14.9:

(1) Locate the point where the central axis intersects the surface and draw a horizontal line (AB) that is perpendicular to the central axis through this point.

---

[2] Khan, F. *The Physics of Radiation Therapy,* Third Edition. Philadelphia: Lippincott Williams & Wilkins, 2003.

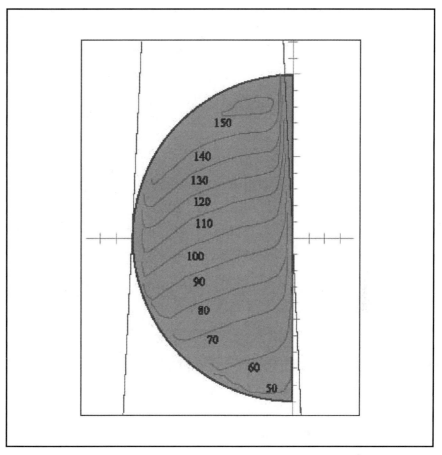

Figure 14.8: The dose distribution produced by a 4 MV beam incident "tangentially" on a semicircular phantom of radius 10 cm. The distance from the source to the center of the semicircle is 100 cm and this is the location where the dose distribution has been normalized to 100%. This dose distribution is characteristic of that which results from tangential irradiation of the human breast. The field size is 10 × 10 cm².

(2) Draw vertical lines parallel to the central axis and spaced about 1 cm apart.

(3) Superimpose the isodose chart with the surface along the horizontal line drawn in step 1.

(4) For each vertical line, shift the isodose lines by an amount $k \times g$, where g is the air gap along the vertical line and k is an empirical constant which depends on the beam energy and is always less than 1.00 (see Table 14.1).

(5) Mark an X along the vertical line where the isodose curves intersect this line.

(6) Repeat steps 4 and 5 for each vertical line.

(7) Connect the X's to trace out the new isodose curve.

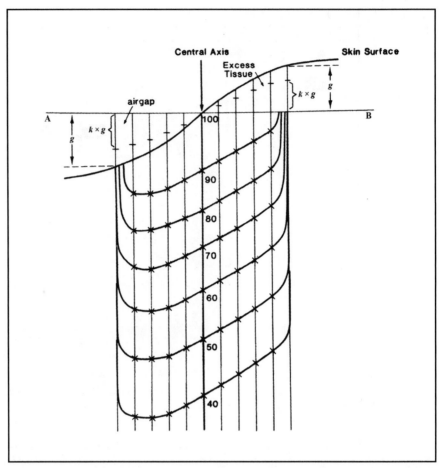

Figure 14.9: Illustration of the isodose shift method. (Adapted from Khan, F. M. *The Physics of Radiation Therapy,* Third Edition, Fig. 12.15, p. 247, © 2003, with permission from Lippincott Williams & Wilkins.)

If you examine Table 14.1, you will see that an approximate value of k for typical megavoltage beams is 2/3. You will also notice that the highest value of k is for the lowest energy range. We should expect this, as lower-energy radiation is attenuated more rapidly and therefore the shift needs to be larger for lower-energy beams. When $k \rightarrow 1.00$, the full shift is applied. This is the case in which the attenuation by matter becomes so rapid that it dominates inverse square changes.

One must remember that patients are three-dimensional. If the patient contour differs significantly in and out of the page, the dose distribution may be different from what the isodose shift method predicts.

The effective SSD and the rTAR methods are useful for calculating the dose to specific points, but the isodose shift method is the easiest method for generating the modified dose distribution.

Table 14.1: Isodose Shift Factors k*

Photon energy (MV)	k
Up to 1	0.8
Co-60–1	0.7
5–15	0.6
15–30	0.4

*Values taken from Khan, F. M. *The Physics of Radiation Therapy*, Third Edition, 2003.

14.2.2 Effective SSD Method

The SSD is taken to be the distance from the source to the point at which the central axis intersects the skin surface. The air gap g is the vertical distance of the skin surface from the plane AB in Figure 14.10. The air gap can be positive (tissue deficit) or negative (tissue excess). The procedure for calculating the PDD at point **P** is as follows:

(1) Place the isodose chart for standard SSD on the skin contour so that the surface on the isodose chart is lined up with surface AB. Shift the isodose chart down by an amount g so that the surface is at A'B'.

(2) Multiply the shifted chart PDD at point **P** by a correction factor described below.

The isodose chart is first shifted down from AB so that the surface is at A'B'. Here we derive the correction factor for the PDD as measured

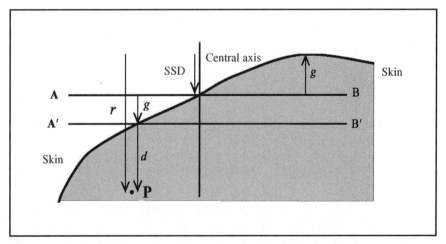

Figure 14.10: Geometry for the effective SSD and ratio of TAR method. Note that this figure is essentially the same as Figure 13.18.

with the surface at A′B′. The PDD takes into account attenuation of radiation by matter and the inverse square effect. When the PDD chart is shifted downward, the shift accounts for the change in attenuation of the matter due to the air gap but does not account for inverse square changes.

The dose at point **P** can be written:

$$D_P = D_{d_0}\left(\text{SSD} + g + d_0, f\right) \times \text{PDD}_P^s, \tag{14.1}$$

where $D_{d_0}\left(\text{SSD} + g + d_0, f\right)$ is the dose at depth d_0 at a total distance from the source of SSD + g + d_0 and for field size f, and PDD_P^s is the value of the PDD at point **P** read from the *shifted* isodose chart. We have neglected the small change in the PDD (i.e., the Mayneord factor) introduced by changing the SSD. The dose at point **P** can also be written as:

$$D_P = D_{d_0}\left(\text{SSD} + d_0, f\right) \times \text{PDD}_P, \tag{14.2}$$

where $D_{d_0}\left(\text{SSD} + d_0, f\right)$ is the dose at depth d_0 at a total source distance of SSD + d_0 and PDD_P is the corrected value of the PDD. The expressions for D_P in equations (14.1) and (14.2) can be equated and the resulting equation solved for PDD_P:

$$\frac{\text{PDD}_P}{\text{PDD}_P^s} = \frac{D_{d_0}\left(\text{SSD} + g + d_0, f\right)}{D_{d_0}\left(\text{SSD} + d_0, f\right)} = \left(\frac{\text{SSD} + d_0}{\text{SSD} + g + d_0}\right)^2, \tag{14.3}$$

so that

$$\text{PDD}_P = \text{PDD}_P^s \left(\frac{\text{SSD} + d_0}{\text{SSD} + g + d_0}\right)^2. \tag{14.4}$$

The correction is seen to be less than 1.00 for positive values of g. Shifting the isodose curves by the full amount g overestimates the correction. This is consistent with the isodose shift method where we shift the isodoses by an amount $k \times g$ where k is less than 1.00.

14.2.3   Ratio of TAR (rTAR) Method

This method provides a means of calculating a modified PDD due to the presence of an air gap. The isodose chart is placed with its surface at AB in Figure 14.10. The isodose line going through point **P** is noted and then this value is corrected. Note that in this method the isodose chart is *not* shifted.

For a flat skin surface (no air gap) the dose at point **P** is given by:

$$D_P^0 = D_{fs}\left(r_P, f\right) \times \text{TAR}\left(d + g, f_d\right), \tag{14.5}$$

where f_d is the equivalent square of the jaw setting as measured at depth d. With a gap present:

$$D_P^g = D_{fs}\left(r_P, f\right) \times \text{TAR}\left(d, f_d\right). \tag{14.6}$$

The correction factor is just the ratio of the dose with the gap to the dose without the gap:

$$\frac{D_P^g}{D_P^0} = \frac{\text{TAR}\left(d, f_d\right)}{\text{TAR}\left(d+g, f_d\right)}, \tag{14.7}$$

and therefore:

$$\text{PDD}_P = \text{PDD}_P^0 \times \frac{\text{TAR}\left(d, f_d\right)}{\text{TAR}\left(d+g, f_d\right)}, \tag{14.8}$$

where PDD_P^0 is the value of the unshifted PDD.

The methods of sections 14.2.1, 14.2.2, and 14.2.3 are acceptable for making approximate corrections of isodose values. For accurate dose calculations or for MU calculations based on dose prescribed to an off-axis point, the method of section 13.4 in chapter 13 is preferred. Example 14.2 illustrates a concrete application of the method in this and the previous section.

Example 14.2

A 10×10 cm^2 4 MV beam incident at a 45° angle is used to treat a patient (see Figure 14.7). The SSD along the central axis is 100 cm. At a point 3.0 cm off the central axis, there is an air gap of 3.0 cm. Calculate the PDD at 3.0 cm off the central axis and at a depth of 5 cm using (a) the effective SSD method and (b) the rTAR method, given that TAR(5,10) = 0.940 and TAR(8,10) = 0.835. Examine Figure 14.7 and read the computer-calculated PDD at point **P** from the figure. Compare this value with the result of your calculations.

If you took a 10×10 cm^2 isodose chart and shifted it downward 3.0 cm, you would find the $\text{PDD}_P^s = 83\%$. The correction factor is [(SSD + d_m)/ (SSD + g + d_m)]^2 = [(100 + 1.2)/(100 + 3 + 1.2)]^2 = 0.943, and therefore PDD_P = 83% × 0.943 = 78%.

When the isodose curve is not shifted down, the PDD_P^0 = 70.4%. The correction is TAR(5,10)/TAR(8,10) = 0.940/0.835 = 1.126, and therefore PDD_P = 1.126 × 70.4% = 79%. This agrees reasonably well with the effective SSD method.

The PDD at point **P** in Figure 14.7 is a little less than 80%.

14.3 Parallel-Opposed Fields

Single beams such as shown in Figure 14.1 are often used to treat superficial anatomical structures. Examples are treatment of the lymph nodes in the supraclavicular fossa, which are at a depth of about 3 cm, and spine treatments; the spinal cord is at a depth of roughly 5 cm from the posterior skin surface.

For deeper targets, a single beam would deliver excessive dose to tissues close to the skin surface and the dose distribution over any extended target at depth would be highly nonuniform. The basic goal of radiation therapy is to deliver as much dose as possible to the target and as little as possible to surrounding normal tissue. For deep targets, multiple beams, intersecting at the target, are used to spread out the dose to normal tissue.

The most simple multiple beam arrangement consists of two beams that are parallel to one another but enter from opposite sides of the body. These beams are said to be *parallel opposed*. Parallel-opposed fields are used to treat metastatic disease in limbs and they are used for a portion of the treatment of brain, head and neck, and lung cancers.

The dose distribution from parallel-opposed beams is remarkably uniform. An example is shown in Figure 14.11 for two 4 MV beams. In Figure 14.1 we see that the dose varies from about 100% to 40% over a depth of 20 cm. In Figure 14.11 the dose varies from approximately 98% to 110%.

For parallel-opposed fields, the dose is highest near the skin surface and then reaches a minimum at mid-depth (see Figure 14.12 and Example 14.3).

The dose uniformity along the central axis for parallel-opposed fields depends on patient thickness—as patient thickness increases, dose uniformity decreases—and on beam energy—as beam energy increases, dose uniformity increases.

If dose uniformity along the central axis is defined as the ratio of the maximum peripheral dose to the dose at the center (Figure 14.12), Table 14.2 can be used to decide on an appropriate beam energy.

Table 14.2: Requirements for ±5% Dose Uniformity Parallel-Opposed Fields (10 × 10 cm²)

Maximum patient thickness	Beam energy
15	Co-60, 4–6 MV
20	10 MV or above

Example 14.3

A 25-cm thick patient is treated with parallel-opposed AP/PA 4 MV, 10×10 cm^2 (open) beams to mid-depth with a total dose of 200 cGy (on the central axis). Each beam delivers 100 cGy. The SSD = 100 cm for both beams.

(a) What is the total dose at an anterior depth of 1.2 cm (d_0) and a posterior depth of 1.2 cm?

   The dose is the same at both of these points because of symmetry. Let us compute the dose at the anterior depth of 1.2 cm.

   There are two beams which contribute, the anterior and posterior, and thus $D_{total} = D_{AP} + D_{PA}$. We will compute the anterior contribution first:

   $$D_{AP} = \frac{D_{AP,mid}}{DD(12.5,10,100)} = \frac{100 \text{ cGy}}{0.534} = 187 \text{ cGy},$$

   where $D_{AP,mid}$ is the dose at mid-depth from the AP beam and DD(12.5,10,100) is found in appendix B.

   The dose from the PA beam can be calculated in two different ways:

   (1) Use the maximum dose from the PA beam (at depth 1.2 cm from the posterior skin surface). This will be 187 cGy (same as maximum for AP beam) because of symmetry.

   $$D_{PA} = D_{PA,maximum} \times DD(23.8,10,100)$$

   $$= 187 \times 0.263 = 49.2 \text{ cGy.}$$

   (2) Use the mid-depth PA dose and a ratio of PDD.

   $$D_{PA} = D_{PA,mid} \times \frac{PDD(23.8,10,100)}{PDD(12.5,10,100)} = 100 \times \frac{26.3\%}{53.4\%} = 49.3 \text{ cGy}$$

   Therefore $D_{total} = D_{AP} + D_{PA} = 187 + 49.3 = 237$ cGy.

(b) If the dose is normalized to 100% at mid-depth, what is the percent depth dose at a depth of 1.2 cm from either skin surface?

   $$PDD = 237/200 = 119\%.$$

   This can be compared with Figure 14.12, which shows a maximum PDD of approximately 113%. The difference is likely due to the fact that the calculation in this example does not include "build-down" (see page 14-16).

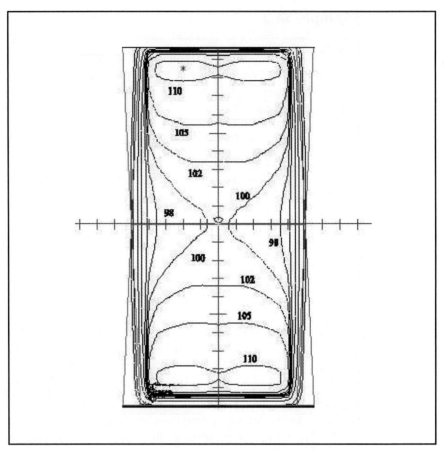

Figure 14.11: Dose distribution from 4 MV parallel-opposed fields. The field size is 10 × 10 cm². The phantom is 20 cm thick and the isocenter is at a depth of 10 cm (i.e., at mid-depth). The 100% isodose line shows an "hourglass" shape, which is characteristic of parallel-opposed beams. The distribution is remarkably uniform.

The PDD values in appendices B and C assume an infinitely deep phantom (or patient). Near the exit surface of a radiation beam, there will be a lack of full scatter (and thus a lack of CPE) because the air beyond the exit surface does not contribute to scatter. This will lead to a reduction in the dose due to scatter. This phenomenon is sometimes referred to as *build-down*. In Example 14.3 we have therefore overestimated the dose at d_0. Some treatment planning systems may not take this into account, nor do the isodose charts displayed in this book (e.g., Figure 14.11). PDD data are acquired with a scanning water phantom as discussed in section 9.4 in chapter 9. In practice, an infinitely deep phantom is clearly not possible nor necessary, provided that there is a sufficient amount of water below the maximum depth at which data are

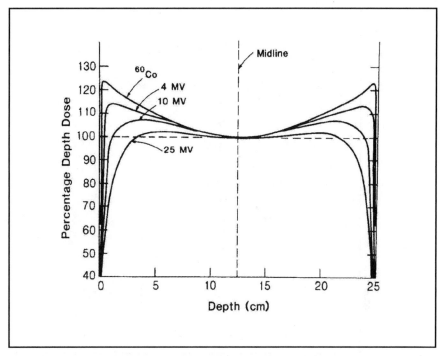

Figure 14.12: Dose distribution along the central axis for parallel-opposed fields of varying energy incident upon a 25 cm thick patient (SSD = 100 cm, field size 10 × 10 cm²). All dose distributions are normalized to 100% at the midline. (Reprinted from Khan, F. M. *The Physics of Radiation Therapy*, Third Edition, Fig. 11.11, p. 211, © 2003, with permission from Lippincott Williams & Wilkins.)

recorded. For megavoltage radiation beams, 5 cm of water is sufficient for this purpose. Any additional water does not increase the scatter dose. So the 5 cm boundary thickness of water effectively gives "infinite depth" conditions.

14.3.1 Adding Isodose Distributions

In the old days, isodose distributions resulting from multiple beams were combined manually. Today, computerized treatment planning systems perform this task automatically. It is still instructive, however, to understand the procedure for carrying out this task.

The dose distribution from a combination of two single beams can be obtained by superimposing the two sets of isodose curves and marking all intersections of the first and second sets with dots. Then connect all the dots having the same numerical values. This is illustrated in Figure 14.13. The resulting dose distribution can be renormalized as desired. For example, the 135% line in Figure 14.13 can be renormalized to 100% by

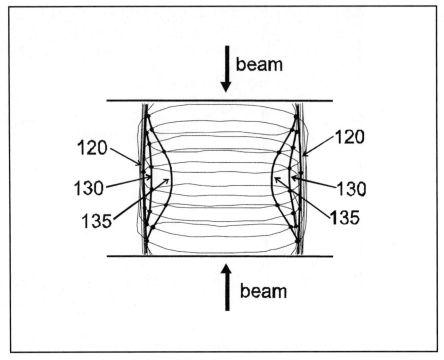

Figure 14.13: Adding isodose curves for parallel-opposed fields. The beam energy is 4 MV, field size 20 × 20 cm², patient thickness is 20 cm, and SSD = 100 cm for both beams. The procedure is to draw the isodose curves for the beam incident from above (shown dashed) and for the beam incident from below (dotted). Everywhere isodose lines intersect draw a dot and label the dot with the total value. Finally, connect all dots having the same value. These are shown as *solid curves*.

dividing all of the new isodose lines by 135%. To combine more than two beams, first combine any two, and then add the combination to the other beams one by one.

14.3.2 Beam Weighting

In Figure 14.11 the dose delivered by both beams is equal. It is advantageous to have one beam deliver more dose than the other when:

(1) the field is directed through a radiosensitive structure such as the spinal cord.
(2) tumor is not at mid-depth. This is illustrated in Figure 14.14. With equal weighting, the dose is high in the anterior normal tissue. Some kind of weighting may be necessary for parallel-opposed fields under these circumstances. If the tumor is closer to one skin surface than the other, weight the beam on that side more than 50% to shift the dose distribution toward the tumor (see Figure 14.15).

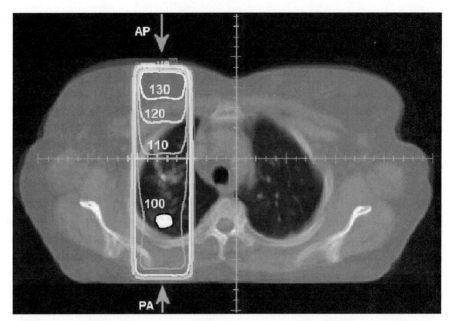

Figure 14.14: Two 6 MV parallel-opposed beams are used to treat a posterior lung tumor (white for visualization). The isocenter is at the center of the tumor. Both beams deliver an equal dose to the isocenter (50%). The dose distribution is normalized to 100% at the isocenter. Because the tumor lies so far posterior, the dose to anterior tissue is high. The maximum dose is 139%. See COLOR PLATE 4.

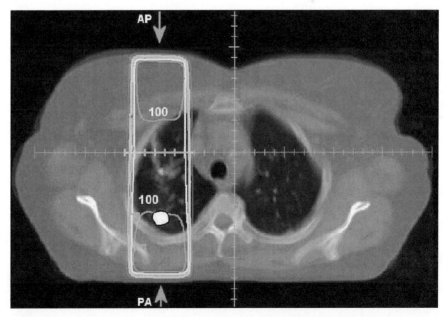

Figure 14.15: This is the same as Figure 14.14 except the beams have now been weighted to reduce the excess dose to the anterior tissue. The PA beam has been weighted 65% and the AP beam 35% at the isocenter. This means that 65% of the dose (at isocenter) is delivered by the PA beam and 35% by the AP beam. The high-dose region in the anterior tissue has now been reduced. See COLOR PLATE 5.

Beam weighting is commonly defined in one of two ways:

(1) relative weighting at d_0.
(2) relative weighting at the isocenter.

An example of beam weighting at the isocenter is shown in Figures 14.14 and 14.15.

14.4 Wedges

Wedges are wedge-shaped pieces of metal that are inserted in the beam to modify the dose distribution delivered by the treatment machine (see Figure 14.16). There are two types of wedges: internal (sometimes called "motorized") and external. Elekta linacs use an internal wedge. Varian and Siemens linacs use external wedges. An internal wedge is a single wedge inside the head of the linac above the collimator jaws. A motor moves the wedge into the beam when desired. External wedges are bolted to a tray that slides into a slot on the collimator of the treatment machine (see Figure 14.17). They are commonly made out of steel or lead. The slot for an external wedge is usually just above or below the slot for cast blocks. The trays are generally coded in some way so that the particular wedge and its orientation have to be properly identified on the treatment console before the machine will produce a beam. This serves as a double check to ensure that the proper wedge has been

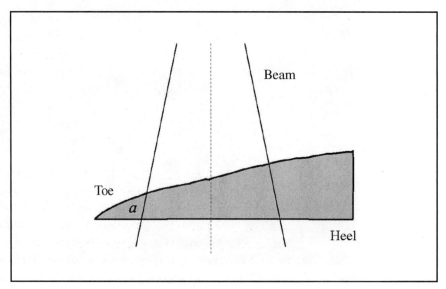

Figure 14.16: The cross section of a 30° wedge supplied by a major manufacturer. The angle a is NOT the wedge angle—see the text. Note that the cross section of the wedge is not precisely triangular.

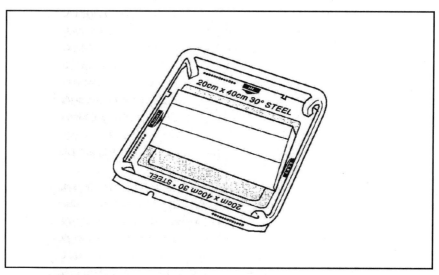

Figure 14.17: A wedge mounted on a tray. This wedge tray can be inserted into the collimator in any one of four different orientations. The maximum field size for this 30° wedge is 20 cm × 40 cm, as written on the tray. (Copyright © 2010, Varian Medical Systems Inc. All rights reserved.

inserted and that the orientation of the wedge is correct. It is also possible to produce a wedged dose distribution by moving one of the jaws while the beam is on. This is called a *dynamic wedge*. The thick end of the wedge is called the "heel" and the thin end is called the "toe." The wedge angle is NOT the physical angle of the wedge. There is no universally agreed upon definition of wedge angle. A common definition is that it is the angle between the isodose curve and the line perpendicular to the central axis (the "normal") at a specified depth (often 10 cm). Another definition is that it is the angle between the 50% isodose curve and the normal to the central axis (θ in Figure 14.18). Varian Medical Systems defines the wedge angle for their wedges as the angle with respect to the normal of the 80% isodose line (presumably for 100% at d_m).

Figures 14.18 and 14.19 show the dose distribution for 30° and 45° wedges for 6 and 15 MV beams, respectively. The isodose curves become less steep with increasing depth, probably due to an increase in the scatter component of the radiation.

Medical linear accelerators and Co-60 units having an external wedge are generally delivered with a set of these by the manufacturer. The wedges provided are usually 15°, 30°, 45°, and 60°. On a dual photon energy machine the same physical object (say the 45° wedge) is used for both energies even though the degree of isodose tilt will not be exactly the same for the two energies. The Elekta internal wedge is a 60° wedge mounted inside the head of the treatment machine. The wedge is either in or out of the beam. If, for example, a 45° wedge angle is desired, then the wedge is inserted into the beam during part of the treatment and withdrawn during the remainder of the treatment.

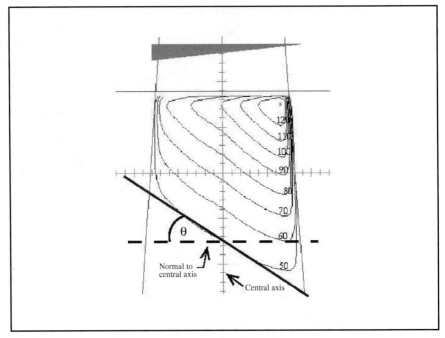

Figure 14.18: Isodose curves for a 6 MV beam (15 × 15 cm², SSD = 100 cm) with a θ = 30° wedge. In this illustration the wedge angle is the angle between the 50% line and the normal to the central axis.

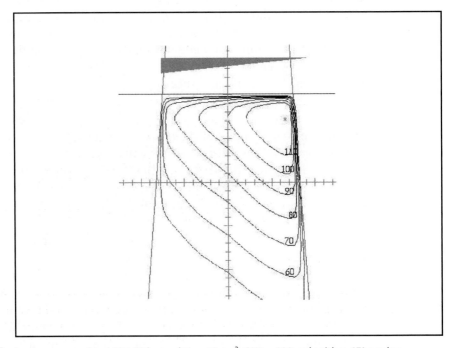

Figure 14.19: Isodose curves for a 15 MV beam (15 × 15 cm², SSD = 100 cm) with a 45° wedge.

Most wedges can be inserted in multiple orientations (toe toward gantry, heel toward gantry, etc.). Collimator rotation can also be used to change the orientation of a wedge. There is a maximum field size (less than the maximum jaw setting) that can be used with a wedge. As an example, for one older model linac, the maximum usable field size is 25 cm in the wedge direction by 30 cm wide (as measured at the isocenter) for all wedges except the 60° wedge for which the maximum field size is 20 cm × 30 cm. Interlocks prevent the field size from exceeding the limits for whichever wedge is inserted.

There are two possible reasons for using a wedge:

(1) *Tissue compensation.* The prime example is breast treatment with opposed tangent fields (see Figure 14.20). The wedges compensate for the tapering of the breast in the anterior direction and produce a much more uniform dose distribution. A wedge will compensate for the tilt in the isodose lines caused by the effects of skin contour, such as shown in Figures 14.7 and 14.8.

(2) *Multiple fields.* For multiple adjacent fields, it may be necessary to correct for a dose nonuniformity created by the overlap of adjacent beams. This topic is discussed in the next section.

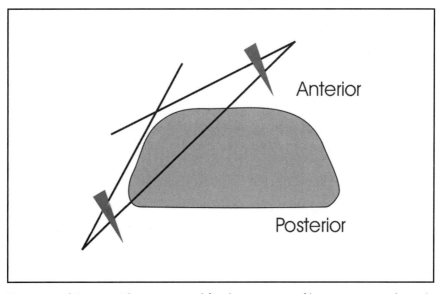

Figure 14.20: Two opposed "tangent" beams are used for the treatment of breast cancer, as shown in this transverse view. Wedges are placed in each beam to compensate for the taper in the breast skin contour shown in the anterior direction. The result is a more uniform dose distribution.

14.4.1 Wedged Fields

Superficial tumors are sometimes irradiated from two different directions (see Figure 14.21) in a cross fire pattern. The cross section of the
phantom used to illustrate this is a square. Most patients are not shaped
like this, although the anterior apex of the neck may not be too different! This shape is chosen so that each beam will be perpendicularly incident on a flat surface. The reason for this is to clearly illustrate the
effects of the adjacent beams without the additional complication from
the effects of a sloping phantom or patient surface. In a real patient,
with adjacent beams there will be sloping skin surface that will also
have an effect on the dose distribution. The dose distribution produced
by such cross irradiation is highly nonuniform. In particular, there is a
pronounced hot spot in the proximal corner where the two beams cross.
Wedges placed in each beam with the heels facing each other as in
Figure 14.22 can significantly improve dose uniformity. When placing
wedges in adjacent beams, the heels must always face one another.

How does one determine the wedge angle to use when there is cross
fire between two adjacent beams? The basic idea is to choose the wedge
angle so that the isodose curves become parallel in the overlap region
(see Figure 14.23). When the isodose curves become parallel, the two
dose distributions add like parallel-opposed fields. We have already
seen that parallel-opposed fields add to produce a surprisingly uniform
dose distribution. The desired wedge angle depends on the angle between
the central axes of the two beams, which is called the hinge angle φ (see
Figure 14.23). For a given hinge angle, the optimum wedge angle is
given by

$$\theta = 90 - \varphi / 2. \tag{14.9}$$

14.4.2 Wedge Transmission Factor

The wedge transmission factor is often simply called the *wedge factor,*
denoted $\mathrm{WF}(d, f_d')$. It is measured on the central axis:

$$\mathrm{WF}\left(d, f_d'\right) = \frac{D_d\left(100, f_d'\right) \text{with wedge}}{D_d\left(100, f_d'\right) \text{without wedge}}. \tag{14.10}$$

Tables of wedge factors for the Mevalac 6 MV and 18 MV beams appear
in appendix C. Typical values of the wedge factor range from 0.3 to 0.8.
The presence of a wedge significantly raises the number of monitor units
(or the time on for Co-60) necessary to deliver the prescribed dose.

The wedge factor depth dependence is a result of "beam hardening."
As the radiation traverses the wedge, the low-energy component of the

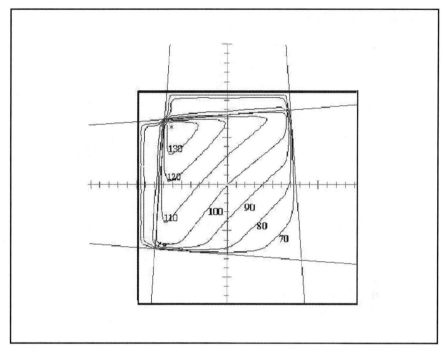

Figure 14.21: The dose distribution from two 4 MV beams at right angles to one another that are incident on a square phantom.

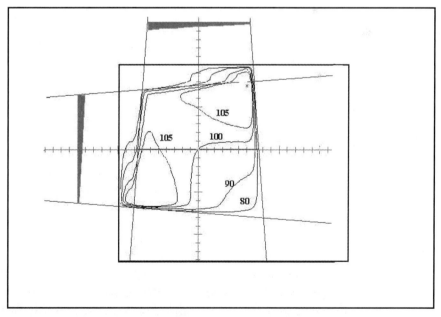

Figure 14.22: This is the same as Figure 14.21 except 45° wedges have been placed in the beams with heels facing one another (sometimes called a "wedged pair"). This eliminates the hotspot in the upper left-hand corner of Figure 14.21 and results in a much more homogeneous dose distribution.

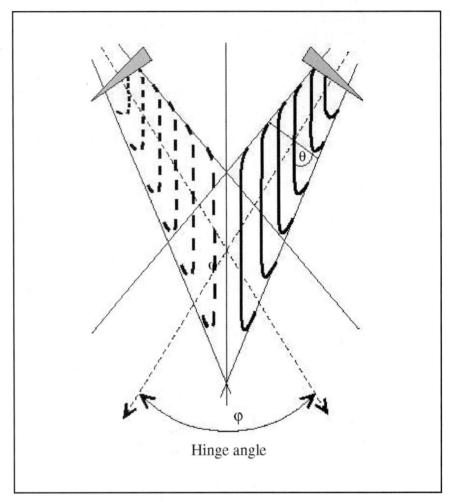

Figure 14.23: Adjacent beams with isodoses tilted by wedges. The hinge angle φ is the angle between the central axes of the two beams. The wedge angle should be chosen so as to tilt the two sets of isodoses so that they are roughly parallel and thus add like parallel-opposed fields. (Adapted from Khan, F. M. *The Physics of Radiation Therapy,* Third Edition, Fig. 11.18, p. 219, © 2003, with permission from Lippincott Williams & Wilkins.)

energy spectrum is preferentially absorbed. When the beam exits the wedge, its average energy is higher than when it entered. Do not confuse the intensity with the energy of the beam. The wedge reduces the number of photons (intensity), but the photons that do come through have a higher average energy. This effect is most pronounced for low-energy beams and thick wedges. The dependence of the wedge factor on field size is due to scattering in the wedge.

As an example, the wedge factor for a 20×20 cm^2 field may be as much as 5% higher than for a 10×10 cm^2 field. The wedge factor selected from the tables in appendix C should be chosen based on the irregular field size.

As previously mentioned, Elekta linacs have a single internal wedge. This is a 60° wedge, which is either in or out of the field. To produce a radiation field with an effective wedge angle other than 60°, the wedge is placed in the field for a portion of the total irradiation time. If MU_t is the total number of monitor units for a field, MU_w is the number of monitor units for which the wedge is in the field, and MU_o is the number of monitor units for which the wedge is withdrawn (out), then the effective wedge factor is

$$\mathrm{WF}_{\mathit{eff}}\left(d, f_d'\right) = \frac{1}{\mathrm{MU}_t}\left(\mathrm{WF}\left(d, f_d'\right) \times \mathrm{MU}_w + \mathrm{MU}_o\right), \qquad (14.11)$$

where $\mathrm{WF}\left(d, f_d'\right)$ is the wedge factor for the 60° wedge.

14.4.3 Dose Rate Calculations with a Wedge Present

When a wedge is inserted in the beam, the dose rate on the central axis is reduced by the wedge factor. The dose rate on the central axis is calculated in the usual way and then multiplied by the wedge factor. For a TMR calculation:

$$\dot{D}_d\left(r, f_d'\right) = \dot{D}_{d_0}\left(100 + d_0, 10\right) \times S_c\left(f\right) \times S_p\left(f_d'\right) \times \left(\frac{100 + d_0}{\mathrm{SSD} + d}\right)^2 \times \mathrm{TMR}\left(d, f_d'\right)$$

$$\times \mathrm{TF} \times \mathrm{WF}\left(d, f_d'\right). \qquad (14.12)$$

This is simply equation (13.1) multiplied by the wedge factor. The number of monitor units is calculated from the dose rate in the usual way: $\mu = D/\dot{D}$, as shown in Example 14.4.

Example 14.4

A patient is to be treated isocentrically on the Mevalac with a 6 MV beam at a depth of 5.0 cm and with a 15 $\times$ 15 cm^2 open (unblocked) field. A 15° wedge is to be used. How many MU should be set to deliver a dose of 180 cGy on the central axis?

The value of WF(5,15) = 0.712, and TMR(5.0, 15.0) = 0.935 is found in the tables in appendix C:

$$\dot{D}_d\left(r, f_d'\right) = \dot{D}_{d_0}\left(100 + d_0, 10\right) \times S_{c,p}\left(f\right) \times \left(\frac{100 + d_0}{\mathrm{SSD} + d}\right)^2 \times \mathrm{TMR}\left(d, f_d\right)$$

$$\times \mathrm{TF} \times \mathrm{WF}\left(d, f_d\right)$$

$$= 1.000 \times 1.030 \times \left(\frac{100 + 1.5}{100}\right)^2 \times 0.935 \times 1.00 \times 0.712$$

$$= 0.706 \text{ cGy/MU}$$

and $\mu = D/\dot{D} = 255$ MU.

Calculations of the dose at points off the central axis in the presence of a wedge require wedge off-axis factors. Although we will not discuss the details here, in principle this is no more difficult than the use of the OAR in chapter 13, section 13.4.

Wedges are one of the single biggest causes of error in radiation therapy—either the wedge is not inserted when it should be (i.e., MU calculation assumes the presence of a wedge), or it is inserted the wrong way (e.g., toe and heel are reversed), or the MU calculations do not take into account the wedge transmission factor even though a wedge is called for in the treatment instructions. Note that if the wedge is inserted the wrong way, the dose delivered to points on the central axis will be as intended. The dose distribution, however, will be worse than if no wedge was used and will be highly nonuniform.

14.5 Multiple Beams

For curative treatment of deep-seated tumors, multiple beams are usually used, generally three or more. Parallel-opposed beams deliver a large dose to subcutaneous tissue, which may be undesirable. Multiple beams maximize the dose to the tumor and spread out the dose to normal tissues and organs. The basic strategy is to use multiple beams in a cross-fire arrangement with the target in the region of overlap. In this region, the dose will be high and elsewhere it will be relatively low. One method for accomplishing this is to use sets of parallel-opposed fields. This implies an even number of beams. The drawback here is that along the entire central axis of the parallel-opposed beams, the dose will be relatively high. Sometimes an odd number of beams is preferable. In this case, the use of wedges may be called for. If the central axes of all the beams lie in the same plane they are said to be coplanar. Non-coplanar beams can be delivered by using a couch rotation (sometimes called a couch "kick"). In choosing multiple beams, there are a number of degrees of freedom available to the treatment planner:

(1) Field size and blocking.
(2) Number of beams or ports.
(3) Beam direction (as determined by gantry and couch angle).
(4) Beam weighting.
(5) Beam energy.
(6) Beam modifiers: wedges, compensators.

A region of relatively uniform high dose occurs where beams overlap one another. The size and shape of the region of overlap can be adjusted by changing the field size and beam angle. An example of a commonly used multiple beam arrangement is a "four-field box," as shown in Figures 14.24 and 14.25. This is essentially two parallel-opposed fields

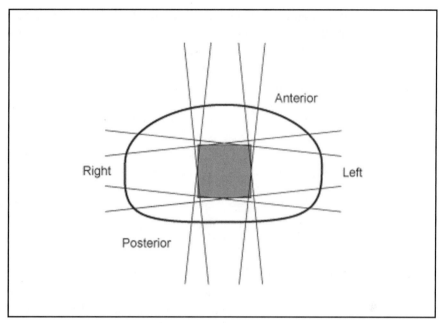

Figure 14.24: A four-field box beam arrangement drawn on an axial slice of a patient. The dose is high in the shaded region where all of the beams overlap, but relatively low elsewhere. This is a beam arrangement that is commonly used for pelvic irradiation, such as for treatment of prostate cancer.

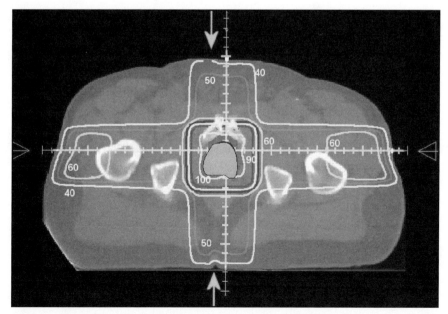

Figure 14.25: A four-field box dose distribution resulting from four beams. The beams are all 15 MV equally weighted. The isocenter is at the center of the coordinate system where the dose has been normalized to 100%. The isodoses are displayed in increments of 10% from 100% down to 40%. Each tick mark on the grid represents 1 cm. This is a prostate treatment. The prostate is represented by the uniformly gray structure at the center of the axial slice. The dose is high and uniform where the beams overlap and relatively low elsewhere. See COLOR PLATE 6.

at right angles to one another. As the dose throughout a parallel-opposed field arrangement is roughly uniform, we expect each set of parallel-opposed fields to contribute about equally to the dose at the center (assuming equal weighting for all beams). This implies that the dose in the periphery of each set of beams should be roughly 50%.

Figure 14.26 shows an example of two opposed pairs of beams at an angle other than 90° (four oblique beams). The shape of the region of overlap where the dose is high is a rhombus.

A wedged pair of beams is two intersecting beams accompanied by the use of wedges. The beams are sometimes orthogonal. The heels must face one another to obtain a uniform dose distribution. Figure 14.22 showed a wedged pair. This type of beam arrangement is used for treatment of the maxillary antrum.

A three-beam arrangement such as used to treat the rectum is shown in Figure 14.27. The two lateral beams must be wedged.

Non-coplanar beams may be useful when it is essential to avoid a critical structure and it is not possible to do so with a coplanar beam arrangement. Care must be taken to avoid a collision between the gantry and the patient or couch. Non-coplanar converging arcs are used in stereotactic radiosurgery (see chapter 20).

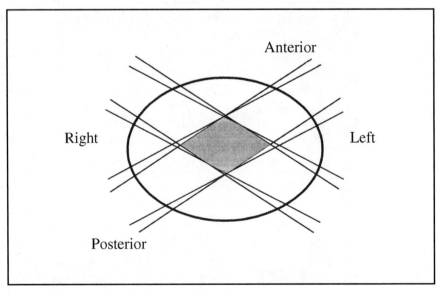

Figure 14.26: A set of four oblique beams. The area of high dose corresponds to the region of overlap—rhombus shaped in this case.

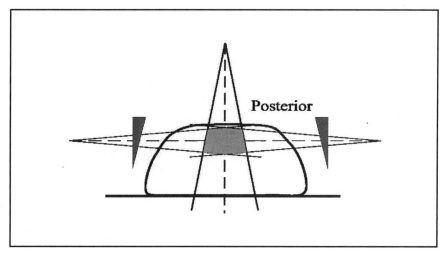

Figure 14.27: A three-field rectum treatment. Wedges are used for the lateral beams; otherwise the dose would be higher in the posterior part of the target volume. The wedge makes the dose more uniform throughout the target.

14.6 Dose-Volume Specification and Reporting

The International Commission on Radiation Units and Measurements (ICRU) recommends standardized methodology for defining tissue treatment volumes and for reporting dose. The references of record are ICRU Report 50 and Report 62.

The target volume is separated into three distinct boundaries: (1) visible tumor (gross tumor volume, or GTV); (2) a region to account for microscopic tumor extension (clinical target volume, or CTV); and (3) a region to account for positional uncertainties (planning target volume, or PTV). See Figure 14.28.

The GTV is the volume of disease that can be either seen with imaging studies (e.g., CT, MRI, etc.) or felt on palpation. The CTV contains the entire GTV plus suspected microscopic disease that extends outside the GTV. The definition of the CTV will involve known routes of spread of the given tumor type. This may include lymph nodes. The CTV must be treated adequately to achieve the goals of therapy. In a specific patient there may be more than one CTV, and these may be treated to different doses.

The PTV includes a margin to be added to the CTV to account for uncertainties or variations in the position of the CTV. There are variations associated with the setup of the patient on a daily basis. The

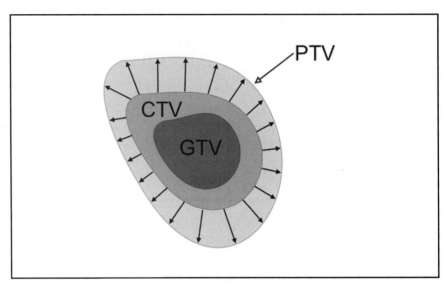

Figure 14.28: GTV, CTV, and expansion of CTV to PTV. The margin between the CTV and PTV may be different in different directions.

patient may not be in precisely the same position every day. In addition, internal organs, including the target, may move inside the patient. An example of this is motion associated with breathing. You can think of the PTV as a bounding envelope in three-dimensional space. The GTV and the CTV move inside this envelope but cannot move through it. The PTV includes all of the uncertainties/variations for the CTV. The purpose of establishing a PTV is to add a margin to ensure that the entire CTV receives the prescribed dose.

For any given beam, the beam aperture is usually made a little larger than the PTV, as seen from that direction, to allow for beam penumbra since, by definition, the edge of the beam corresponds to only the 50% isodose line. It may be necessary to set the beam edges as much as 7 mm outside the PTV to make such an allowance. A compromise may be necessary between the need for adequate margin coverage and the desire to spare organs at risk.

The treated volume is the volume enclosed by an isodose surface specified by the radiation oncologist; e.g., 95% isodose surface. The irradiated volume receives a dose considered significant in relation to normal tissue tolerance (e.g., 50% isodose surface).

Normal tissues whose radiation sensitivity may significantly influence treatment planning, perhaps limiting the prescribed dose, are called *organs at risk*. Examples are the spinal cord, optic chiasm, kidneys, liver, lens of the eye, etc. Like the GTV, the size, shape, and position of organs at risk vary and this leads to a margin analogous to the PTV called the *planning organ at risk volume (PRV)*. If the PTV and PRV overlap, it becomes necessary to make a difficult clinical choice or a compromise of some sort. A *serial* organ at risk is one in which radiation damage to even a small volume will cause serious disruption or total loss of function. The prime example is the spinal cord. A *parallel organ* is one is one in which radiation damage to a part of the organ may cause some loss of function but does not incapacitate the entire organ. For a parallel organ the degree of damage is related to the size of the irradiated region of the organ that receives a dose above the threshold level. Lungs and kidneys are parallel organs. Some organs cannot be easily categorized. A serial organ is like a string of Christmas light bulbs wired in series. If one bulb fails, the whole string will fail because electrical current must pass through the filament of each bulb to reach the next bulb. When the bulbs are connected in parallel, one bulb can fail and the rest of the bulbs will continue to be illuminated.

One must distinguish between positional uncertainties, or errors, and mistakes. The word "error" is often used to describe uncertainties. This is unfortunate terminology because the term "error" implies a mistake or blunder. This is not what the word "error" means in this context. To avoid this confusion, we shall use the word uncertainty. Careful quality assurance should eliminate almost all mistakes. *Uncertainties* are variations in CTV position inherent in the process of treatment planning and delivery that are left over after mistakes are eliminated.

There are two contributions to the overall margin or uncertainty: (1) uncertainties in the position of the patient's bony anatomy with respect to a coordinate system fixed in the treatment room, called the *setup margin* and (2) changes in position or shape with respect to the patient's bony anatomy, called the *internal margin*. These uncertainties can be random or systematic.

Uncertainties in the position of the patient's bony anatomy are caused by daily setup variations, mechanical variations in the treatment unit such as couch sag, gantry angle uncertainty, systematic differences between the simulator and treatment unit, etc. These uncertainties require a setup margin. Some positioning aids and immobilization devices can help reduce setup uncertainties.

The *internal margin* is the margin to be added to the CTV to account for variations in size, shape, or position with respect to bony anatomy. The internal margin will usually be asymmetric. The internal margin is associated with physiological processes such as respiration, heartbeat, swallowing, bladder and rectal filling, etc. Such motion is not easily controllable. The volume expansion of the CTV to accommodate the internal margin is sometimes called the *internal target volume (ITV)*.

Interfractional uncertainties are variations in position occurring between separate fractions. These are due to daily setup variations or physiological factors (degree of bladder filling, bowel gas, etc.). Additional factors are tumor shrinkage or weight loss. Intrafractional uncertainties are associated with motion, either motion of the patient as a whole or internal motion associated with physiological processes such as respiration.

The total margin to be added to the CTV to form the PTV should ideally be based on data reported in the literature or collected in the user's clinic.

14.7 Evaluation of Patient Dose Distributions

Evaluation of a patient's treatment plan must include a thorough examination of the isodose distribution in three dimensions. The sagittal and coronal planes should be examined as well as the axial planes. The amount of information contained in the isodose distribution is huge, and it is helpful to have various tools that condense or summarize these data and facilitate comparison of rival treatment plans.

Cumulative dose-volume histograms (DVHs) are a treatment planning tool used in conjunction with 3-D dose distributions to evaluate dose to normal tissue and tumors. Let us introduce the idea of the dose-volume histogram by first calculating a cumulative dose-*area* histogram. Figure 14.29 shows an axial CT slice of a patient's treatment plan. This particular slice goes through the center of the patient's stomach. The stomach is an organ at risk and we wish to evaluate the dose distribution by calculating a cumulative dose-area histogram for the stomach.

In Figure 14.30 the image of the stomach has been divided up into square boxes. The dose is assumed to be constant in each box. This is a reasonable approximation to the extent that the boxes are small enough. In Figure 14.30 the boxes are not very small and the calculations may

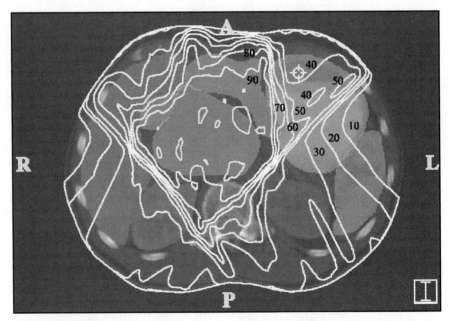

Figure 14.29: The dose distribution on an axial CT slice. We are concerned with the dose distribution in the patient's stomach, which is anterior and on the patient's left (your right). The isodose lines are labeled in this region (in percent). In section 4.7, we calculate the "dose area histogram" for the stomach. See COLOR PLATE 7.

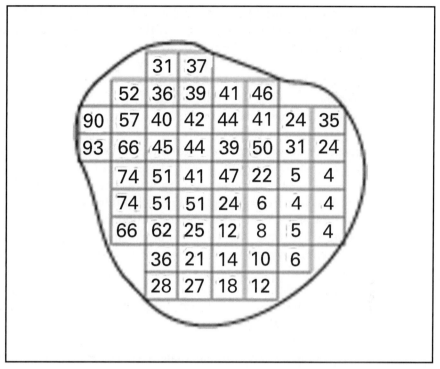

Figure 14.30: The image of the stomach in Figure 14.29 has been divided up into square boxes. Each box is labeled with a dose (in percent), which is assumed to be constant within the box.

not be very accurate, but it is acceptable for the purpose of illustration. We could make it more accurate by making the boxes smaller.

The dose distribution data displayed in Figure 14.30 is tabulated in Table 14.3. The first column of the table lists the percent dose. The second column is the number of boxes that have a percent dose equal to or

Table 14.3: Dose-Area Histograms

Dose (%)	Number of boxes equal to or above[a]	Percentage of total[b]
100	0	0.0
90	2	3.8
80	2	3.8
70	4	7.5
60	7	13.2
50	13	24.5
40	23	43.4
30	31	58.5
20	39	73.6
10	44	83.0
0	53	100.0

[a]Number of boxes that have a percent dose equal to or above the value in column 1.
[b]Percentage of the total number of boxes that have dose equal to or above the value in column 1.

above the value in the first column. The third column has the percentage of the total number of boxes that have dose equal to or above the value in the first column. As an example of the counting, look at the second row in the table. There are two boxes in Figure 14.30 that have a dose of 90% or above. There are a total of 53 boxes in Figure 14.30. Two boxes represents about 4% of the total. You should try to verify the rest of the rows in the table.

The data in Table 14.3 are plotted in Figure 14.31. This is a cumulative dose-area histogram. It shows the percentage of the area that is above a given dose. We see that 100% of the area of this organ has a dose of 0% or above. The maximum dose is a little above 90% (i.e., 93%).

When a treatment planning computer calculates dose, it divides the volume up into little boxes called *voxels* (short for volume elements). The dose is assumed to be constant inside each box. This is an acceptable approximation provided that the boxes are small enough. The collection of all of the dose values in the voxels is called the *dose matrix*.

A cumulative dose volume histogram (cDVH, or just DVH for short) shows the volume (usually in percent) receiving at least dose D. The dose is sometimes given in percent and sometimes in centigray (cGy) or gray (Gy). To calculate a DVH for a structure, that structure must be outlined ("contoured") in the treatment planning system so that the computer "knows" which voxels belong to that structure.

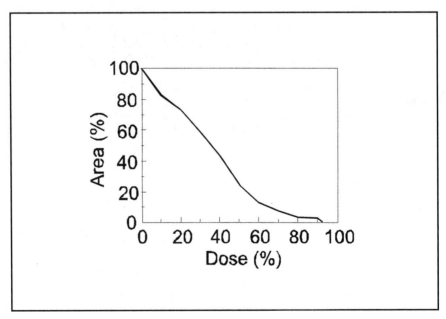

Figure 14.31: A cumulative dose area histogram for the dose distribution in the stomach shown in Figures 14.29 and 14.30.

Figure 14.32 shows an example of a DVH for an organ at risk. The vertical axis shows the volume as a percentage of the whole. Sometimes the absolute volume (in cubic centimeters) is shown. This is useful when the entire structure is not contoured, such as might be the case with the spinal cord. The horizontal axis shows the dose as a percentage, where the dose has been normalized to 100% at some location. Often the absolute dose is shown on the horizontal axis to remove any confusion about normalization. It is always true that 100% of the volume receives at least zero dose, and therefore all DVHs start at 100% on the vertical axis. The dotted lines in the figure show that 50% of the volume receives at least 40% of the dose. The maximum dose received by this organ is 90%. If the prescription calls for a dose of 45 Gy delivered to the 100% dose surface, then 50% of the volume of this organ receives at least 0.40×45 Gy = 18 Gy.

It is common to encounter the notation V_D where V is the percentage of the volume receiving a dose of at least D (usually in Gy). Likewise D_V is the dose (in Gy or percent) received by at least $V(\%)$ of the volume. As an example V_{66} is the percentage of the volume that receives at least 66 Gy. $D_{95\%}$ is the dose received by 95% of the volume. In Figure 14.32, $V_{40\%} = 50\%$; that is, 50% of the volume receives over

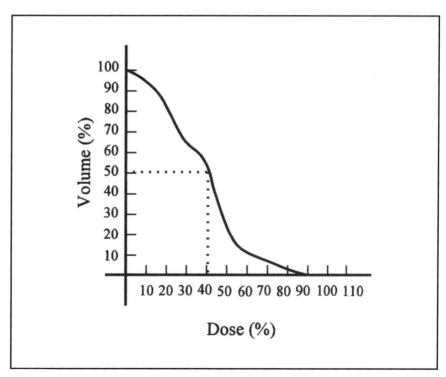

Figure 14.32: A cumulative DVH for a normal organ. This shows the volume (in percent of the total) receiving at *least* dose D (in percent, normalized to 100% at some convenient location).

40% of the prescribed dose (assumed to be 100%). The mean dose to a structure is 0.01 times the area under the DVH when the DVH is in the form of volume (%) versus dose (absolute, not percent).

If the dose is uniform (the same) throughout the volume, then the DVH will appear as in Figure 14.33. This is an ideal dose volume histogram for a target because 100% of the volume receives the full prescription dose and none of the target receives more than or less than the prescription dose. A realistic DVH for a target volume (either CTV or PTV) appears in Figure 14.34. In this figure the minimum dose is about 80%—that is to say that 100% of the volume receives 80% of the dose or more. This is a "cold" spot of 80%; it is the lowest dose in the target volume. The maximum dose in the target is a little bit above 110%. This is the "hot" spot. A common treatment planning goal is that 100% of the PTV receive at least 95% of the dose ($V_{95\%} = 100\%$) or perhaps even 98% ($V_{98\%} = 100\%$) of the prescribed dose.

Figures 14.35 and 14.36 show DVHs for an organ at risk from rival treatment plans. When comparing the dose to organs at risk in rival treatment plans, the target coverage should be the same for each plan. In Figure 14.35 DVH ① is clearly superior to DVH ②. The volume receiving any given dose is always less for plan ①. In Figure 14.36 the situation is not so clear, since the DVHs cross one another. The volume receiving low dose is less for DVH ①, but the volume receiving a high

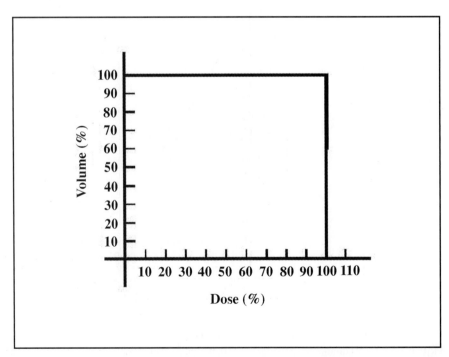

Figure 14.33: A DVH in which the dose is uniformly 100% throughout the entire volume. This is an ideal DVH for a target.

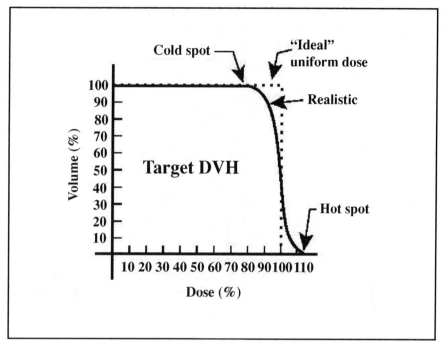

Figure 14.34: A realistic target DVH. The cold spot in the target is about 80% of the prescribed dose and the hot spot is a little over 110%.

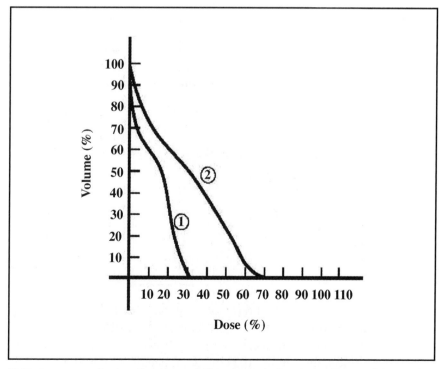

Figure 14.35: DVHs for a normal organ from two different treatment plans. The DVH labeled ① is clearly preferred to the other DVH (labeled ②) because ① lies entirely below ②.

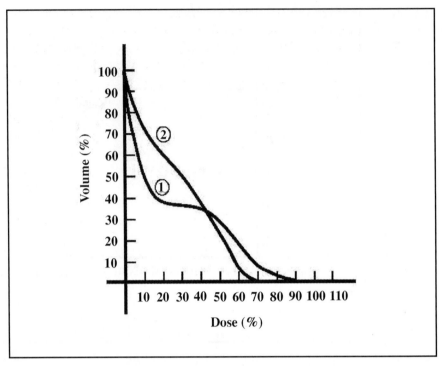

Figure 14.36: DVHs for a normal organ from two different treatment plans. Which DVH is better? When DVHs cross, it is not always clear which one is preferred.

dose is more for DVH ①. The question is: "Which is preferable, for a large amount of an organ to receive a low dose or for a small amount of an organ to receive a high dose?" For organs such as the spinal cord, optic nerves and optic chiasm (so called serial organs) the choice is clear, since damage to even a small amount of these organs will have serious consequences. In this case, DVH ② is preferred because the maximum dose is lower. For some organs at risk however, the answer to this question may not be clear and only additional biological or clinical data can settle the question. Biological indices include the tumor control probability (TCP), the normal tissue complication probability (NTCP), the equivalent uniform dose, (EUD) and the probability of uncomplicated control.

DVHs are not a substitute for the entire dose distribution. The single biggest drawback of DVHs is a loss of spatial information. DVHs do not tell us the location of the hot spot or the cold spot. If the hot spot is at the center of the tumor, that may be acceptable, perhaps even desirable. If the hot spot is on the periphery of the tumor, particularly if it is near a critical organ at risk, that may be unacceptable. The same considerations apply to a cold spot. A cold spot at the center of the target is probably unacceptable. A cold spot at the periphery of a target may be acceptable, provided that it is not too cold.

The integral dose is a measure of the total energy absorbed by the patient from radiation. This quantity is not generally calculated for most treatment plans. but it is nonetheless a useful concept to understand. Let us start by supposing that the dose throughout some volume is completely uniform (i.e., the same everywhere throughout the volume). Under these circumstances the integral dose to this volume would be the dose multiplied by the mass of this volume. For example, if the dose is 60 Gy and the mass of the volume is 2 kg, then the integral dose is 60 J/kg × 2 kg = 120 J. If the dose varies throughout a volume (as it always does), then the integral dose may be found by dividing the volume into voxels. The voxels need to be small enough so that the dose is approximately constant in each voxel. The integral dose in each voxel can be computed by multiplying the mass of the voxel by the dose in that voxel. The total integral dose received by a patient can then be calculated by summing the integral dose for all of the voxels. In designing a treatment for a patient, one would like to minimize the integral dose to the patient while maintaining a fixed dose to the PTV.

14.8 Arc or Rotation Therapy

In arc or rotation therapy the gantry rotates continuously around the patient while the beam is on. This can produce dose distributions that are very conformal in an axial plane. Practical restrictions may make it impossible to deliver a full 360° rotational treatment. For example, it may not be possible to treat through the edges of the couch because of the presence of metallic bars. Sometimes partial arcs are delivered where the angular rotation of the gantry is less than the full 360°.

Figure 14.37 shows the dose distribution for various arcs. For the full 360° rotation, the dose maximum is at the isocenter. For the partial arcs, the dose maximum is displaced toward the irradiated sector. For this reason, one should point the beam past (or beyond) the desired position of the dose maximum. This technique is called "past pointing."

For a full 360° rotational treatment, the average dose rate is calculated as follows:

(1) Locate the desired position of the isocenter on an axial contour of the patient.
(2) Draw radial spokes (in the same way as for Clarkson integration) from the isocenter to the skin surface. These should be drawn at regular angular intervals (see Figure 14.38 in which the radial spokes are drawn at 20° intervals).
(3) Determine the appropriate field size to cover the target.
(4) Compute the average TAR or TMR as follows:

$$\overline{\text{TMR}} = \frac{1}{n}\left[\text{TMR}\left(d_1, f\right) + \text{TMR}\left(d_2, f\right) + \cdots + \text{TMR}\left(d_n, f\right)\right], \quad (14.13)$$

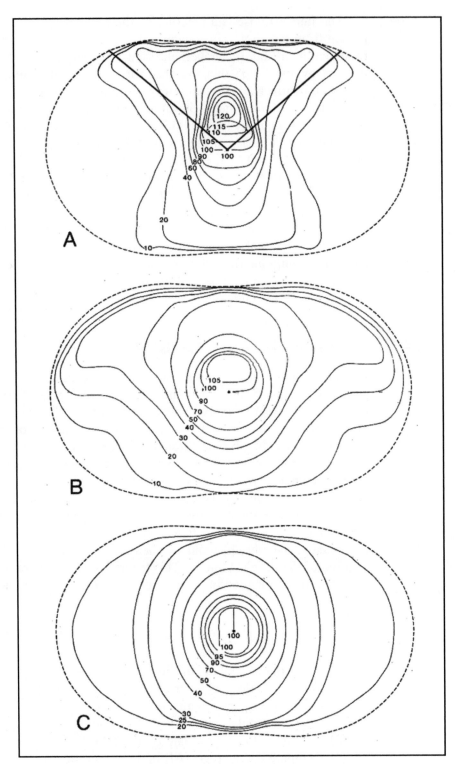

Figure 14.37: Dose distribution for a rotational arc therapy. A 100° arc is shown in (a). A 180° degree arc is shown in (b) and a full 360° arc is shown in (c). Notice that the maximum dose is shifted toward the irradiated sector for the partial arcs. (Reprinted from Khan, F. M. *The Physics of Radiation Therapy,* Third Edition, Fig. 11.16, p. 218, © 2003, with permission from Lippincott Williams & Wilkins.)

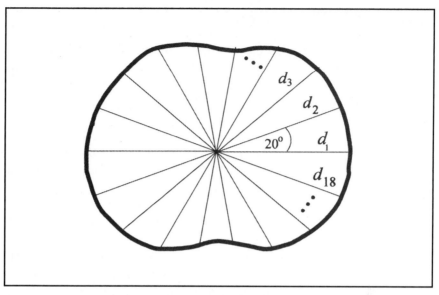

Figure 14.38: The setup for a calculation of a 360° rotational treatment. Radial spokes have been drawn every 20° from the isocenter to the skin surface. There are a total of 18.

where $\overline{\text{TMR}}$ is the average TMR and n is the number of radial spokes. An alternative is to calculate the average TAR in the same way.

(5) The average dose rate at the isocenter is:

$$\dot{D}_{iso} = \dot{D}_{fs}\left(\text{SAD}, f\right) \times \overline{\text{TAR}}$$

or   (14.14)

$$\dot{D}_{iso} = \dot{D}_{d_0}\left(\text{SAD}, f\right) \times \overline{\text{TMR}}.$$

The number of MU to set is calculated in the usual way: $\mu = D / \dot{D}_{iso}$.

Rotational treatments are no longer routinely used. To the extent that the patient skin contour does not change dramatically above (superior) or below (inferior) the axial central plane (plane through the geometric center), the dose distribution will be the same on axial slices above and below this plane. The dose distribution will therefore be cylindrical. Most target volumes are not cylindrical in shape; they tend to taper away from the central axial plane. For this reason, rotational treatments have largely been replaced by static custom-shaped fields. An exception to this is stereotactic radiosurgery (linac based) in which multiple arcs are used in different planes (by using a couch rotation) to deliver highly conformal dose distributions to targets in the brain. Intensity-modulated arc therapy (IMAT) and tomotherapy are sophisticated extensions of simple rotational therapy (see chapter 20).

14.9 Surface Dose

Skin sparing for megavoltage photon beams was discussed in chapter 7, section 7.5. The reasons for skin sparing were also addressed in that section. There was also a discussion of reasons that there is any skin dose at all. We repeat those reasons here:

(1) Electron contamination of the beam. Electron contamination is due to photon interactions in the head of the treatment machine. This is unavoidable. Electron contamination is also introduced by accessory trays, such as block or compensator trays. Electrons are set in motion inside the tray by photon interactions there, and some of these electrons will "spray" off the bottom of the tray.

(2) Backscattered electrons and photons from deeper layers. This is an unavoidable consequence of the basic physics of the interaction of radiation with matter.

In the build-up region, the dose increases rapidly in the first few millimeters (see Figure 14.39). Any material on a patient's skin can lead to a dramatic increase in skin dose.

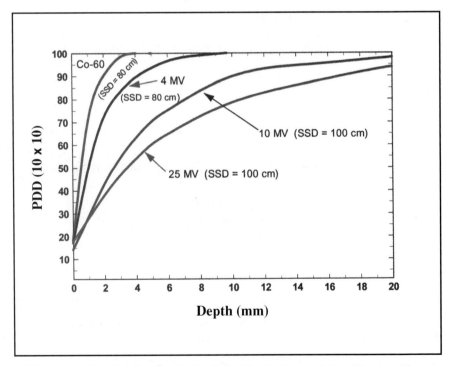

Figure 14.39: Build-up curves for 10 × 10 cm² radiation fields. The depth scale is in millimeters. The specific values of the surface dose vary from machine to machine. The important point here is the rapid rise in dose in the first few millimeters. (Data taken from Khan, F. M. *The Physics of Radiation Therapy,* Third Edition, 2003.)

In the build-up region, the dose distribution depends on:

(1) Beam energy.
(2) SSD.
(3) Field size.
(4) Tray distance from skin.
(5) Angle of beam incidence.

The relative surface dose reaches a shallow minimum at an energy of about 10 MV, where its value is 10% to 15% for a 10×10 cm^2 field. The surface dose depends sensitively on the field size (see Figure 14.40). The surface dose rises as the field size goes up. This is probably due to increased electron contamination from the collimator and the air.

A tray in the beam becomes a source of electron contamination. As the tray-to-skin distance decreases, the skin dose increases. This can be seen in Figure 14.41. This figure shows that when the distance between the tray and the skin surface becomes less than about 30 cm. the surface dose begins to rise rapidly. It is advisable to keep trays at least 15 to 20 cm away from the skin if possible.

When a beam enters the skin obliquely, the skin dose is higher than for perpendicular incidence (see Figure 14.42). For a beam that grazes

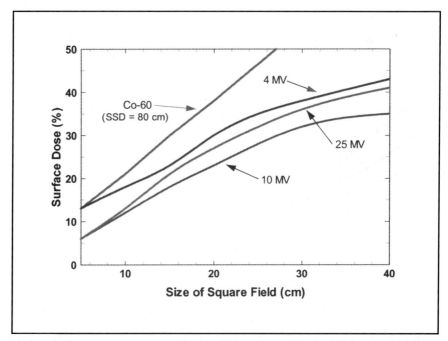

Figure 14.40: Surface dose as a function of field size for different energy beams. The SSD = 100 for all beams except Co-60. The 10 MV curve is below the 25 MV curve. (Data taken from Jani, S.K. *Handbook of Dosimetry Data for Radiotherapy,* 1993.) See COLOR PLATE 8.

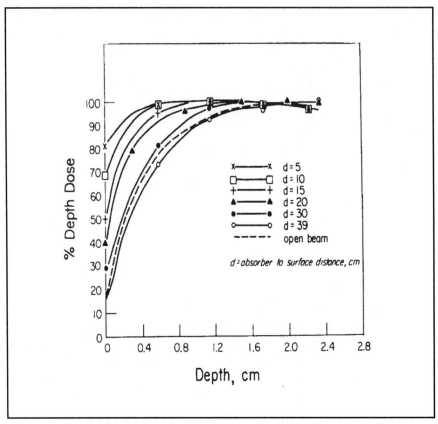

Figure 14.41: The effect of an acrylic accessory tray in proximity to the skin surface. The PDD in the build-up region has been plotted for various tray-to-skin surface distances. This is for 10 MV, $f = 15 \times 15$ cm^2, SSD = 100 cm, tray thickness 1.5 g/cm^2. (Reprinted from Khan, F. M. *The Physics of Radiation Therapy,* Third Edition, Fig. 13.6, p. 282, © 2003, with permission from Lippincott Williams & Wilkins.)

the skin tangentially, there is an approximate formula for estimating the skin dose:

Percent skin dose ≈

$$\frac{1}{2}\left(100\% + \text{Entrance \% dose for perpendicular incidence}\right), \qquad (14.15)$$

where perpendicular incidence corresponds to 0° and 90° is tangential incidence. Equation (14.15) is sometimes referred to as the "Jackson formula."

14.10 Bolus

There are clinical situations in which skin sparing is not desirable. This is the case for superficial tumors or for tumors that have invaded the skin. Under these circumstances it may be beneficial to have an enhanced surface dose. A lower beam energy could be used, but this

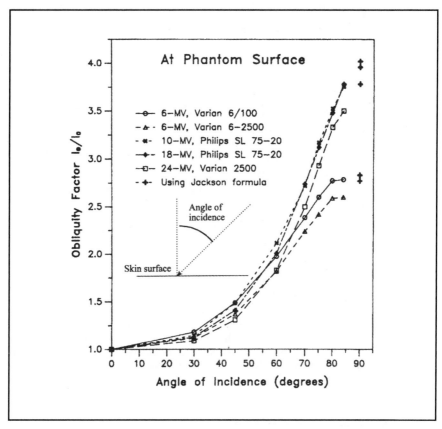

Figure 14.42: The enhancement in dose due to oblique beam incidence for 10 × 10 cm² fields. The obliquity factor is a multiplier: whatever the value of the dose at the surface for perpendicular incidence, multiply it by this factor for oblique incidence. An angle of incidence of 0° corresponds to a beam that is perpendicularly incident upon the surface. As the angle of incidence rises, the dose rises steeply by up to a factor of 4. The "+" marks at 90° are from equation (14.15). (Adapted from Khan, F. M. *The Physics of Radiation Therapy*, Third Edition, Fig. 13.11, p. 286, © 2003, with permission from Lippincott Williams & Wilkins.)

may not be advisable if it is also necessary to have a high dose at depth. One strategy to bring the surface dose up without appreciably reducing the penetration of the beam is to add a layer of material over the skin surface. This material is called *bolus*. The use of bolus brings d_m closer to the skin surface. Even a small thickness of bolus can dramatically raise the surface dose, as shown in Figure 14.43.

Bolus material should be approximately tissue equivalent. It should be pliable and flexible so that it conforms to the skin surface without any gaps. Large gaps between bolus material and the skin surface may negate the effect of the bolus.

A gelatinlike commercial product called "Superflab" is sold in different thicknesses, lengths, and widths. Sometimes, wet gauze or a wet washcloth is used. You can make your own bolus material by mixing 200 mL of water, 100 mL of glycerin and 100 g of gelatin. Propylparaben can be added, if desired, to prevent deterioration.

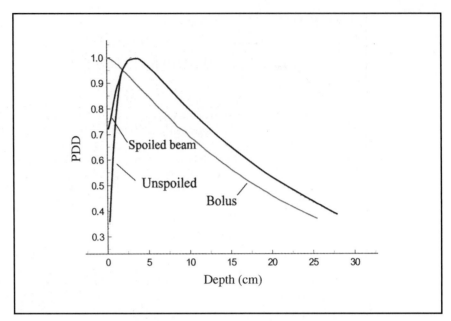

Figure 14.43: The effect of bolus and the effect of a beam spoiler on the percent depth dose. Bolus of thickness d_m eliminates the build-up region in the skin but slightly reduces the beam penetration. A beam spoiler adds electron contamination to the beam. This raises the surface dose but does not affect the beam penetration.

14.11 Beam Spoilers

Sometimes, bolus placement is inconvenient due to a very highly contoured skin surface. Instead, a beam "spoiler" may be used, which spoils the skin sparing. A beam spoiler is usually one or more solid plastic trays that are placed in the beam and close to the skin surface. A spoiler will increase the skin dose without diminishing beam penetration. Bolus will diminish beam penetration to a small degree (see Figure 14.43.)

14.12 Tissue Compensators

A wedge is a crude compensator—it compensates in one direction only, and is not custom-made for the individual patient. A compensator is a custom-made beam modifier that "compensates" for a patient's skin contour in two directions. Compensators are useful for treatment of any anatomical locations that involve significant skin sloping, such as head and neck, mantle fields, and AP lung and breast treatments. See Figure 14.44. There are two major types of compensators:

(1) *Missing tissue compensator:* Relatively easy to design, produces uniform dose distribution when sloping or contoured skin surface is present.

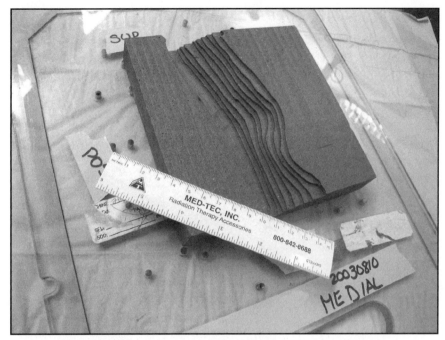

Figure 14.44: A photo of a compensator attached to a tray. This compensator has been designed for a breast treatment. It has over a half dozen steps in thickness. The steps have been cut from a template using a milling machine. The compensator becomes thicker toward the right, which corresponds to the anterior portion of the breast where there is "missing" tissue. The composition of this compensator is 81% bismuth and 19% polyethylene.

(2) *Dose compensation:* More general, compensates for missing tissue and inhomogeneities.

Compensator design requires a knowledge of the individual patient's skin topography. In the old days, this information was obtained from a mechanical pointer or a Moiré fringe camera. Today, skin topography is obtained from CT data. Compensators are composed of high-density materials such as Cerrobend or "PolyLead®." The compensator material is machined on a milling machine to produce the appropriate thickness at various locations. Factors that affect the thickness of compensator material are: beam divergence, the relative linear attenuation coefficient of compensator material and tissue, and the reduction in scatter at various depths because the compensator material is placed at a distance from the skin.

Figure 14.45 shows a missing tissue compensator. The approximate thickness t of material needed along any ray is given by:

$$e^{-\mu_{eff}t} = \frac{\text{TAR}(d,f)}{\text{TAR}(d-h,f)}, \tag{14.16}$$

where h is the tissue thickness deficit, d is the depth at which dose uniformity is to be achieved, and μ_{eff} is an effective linear attenuation

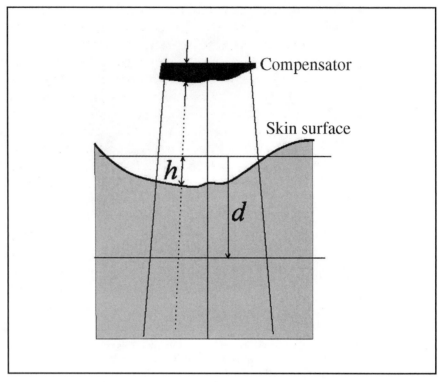

Figure 14.45: A missing tissue compensator.

coefficient for polyenergetic broad beam radiation as discussed in chapter 5, section 5.5.2.

When a compensator is used, dose rate calculations must include a transmission factor for the compensator and the tray. Compensators have largely been replaced by the use of IMRT. The advantages of IMRT over compensators are discussed in chapter 20.

14.13 Tissue Inhomogeneities

The dose distributions that we have calculated so far are based on the assumption of uniform-density tissue (assumed to have a density of 1 g/cm^3). In real patients there are a variety of tissues and structures that have densities that depart significantly from this. These include: fat, bone, lungs, air cavities (sinuses, trachea), metal prostheses (e.g., hip), etc. When such structures are present, accurate dose calculations require accounting for departures from unit density.

There are three effects of the presence of inhomogeneities:

(1) There is a change in the absorption of the primary beam.
(2) The dose due to scatter radiation will be affected by nearby inhomogeneities. The farther away a particular point is from an

inhomogeneity, the less important this becomes. This may be less important for higher-energy beams where the scatter component of the dose is less significant.

(3) When photons interact with matter, they set electrons in motion. The fluence of these electrons plays a key role in the buildup of dose at boundaries (at exit boundaries there is a build-down effect). When a photon beam traverses a large air cavity, there may be a loss of charged particle equilibrium. At the distal side of the cavity, the dose may have to build up again as it reenters tissue. These effects are called *interface effects*. None of the correction methods described below take account of this effect.

Examine Figure 14.46.[3] At point A the primary component of the dose is unaffected by the inhomogeneity. The scatter component will be reduced and therefore the total dose will be reduced slightly. At point B there will be a slight decrease in attenuation of the primary dose, which will lead to an *increase* in the primary dose. However there will also be

---

[3] Refer to Johns and Cunningham, Chapter 11, pp. 391–392, *The Physics of Radiology,* Charles C Thomas, 1983.

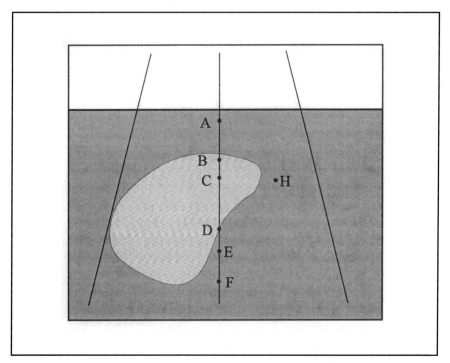

Figure 14.46: The lightly shaded structure has a low density. In the text, there is a discussion of the dose at the labeled points.

decreased scatter dose. Near the interface there will be a reduction in dose. At point C there will be a significant decrease in primary attenuation. Although the scatter will decrease, the total dose is likely to be enhanced over what it would be in the absence of the inhomogeneity. At point D on the interface there may be a loss of CPE because of the large volume of low-density material that the beam has traversed in reaching this point. Opposing this is an increase in the primary component of the dose due to a decrease in attenuation. The net effect is likely to be an increase in dose. At both E and F the primary component will be increased by the same amount, but the change in the scatter component will be different. At point H there is no change in the primary component, but the scatter contribution will be lower and therefore the dose will be reduced.

At megavoltage beam energies the dominant photon interaction in tissue is Compton scattering. Compton scattering in a medium depends on the electron density (number per cubic centimeter) of the medium. In this section the electron density relative to water will be given the symbol ρ_e. As this is a relative value, it has no units or dimensions. As an example, a typical value of the electron density of lung tissue is 0.25 times that of water, therefore $\rho_e = 0.25$. The relative electron density of cortical bone can be as high as 1.7.

We next turn our attention to methods for dose correction in the presence of inhomogeneities. There are two major classes of correction techniques. The first class is based on the effective path length. These are one-dimensional methods that take account of electron density information along a ray path from the source to the point in question. Corrections of this type are the ratio of TAR (rTAR) method and the power law method. The second class of methods is three-dimensional corrections, which are based on full 3-D density data acquired from CT images. Relative electron density values can be derived from standard CT images (see chapter 19, section 19.4.3). These methods perform a ray trace to determine the change in the primary photon fluence (as in the 1-D methods) and calculate the scatter dose based on the 3-D density data. An example of this type of correction is the equivalent tissue-air ratio (ETAR) method.

For all of these methods the corrected dose D' (or dose rate) is found by multiplying the uncorrected dose D (calculated ignoring inhomogeneities) by a correction factor CF:

$$D' = D \times \text{CF}. \tag{14.17}$$

In Figure 14.47 there are three distinct layers having relative electron density: ρ_1, ρ_2, and ρ_3. The effective or radiological depth d_{eff} of

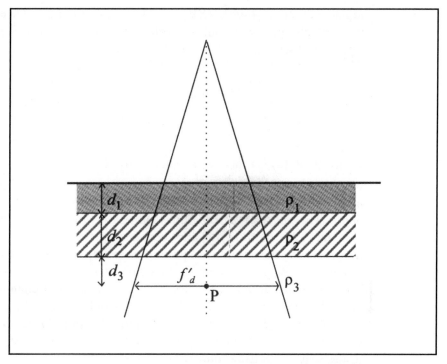

Figure 14.47: A slab phantom with three distinct regions with different relative electron densities.

point **P,** is given by a sum of the depths weighted by the relative electron density:

$$d_{eff} = \rho_1 d_1 + \rho_2 d_2 + \rho_3 d_3. \tag{14.18}$$

The actual physical depth of point **P** is $d_1 + d_2 + d_3$.

In the ratio of TAR method, the correction factor (at point **P**) is:

$$CF_P = \frac{TXR\left(d_{eff}, f'_d\right)}{TXR\left(d, f'_d\right)}, \tag{14.19}$$

where TXR stands for either TAR, TMR, or TPR and f'_d is the equivalent square of the blocked field size in the patient at depth d (see chapter 13). Notice that regardless of whether we use TAR or TMR, the result is formally the same since the PSF [see equation (10.16)] simply divides out. The effect of multiplying the equation for the dose rate [see for example equation (14.12)] by the correction factor in equation (14.19) is to simply replace $\mathrm{TXR}(d,f'_d)$ with $\mathrm{TXR}(d_{eff},f'_d)$ because the term $\mathrm{TXR}(d,f'_d)$ simply cancels out. One could therefore, write the (corrected) dose rate equation (14.12) as:

$$\dot{D}_d\left(r,f_d\right)=\dot{D}_{d_0}\left(100+d_0,10\right)\times S_c\left(f\right)\times S_p\left(f'_d\right)\times\left(\frac{100+d_0}{\mathrm{SSD}+d}\right)^2$$
$$\times\mathrm{TMR}\left(d_{eff},f'_d\right)\times\mathrm{TF}\times\mathrm{WF}\left(d,f'_d\right),$$

(14.20)

where $\mathrm{TMR}\left(d,f'_d\right)$ has been replaced by $\mathrm{TMR}\left(d_{eff},f'_d\right)$. Tabular values of TMR such as those that appear in appendices B and C of this book are measured for water. The quantity d_{eff} is like an equivalent water depth. This quantity is sometimes called the "radiological depth."

The rTAR method does not account for the proximity of the inhomogeneity to the calculation point. For example. suppose that $\rho_1 = \rho_3 = 1.0$ and that $d_1 = d_3 = 5$ cm. In this case, $d_{eff} = 10 + \rho_2 d_2$. Now suppose that we move the interface closer to point **P** without changing either d or d_{eff} by making $d_3 = 1$ and $d_1 = 9$. We would expect the correction to change, but it doesn't. The rTAR method correctly accounts for the change in the attenuation of the primary component of the dose but not in the scatter contribution.

Example 14.5

In the diagram at the right, find the correction factor for the inhomogeneity at points A and B for a 10 × 10 cm² Co-60 beam.

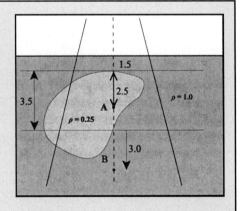

At point A: $d_{eff} = 1.5 + 0.25 \times 2.5 = 2.1$ cm, whereas $d = 4.0$ cm. $\mathrm{CF_A} = \mathrm{TAR}(2.1,10)/\mathrm{TAR}(4,10) = 1.02/0.957 = 1.07$.

At point B: $d_{eff} = 1.5 + 0.25 \times 3.5 + 3.0 = 5.4$ cm and $d = 8.0$ cm. $\mathrm{CF_B} = \mathrm{TAR}(5.4,10)/\mathrm{TAR}(8,10) = 0.906/0.805 = 1.13$.

The power law method (sometimes called the "modified Batho method") uses (at point **P** in Figure 14.47):

$$CF_P = \frac{\left[TXR\left(d_3, f_d'\right)\right]^{\rho_3 - \rho_2}}{\left[TXR\left(d_2 + d_3, f_d'\right)\right]^{1 - \rho_2}},$$

(14.21)

where d_3 is the depth within the medium and $d_2 + d_3$ is the distance to the upper surface of the overlying medium. The density of the medium at point **P** is ρ_3, and ρ_2 is the density of the overlying material. Equation (14.21) assumes that $\rho_1 = 1.0$. Once again TXR stands for either TAR, TMR, or TPR. This expression for the correction factor is by no means expected to be obvious. The power law correction factor does depend on the proximity of the calculation point to the inhomogeneity.

Example 14.6

Repeat Example 14.5 using the power law correction.

Point B: Use equation (14.21) for CF_P: In this case, put $d_3 = 3.0$ cm, $\rho_3 = 1.00$, and $d_2 + d_3 = 6.5$ cm and $\rho_2 = 0.25$; TAR(3,10) = 0.992 and TAR (6.5,10) = 0.865 for Co-60.

$$CF_B = \frac{\left[TAR\left(3.0, 10\right)\right]^{1.00 - 0.25}}{\left[TAR\left(6.5, 10\right)\right]^{1.00 - 0.25}} = 1.11$$

This is a few percent lower than the CF derived from the rTAR method in Example 14.5.

Point A: In this case, $d_3 = 2.5$ (it is the depth in the medium of calculation), $d_2 + d_3 = 4.0$ (distance to the top of the interface of the medium above), $\rho_3 = 0.25$, $\rho_2 = 1.0$, TAR(2.5,10) = 1.008 for Co-60.

$$CF_A = \frac{\left[TAR\left(2.5, 10\right)\right]^{0.25 - 1.00}}{\left[TAR\left(4.0, 10\right)\right]^{1 - 1}} = 0.994$$

The correction factor is close to 1.00 at this depth and it is less than the CF from the rTAR method. The rTAR method does not work well inside an inhomogeneity and the power law result is probably more accurate.

The rTAR method results in an overcorrection when $\rho_e < 1$ and an undercorrection when $\rho_e > 1$.

The ETAR method takes account of the full three-dimensional nature of the material. It accounts for changes in scatter by scaling the field size parameter. The correction factor is:

$$CF = \frac{TAR\left(d_{eff}, \tilde{f}\right)}{TAR\left(d, f_d'\right)}, \tag{14.22}$$

where d_{eff} is the equivalent depth (as before), d is the actual depth, f_d' is the field size at depth d, and $\tilde{f} = f_d' \times \tilde{\rho}$ is an effective field size with $\tilde{\rho}$ a weighted average density over the irradiated medium. The value of $\tilde{f}$ is calculated by a treatment planning computer. The volume elements are weighted according to their relative contribution to the scattered dose. We will not discuss how this is done here, suffice it to say that $\tilde{f} < f_d'$ when there are low-density inhomogeneities present.

The presence of inhomogeneities is more important at low energies because lower-energy beams are attenuated more rapidly and because the scatter contribution to the dose is more important at low energy. This is illustrated in Figure 14.48.

Figures 14.49 and 14.50 illustrate the effects of inhomogeneity corrections on the dose distribution in a patient's lung.

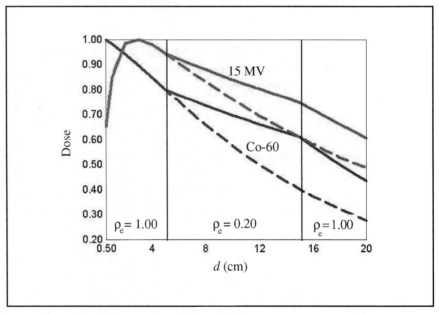

Figure 14.48: The depth dose as a function of the geometric depth for a 10 × 10 cm² Co-60 beam and for a 10 × 10 cm² 15 MV beam in the presence of an inhomogeneous (solid curves) slab 10 cm thick with a relative electron density of 0.20. The dashed curves are the depth dose values, assuming a homogeneous water phantom. The corrected depth dose is based on equation (14.19). The effect of the inhomogeneity on the Co-60 beam is greater than for the 15 MV beam because the Co-60 beam has a steeper gradient and is therefore affected more by the absence of matter. Nonequilibrium effects are not included in this figure. See COLOR PLATE 9.

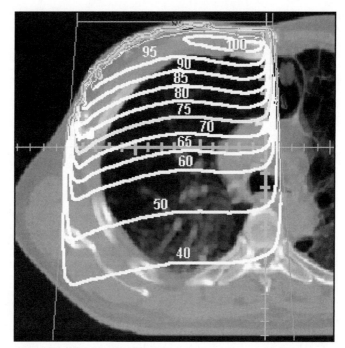

Figure 14.49: A CT axial slice of the thorax with the uncorrected dose distribution from an AP beam superimposed. The beam is 4 MV, 15 × 15 cm², SSD = 100 cm. The tick marks are 1 cm apart.

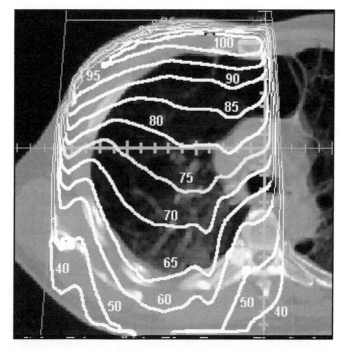

Figure 14.50: The dose distribution corrected for the presence of the low-density lung. The correction is based on the power law method. Note how the isodose curves have been stretched considerably in the posterior direction.

Table 14.4: Approximate Correction Factors

Energy	CF (% per cm)*	
	Lung	Bone
Co-60	+4.0%	−2.5%
4–6 MV	+3.0%	−2.0%
10 MV	+2.5%	−1.5%
18–25 MV	+1.5%	−1.0%

*This is the percent change in dose per centimeter of tissue traversed. (Adapted from AAPM Report No. 85, Table 8, p. 34, © 2004, with permission from American Association of Physicists in Medicine.)

Table 14.4 gives approximate values for the correction necessary for different energy beams traversing either lung or bone tissue at points beyond the inhomogeneity.

14.14 Field Matching

When radiation fields are adjacent to one another, they can overlap and diverge into one another. In such a case the field geometry should be arranged so that the edges of the adjacent fields cross at some preselected appropriate depth in the patient. However, it will be shown that simply matching the edges of the beams in this way can lead to undesirable "hot" or "cold" spots. To overcome these, it is better, if possible, to arrange adjacent beams so that their edges never overlap at all. There are numerous techniques to match adjacent fields and some of these will be discussed here. The techniques described are based on ideal geometry and in some cases approximations. *All field matching should be verified clinically using imaging and using the treatment planning system.*

Figure 14.51 shows two adjacent fields such as might be used to irradiate a patient's spine. These two fields are to be matched so that they overlap at the depth d as shown. The gap length G on the skin surface required to accomplish this is:

$$G = d\left(\frac{L_1}{SSD_1} + \frac{L_2}{SSD_2}\right),$$ (14.23)

where L_1 and L_2 are the distances from the central axis to the field edge of the two fields *at the patient surface, d* is the match depth, and SSD_1 and SSD_2 are the two SSDs for the beams. For an asymmetric jaw setting, L_1 and L_2 are *not* half the total field size. Gap settings should always be verified clinically using a simulator and by taking films or using fluoroscopy. It is common to move the match point (migrate or feather) horizontally several times during the entire course of treatment by making one field larger and the other smaller.

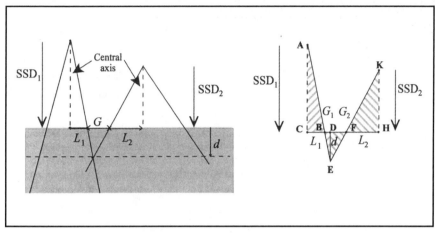

Figure 14.51: The gap setting G on the skin surface necessary to match adjacent fields at a depth d in a patient. The geometry is shown on the right-hand side. An application of similar triangles discussed in the text is used to derive equation (14.23) for G.

Equation (14.23) can be easily derived by considering similar triangles. Refer to Figure 14.51. The total gap G is divided into two parts G_1 (line segment BD) plus G_2 (line segment DF). We will find each of these contributions separately and then add them. Triangle ABC is similar to triangle BDE and therefore $G_1/L_1 = d/\text{SSD}_1$. Triangle KHF is similar to triangle DFE and therefore $G_2/L_2 = d/\text{SSD}_2$. Adding the two contributions $G = G_1 + G_2$ results in equation (14.23).

Figure 14.52 shows the dose distribution for two 6 MV beams matched at a depth of 5 cm. The gap between the two fields is 1 cm [calculated using equation (14.23)]. Note the hot and cold spots mentioned earlier. These could be eliminated by using independent jaws to make L_1 and $L_2 = 0$; that is, by matching the two field edges along their respective central axes.

Orthogonal field junctions are present whenever adjacent fields are perpendicular to one another. The prime example of this is craniospinal irradiation. In craniospinal irradiation the patient is prone and there are a posterior spinal field and two lateral brain fields (see Figure 14.53). These fields involve divergence of the beams in multiple directions. The goal is to angle the beams to prevent overlaps leading to hot spots (or cold). Figure 14.53 shows how a couch rotation can be used to match the divergence of the right lateral field with the PA spinal field. The foot of the couch (farthest from the gantry stand) is rotated toward the gantry through an angle θ_1.

The geometry is shown in more detail in Figure 14.54. This diagram shows that:

$$\tan \theta_1 = \frac{\text{W}_1}{\text{SAD}}, \tag{14.24}$$

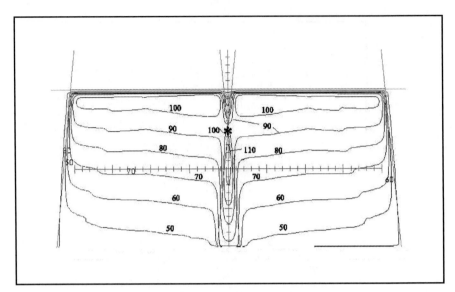

Figure 14.52: Matching of adjacent beams. Two 20 × 20 cm², 6 MV, SSD = 100 cm beams are matched at a depth of 5 cm (at the location of the asterisk on the central axis). Note that there is a cold spot above the match depth where the beams "underlap" and a hot spot of 116% below where the beams overlap. The tick marks are 1 cm apart.

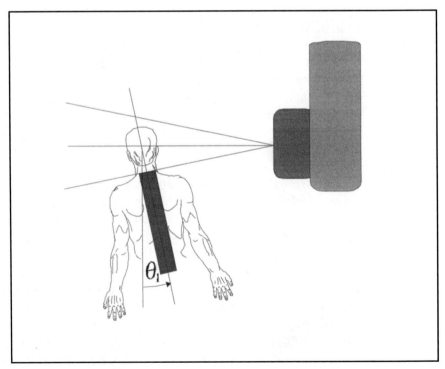

Figure 14.53: Craniospinal irradiation. One of the lateral fields is shown along with the posterior field (shaded). The other lateral field is not shown for simplicity. A couch rotation through an angle θ_1 is necessary to match the divergence of the lateral field with the edge of the posterior field. When the opposite lateral field is delivered, the couch must be rotated in the opposite direction.

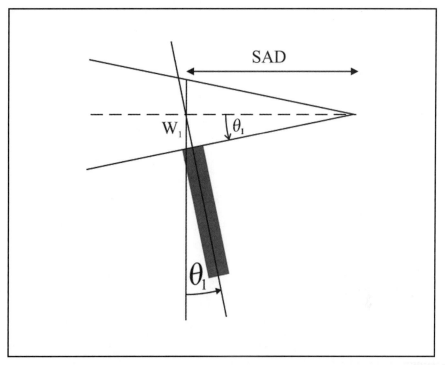

Figure 14.54: The geometry for matching the divergence of a lateral field to the posterior spine field for craniospinal irradiation.

where W_1 is the distance from the central axis of the lateral field to the inferior field edge and the SAD is usually 100 cm. If the field is symmetric, then W_1 is half the field size. A typical angle of rotation is about 5°.

Figure 14.55 shows how the divergence of the PA field is matched with the lateral field. The collimator is rotated for the lateral field through an angle θ_2 given approximately by:

$$\tan \theta_2 = \frac{W_2}{SAD}, \qquad (14.25)$$

where W_2 is the distance from the central axis of the posterior field to the superior border at the isocenter. If the PA field is symmetric, then W_2 is half the field size. Note that the couch rotation of Figure 14.53 does affect the lateral field; but since the couch rotation is small, the effect is relatively small.

The junction between fields is usually moved ("feathered") by about 1.0 cm (perhaps every 1000 cGy) to smooth any mismatch between fields and thus to minimize hot spots and cold spots. This can be accomplished by decreasing the size of the cranial (lateral) fields and increasing the size of the PA field by an equal amount.

The most complex field-matching problem routinely encountered in radiation therapy is associated with the treatment of breast cancer when

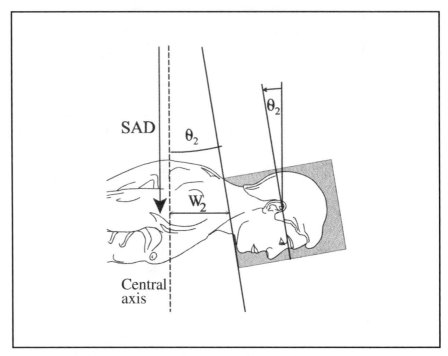

Figure 14.55: Matching the divergence of the posterior field with the lateral field by rotation of the collimator for the lateral field.

it is necessary to treat the entire involved breast and chest wall. Depending on regional lymph node involvement, it may also be necessary to treat the supraclavicular and possibly the axillary and internal mammary lymph nodes. This requires several adjacent fields that must be arranged so as to avoid overlap. The patient is supine with the arm on the involved side raised above the head (see Figure 14.56). The breast and the chest wall are treated with tangential fields (see the fields labeled II and III in Figure 14.56). The supraclavicular lymph nodes are treated with a single anterior field adjacent to the tangent fields (see the field labeled I in Figure 14.56). Matching these fields so that they do not overlap is challenging and many techniques have been invented for this purpose. The reader is referred to the excellent discussions in the books by Bentel and by Khan and Potish.[4]

Let us begin by assuming that the tangential fields have their central axes in a horizontal plane (gantry angle of 90° or 270°) and that the anterior supraclavicular field has its central axis in a purely vertical plane (gantry angle 0°). The supraclavicular field is usually "half-beam blocked" (see Figure 14.57). The central axis of this field is located at the inferior border of the field so that there is no divergence of this field

---

[4] Bentel, G. C., *Radiation Therapy Planning,* Second Edition, New York: McGraw-Hill, 1996 and Khan, F., and R. A. Potish (eds.), *Treatment Planning in Radiation Oncology,* Baltimore: Williams & Wilkins, 1998.

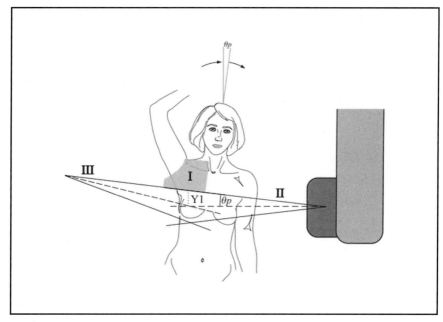

Figure 14.56: A patient treated for breast cancer with a supraclavicular field (I) and two tangent fields [II (medial) and III (lateral)]. The supraclavicular field is an anterior field which is half-beam blocked, forming a transverse matchline at the inferior border of this field. The couch is rotated to match the superior border of the tangent fields with the supraclavicular field. The gantry is shown in position to treat the medial (II) field.

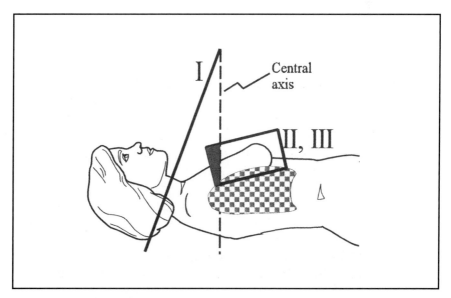

Figure 14.57: Sagittal view of the supraclavicular beam (I) and the two tangential beams (II and III). The tangential beams are angled by using a collimator rotation so that the posterior border will be roughly parallel with the chest wall. The superior borders of the tangential fields are blocked so that they will match the supraclavicular field.

into the tangential fields. This creates a transverse match line with the tangential fields (see Figure 14.57).

To match the tangential fields with the supraclavicular field, the couch (pedestal) is rotated by turning the foot of the couch away from the collimator through an angle θ_p as shown in Figure 14.56. This angle is given by:

$$\tan\theta_p = \frac{Y1}{SAD},\qquad(14.26)$$

where Y1 is the partial tangential field size from the central axis to the superior border of the field at isocenter. If the field is symmetric, this is simply half the field size. This angle is typically about 5°. This field match would be perfect if the tangential gantry angles for fields I and II were at 90° and 270° and if the supraclavicular field gantry angle were zero.

The supraclavicular field is usually angled about 10° to 15° to avoid the esophagus, trachea, and spinal cord (see Figure 14.58). The tangential fields are not horizontal but rather oblique as in Figure 14.58. This obliquity causes a slight overlap between the superior border of the tangential field and the inferior border of the supraclavicular field.

The posterior borders of the tangential fields are often arranged so that they do not diverge into the patient's lung (see Figures 14.58 and 14.59). The angle between the two central axes departs from 180° so that the posterior borders of the two beams are parallel. The departure

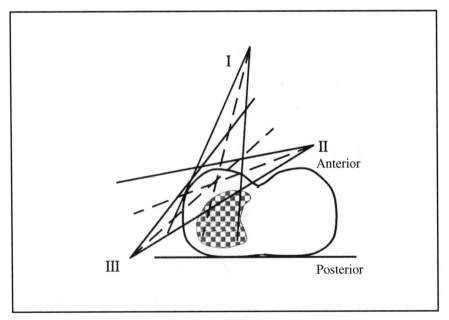

Figure 14.58: An axial view of the supraclavicular beam (I), the tangential medial beam (II), and the tangential lateral beam (III). The gantry angles of the two tangential beams are arranged so that the posterior borders of these beams are parallel. This reduces divergence of the beams into the lung.

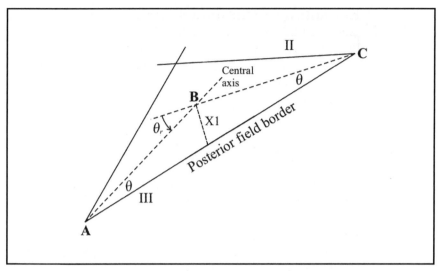

Figure 14.59: The posterior border of the two tangential fields are matched by departing from an angle of 180° between these two beams. The departure angle θ_r is twice the half-beam angle θ. The line representing X1 is perpendicular to the central axis of beam II.

angle θ_r is shown in Figure 14.59. It is twice the half angle θ of the beam, as we now demonstrate. The departure angle θ_r is the exterior angle of triangle ABC in Figure 14.59, and therefore it is equal to the sum of the two remote interior angles (i.e., $\theta_r = \theta + \theta$). The tangent of the angle θ is equal to X1/SAD and therefore the departure angle is:

$$\theta_r = 2\tan^{-1}\frac{X1}{SAD}, \qquad (14.27)$$

where X1 is the distance from the posterior border of the field to the central axis.

Example 14.7

A patient is treated for breast cancer with two tangent beams and a supraclavicular beam using the 6 MV Mevalac. The medial (beam II in Figure 14.56) portal (beam's-eye view) is shown in the figure at right. The MLC is used to shape the field. The gantry angle for this beam is 50°.

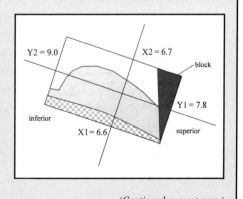

(Continued on next page)

Example 14.7 (continued)

(a) What is the approximate angle of the pedestal rotation necessary to match the superior border of the tangential fields with the inferior border of the supraclavicular field (field I in Figure 14.56)?

The angle is given by equation (14.26), thus: $\tan \theta_p = Y1/SAD = 7.8/100 = 0.078$ and therefore $\theta_p = 4.5°$.

(b) Calculate the approximate lateral gantry angle necessary to avoid posterior divergence of the tangential beams into the patient's lungs.

The angle of departure is given by equation (14.27): $\theta_r = 2 \tan^{-1} X1/SAD = 2 \tan^{-1} 6.6/100 = 7.6° \approx 8°$. If the lateral gantry angle were set so that the lateral field was exactly parallel opposed to the medial field, the angle would be $50° + 180° = 230°$. To achieve field matching, the numerical value of the angle has to be reduced by $8°$ and therefore the needed gantry angle is $222°$.

(c) For the medial field, the dose to be delivered is 90 cGy at the isocenter, which is at a depth of 9.0 cm. A 15° wedge is used with heel anterior. Using the data for the Mevalac in appendix C, calculate the number of MU needed. The dose rate is given by equation (14.12):

$$\dot{D}_d\left(r,f_d'\right) = \dot{D}_{d_0}\left(100+d_0,10\right) \times S_c\left(f\right) \times S_p\left(f_d'\right) \times \left(\frac{100+d_0}{\text{SSD}+d}\right)^2$$
$$\times \text{TMR}\left(d,f_d'\right) \times \text{TF} \times \text{WF}\left(d,f_d'\right).$$

First determine the equivalent field size of the open (unblocked) field f. We need to find the equivalent field size of the rectangle with dimensions (X1+X2) by (Y1+Y2) = 13.3 cm by 16.8 cm. This is 14.8 cm. Next, find the equivalent square of the blocked field in the patient, f_d'. The triangular blocked area is about 6% of the area of the rectangle. The flash represents about 40% of the area. The total area reduction is therefore about 45% and $f_d' = 14.8\sqrt{1-0.45} = 11$ cm.

Example 14.7 (continued)

We can now begin to evaluate the terms in the equation for the dose rate:

$$\dot{D}_d\left(r,f_d\right)=\dot{D}_{d_0}\left(100+d_0,10\right)\times S_c\left(f\right)\times S_p\left(f_d'\right)\times\left(\frac{100+d_0}{\text{SSD}+d}\right)^2$$

$$\times\text{TMR}\left(d,f_d'\right)\times\text{TF}\times\text{WF}\left(d,f_d'\right)$$

$$=1.000\times S_c\left(14.8\right)\times S_p\left(11\right)\times\left(\frac{100+1.5}{100}\right)^2$$

$$\times\text{TMR}\left(9,11\right)\times\text{TF}\times\text{WF}\left(9,11\right)$$

$$=1.000\times1.014\times1.003\times1.030\times0.820\times1.0\times0.709$$

$$=0.609\text{ cGy/MU}$$

The number of monitor units necessary is $\mu = D\big/\dot{D} = 90\big/0.609$ = 148 MU.

14.15 Patient Positioning and Immobilization Devices

A patient should be in the same position during treatment as during simulation when data were collected for treatment planning (see chapter 19). In addition, it is important that patients be positioned reproducibly on the couch each day for treatment. Once positioned, a patient's position should not change during treatment and therefore some sort of immobilization may be necessary. The use of IMRT and stereotactic radiosurgery has heightened the need for precise positioning and rigid immobilization. Both of these therapies are associated with very high dose gradients, often in proximity to critical organs. The fabrication of custom treatment devices requires careful training. Improperly constructed devices can be responsible for significant geometric errors in radiation therapy treatment. The number of devices designed over the years for patient positioning and immobilization is huge. For an in-depth discussion, the reader is referred to the bibliography at the end of this chapter.

Positioning and immobilization devices have been classified in terms of: position aids, simple immobilization devices and complex immobilization devices.[5] Position aids are designed to place a patient in

---

[5] Keller, R. "Immobilization Devices," Chapter 7 in *Principles and Practice of Radiation Therapy.* C. M. Washington and D. T. Leaver (eds.). New York: Mosby, 1996.

a specific position for treatment and may provide some support to specific areas of the body. They may be used to position extremities so that they do not interfere with treatment of other areas. These devices are usually not custom made nor do they provide immobilization. Simple immobilization devices are generic devices that provide some immobilization and usually require patient cooperation. Complex immobilization devices significantly restrain patient movement and ensure reproducibility of patient position. These devices are usually custom-made for individual patients. The type of device used clearly depends on the anatomical treatment site.

With any of these devices there are questions about whether the radiation beam will traverse the device and if so the effect of this on the patient. It may be necessary to know the transmission factor and to understand that there will be a loss of buildup leading to a higher skin dose. One must keep in mind patient comfort, not simply because this will make treatment more pleasant but also because a comfortable patient is less likely to move during treatment.

Positioning aids include various types of head holders, tilt boards, foam rubber wedges for knee support, etc. Head holders or headrests are used to position and support a patient's head. These come in a variety of sizes and shapes used to position head height and to support various neck contours. They are typically labeled with letters A–F for identification. See Figure 14.60. A breast board is another example of a positioning device (see Figure 14.61 and Figure 19.11 in chapter 19). A breast board serves a number of purposes. It provides an armrest so that the arm may be comfortably raised above the shoulder and out of the way of the lateral beam (see beam III in Figure 14.56). The armrest can be moved to various indexed positions for comfort and reproducibility. It allows the patient to be tilted up so that the chest wall is horizontal, eliminating the need for a collimator rotation for the lateral fields (see

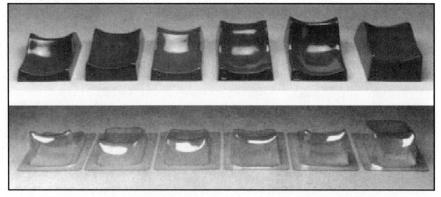

Figure 14.60: Head holders come in a variety of types and sizes, available in solid foam ("Timo" along the top row) or clear hard plastic ("Silverman," along the bottom row). (Courtesy of Best Medical, Springfield, VA, www.TeamBest.com)

Figure 14.57). In addition, the tilt of the board pulls the breast down into (what may be) a better treatment position. The tilt angle is adjustable and indexed for reproducibility.

Foam polyurethane casts which go by the trade name Alpha Cradle® are very commonly used for positioning breast and lung patients and for patients who are having treatment to the lower extremities. These are custom-made for each patient. A thin Styrofoam base is placed inside a large plastic bag. Two different liquid chemicals are mixed and then poured into the bag. The patient then lies on the bag. A chemical reaction causes the liquid to expand and foam up. The foam conforms to the patient's shape and then hardens in about 10 minutes. See Figure 14.62.

A vacuum bag device plays a role that is similar to an Alpha Cradle®. A thick plastic bag containing Styrofoam pellets is placed under the patient. The pellets mold to conform to the patient's contour. The air is then evacuated from the bag leaving a mold of the patient's body. The patient then lies in this mold each day for treatment. At the end of the treatment course, the bag can be reused by allowing air to enter the bag.

A "belly board" is a mattress designed to support a patient in a prone position (see Figure 14.63). There is a window cut out of the middle of the board that permits the abdomen to hang down. This reduces the amount of intestine intercepted by lateral radiation fields of the type shown in Figure 14.27.

Thermoplastic materials are commonly used for custom immobilization. A common trade name is Aquaplast®. These come in sheets of varying thickness, which are either solid or in the form of a mesh. For treatment of the brain and head and neck, it is common to use thermoplastic masks combined with a headrest and a baseplate (see Figure 14.64). The headrest is of the type discussed above. The thermoplastic material is in a frame that can be secured to the baseplate, thus effectively limiting motion of the head and neck. The plastic sheet may have holes cut out for the patient's eyes and mouth. The thermoplastic becomes soft when it is immersed in warm water. The preparation of these devices requires a temperature-regulated water bath. The water temperature should be between 70 °C and 80 °C (160 °F to 180 °F). This is warm but not intolerable for most patients. When the thermoplastic is heated, it changes from opaque to translucent. When this occurs, it is ready to be molded. The material is stretched over the patient's head and then snapped into a plastic baseplate under the patient. It is then molded and smoothed to follow the contours of the patient's face and head. The bridge of the nose should be pinched. It is best to have two people on hand. The mask requires about 10 minutes to cool and harden. It becomes opaque again as it hardens. It is important to let the mask fully cool before removing it from the patient. Impatience can lead to problems later. The construction of thermoplastic masks is an art. To ensure good results, the technician should receive careful training. Another type of immobilization used for brain treatments are stereotactic frames. These will be discussed in the context of radiosurgery in chapter 20.

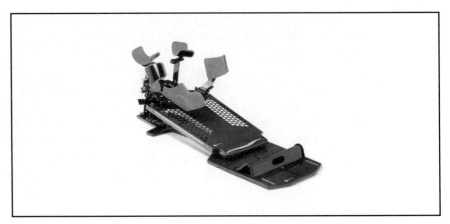

Figure 14.61: A breast board provides an arm holder and a headrest. It also allows the patient to be tilted upward. (Courtesy of Civco Medical Solutions, Kalona, IA)

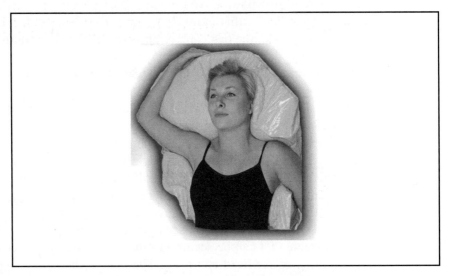

Figure 14.62: A custom-made polyurethane foam "Alpha Cradle®" for a breast patient. (Courtesy of Smithers Medical Products Inc., North Canton, OH. Alpha Cradle® is a registered trademark of Smithers Medical Products, Inc.)

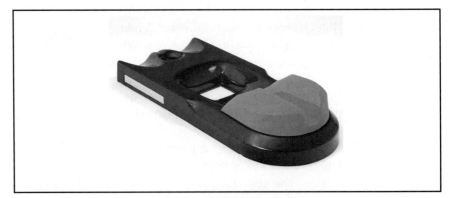

Figure 14.63: A "bellyboard" for treating a prone patient. The opening in the center of the board allows the abdomen to hang down. This reduces the amount of intestine in the treatment field for lateral pelvis treatments. (Courtesy of Civco Medical Solutions, Kalona, IA)

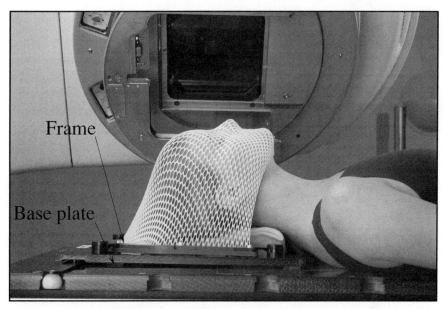

Figure 14.64: Thermoplastic mask for brain or head & neck treatment. Masks are available that extend down over and cover the shoulders. (Courtesy of Civco Medical Solutions, Kalona, IA)

Chapter Summary

- **Isodose charts:** Like topographical maps, each line is a line of constant dose, usually expressed as a percentage of the dose at the normalization point or of the prescribed dose.

- **Skin contour:** How does it affect dose distributions? Isodose lines are roughly parallel to skin surface. Three methods for manually adjusting isodose charts: (1) isodose shift method, (2) effective SSD method, and (3) ratio of TAR method.

- **Wedges:** Thick end is called *heel* and thin end is called *toe*. Used for (1) tissue compensation (e.g., tangential breast treatment) and (2) multiple fields.

  – Wedge angle: No universal definition, see diagram at right for one commonly used definition

  – Multiple fields: Hinge angle φ is the acute angle between the central axes of the beams, optimum wedge angle is given by $\theta = 90 - \varphi/2$.

– Wedge transmission (factor): WF(d, f'_d) ranges from 0.3 to 0.8, depends on wedge angle, field size, and depth.

– Dose rate on the central axis for shaped fields with a wedge:

$$\dot{D}_d\left(r, f'_d\right) = \dot{D}_{d_0}\left(100 + d_0, 10\right) \times S_c\left(f\right) \times S_p\left(f'_d\right) \times \left(\frac{100 + d_0}{\text{SSD} + d}\right)^2 \times \text{TMR}\left(d, f'_d\right)$$

$$\times \text{TF} \times \text{WF}\left(d, f'_d\right). \tag{14.12}$$

- **Dose-volume histograms:** Cumulative histogram; percent of volume receiving dose D (or percent of prescribed dose) or above. Always starts at 100% volume receiving 0 dose or above (see diagram at right).

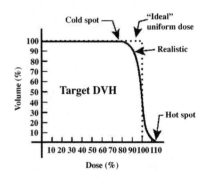

  – Does not tell distribution of dose: where hot spots and cold spots are.

  – V_D is the percentage of the volume receiving a dose of at least D (usually in Gy). D_V is the dose (in Gy or percent) received by at least $V(\%)$ of the volume.

- **Dose-volume specifications:**

  – GTV: Gross tumor volume; either seen on imaging or felt on palpation.

  – CTV: Contains entire GTV plus margin for microscopic disease.

  – PTV encompasses entire CTV plus margin for uncertainties in position of CTV and setup variations/organ motion; aperture must be larger than PTV to account for penumbra.

- **Skin dose:** Dose rises rapidly in first few millimeters.

  – Reasons for surface dose

    ○ Electron contamination of the beam

      (a) Photon interactions in air, collimator, etc.

      (b) Beam modifying devices, e.g., electrons set in motion in block tray; keep trays 15 to 20 cm away if possible.

    ○ Backscattered electrons and photons from deeper layers.

  – Systematic dependences:

    ○ Beam energy ↑ Skin dose ↓   Tray distance ↓ Skin dose ↑

    ○ Field size ↑ Skin dose ↑   Angle of incidence ↓ Skin dose ↓

– For tangential beams: % skin dose $\approx$ 1/2 (100% + % entrance dose for perpendicular incidence).

- **Bolus:** Tissue equivalent material placed on skin to raise surface dose.

- **Beam spoiler:** "Spoil" skin sparing by putting plastic tray in beam near skin; increases skin dose by increasing electron contamination but does not reduce penetration.

- **Tissue inhomogeneities:** Dose distributions discussed so far based on homogeneous medium. Relative electron density ρ_e is the electron density relative to water. Water has $\rho_e = 1.00$.

  – Inhomogeneities: Bone, air, lung, metal prostheses (e.g., hip) etc. Lung: density $\rho_e \sim 0.25$, but can vary substantially. Cortical bone: $\rho_e \sim 1.7$

  – Effects:

    ○ Changes in absorption of primary beam; especially important beyond inhomogeneity

    ○ Changes in scatter conditions

    ○ Lack of CPE at boundaries; build-up, build-down

  – Electron density is important quantity (Compton dominates), electron density relative to water ρ_e

  – Methods of Correction: $D' = D \times \text{CF}$

    ○ Ratio of TAR (rTAR): $\text{CF} = \dfrac{\text{TXR}\left(d_{\mathit{eff}}, f_d'\right)}{\text{TXR}\left(d, f_d\right)}$, where TXR represents either TAR or TMR and $d_{\mathit{eff}} = \rho_1 d_1 + \rho_2 d_2 + \rho_3 d_3$ is the effective pathlength.

    ○ Power law ratio (extension of Batho power law):

    $$\text{CF} = \frac{\text{TXR}\left(d_3, f_d'\right)^{\rho_3 - \rho_2}}{\text{TXR}\left(d_2 + d_3, f_d'\right)^{1 - \rho_2}}, \text{ where } \rho_1 = 1.0.$$

    ○ Effective TAR (ETAR) (3-D): Method that attempts to account for shape and proximity of structure, adjust field size for modified scatter conditions: $\text{CF} = \dfrac{\text{TAR}\left(d_{\mathit{eff}}, \tilde{f}\right)}{\text{TAR}\left(d, f_d'\right)}$, where d_{eff} is the effective depth and $\tilde{f}$ is an effective field size determined from CT data.

  – Ratio of TAR method does not work well inside inhomogeneity.

- **Field Matching**

  - **Adjacent field** (e.g.. cord irradiation): Match fields at depth *d*. Find necessary gap length on skin *G*.

    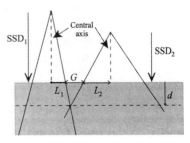

    $$G = d \left(\frac{L_1}{SSD_1} + \frac{L_2}{SSD_2} \right)$$

    Note that L_1 and L_2 are the distances from the central axis to the field edge of the two fields (not the field length) as measured on the surface.

  - **Orthogonal fields** (craniospinal):

    ○ $\tan \theta_1 = \dfrac{W_1}{SAD}$, pedestal rotation angle to match divergence of lateral field with PA field, where W_1 is the distance from the central axis of the lateral field to the inferior field edge.

    ○ $\tan \theta_2 = \dfrac{W_2}{SAD}$, collimator rotation necessary to match the divergence of the PA field with the lateral field, where W_2 is the distance from the central axis of the posterior field to the superior border.

  - **Breast**

    ○ $\tan \theta_P = \dfrac{Y1}{SAD}$, pedestal rotation angle necessary to match divergence of tangent field to supraclavicular fields, where Y1 is the distance from the central axis to the superior border of the tangential field.

    ○ $\tan \theta_r = 2 \tan^{-1} \dfrac{X1}{SAD}$, the "departure" angle between the central axes of the tangential fields when the posterior borders are matched (Figure 14.59), and X1 is the distance from the central axis to the posterior border of the tangential fields.

Problems

1. Refer to Figure 14.1. Locate the depth of the following isodose lines on the central axis: 90%, 80%, 70%, and 50%. Look up the PDD at these depths in appendix B and compare.

2. Recall that the beam width is defined as the distance between the 50% lines. Examine Figure 14.2.
    a. Use the scale in this figure to find the field size.
    b. If the field size is set to 20×20^2 at the isocenter (distance of 100 cm), calculate the expected field size at a depth of $d_m = 1.2$ cm (SSD = 100 cm). Does the answer agree with what you found in part a?
    c. Determine the size of the physical penumbra in the in-plane direction and in the cross-plane direction. Use the definition of penumbra given in chapter 9, section 9.4.

3. In Figure 14.3 the dose delivered to a depth of 10 cm on the central axis is 100 cGy. Approximately what dose is delivered to a depth of 10 cm and at a distance of 5 cm off the central axis?

4. A patient is treated with two beams having a hinge angle of 60°. What is the optimum wedge angle neglecting the effects of skin contour?

5. One of the beams in a patient's treatment is 6 MV with a 45° wedge (Mevalac). The field is unblocked and the field size is 15×15 cm^2. The treatment is isocentric and the prescription calls for 90 cGy from this beam to be delivered to a depth of 5.0 cm on the central axis. Refer to appendix C for beam data.
    a. Calculate the required MU setting.
    b. The patient is treated with the MU calculated in part a, but the therapist forgets to put the wedge in. What dose does the patient actually receive from this beam?

6. Draw in the correct orientation for wedges (if any) to be used in the figures below.

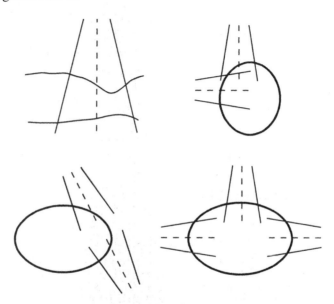

7. Assume that the surface dose for a 10 MV, 15×15 cm^2 field (incident perpendicularly) at SSD = 100 cm (no tray) is 14% of the dose at d_m.
   a. Calculate the percent surface dose for tangential incidence using equation (14.15).
   b. A tray is placed in the beam at a distance of 15 cm from the skin. For perpendicular beam incidence, what is the percent surface dose?

8. How do each of the following factors influence the construction of a PTV from a CTV?
   a. Patient setup uncertainty.
   b. Organ motion.
   c. Microscopic disease.
   d. Proximity of critical structures.
   e. Penumbra.

9. An isocentric "four-field box" is delivered to a patient's pelvis with the Mevalac. The patient is 22 cm thick in the anterior-posterior direction and 34 cm thick in the lateral direction. All beams are open field 10×10 cm^2, 18 MV. The total prescribed dose to the isocenter (at the center of the patient) is 200 cGy. All beams are to be weighted equally. Calculate the number of MU necessary for the lateral beams and the anterior-posterior beams. Refer to appendix C for beam data.

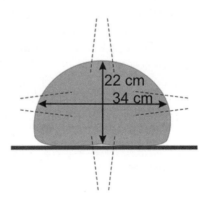

10. What are the limitations of the use of dose-volume histograms in the evaluation of treatment plans?

11. Refer to the "realistic" DVH in Figure 14.34. A dose of 100% represents 72 Gy and 100% of the volume corresponds to 200 cm^3.
    a. What is the value of $D_{95\%}$ (in Gy)?
    b. What is the value of $V_{95\%}$ (in cm^3)?

12. a. Repeat Example 14.5 using TMR values for the 6 MV Mevalac beam.
    b. Repeat Example 14.6 using TMR values for the 6 MV Mevalac beam.

13. Refer to Figures 14.49 and 14.50. The tick marks in these figures are 1 cm apart. Compare the corrected dose distribution with the uncorrected dose distribution at the posterior border of the lung. Measure the amount of lung traversed by the beam and apply the correction indicated in Table 14.4. Does the table give a depth dose in agreement with Figure 14.50?

14. A patient is treated at 120 cm SSD with two adjacent symmetric fields of length 20 cm and 16 cm as measured at isocenter, *not at 120 cm*. Calculate the gap required on the skin surface for the beams to match at a depth of 10 cm.

15. A patient with medulloblastoma is treated with two lateral opposed brain fields and a posterior spinal field as in Figure 14.53. A collimator rotation of the lateral fields is used to match the divergence of the posterior field as in Figure 14.55. If the posterior field is symmetric and 30 cm in length, what collimator rotation angle is necessary for the match?

16. A patient is treated for breast cancer with non-opposed tangents to the left breast. The gantry angle for the lateral beam is 131°. If the medial beam were parallel opposed, the gantry angle would be 311°. The distance from the central axis to the posterior border of the medial field is 7.0 cm. What gantry angle should be set for the medial field so that the posterior borders of the two tangent fields are parallel?

Bibliography

American Association of Physicists in Medicine (AAPM) Report No. 72. Basic Applications of Multileaf Collimators, Report of the AAPM Radiation Therapy Committee Task Group No. 50. Madison, WI: Medical Physics Publishing, 2001.

American Association of Physicists in Medicine (AAPM) Report No. 85. Tissue Inhomogeneity Corrections for Megavoltage Photon Beams, Report of the AAPM Radiation Therapy Committee Task Group No. 65. Madison, WI: Medical Physics Publishing, 2004.

Bentel, G. C. *Radiation Therapy Planning,* Second Edition. New York: McGraw-Hill Professional, 1995.

International Commission on Radiation Measurements and Units (ICRU) Report 50. Prescribing, Recording and Reporting Photon Beam Therapy. Bethesda, MD: ICRU, 1993.

International Commission on Radiation Measurements and Units (ICRU) Report 62. Prescribing, Recording and Reporting Photon Beam Therapy. (Supplement to ICRU Report 50). Bethesda, MD: ICRU, 1999.

Hendee, W.R. *Medical Radiation Physics.* 1st edition. Chicago, IL: Year Book Medical Publishers, 1970.

Hendee, W. R., G. S. Ibbott, and E. G. Hendee. *Radiation Therapy Physics,* Third Edition. Hoboken, NJ: John Wiley & Sons, Inc., 2005.

Jani, S.K. *Handbook of Dosimetry Data for Radiotherapy.* Boca Raton, FL: CRC Press, 1993.

Johns, H. E., and J. R. Cunningham. *The Physics of Radiology,* Fourth Edition. Springfield, IL: Charles C Thomas, 1983.

Keller, R. "Immobilization Devices," Chapter 7 in *Principles and Practice of Radiation Therapy.* C. M. Washington and D. T. Leaver (eds.). New York: Mosby, 1996.

Khan, F. M. (ed.). *Treatment Planning in Radiation Oncology.* Philadelphia: Lippincott Williams & Wilkins, 2006.

Khan, F. M. *The Physics of Radiation Therapy,* Fourth Edition. Philadelphia: Lippincott Williams & Wilkins, 2009.

Khan, F. M. *The Physics of Radiation Therapy,* Third Edition. Philadelphia: Lippincott Williams & Wilkins, 2003.

Khan, F. M., and R. A. Potish (eds.). *Treatment Planning in Radiation Oncology.* Baltimore, MD: Williams & Wilkins, 1998.

Stanton, R., and D. Stinson. *Applied Physics for Radiation Oncology, Revised Edition.* Madison, WI: Medical Physics Publishing, 2009.

Van Dyk, J. (ed.). *The Modern Technology of Radiation Oncology.* Madison, WI: Medical Physics Publishing, 1999.

Washington, C. M., and D. T. Leaver. *Principles and Practice of Radiation Therapy,* Second Edition. St Louis, MO: Mosby, 2003.

Williams, J. R., and D. I. Thwaites (eds.). *Radiotherapy Physics: In Practice,* Second Edition. New York: Oxford University Press USA, 2000.

15 Electron Beam Dosimetry

15.1 Introduction

The energy of the electrons in a linear accelerator electron beam is almost monoenergetic. For this reason, electron beam energies should be referred to in units of MeV rather than MV as for photon beams. The average energy of the photons in a photon beam changes little with depth as it traverses matter. In contrast, electrons continually lose energy as they traverse matter. The stated energy of an electron beam is the energy at the phantom or patient surface.

The widespread use of electron beam therapy began in the 1970s when linacs capable of producing a range of electron energies became common. The most useful energies are between 6 and 20 MeV. The short, well-defined range of electrons makes them advantageous for treating superficial tumors at a depth of about 5 cm or less. Electron beam treatments have now replaced most superficial energy x-ray treatments (at least in the United States). This may be, in part, due to reimbursement patterns. Electrons are commonly used to treat skin and lip cancer, for scar boosts for breast cancer, lymph node boosts, for posterior neck boosts to spare the spinal cord, and for total skin electron irradiation for a rare skin disease known as mycosis fungoides.

The intensity of a photon beam falls off gradually as it penetrates matter. Photons have no specific range in matter. Electrons, however, have a fairly well defined range (see chapter 6, section 6.2). This can be seen by examining the percent depth dose curves in Figure 15.1. This figure shows percent depth dose curves for electron beams with energies ranging from 6 to 18 MeV. The percent depth dose for a 4 MV photon beam is also shown in the same graph for comparison. Note the short and relatively well-defined range of the electron beams in comparison to the 4 MV x-ray beam. A table of percent depth doses for the Mevalac electron beams appears in appendix C. Recall that the Mevalac is a fictitious linear accelerator with five electron beam energies.

The range of an electron beam as defined in Figure 15.2 is called the practical range R_p. Electrons lose energy by colliding (scattering) with "stationary" electrons in the medium. Electrons can scatter through large angles because the electron mass is so small.

The dependence of the energy on depth is:

$$E_d = E_0 \left(1 - \frac{d}{R_P} \right), \tag{15.1}$$

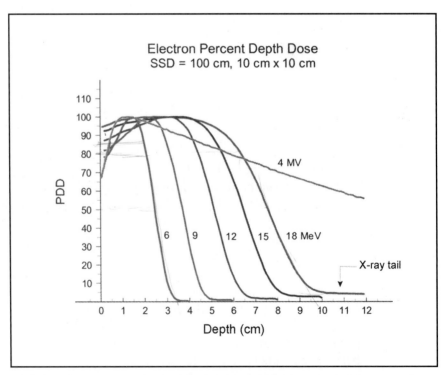

Figure 15.1: Electron depth dose curves for the Mevalac. An x-ray depth dose curve for a 4 MV beam is shown for comparison. Note: (1) Electron beams have less skin sparing than photon beams (80% to 90% surface dose); (2) The surface dose increases as the energy increases; (3) There is an increase in range with increasing energy; (4) There is an x-ray "tail" which increases in amplitude as the energy increases.

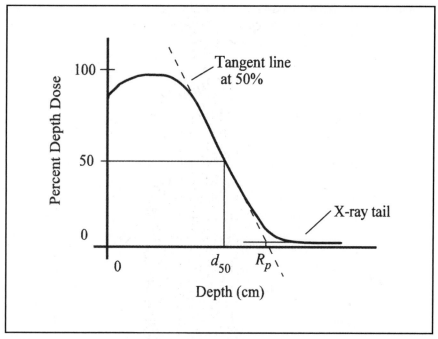

Figure 15.2: An illustration of the definition of the practical range of an electron beam. A tangent is drawn to the PDD curve at a depth where the PDD = 50% (d_{50}). A horizontal line is drawn which coincides with the x-ray tail. At the intersection of these two lines, drop a vertical line down to the horizontal axis. Read off the value of R_p where the vertical line intersects the horizontal (depth) axis.

where E_d is the energy of the electrons at depth d, E_0 is the kinetic energy of the electrons at the surface, and R_p is the practical range. When $d = 0$, $E_d = E_0$ as expected, and when $d = R_p$, $E_d = 0$, the electrons have lost all of their kinetic energy.

The rate of energy loss depends on the electron density of the medium. For electrons in the MeV energy range, the energy loss rate in water is about 2 MeV/cm (see chapter 6, section 6.2). For this reason, the electrons will lose all of their kinetic energy in a distance R_p(cm) ≈ (E_0 MeV)/(2 MeV/cm) = E_0/2.

As an example, 6 MeV electrons have a range of about 6/2 = 3 cm in water (see Figure 15.1).

 Rule of thumb: The practical range of electrons in water is given by:

$$R_p\left(\text{cm}\right) \approx \frac{E_0\left(\text{MeV}\right)}{2},$$

where E_0 is the incident electron energy in units of MeV.

Table 15.1: Electron Beam Bremsstrahlung Tail*
(Normalized to 100% at d_m for 10 × 10 to 15 × 15 cm² fields)

Energy (MeV)	Amplitude of x-ray tail
6–12	0.5–2%
12–15	2–4%
15–20	4–5%

*Data from Jani, S. K. *Handbook of Dosimetry Data for Radiotherapy*, Table 2.B2, p. 86, 1993.

Electrons exhibit less skin sparing than photons. The percent depth dose at the surface is 80% to 90% as opposed to a typical value of about 30% for a photon beam. The relative surface dose increases with energy, just the opposite of photons. There is an increase in range with energy. There is a small residual "tail" to the PDD curves that increases in amplitude with increasing energy. The tail is due to bremsstrahlung x-ray production by the electrons. The electrons interact with the scattering foil, applicator, and collimator, producing a small x-ray contamination component. It is generally of no clinical significance except for total skin electron irradiation for mycosis fungoides. Table 15.1 lists nominal values of the amplitude of the x-ray (bremsstrahlung) tail.

The prescription point is usually to the deepest point of the tumor. Physicians usually want the 80% to 90% line to cover the deepest extent of the target.

Rule of thumb:

$$d_{80}\left(\text{cm}\right) \approx \frac{E_0\left(\text{MeV}\right)}{3},$$

where d_{80}(cm) is the central axis depth (in cm) of the 80% isodose and E_0 is the incident energy (in MeV) of the electron beam.[1]

Examine Figure 15.1 to see how well this approximate relationship works.

Table 15.2 lists the values of the depth of maximum build-up d_m for the Mevalac. Examination of the table shows that the value of d_m generally rises as the energy goes up. For high-energy electrons the percent depth dose maximum is very broad. The value of d_m actually declines from 3.4 cm at 15 MeV to 1.9 cm at 18 MeV. There is a very broad plateau near d_m for the 18 MeV beam (see Figure 15.1).

A table of depth dose values for the Mevalac linear accelerator appears in appendix C.

---

[1] Some people use the rule of thumb that d_{90} is approximately equal to $E_0/4$, but this rule is not very accurate.

Table 15.2: Mevalac Electron d_m Values*

Energy (MeV)	6	9	12	15	18
d_m(cm)	1.3	2.2	2.8	3.4	1.8

*The Mevalac is a fictitious linear accelerator introduced in chapter 12 (Table 12.1 and appendix C).

15.2 Electron Applicators

Electrons are easily scattered by all of the objects that they encounter after emerging from the waveguide, such as the scattering foil, monitor chambers, collimator jaws, and the intervening air. It is therefore necessary to collimate the beam down close to the patient skin surface. This is accomplished by using an attachable applicator that extends down close to the isocenter (see Figure 9.21). These are sometimes called "cones" even though they are not cone shaped. Linac manufacturers provide a variety of applicator sizes; usually a set of square aperture applicators with sizes 10 × 10, 15 × 15, (14 × 14 for Elekta), 20 × 20, and 25 × 25 (in centimeters) and a circular aperture of diameter 5 to 6 cm. An interlock will prevent electron beam production unless an applicator is attached. The potential for injury exists due to a collision because the end of the applicator is near the patient's skin surface. The cones are spring-loaded or padded at the bottom to help avoid injury if the cone should contact the patient. There are collision avoidance sensors (touch pad or touch sensor) in the end of the cone that shut off all motor controls on the linac when there is excessive pressure. The end of the applicator is usually at a distance of 95 cm from the source.

When an applicator is inserted, the secondary collimator jaws must be set to a specific field size that is larger than the size of the applicator aperture. As an example, for one particular linac, the 10 × 10 cm^2 cone requires the jaws to be set to 19 × 19 cm^2. On older linacs this field size must be set by the operator. On newer machines the field size is automatically set once the applicator is attached to the collimator. The necessary field size depends on the applicator size and perhaps on energy. There is an interlock that will only allow the linac to produce a beam if the correct jaw setting is established. If the jaw setting is not the standard value, the dose rate would be affected and the beam might not meet specification for flatness and symmetry.

The PDD of electron beams is generally independent of applicator size for applicators of 10 × 10 and larger and for beam energy of approximately 20 MeV and less. Electrons have a short range and scattered electrons have an even shorter range. For field sizes larger than 10 × 10 no additional scattered electrons can reach the central axis. Therefore the PDD remains unchanged for applicators larger than 10 × 10 unless the electron energy is above 20 to 25 MeV.

15.3 Field Shaping

The shaping of electron field portals is accomplished with the use of small blocks put into the end of the applicator (see Figure 15.3). These are sometimes called *electron cutouts*. There is an empirical relation for the necessary block thickness; for lead:

$$t_{Pb}\,(\mathrm{mm}) \cong 0.5 E_0\,(\mathrm{MeV}) + 1, \tag{15.2}$$

where t_{Pb}(mm) is the thickness of the lead in millimeters. This amount of lead is sufficient to completely stop the electrons. Some of the x-ray contamination may however penetrate the cutout. For the same transmission, Cerrobend® cutouts need to be a little bit thicker:

$$t_C\,(\mathrm{mm}) = 1.2\, t_{Pb}\,(\mathrm{mm}), \tag{15.3}$$

where t_C(mm) is the thickness of Cerrobend in millimeters.

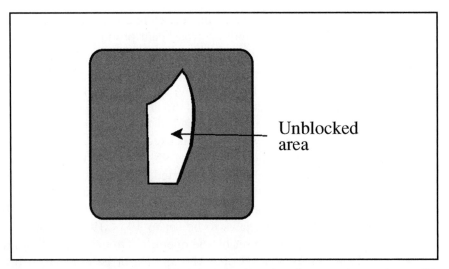

Figure 15.3: Beam's-eye view of an electron block ("cutout") used to shape an electron beam. This block is shaped for a posterior neck boost. The block fits into the end of the electron applicator. (Adapted from Stanton, R., and D. Stinson, *Applied Physics for Radiation Oncology, Revised Edition*, Fig. 13.5, p. 212, © 2009, with permission.)

Example 15.1

What is the necessary thickness of a Cerrobend® block for shaping a 22 MeV electron beam?

$$t_{Pb} = 0.5(22) + 1 = 12 \text{ mm}$$

$$t_C = 1.2\,(12) = 14 \text{ mm} = 1.4 \text{ cm}$$

As mentioned earlier, the percent depth dose for electron beams with energies below 20 MeV is relatively unaffected by field size (either applicator size or blocking) for applicators of size 10×10 cm^2 and larger. A single table of depth dose values for applicators of size 10×10 cm^2 and larger (e.g., 15×15, 20×20, and 25×25) is usually adequate. For applicators of size less than 10×10 cm^2, the depth dose can be significantly affected by the field size (see Figure 15.4), and separate tables may be necessary for small field sizes. For small field sizes the depth dose curve shifts toward the surface and the output can be reduced. These effects are illustrated in Figures 15.4 and 15.5.

These effects can be explained in terms of side scatter or lateral equilibrium. For a small volume on the central axis when the field is very small, there is a loss of side scatter equilibrium—there is more radiation scattered out of the volume than into the volume and therefore a reduction in dose and a reduction in PDD. This is illustrated in Figure 15.6.

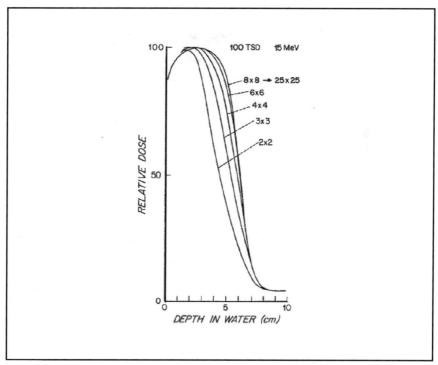

Figure 15.4: The effect on the PDD curve of blocking for a 15 MeV electron beam. The largest field size is 25×25 cm^2. The PDD curve does not change much until the field size is reduced to 6×6 cm^2. As the field size is reduced from 6×6 cm^2, the PDD curve becomes less steep and d_m shifts toward the surface. (Reprinted from AAPM TG-25, Figure 14, "Clinical electron-beam dosimetry: Report of AAPM Radiation Therapy Committee Task Group No. 25." *Med Phys* 18:73–109, © 1991; Redrawn from Meyer, J. A., J. R. Palta, and K. R. Hogstrom, "Demonstration of relatively new electron dosimetry measurement techniques on the Mevatron 80." *Med Phys* 11:670–677, © 1984. With permission from American Association of Physicists in Medicine (AAPM).)

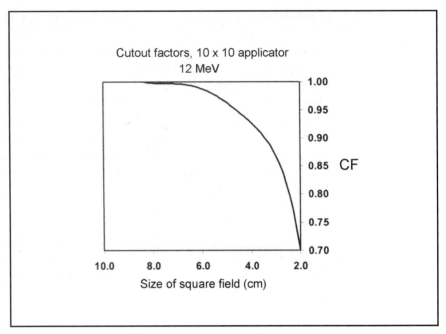

Figure 15.5: The effect of blocking on the dose rate (at d_m) for a 12 MeV electron beam. Note the inverted horizontal scale. For shaped fields of side length less than about 6 cm, there is a sharp decline in dose rate because of a departure from lateral equilibrium. The cutout factor (CF) is the reduction in the dose rate due to the presence of blocking [see equation (15.5)].

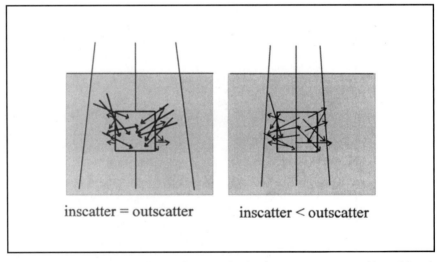

Figure 15.6: A small volume element resides on the central axis. Electrons are scattered into this volume element through the sides, provided that the total volume irradiated is large enough. Electrons are also scattered out through the sides. If the number scattered out is equal to the number scattered in, then there will be lateral scatter equilibrium. If the field size is reduced sufficiently, then there will be a decrease in the fluence of electrons scattered in through the side. The number scattered out however will remain the same and *the dose rate will therefore decrease.*

15.4 Dose Rate Calculations for Electron Beams

The basic principle of monitor unit calculations for electrons is no different than for photons. The number of monitor units required to deliver a dose D is $\mu = D/\dot{D}$, and therefore the problem reduces to one of finding the dose rate. Just as for photons, it is important to understand the normalization conditions. Common normalization conditions are: 10×10 applicator, SSD = 100 cm, dose rate is set to 1.000 cGy/MU at d_m on the central axis for each beam energy. Symbolically, this is written $\dot{D}_{d_m}(100+d_m,10) = 1.000$ cGy/MU. This dose rate is established at the time of TG-51 protocol electron beam calibration. If, for a given energy electron beam, the dose rate is not 1.000 cGy/MU under these conditions, then the sensitivity of the monitor chambers is adjusted so that the dose rate will be 1.000 cGy/MU. These are the conditions that will be assumed in this book for the Mevalac linear accelerator. One then measures the relative dose rate for other size applicators. We define the quantity $S_e(f_a)$:

$$S_e(f_a) = \frac{\dot{D}_{d_m}(100+d_m,f_a)}{\dot{D}_{d_m}(100+d_m,10)}, \qquad (15.4)$$

where f_a represents the applicator size. This data is given in Table 15.3 for the Mevalac.

The dose rate at a total distance r from the source, at depth d, for applicator size f_a is:

$$\dot{D}_d(r,f_a) = \dot{D}_{d_m}(100+d_m,10) \times S_e(f_a) \times CF(f_a,f') \times ISF \times DD(d,f_a,f') \qquad (15.5)$$

where $CF(f_a,f')$ is the "cutout factor" that accounts for the reduction in dose rate due to the presence of a cutout with equivalent field size f', ISF is an inverse square correction (factor) that is necessary when the SSD is not equal to 100 cm, and DD is the depth dose. These quantities

Table 15.3: Mevalac Electron Applicator Factors $S_e(f_a)$

E (MeV)	6×6	10×10	15×15	20×20	25×25
6	0.962	1.000	1.004	1.009	0.997
9	0.981	1.000	1.000	0.984	0.963
12	0.987	1.000	0.997	0.974	0.946
15	0.992	1.000	0.991	0.968	0.934
18	1.002	1.000	0.982	0.962	0.927

d_m values are those listed in Table 15.2.

are discussed further below. If we drop the functional notation, equation (15.5) can be written in compact form as:

$$\dot{D}_d = \dot{D}_{d_m} \times S_e \times \text{CF} \times \text{ISF} \times \text{DD}. \tag{15.6}$$

Electron cutouts are almost always used to shape electron fields. If a cutout is not used, CF = 1.000. If the aperture of the cutout is sufficiently small, the value of CF may be a significant correction to the dose rate. This occurs as a result of a lack of lateral equilibrium. Khan[2] has shown that the condition for lateral equilibrium is that the distance from any field boundary $R > 0.88 \sqrt{E}$, where R is in centimeters and E is in units of MeV. A conservative guideline for the establishment of lateral equilibrium is that all field edges be at a distance greater than $R = \sqrt{E}$ from the point of calculation. In this case, the cutout factor may be assumed to have a value of 1.00 without making an error of more than a few percent in the dose rate. As an example, for a point at the center of a square field with beam energy of 9 MeV, $\sqrt{E} = 3$ and therefore the cutout factor may be neglected for a field size of 6 × 6 cm² and larger. For an irregular field, a cutout can be evaluated as follows: At the point of dose calculation, draw the largest circle around this point, which is completely circumscribed by the boundaries of the cutout. If $R > \sqrt{E}$, no cutout factor correction is needed (see Figure 15.7).

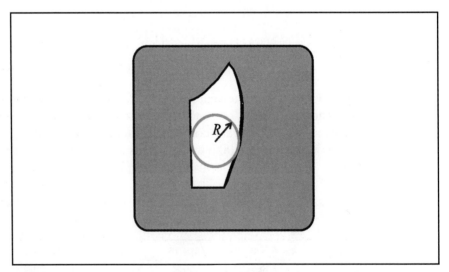

Figure 15.7: Evaluation of an electron cutout. Draw the largest circle around the point of calculation that is completely enclosed by the boundaries of the cutout. If $R > \sqrt{E}$, where R is in centimeters and E is in units of MeV, an electron cutout factor correction is unnecessary.

---

[2] Khan, F. M. *The Physics of Radiation Therapy,* Third Edition, 2003.

Most treatment planning systems are not very good at calculating cutout factors. If a cutout correction factor is necessary, it can be measured for the individual patient's cutout or it can be estimated from a table of previously measured values. One method involves compilation of a table of cutout factors for square fields. If the field has an irregular shape, one first draws an equivalent rectangle as in chapter 13, section 13.3 for photon fields. The cutout factor for the rectangular field of dimensions $L \times W$ can be related to the tabulated cutout factors for the square fields as follows:

$$\mathrm{CF}\left(f_a, f'\right) = \sqrt{\mathrm{CF}\left(f_a, L\right) \times \mathrm{CF}\left(f_a, W\right)}. \tag{15.7}$$

Example 15.2

A prescription calls for 200 cGy of 15 MeV electrons using a 20 × 20 applicator. The dose is to be delivered to depth d_m with SSD = 100 cm. The cutout is large and therefore CF can be assumed to be 1.000. Calculate the required MU. The applicator factor is $S_e(20) =$ 0.968. The DD = 1.00 since $d = d_m$.

$$\dot{D}_d\left(r, f_a\right) = \dot{D}_{d_m}\left(100 + d_m, 10\right) \times S_e\left(f_a\right) \times \mathrm{CF}\left(f_a, f'\right) \times \mathrm{ISF} \times \mathrm{DD}\left(d, f_a, f'\right)$$

$$= 1.000 \times 0.968 \times 1.0 \times 1.0 \times 1.00$$

$$= 0.968 \text{ cGy/MU}$$

$$\mu = \frac{D}{\dot{D}} = \frac{200 \text{ cGy}}{0.968 \text{ cGy/MU}} = 207 \text{ MU}$$

When a linac operates in x-ray mode, the majority of the photons produced in the target travel directly from the target to the patient without undergoing significant scattering or absorption. In this case, only geometrical divergence causes beam attenuation and thus x-ray beams closely follow the inverse square law described in chapter 5, section 5.5. In contrast to x-ray photons, a significant fraction of the electrons reaching the patient have been scattered by objects closer to the patient than the source. For this reason, electrons do not generally follow a simple inverse square law. Electrons scattering may give rise to an apparent or "virtual" source, which is distinct from the actual source. The distance from the apparent source is called the virtual source distance or VSD for short. The VSD is kind of an "average" source distance. Electrons obey a modified inverse square law over a limited range when the VSD is used instead of the actual source distance. The modified inverse square correction depends on the VSD and the air gap $g = \mathrm{SSD} - 100$ cm (see Figure 15.8).

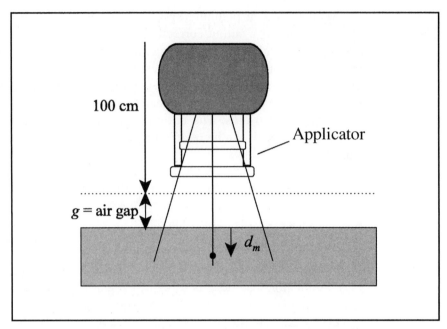

Figure 15.8: The air gap for an electron applicator is usually measured from a distance of 100 cm, not from the end of the applicator. For example, if the SSD = 105 cm, then g = 5 cm.

The value of the VSD usually depends on the energy and the applicator size and can be determined as follows. It is expected that $\dot{D}_{d_m}\left(100+d_m+g,f_a\right)$ will follow an inverse square law:

$$\dot{D}_{d_m}\left(100+d_m+g,f_a\right) \propto \left(\frac{1}{\mathrm{VSD}+d_m+g}\right)^2, \tag{15.8}$$

where the symbol $\propto$ means proportional to. In the absence of a gap (g = 0):

$$\dot{D}_{d_m}\left(100+d_m,f_a\right) \propto \left(\frac{1}{\mathrm{VSD}+d_m}\right)^2, \tag{15.9}$$

and the inverse square correction for a gap is then

$$\mathrm{ISF} = \frac{\dot{D}_{d_m}\left(100+d_m+g,f_a\right)}{\dot{D}_{d_m}\left(100+d_m,f_a\right)} = \left(\frac{\mathrm{VSD}+d_m}{\mathrm{VSD}+d_m+g}\right)^2. \tag{15.10}$$

For a given energy and applicator size, measure the dose rate $\dot{D}_{d_m}\left(100+d_m+g,f_a\right)$ at depth d_m on the central axis for a range of values of the air gap from 0 to about 20 cm (see Figure 15.8). A graph of

$\sqrt{1/\text{ISF}}$ versus g is shown in Figure 15.9. From equation (15.10) we may write:

$$\sqrt{\frac{1}{\text{ISF}}} = \frac{\text{VSD}+d_m+g}{\text{VSD}+d_m} = 1+\left(\frac{1}{\text{VSD}+d_m}\right)g\,.$$

$$\begin{array}{ccccc} \updownarrow & & \updownarrow & \updownarrow & \updownarrow \\ y & & =b+ & m & x \end{array}$$

(15.11)

Equation (15.11) is the equation for a straight line $y = mx + b$: the square root term on the left hand side is y, on the right hand side the intercept $b = 1$, the slope m is the term in parentheses, and x is g. If we make a graph of y versus x (Figure 15.9), we can measure the slope, set it equal to $(\text{VSD} + d_m)^{-1}$ and solve for the value of VSD. Typical values of the VSD range from about 80 to 90 cm.

If the air gap is larger than about 10 cm, the expression for the inverse square correction in equation (15.10) may become unreliable. If there is any doubt, the dose rate should be measured by a physicist. An alternative to the use of a virtual source distance is to use only fixed values of the SSD, say 100, 105, 110, etc., clinically and to measure the applicator output at these SSDs and make a table of them. For air gaps less than about 10 cm, the depth dose is relatively independent of SSD.

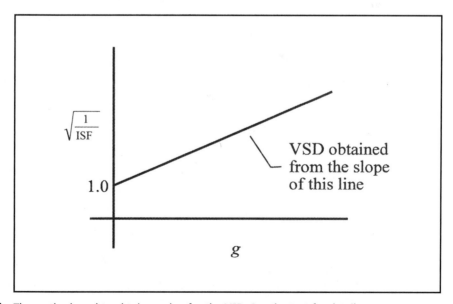

Figure 15.9: The method used to obtain a value for the VSD. See the text for details.

Example 15.3

A posterior neck boost calls for the 9 MeV beam on the Mevalac using a 15 × 15 applicator. The prescription calls for 180 cGy delivered to a depth of d_m on the central axis. The average air gap over the field is 4.5 cm. Calculate the MU using VSD = 86.0 cm. Assume CF = 1.00, $S_e(15) = 1.000$, $d_m = 2.2$ cm.

$$\dot{D}_d\left(r, f_a\right) = \dot{D}_{d_m}\left(100 + d_m, 10\right) \times S_e\left(f_a\right) \times CF\left(f_a, f'\right) \times ISF \times DD\left(d, f_a, f'\right)$$

$$ISF = \left(\frac{86.0 + 2.2}{86.0 + 2.2 + 4.5}\right)^2 = 0.905$$

$$\dot{D}_{d_m}\left(100 + d_m + 4.5, 15\right) = 1.00 \times 1.00 \times 1.000 \times 0.905 \text{ cGy/MU}$$

$$\mu = \frac{D}{\dot{D}_d} = \frac{180 \text{ cGy}}{0.905 \text{ cGy/MU}} = 199 \text{ MU}$$

15.5 Internal Blocking

Lead is used to protect the oral mucosa, tongue, or eye, etc. This raises a problem, however, because of electron backscatter from lead. The dose at the tissue/lead interface can be up to 68% greater than without the lead. The backscattered electrons have much lower energy. The *electron backscatter factor (EBF)* is defined as the dose (in the tissue) at the interface between tissue and another material divided by the dose in the absence of the other material. For a lead/polystyrene interface:

$$EBF = 1.0 + 0.735 e^{-0.052 E_d}, \tag{15.12}$$

where E_d = the energy at the depth of the interface in MeV.[3] Polystyrene is approximately tissue equivalent. To reduce the dose to the tissue at the interface, a low Z material is placed in front of the lead. Common materials are aluminum, wax, plastic, and so forth. Oral stents are made out of dental acrylic.

---

[3] Khan, F. M. *The Physics of Radiation Therapy,* Third Edition, 2003.

Example 15.4[4]

A mucosal lesion is to be treated with 9 MeV electrons externally on the cheek. The cheek thickness including the lesion is 2 cm.

a. Compute the thickness of lead required to shield oral structures beyond the cheek.

We can use the equation $t_{Pb}(\text{mm}) = 0.5\ E_0(\text{MeV}) + 1$, but we must be careful to use the value of the electron energy at the surface of the lead for E_0. If the cheek is 2 cm thick, then the electrons will lose an energy of 4 MeV in penetrating to the surface of the lead. Therefore $E_0 = 9 - 4 = 5$ MeV and the lead thickness necessary is $t_{Pb} = 0.5(5) + 1 = 3.5$ mm.

b. Compute the magnitude of the electron backscatter enhancement to the dose at the lead/tissue interface.

$$\text{EBF} = 1.0 + 0.735\,e^{-0.052 E_d}$$
$$= 1.0 + 0.735\,e^{-0.052(5)} = 1.57$$

This is a 57% enhancement.

c. Compute the thickness of the bolus necessary to absorb the backscatter.

According to Table 15.4, the HVL for the backscattered electrons in polystyrene is approximately 4 mm. A thickness of about 1 cm would be 2.5 HVL, which would reduce the backscatter from 57% enhancement to about 10%. Note that once the bolus is inserted, the energy of the electrons at the lead surface will decrease and the thickness of the lead required will decrease accordingly.

Table 15.4: Dose Enhancement at Tissue/Lead Interface

Electron energy (MeV)	Dose enhancement at tissue/lead interface	HVL of backscattered electrons in polystyrene
14	35%	6 mm
10	45%	5 mm
6	55%	4 mm

HVL = Half-value layer.

---

[4] Adapted from Khan, F. M. *The Physics of Radiation Therapy*, Third Edition, 2003.

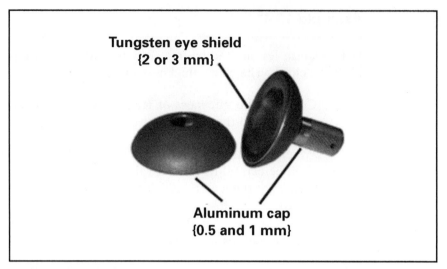

Tungsten eye shield
{2 or 3 mm}

Aluminum cap
{0.5 and 1 mm}

Figure 15.10: Tungsten eye shields used for protecting the eye during electron beam treatments. The shields fit over the eye like a contact lens. An aluminum cap can be added to reduce the backscatter dose. (Courtesy of Radiation Products Design, Inc., Albertville, MN)

For electron treatments in the vicinity of the eye, it is common to shield the eye using tungsten eye shields. It is particularly important to shield the lens, which is at a depth of approximately 3 mm from the surface of the eye. An eye shield is shown in Figure 15.10. Eye shields are applied to the patient's eye like a contact lens. The electron shielding is provided by tungsten, which is 2 to 3 mm thick. If the shield is to go underneath the eyelid, then an aluminum cap (either 0.5 or 1 mm thick) may be added to reduce the backscatter dose to the eyelid. As an example of the use of these eye shields consider a 9 MeV beam incident upon a 2 mm tungsten eye shield with a 0.5 mm aluminum cap. Measurements show that the dose at a depth of 3 mm is 4.8% and the backscatter dose at the inner aluminum surface is 106%.[5,6]

15.6 Isodose Curves

Isodose lines are shown in Figures 15.11 through 15.13 for 10×10 cm^2 electron beams with energies of 6, 9, and 22 MeV. For low energies all isodose curves show some lateral expansion with depth (see Figures 15.11 and 15.12). For high energies, only low-value isodose curves bulge out (see the 10% line in Figure 15.13), whereas high-value isodose curves are laterally constricted inward with increasing depth. At depth d_m, the 90% isodose line is approximately 1 cm from the geometric field edge (see Figure 15.12). It is common to laterally include a 1 cm margin at the surface around the target volume for this reason.

---

[5] Doses are normalized to d_m without the eye shield.
[6] Data from Cardinal Health catalog, Cardinal Health, Inc., Dublin, OH.

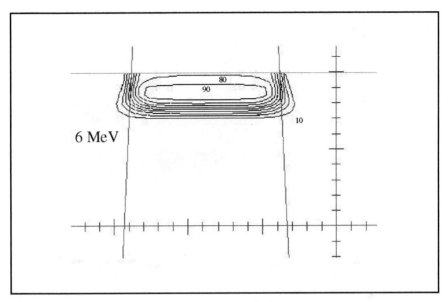

Figure 15.11: Dose distribution for a 6 MeV 10 × 10 electron beam with SSD = 100 cm. The distance between tick marks is 1 cm.

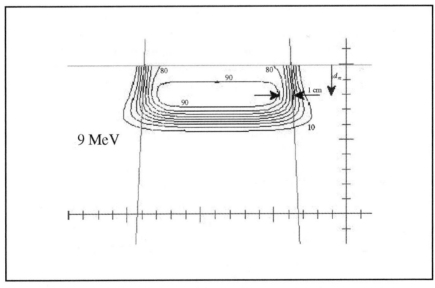

Figure 15.12: Dose distribution for a 9 MeV 10 × 10 electron beam with SSD = 100 cm. At a depth of d_m, the distance between the 90% line and the field edge is about 1 cm.

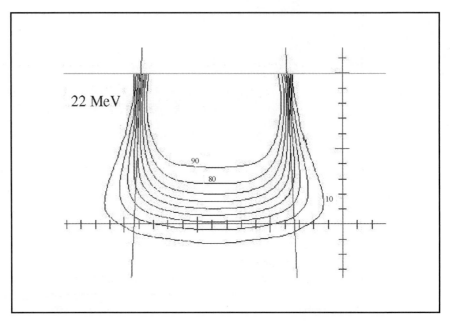

Figure 15.13: Dose distribution for a 22 MeV 10 × 10 cm² electron beam with SSD = 100 cm. Low-dose isodose lines bulge out whereas high-dose lines are "pinched" inward.

15.7 Inhomogeneities

Anatomical regions irradiated with electrons may include bone, lung, and air cavities. Electrons interact with atomic electrons and nuclei in the medium as discussed in chapter 6, section 6.2. The effects of inhomogeneities on electron dose distributions depend on the beam energy and the shape, size, electron density, and effective atomic number of the inhomogeneity.

Large slab inhomogeneities may be crudely treated somewhat like photons by introducing an effective depth. For electrons, we introduce the coefficient of equivalent thickness (CET). The water-equivalent thickness of a slab inhomogeneity (see Figure 15.14) of thickness z is $z \times$ CET. The thickness of the water-equivalent tissue is $d - z$, where d is the depth of the point of interest. Therefore the total effective thickness is $d - z + z \times$ CET or:

$$d_{eff} = d - z\left(1 - \mathrm{CET}\right). \qquad (15.13)$$

The CET is related to the stopping power and therefore depends on energy as well as depth. For compact bone CET = 1.65, for spongy bone CET is approximately 1.00, for lung tissue CET is approximately equal to the relative electron density (about 0.20 to 0.25). The depth dose is to be looked up for the effective depth. The CET method of correction is not very accurate and is not widely used clinically. In a low-density cavity such as lung tissue, scattered electrons can travel a long distance and the dose will spread out significantly in the lateral direction.

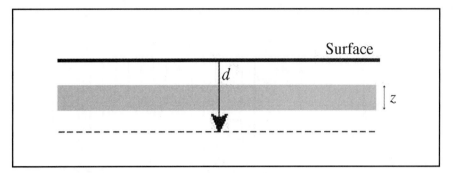

Figure 15.14: The shaded region is an inhomogeneity with thickness z. The dose is to be evaluated at depth d.

For small inhomogeneities, effects due to edges can be surprising. A small high-density inhomogeneity either on top of or inside the patient leads to a lobe of high dose in the low-density material and a corresponding region of low dose under the high-density material. This is illustrated in Figure 15.15.

This is due to additional scattering away from the high-density material toward the low-density material, as illustrated in Figure 15.16.

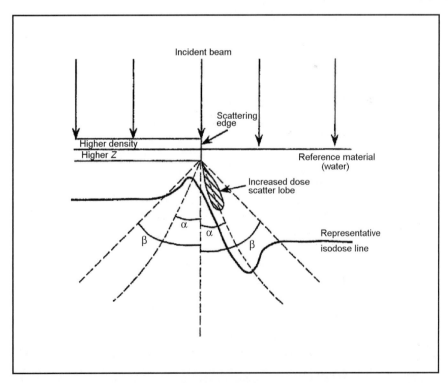

Figure 15.15: The edge effect caused by the edge of a high-density, high-Z inhomogeneity. A high-dose lobe residing at approximately angle α appears to the side of the edge due to increased scatter. Beyond angle β there is negligible effect due to the edge. (Reprinted from Williams, J. R., and D. I. Thwaites (eds.). *Radiotherapy Physics: In Practice,* Second Edition, Figure 10.6, page 212, © 2000. By permission from Oxford University Press.)

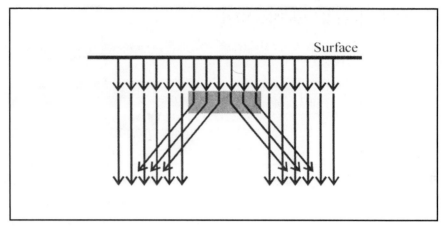

Figure 15.16: Schematic depiction of the effects of a small high-density inhomogeneity. This could be lead used for blocking. Electrons are scattered out of the high-density material. There will be a hot spot outside the edge of the high-density material (After Khan, F. M. *The Physics of Radiation Therapy,* Third Edition. Philadelphia: Lippincott Williams & Wilkins, © 2003.)

In this diagram the arrows represent fluence. If the dose is proportional to the fluence, then it is apparent that the dose will be enhanced just lateral to and downstream of the edge of the high-density material.

The dose perturbation due to the presence of the inhomogeneity has been described in terms of angles α and β. The angle α is the angle along which the maximum dose increase or reduction occurs. Beyond an angle β the effect of edge scatter is negligible. Outside the angle β and underneath the inhomogeneity, the dose may be computed using the CET. The influence of an edge increases with increasing energy. See Table 15.5.

Edge effects are important at the interface between different media (lung, bone, air cavities, etc.) and at the edges of pronounced surface irregularities such as the nose, ear canal, and bolus, and especially at the edge of lead that is used on the surface for beam shaping/shielding.

Table 15.5: Edge Effect Parameters: Approximate Values*

Energy at interface (MeV)	α	β	Maximum increase (bone/water interface)
5	60°	--	4%
10	30°	70°	8%
20	15°	35°	14%

*Data from Williams, J. R., and D. I. Thwaites (eds.). *Radiotherapy Physics: In Practice,* Second Edition, p. 212, 2000.

15.8 Field Matching

Adjacent electron fields may be necessary under the following circumstances:

1. Provision for varying penetration by using different energy electron beams for adjoining areas.
2. Treatment of a larger area than the standard applicators allow.
3. When an adjacent area has had previous treatment.

As electrons are usually used to treat superficial tissue, electron beams are usually abutted on the surface; otherwise there would be a cold spot near the surface. Abutting electron beams gives a hot spot, but you live with it (see Figure 15.17). Use field migration if necessary. Extended SSD will give a broadened penumbra.

Figure 15.18 shows an example of electron/photon beam matching. When an electron field is abutted, at the surface, with a photon field, a hot spot develops on the side of the photon field.

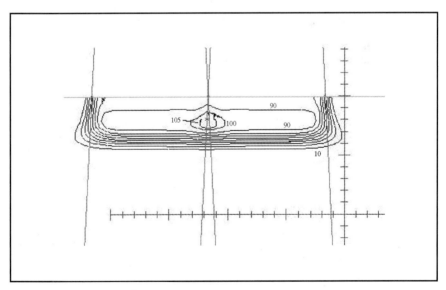

Figure 15.17: Two adjacent 10 × 10 cm² 9 MeV electron beams (SSD = 100 cm) matched at the surface. The hot spot is 110%. The tick marks on the scale are 1 cm apart. This dose distribution was calculated with treatment planning software.

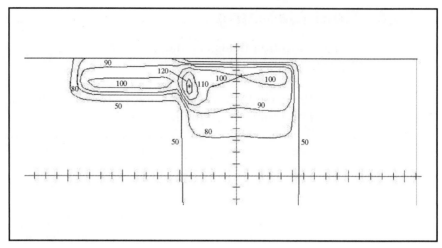

Figure 15.18: Calculated dose distribution for abutting electron and photon fields. The electron field is a 9 MeV 10 × 10 cm² field with SSD = 100 cm. The photon beam is 6 MV, 10 × 10 cm², SSD = 100 cm. The fields are matched at the surface. The hotspot is 125% at the location of the asterisk. The tick marks are spaced 1 cm apart.

Chapter Summary

- Electron beams are roughly monoenergetic; refer to beam energy in MeV; beam loses energy as it moves into matter.

- Photon beam intensity falls off gradually in matter; no specific range; electron beams have relatively well-defined range; useful for superficial treatment.

 Rule of thumb: The practical range of electrons in water is given by:

$$R_p\left(\text{cm}\right) \approx \frac{E_0\left(\text{MeV}\right)}{2},$$

where E_0 is the incident electron energy in units of MeV.

- **Depth Dose:** Surface doses are in the range of 80% to 90%. Relative surface dose increases with increasing energy, just the opposite of photons. Depth dose is little affected by field size until the field size is reduced to about 6 × 6 cm² or smaller. For air gaps less than 10 cm, the depth dose is relatively independent of SSD.

- **Bremsstrahlung Tail:** Electrons interact with scattering foil, cones, collimator to produce x-rays; small x-ray contamination component, generally not significant except for total skin electron irradiation treatment.

Table 15.1: Electron Beam Bremsstrahlung Tail*
(Normalized to 100% at d for 10 × 10 to 15 × 15 cm² fields)

Energy (MeV)	Amplitude of x-ray tail
6–12	0.5–2%
12–15	2–4%
15–20	4–5%

*Data from Jani, S. K. *Handbook of Dosimetry Data for Radiotherapy*, Table 2.B2, p. 86, 1993.

Table 15.2: Mevalac Electron d_m Values*

Energy (MeV)	6	9	12	15	18
d_m(cm)	1.3	2.2	2.8	3.4	1.8

*The Mevalac is a fictitious linear accelerator introduced in chapter 12 (Table 12.1 and appendix C).

- Prescription dose is usually delivered to deepest point of tumor, usually depth of 80% to 90% PDD.

 Rule of thumb:

$$d_{80}\left(\text{cm}\right) \approx \frac{E_0\left(\text{MeV}\right)}{3},$$

where d_{80}(cm) is the central axis depth (in cm) of the 80% isodose and E_0 is the incident energy (in MeV) of the electron beam.

- **Isodose Curves:** For low energies, all isodose curves show some lateral expansion with depth. For high energy, only low-value isodose curves bulge out and high isodose lines curve in. It is common to laterally include 1 cm margin at the surface around the target volume.

- **Electron Applicators:** Electrons are easily scattered in the linac head and intervening air and must collimate almost down to patient skin surface.

- **Field Shaping:** Accomplished with small blocks put into the end of the applicator—called "cutouts"—thickness necessary:
  —Lead: $t_{Pb}(\text{mm}) = 0.5\, E_0(\text{MeV}) + 1$
  —Cerrobend®: $t_C(\text{mm}) = 1.2\, t_{Pb}(\text{mm})$

- **Blocking** can have a significant effect on output and depth dose distribution for electrons
  —depth dose curve shifts toward surface
  —output is reduced.
  Blocking may be important when the smallest distance from the point of dose calculation to the block edge is less than $\sqrt{E}$ in centimeters. For heavily blocked fields (and or large air gap) a physicist may need to measure output.

- **Monitor Unit Calculations:** As for all MU calculations: $\mu = D/\dot{D}$. The dose rate is given by

$$\dot{D}_d\left(r, f_a\right) = \dot{D}_{d_m} \times S_e\left(f_a\right) \times \text{CF}\left(f_a, f'\right) \times \text{ISF} \times \text{DD}\left(d, f_a, f'\right),$$

  where

  $\dot{D}_{d_m} = 1.00$ cGy/MU is the dose rate in phantom at d_m for SSD = 100 cm and for a 10 × 10 applicator,
  $S_e(f_a)$ is the applicator factor (f_a represents the applicator size),
  CF is the cutout factor for a cutout with an equivalent field size f',
  ISF = 1 if SSD = 100 cm (otherwise see ISF below),
  DD is the depth dose at desired treatment depth.

- **ISF:** For photons, only geometrical divergence (inverse square law) causes beam attenuation in air. In contrast, electrons are easily scattered by matter in between the source and the patient and therefore do not follow an inverse square law in a simple fashion. Electron scattering gives rise to an "apparent" source that is not at location of actual source; distance from apparent source is called *virtual source distance* (VSD). Electrons obey inverse square law (over limited range) when VSD is used instead of actual source distance:

$$\text{ISF} = \frac{\dot{D}_{d_m}\left(100 + d_m + g, f_a\right)}{\dot{D}_{d_m}\left(100 + d_m, f_a\right)} = \left(\frac{\text{VSD} + d_m}{\text{VSD} + d_m + g}\right)^2, \qquad (15.10)$$

  where $g = \text{SSD} - 100$ cm is the air gap. The value of the VSD depends on the energy and the cone size and is generally between 80 and 90 cm.

Problems

1. What is the typical surface dose for electron beams? How does this change as the beam energy increases?

2. a. Examine Figure 15.1. Give the approximate values for R_p and d_{80} for the 6 and 18 MeV beams by reading the graph.
   b. How do the values from a. compare with those expected, based on the rules of thumb given in the chapter?

3. A planning target volume (PTV) extends to a depth of 5.0 cm. At its widest, the tumor is 9 cm in lateral extent. The SSD = 100 cm.

   Skin

   5.0 cm

   9 cm

   a. What energy electron beam should be used to treat this tumor?
   b. What is the smallest applicator size that should be used (assuming no collimator rotation)?
   c. The prescribed dose is 180 cGy to d_m on the central axis. If the SSD = 100 cm, how many MU are required for the Mevalac? Assume the cutout factor is 1.00.

4. A dose of 200 cGy is to be delivered to the 90% isodose depth on the central axis with the 9 MeV beam from the Mevalac. The applicator is 6 × 6 cm^2, the SSD = 100 cm, and the cutout factor is 1.00. Calculate the required number of MU.

5. a. A posterior neck boost is to be given with two lateral 9 MeV electron beams using a 10 × 10 applicator on the Mevalac. The average air gap is 5.0 cm and the cutout factor is 1.00. The prescribed dose is 180 cGy for each beam delivered to d_m. Assume VSD = 86.0 cm. Compute the MU required.
   b. Approximately what dose does the spinal cord receive from this bilateral treatment? Assume the spinal cord is at a depth of 3.5 cm for both beams. A percent depth dose table can be found in appendix C.

6. What thickness of lead is desired to shield the eye from 6 MeV electrons?

7. Describe the dose distribution when a 9 MeV electron field is abutted at the surface with a 6 MV photon field.

Bibliography

AAPM TG-25. (1991). Khan, F. M., K. P. Doppke, K. R. Hogstrom. G. J. Kutcher, R. Nath, S. C. Prasad, J. A. Purdy, M. Rozenfeld, and B. L. Werner. "Clinical electron-beam dosimetry: Report of AAPM Radiation Therapy Committee Task Group No. 25." *Med Phys* 18:73–109. Also available as AAPM Report No. 32.

AAPM TG-51. Almond, P. R., P. J. Biggs, B. M. Coursey, W. F. Hanson, M. Saiful Huq, R. Nath, and D. W. O. Rogers. (1999). "AAPM's TG-51 protocol for clinical reference dosimetry of high-energy photon and electron beams." *Med Phys* 26(9): 1847–1970. Also available as AAPM Report No. 67.

Bentel, G. C. *Radiation Therapy Planning,* Second Edition. New York: McGraw-Hill Professional, 1995.

Jani, S. K. *Handbook of Dosimetry Data for Radiotherapy.* Boca Raton, FL: CRC Press, 1993.

Khan, F. M. *The Physics of Radiation Therapy,* Third Edition. Philadelphia: Lippincott Williams & Wilkins, 2003.

Khan, F. M. *The Physics of Radiation Therapy,* Fourth Edition. Philadelphia: Lippincott Williams & Wilkins, 2009.

Khan, F. M., and R. A. Potish (eds.). *Treatment Planning in Radiation Oncology.* Baltimore, MD: Williams & Wilkins, 1998.

Klevenhagen, S. C. *Physics and Dosimetry of Therapy Electron Beams.* Madison, WI: Medical Physics Publishing, 1993.

Metcalfe, P., T. Kron, and P. Hoban. *The Physics of Radiotherapy X-Rays and Electrons.* Madison, WI: Medical Physics Publishing, 2007.

Meyer, J. A., J. R. Palta, and K. R. Hogstrom. (1984). "Demonstration of relatively new electron dosimetry measurements techniques on the Mevatron 80." *Med Phys* 11: 670–677.

Stanton, R., and D. Stinson. *Applied Physics for Radiation Oncology, Revised Edition.* Madison, WI: Medical Physics Publishing, 2009.

Williams, J. R., and D. I. Thwaites (eds.). *Radiotherapy Physics: In Practice,* Second Edition. New York: Oxford University Press USA, 2000.

16 Brachytherapy

16.1 Introduction

The prefix *brachy* means short. Brachytherapy is a form of short-distance therapy in which radioactive sources are implanted on or inside patients' bodies. This method of radiation therapy allows very high doses to be delivered to the target with rapid falloff in surrounding normal tissue. The dose distributions are not as uniform as they are for external beam therapy; in fact, they are highly non-uniform, with very high doses near sources. Brachytherapy has been used to treat almost every anatomical site. Common sites are cervix and prostate. The subject of brachytherapy is huge. It is a very mature form of treatment, about 100 years old. Consequently, there is a vast literature on this topic and the reader is advised to consult the bibliography at the end of this chapter for more information.

Some brachytherapy implants are permanent, while others are only temporary. Treatment of cervical cancer involves temporary implants. The sources remain in place for a period of time until the desired dose has been delivered and then the radioactive material is removed. Prostate I-125 implants are permanent—the "seeds" remain inside the patient permanently. Prostate implants became quite popular in the late 1990s, especially after a widely influential article by Andy Grove (former CEO of Intel Corporation) was published in *Fortune* magazine describing his search for the best treatment for his prostate cancer.

There are three major types of brachytherapy: intracavitary, interstitial, and intraluminal. In *intracavitary* brachytherapy radioactive sources are placed inside body cavities such as the vagina and cervix. Intracavitary implants are always temporary. The sources stay inside the patient for a period ranging from a few minutes to several days. In *interstitial* brachytherapy the sources are actually embedded in tissue (or placed on the tissue surface for superficial treatments). This can be accomplished with the use of hollow needles. Interstitial implants can be temporary or permanent. Image-guided implants are becoming more common; these include stereotactic brain implants and ultrasound-guided prostate implants. *Intraluminal* brachytherapy involves the placement of sources in a linear array (along a line) inside the pulmonary bronchus, esophagus, etc. The purpose of this is to reduce the size of tumors that are obstructing these structures. Catheters are placed in the lumen by endoscopy and then radioactive sources are placed in the catheter (afterloaded).

Radioactive sources can be placed (loaded) manually or by remote control using a remote afterloader machine. The most common type of remote afterloader is a high dose rate (HDR) remote afterloader.

Radiation from brachytherapy sources can be delivered at low dose rates (LDR) or high dose rates (HDR). Low dose rates range from 40 to 80 cGy/h, whereas high dose rates are defined as dose rates exceeding 20 cGy/min. HDR remote afterloaders deliver dose at a rate on the order of 300 cGy/min, which is approximately the dose rate delivered by linear accelerators for external beam therapy. For pulsed dose rate (PDR) remote afterloaders the instantaneous dose rates are 200 to 1200 cGy/h, but the dose is only delivered for several minutes at a time and then repeated after an hour or some other fixed interval of time.

Isotopes used for brachytherapy (except radium) are classified as "byproduct materials". Use of such materials requires a "medical use license" from the U.S. Nuclear Regulatory Commission (NRC) or an Agreement State. This is discussed in more detail in chapter 17.

16.2   Review of Radioactivity

Here we briefly review some of the material in chapter 3. The rate of decay of a radioactive material is called the *activity*. The SI unit of activity is the becquerel (Bq); 1 Bq = 1 decay/second. An older unit of activity is the curie; 1 Ci = 3.7×10^{10} Bq. A curie is the approximate activity of 1 gram of radium. A curie is a large unit and therefore activity is frequently given in terms of mCi (10^{-3} Ci) and μCi (10^{-6} Ci). Note that 1 mCi is 37 MBq.

The equation for radioactive decay is $A = A_0 e^{-\lambda t} = A_0 (1/2)^n$, where A is the activity at time t, A_0 is the initial activity, λ is the decay constant, and n is the number of half-lives. The half-life $T_{1/2} = (\ln 2)/\lambda \approx 0.693/\lambda$. The mean life $\tau = 1/\lambda \approx 1.44\ T_{1/2}$. The total number of radioactive atoms in a sample is $N_0 = A_0 \tau$. Specific activity is the activity of a radioactive sample divided by the total mass of the element present.

16.3 Radioactive Sources

Radioisotopes used for brachytherapy are x-ray or gamma emitters, except in the case of very localized therapy (Sr-90). Sources used for permanent implants should have a relatively short half-life to minimize the radiation hazard presented by the patient to the public. These isotopes should also have low-energy radiation so that the radiation cannot easily escape the patient's body. Temporary sources utilize longer-lived isotopes so that the sources do not have to be replaced frequently. A shielded room or isolation can be arranged for a temporary "in-patient" implant.

There are two factors to consider when discussing sources: the isotope used and the physical form of the source. The isotope determines the energy of the radiation, the half-life, the HVL, etc. The physical form of the source concerns such attributes as the source encapsulation. If encapsulated, what are the properties of the encapsulation, the dimensions of the source, what activities are available? Most sources used for brachytherapy are sealed sources. One exception to this is I-131, which is used for treatment of thyroid cancer. Sealed sources are doubly encapsulated. Activities for LDR sources range from about 0.1 to 100 mCi. For HDR afterloader units the activity can be as high as 10 Ci.

Radium (Ra-226) is the original radioisotope upon which brachytherapy was developed. Although Ra-226 is no longer used, it is important because it is the foundation upon which modern brachytherapy was developed. Modern techniques of brachytherapy are based on those developed for radium. Ra-226 occurs naturally as part of the decay chain of U-238. U-238 has a half-life of 4.5×10^9 years, and therefore there is still plenty of it around. Radium decays to radon: $^{226}_{88}\text{Ra} \rightarrow {}^{222}_{86}\text{Rn} + {}^{4}_{2}\text{He}$, with a half-life of 1600 years. Rn-222 is a radioactive gas with a half-life of 3.8 days (see chapter 3, section 3.14.1 on secular equilibrium). The emitted alpha particles are absorbed by the encapsulation. The decay of radium is associated with a complex gamma spectrum, which is the therapeutic radiation. The average energy of these gammas is $\bar{E}_\gamma = 0.83$ MeV, but the maximum energy is $(E_\gamma)_{max} = 2.45$ MeV. The high-energy gamma makes it difficult to shield radium sources.

The disadvantages of the use of radium are that it is hard to shield (HVL = 16 mm of lead), that there is the potential for radon gas leakage, and that the helium nuclei emitted can lead to a buildup of helium gas pressure in the sealed radium capsule. This could potentially cause the capsule to burst, although documented cases of this are rare. One gram of radium has an activity of 0.988 Ci and therefore 1 mg of radium has an activity of approximately 1 mCi. The specific activity of radium is therefore approximately 1 Ci/g.

Cesium-137 has replaced radium. It is predominantly used for LDR treatment of cervical cancer, although the use of this isotope is itself now clearly waning. Advantages of Cs-137 over radium are that it requires less shielding and there is no radon hazard. Cs-137 is a byproduct material, which means that it is produced as a byproduct of nuclear fission in a nuclear reactor. It is separated from other isotopes during nuclear fuel reprocessing. It has a half-life of 30 years and emits a single gamma with an energy of 0.662 MeV (see the decay diagram in chapter 3, section 3.13). The HVL in lead for Cs-137 is 5.5 mm.

Cs-137 sources are available in the form of tubes such as the one shown in Figure 16.1. This model is fairly typical. It is 20 mm long and the activity is spread over the central 13.5 mm. The dose distribution

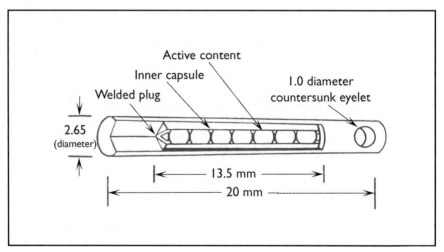

Figure 16.1: A cutaway view of a 20 mm long Cs-137 source tube. The tube is doubly encapsulated stainless steel. Both the inner and outer capsules are welded to prevent leakage of Cs-137. The Cs-137 is incorporated into beads. The "active" length of the radioactive material is 13.5 mm. The entire length of the tube is 20 mm. These sources are used for low dose rate treatment of cervical cancer. This is a CDCS J-type source available in activities ranging from 12.5 mCi to 62.5 mCi. (Adapted with permission from *Brachytherapy Physics*, J. F. Williamson, B. R. Thomadsen, and R. Nath (Eds), Fig. 1b, p. 187. © 1995 American Association of Physicists in Medicine (AAPM).)

around Cs-137 sources (see Figure 16.2) is almost identical to radium within a distance of 10 cm of the source. The reason is that the dose distribution near the source is dominated by inverse square effects, which of course are the same for both isotopes (see Figure 16.11).

Iodine-125 is produced by neutron irradiation of xenon-124 (Xe-124), which is placed in a nuclear reactor. I-125 is used for permanent implants of the brain and prostate and for temporary eye plaques. Its short half-life of 59.5 days along with its small HVL (0.025 mm-lead) make it an ideal isotope for permanent implants. It is both easy to shield and it does not last very long. I-125 decays by electron capture: $^{125}_{53}I + ^{0}_{-1}\beta \rightarrow ^{125}_{52}Te + \nu$, where 93% of the Te-125 decays by internal conversion and 7% by emission of a 35.5 keV gamma ray. Following the electron capture, characteristic x-rays are emitted with energies of 27 and 31 keV. The dose distribution around I-125 seeds is highly anisotropic because of the low energy of the radiation. Seed models

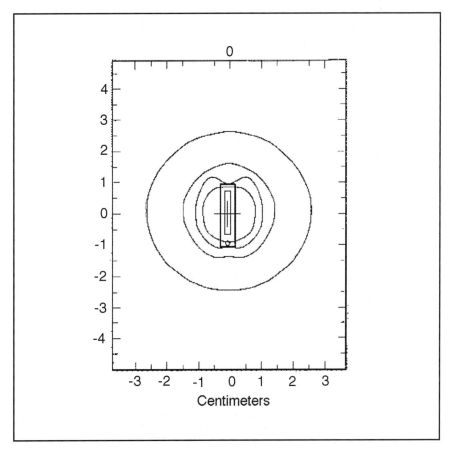

Figure 16.2: Relative dose distribution in water for source shown in Figure 16.1. The isodose lines are 180%, 100%, 60%, and 20%. Note the relatively low dose near the ends of the capsule. This is due to absorption of radiation by the source itself and by the encapsulation. Far from the source the isodose lines are circles concentric with the center of the source.

6702 and 6711 are both constructed with a 0.05 mm thick titanium tube enclosure that is welded at both ends (see Figure 16.3).

Iridium-192 is produced by placing Ir-191 in a nuclear reactor where it is bombarded by neutrons. Iridium-192 is commonly used for HDR afterloaders and for temporary interstitial implants. The half-life of Ir-192 is 73.8 days. When used in an afterloader, the source must be changed about four times per year. Ir-192 undergoes beta decay to various excited states of platinum-192 (Pt-192) and osmium-192 (Os-192), which emit a variety of gamma rays. Ir-192 has a complex gamma spectrum with an average energy of 0.38 MeV. In lead the HVL is 2.5 mm. Ir-192 has a specific activity of approximately 450 Ci/g and a surprisingly high density of 22.4 g/cm^3. This density is higher than almost any other element except platinum and osmium, which both have about the same density as iridium. The combination of high specific activity and high density makes it possible to fabricate physically small, high activity sources. It is possible to make a 10 Ci (Ci, not mCi!) source that is about 5 mm long and 2 mm in diameter. This isotope is well suited for use in HDR units. Ir-192 is also available in the form of "ribbons" (see Figure 16.4). These are seeds that are embedded in a strand of nylon with an outside diameter of 0.8 mm. The seeds are 3 mm long by 0.5 mm in diameter. They are available in source strengths of 0.4 to 1.8 mCi.[1]

Strontium-90 is a pure beta emitter used for eye applicators. It is a long-lived fission fragment with a half-life of 28 years (see chapter 3, section 3.15). Sr-90 emits a low-energy β⁻ decaying to Y-90 (yttrium, see chapter 3, section 3.12.3). In turn, Y-90 undergoes beta decay (maximum energy 2.27 MeV) and it is the beta decay that is the therapeutic radiation (see section 3.12.3).

[1]Meigooni, A. S., and J. F. Williamson. "Single-Source Dosimetry for Interstitial Brachytherapy, pp. 209–233, in 1994 AAPM Summer School Proceedings (*Brachytherapy Physics,* Thomadsen et al. 1994).

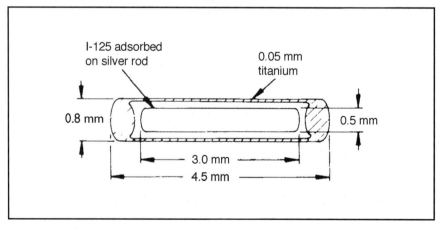

Figure 16.3: Model 6711 I-125 seed. These seeds are supplied with apparent activities from 0.2 to 20 mCi. (Courtesy of GE Healthcare Life Sciences)

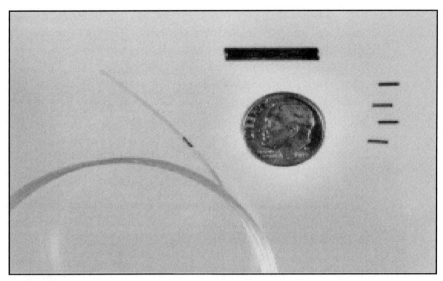

Figure 16.4: Size and appearance of some common sources. Cs-137 tube at the top, I-125 seeds on the right, and an Ir-192 source in a ribbon.

Table 16.1: Brachytherapy Isotopes[a]

Isotope	Half-life	Mean energy (keV)	Maximum energy (keV)	HVL (mm-lead)	Γ[b] (R cm² h⁻¹ mCi⁻¹)	f (cGy/R)
Ra-226	1600 y	830	2450	16	8.25[c] (R cm² h⁻¹ mg⁻¹)	--
Cs-137	30.0 y	662	662	5.5	3.28	0.973
Ir-192	73.8 d	380	1060	2.5	4.69	0.970
I-125	59.5 d	28	35	0.025	1.51	0.910
Pd-103	17.0 d	21	23	0.008	1.48	0.886
Au-198	2.7 d	416	1090 (0.2%)	2.5	2.38	--

y = years; d = days
[a] Some of the values in this table were taken from the AAPM TG-43 report (1995).
[b] Ir-192, I-125, Pd-103, and Au-198 values are for an ideal unfiltered point source.
[c] For 0.5 mm platinum filtration.

Palladium-103 is a reactor-produced isotope with a short half-life of 17 days. It decays by electron capture, which is followed by characteristic x-ray emission in the range 20 to 23 keV. Its low photon energy and short half-life make it ideal for permanent implants.

Table 16.1 lists some key properties of isotopes commonly used in brachytherapy.

16.4 Brachytherapy Applicators

An applicator is a device designed to hold radioactive sources in a specific configuration for treatment of a given anatomical site. There are four major categories of brachytherapy applicators: intraluminal, intra-cavitary, interstitial, and surface mold. They can be as simple as a single, hollow, thin plastic tube (called a *catheter*). A single catheter may be used for intraluminal treatment of the lungs (endobronchial) or esophagus. Catheter diameters are sometimes specified in terms of a peculiar unit called the *French*. A common size is a 6 French catheter, which has a diameter of 2 mm. Intracavitary applicators are used for treatment of the vagina or cervix, such as vaginal cylinders, tandem and ovoids (Fletcher-Suit), Henschke, tandem and ring, etc. For interstitial application, needles or arrays of catheters are used. Sometimes a template is used to guide the insertion of the needles (MUPIT[2], Syed-Neblett device). Older applicators may not be suitable for imaging with CT or MRI because of their metal content. For permanent implants, I-125 seeds are inserted through a needle using a seed "applicator." Common seed applicators are the Mick®, Henschke, and Scott. See Figures 16.5 through 16.8.

---

[2] Martinez Universal Peritoneal Interstitial Template (MUPIT).

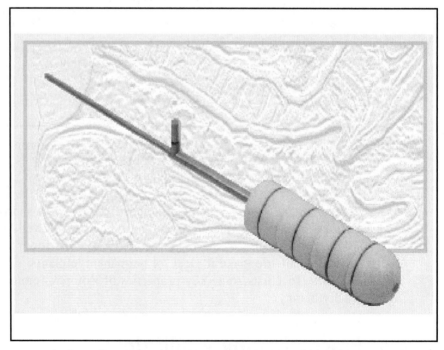

Figure 16.5: A vaginal cylinder for treatment of the vagina, cervix, or endometrium. Cylinders come in a variety of diameters ranging from 20 to 40 mm. The cylinders are put together in sections each 25 mm long. (Courtesy of Nucletron B.V., Veenendaal, The Netherlands)

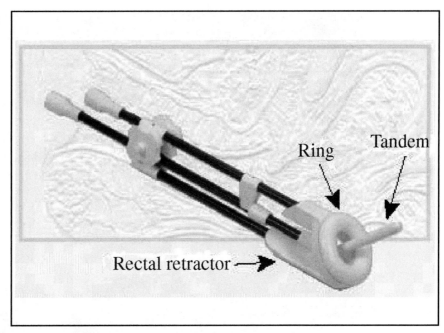

Figure 16.6: A ring and tandem applicator set for the treatment of cervical or endometrial cancer. The tandem extends up into the uterus. This model is designed for imaging with CT or MRI. There is a rectal retractor attached behind the ring. This type of applicator set is available with different size rings, tandem lengths, and tandem angles. (Courtesy of Nucletron B.V., Veenendaal, The Netherlands)

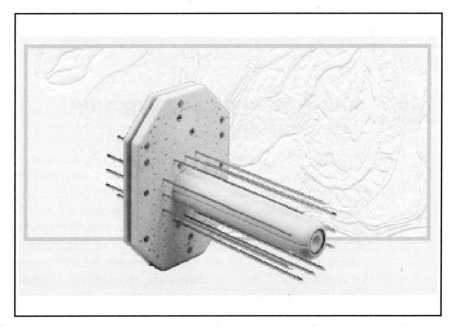

Figure 16.7: The MUPIT perineal interstitial template for the treatment of prostate cancer. (Courtesy of Nucletron B.V., Veenendaal, The Netherlands)

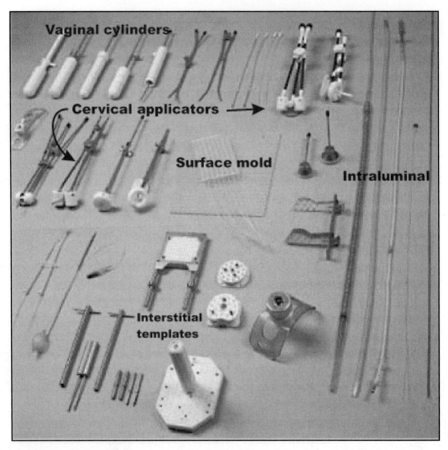

Figure 16.8: A wide array of applicators is available for brachytherapy. (Courtesy of Nucletron B.V., Veenendaal, The Netherlands) See COLOR PLATE 10.

16.5 Source Strength and Exposure Rate Constant

We expect the exposure rate (in air) due to the presence of a radioactive source to be directly proportional to the activity of the source and inversely proportional to the square of the distance from the source (assuming a point source, see chapter 5, section 5.5.1).[3] We will use the symbol $\dot{X}$ to represent the exposure rate, usually expressed in units of R/h or mR/h.[4] We may therefore write the proportionality $\dot{X} \propto A/r^2$ where A is the activity and r is the distance from the source to the point of measurement. We may change the proportional symbol μ to an equal sign by inserting a proportionality constant. This constant is given the

---

[3] Recall that exposure is only defined for photons. This discussion is therefore not relevant for beta emitters such as Sr-90.

[4] A dot over a physical quantity usually represents a rate of change with respect to time.

symbol Γ (upper case gamma) and it is called the *exposure rate constant*. The equation for the exposure rate is therefore:

$$\dot{X} = \Gamma \frac{A}{r^2}. \tag{16.1}$$

As you might expect, the value of Γ depends on the specific radioisotope. In particular, the values depend on the number and energies of gamma rays and x-rays emitted by the source. Perhaps less obvious is that the value of Γ depends on the source encapsulation. Values of Γ can be found in Table 16.1. Typical (non SI) units for gamma are $[\Gamma] = $ R cm^2 h^{-1} mCi^{-1}. Other possibilities are mR cm^2 h^{-1} mCi^{-1} or R m^2 h^{-1} mCi^{-1}. In the case of radium, the units are specified in terms of the number of milligrams present: $[\Gamma_{Ra}] = $ R cm^2 h^{-1} mg^{-1}. The units of Γ are a crazy mixture. When looking up values of Γ, be careful to make sure you know what the units are.

Example 16.1

(a) What is the exposure rate at a distance of 0.5 m from a 50 mCi capsule of Cs-137?

The value of $\Gamma = 3.3$ R cm^2 h^{-1} mCi^{-1} for Cs-137 with standard encapsulation is obtained from Table 16.1:

$$\dot{X} = \Gamma \frac{A}{r^2}$$

$$\dot{X} = 3.3 \text{ R } \cancel{\text{cm}^2} \text{ h}^{-1} \cancel{\text{mCi}^{-1}} \frac{50 \cancel{\text{ mCi}}}{(50)^2 \cancel{\text{ cm}^2}}$$

$$\dot{X} = 0.066 \text{ R h}^{-1} = 66 \text{ mR/h}$$

Slashes have been drawn through units that cancel. It is advisable when solving such problems to write out all of the units to ensure that they combine properly. Note that the distance was converted into centimeters before substituting the value into equation (16.1). This was necessary because the value of Γ is given in terms of cm.

(b) Given that the roentgen-to rad-conversion factor for Cs-137 radiation (for water) is $f_{med} = 0.973$ cGy/R (see Table 16.1), what is the dose rate in free space neglecting attenuation? In chapter 7, section 7.7 we introduced the equation $D_{med} = f_{med} X(R)$ (neglecting attenuation). This equation can be turned into a rate equation by putting dots over the D and X: $\dot{D}_{med} = f_{med} \dot{X}(R)$. The dose rate in free space is therefore $\dot{D}_{water} = 0.973 \times 0.066 = 0.06$ cGy/h.

Equation (16.1) cannot be used to calculate exposure rate near sources such as the ones shown in Figures 16.1 and 16.3. There are two reasons for this: these sources are not point sources and the emission is not isotropic.[5] The dose distribution (which is related to the exposure rate) shown in Figure 16.2 cannot be calculated assuming the source to be a point source because the size of the source is significant in comparison to the distances involved and the source and encapsulation absorb some of the radiation. For the purposes of radiation protection estimates, equation (16.1) may be used to estimate the exposure rate without worrying about these subtleties. This is not the case however for patient dose calculations, which are required to be highly accurate.

The point dose approximation can be reliably used far away from the source (at a distance large compared to the size of the source). The isodose lines for an isotropic point source are circles centered on the source (see Figure 16.2 far from the source). For sources such as those shown in Figures 16.1 and 16.3, radiation is absorbed in the source material itself (self absorption) and in the encapsulation. This can be seen in Figure 16.2. The dose near the end of the tube is relatively low because the radiation has to penetrate the relatively thick end plug. Source and encapsulation absorption is particularly important for low-energy isotopes such as I-125 and Pd-103. The amount of source absorption will depend on the direction of travel of the radiation. A source that does not radiate equally in all directions is said to be anisotropic.

The activity of radioactive sources (particularly Cs-137 and sometimes Ir-192) is sometimes quoted in terms of the equivalent mass of radium, M_{Ra}, often written "mgRaEq." The reasons for this are historical; intracavitary brachytherapy procedures were developed using radium. The equivalent mass of radium for a particular radioisotope is the mass of radium that would lead to the same exposure rate. The equivalent mass of radium for radioisotope x is given by:

$$M_{Ra} = \frac{\Gamma_x}{\Gamma_{Ra}} A_x.$$ (16.2)

This is easily derived as follows:

$$\dot{X}_{Ra} = \dot{X}_x$$

$$\Gamma_{Ra} \frac{M_{Ra}}{r^2} = \Gamma_x \frac{A_x}{r^2}$$

$$\Gamma_{Ra} M_{Ra} = \Gamma_x A_x$$

$$M_{Ra} = \frac{\Gamma_x}{\Gamma_{Ra}} A_x.$$

---

[5] The same in all directions.

Example 16.2

Many years ago a radiation therapy department changed from radium sources to Cs-137 sources for brachytherapy. A 10 mg radium source was replaced by a _____?_____ Cs-137 source.

$$A_x = \frac{\Gamma_{Ra}}{\Gamma_x} M_{Ra} = 10 \; \cancel{mg} \; \frac{8.25 \; \cancel{R} \; \cancel{cm^2} \; \cancel{h^{-1}} \; \cancel{mg^{-1}}}{3.3 \; \cancel{R} \; \cancel{cm^2} \; \cancel{h^{-1}} \; mCi^{-1}}$$

$$= 25 \; mCi$$

This leads to a rule of thumb.

 Rule of thumb: 2.5 mCi of Cs-137 is equivalent to 1 mg of Ra-226 (i.e., 1 mgRaEq).

16.6 Dose Rate Calculations from Exposure Rate

Let us start with the simplest case. We wish to compute the dose rate from a single point source. In the previous section we discussed computation of the exposure rate and in Example 16.1 we computed the dose rate in the absence of any attenuation.

Let us construct a formula in steps for the dose rate in a medium due to a point source at a distance r. This process is illustrated in Figures 16.9 and 16.10. First calculate the exposure rate: $\dot{X}_a = \Gamma A/r^2$ at the observation point in the absence of any nearby scattering medium except air.[6] In step 2: place the source and the observation point in the medium and carve out a small cavity around the observation point. Calculate the exposure rate at the observation point taking into account absorption and scattering. The modification of the exposure rate by absorption and scattering depends on the distance r. We introduce a function $T(r)$ to describe this. The definition is $T(r) = \dot{X}_m/\dot{X}_a$ where $\dot{X}_m$ is the exposure rate at the observation point (surrounded by the air cavity) in the medium.

Functions for $T(r)$ can be found in the literature. As it is a ratio, this quantity has no units. It is somewhat like a TAR. In step 3: convert the exposure rate to the dose rate in the medium by multiplying by f_{med} (see chapter 7, section 7.7). We also introduce a factor to account for anisotropic emission, $\bar{\phi}_{an}$. (the anisotropy factor). This is a correction

---

[6]Recall that exposure is only defined in air.

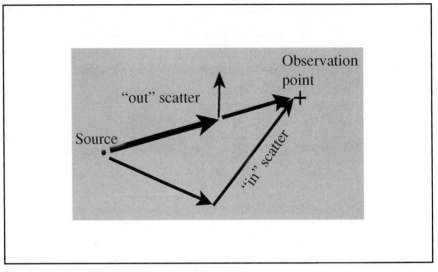

Figure 16.9: The dose rate at an observation point in a medium due to a point source. Some of the radiation traveling toward the observation point is scattered away from the observation point and some of it is absorbed. Some of the remainder will deposit dose at the observation point. The "out" scattered radiation does not reach the observation point (unless it is scattered again). It deposits dose elsewhere. Some of the radiation from the source that is not initially traveling toward the observation point is "in" scattered and deposits dose at the observation point.

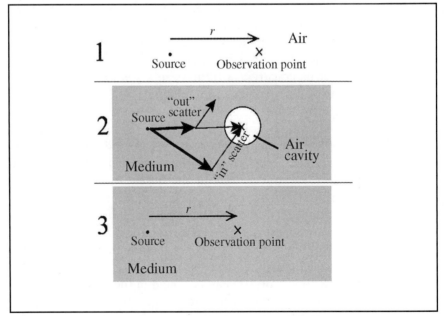

Figure 16.10: Steps in the construction of a formula for the dose at an observation point in a medium from a radioactive source in the medium. In step 1, the exposure is calculated in the absence of any scattering medium other than air. In step 2, the source and observation point are placed in the medium. A small air cavity is carved around the observation point and the exposure is calculated at that point, taking into account scattering and absorption by the medium. In step 3, the dose in the medium is computed by multiplying by f_{med}.

correction averaged over all directions. We may finally put the pieces together to get an expression for the dose rate in the medium:

$$\dot{D} = \Gamma \frac{A}{r^2} f_{med} T(r) \overline{\phi}_{an}. \tag{16.3}$$

For the higher-energy isotopes (Ra-226, Cs-137, Ir-192) at distances less than about 10 cm, absorption and "out" scattering is compensated for by "in" scatter and $T(r) \approx 1$. In this case, the relative dose distribution is dominated by inverse square effects and all point source high-energy isotopes will have approximately the same dose distribution. This is illustrated in Figure 16.11, which shows that Cs-137, Ir-192, and Ra-226 have the same relative dose distribution within a distance of about 10 cm of the sources (assuming a point source). This is *not* true for low-energy isotopes such as I-125. For these low-energy isotopes, absorption and scattering is significant even at short distances.

Now suppose that instead of a single source we have multiple point sources. We can simply compute the dose rate at the point of interest from each one separately and then add the dose rates.

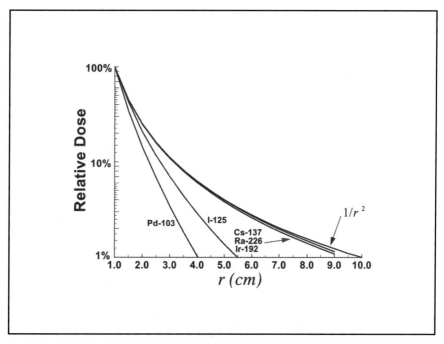

Figure 16.11: The dose distribution in water as a function of distance from a point source for various isotopes. The dose has been normalized to 100% at a distance of 1.0 cm. Note that the vertical scale is a log scale. The higher-energy isotopes (Cs-137, Ra-226, and Ir-192) depart very little from inverse square behavior. The lower-energy isotopes however show significant absorption over a short range.

Example 16.3

Four 3 mCi I-125 seeds are arranged at the corners of a square of side length of 4 cm. Neglecting tissue scattering, absorption, and anisotropic effects, calculate the dose rate at the center of the square using $f_{med} = 0.9$ for I-125 in water.

As all of the sources are equally distant from the center of the square, the contribution to the dose rate at the center of the square from each of them is equal. Therefore we can calculate the dose rate from any one of them and then multiply by 4. The length of the diagonal of the square is given by: $c^2 = a^2 + b^2 = 4^2 + 4^2 = 32$ and therefore $c = \sqrt{32}$ cm. The distance of each source from the center is

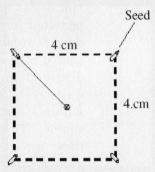

$r = \sqrt{32}\,/2 \approx 2.8$ cm. If we assume that the active length of the seeds is 3 mm (see Figure 16.3), then the distance $r = 28$ mm is roughly 10 times the size of a seed. In this case, the seeds can be treated as point sources.

The dose rate at the center from a single seed is:

$$\dot{D} = \Gamma \frac{A}{r^2} f_{med} T(r)$$

$$= 1.51\ \text{R cm}^2\ \text{h}^{-1}\ \text{mCi}^{-1}\ \frac{3\ \text{mCi}}{(2.8)^2 \text{cm}^2}\ 0.9 \frac{\text{cGy}}{\text{R}}$$

$$= 0.52\ \text{cGy h}^{-1}$$

For all four seeds, the total is $\dot{D} = 4 \times 0.52 = 2.1\,\text{cGy h}^{-1}$.

We have seen how to handle the situation in which we have multiple point sources and we wish to compute the dose at some point in tissue due to these point sources. Now suppose we have a distributed source such as shown in Figure 16.2. Far away from this source we can treat it like a point source; but if we wish to compute the dose distribution nearby (as shown in the figure), we cannot treat the source as a point.

Physicists and mathematicians often approach new problems by attempting to turn them into old problems that they already know how to solve. If we have a distributed source, let us imagine that we build that source from a large number of very small (point) sources. At any location in the medium we can then calculate the dose from each one of the point sources and add all of the contributions to get the total dose due to the distributed source at that point. If you have studied calculus (ugh!), you may recognize this as the process of integration—the dose is given by an integral. For a distributed source like a line (a tube or seed) this integral is called the *Sievert integral*.

16.7 Specification of Source Strength

Due to the problem of self-absorption, the real absolute activity of a source may be difficult to ascertain. Therefore, absolute activity is of limited use in brachytherapy dosimetry. Instead, the activity values that are actually quoted are "apparent" activities. The apparent activity is always less than the actual activity of the encapsulated source. The quantity that is really measured is the *exposure rate*. This is then converted to apparent activity by using equation (16.1). The user must then multiply the quoted activity by a value of Γ to calculate the exposure. Note that the manufacturer divides out the value of Γ to get the apparent activity and the user then multiplies the apparent activity by a value of Γ to calculate the exposure. We see that Γ is therefore a "dummy" variable. Furthermore, it is a dangerous dummy variable, because if the user does not use the same value as the manufacturer, the user will calculate an incorrect value of the exposure. Different references may quote different values of Γ. As an example, prior to 1978, values of Γ for Ir-192 ranged from 3.9 to 5.0 R cm^2 h^{-1} mCi^{-1}.[7] This causes confusion and can be a real headache to users (not to speak of textbook authors). If you are using the manufacturer's apparent activity values to calculate dose, *you must use the same value of Γ that they use.*

It is now recommended that the quantity air kerma strength (S_k) be used to specify the strength of brachytherapy sources. This quantity is directly related to the exposure rate. The procedure for measurement is illustrated in Figure 16.12. This is measured by a calibration lab, not the

---

[7] AAPM TG-43. "Dosimetry of interstitial brachytherapy sources: Report of the AAPM Radiation Therapy Committee Task Group #43" (1995).

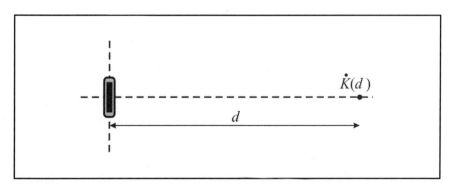

Figure 16.12: Illustration of the definition of air kerma strength. The air kerma rate is measured on the perpendicular bisector at d = 1 m from the source.

user. The air kerma strength is the kerma rate (kerma per unit time, see chapter 7, sections 7.4 and 7.6) measured along the transverse bisector of the source in free space (air, with no scattering medium nearby) at a distance of 1.0 meter. The air kerma rate is then multiplied by the square of the distance, thus the definition of air kerma strength is:

$$S_k = \dot{K}(d) \times d^2. \tag{16.4}$$

The units of S_k are the units of kerma multiplied by distance squared and divided by time. Commonly used units are [S_k] = cGy h^{-1} cm^2. This combination of units gets the special designation "U"; that is, 1 U = 1 cGy h^{-1} cm^2.

16.8 Task Group 43 Dosimetry

The AAPM Task Group 43 (TG-43) formalism is now recommended for interstitial brachytherapy. This is a newer formalism for computing dose based on air kerma strength. The coordinate system used is shown in Figure 16.13. The distance from the center of the source to the point of dose calculation (P in the diagram) is r, the angle θ is as shown in the diagram. In this formalism, air kerma strength replaces apparent activity. The exposure rate constant is replaced by Λ, the dose rate constant. The dose rate constant converts air kerma strength to dose rate. The definition of the dose rate constant is: the dose rate to water at 1 cm on the transverse axis of a unit source (1 U) in a water phantom. The units are: [Λ] = cGy/h/U. It is important to understand that Λ depends on the particular seed model because it includes the effects of source geometry, self-absorption, encapsulation, etc. Values for some common sources are listed in Table 16.2.

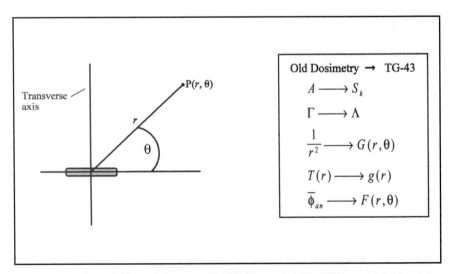

Figure 16.13: Illustration of the geometry for the TG-43 dose calculation formalism.

Table 16.2: Values of Λ*

Seed (model)	cGy h^{-1} U^{-1}
Ir-192 (Fe clad)	1.12
I-125 (6702)	0.93
I-125 (6711)	0.88
Pd-103 (200)	0.74

*Values from AAPM TG-43 report.

$G(r,\theta)$ is the called the *geometry factor*. It describes the relative dose distribution due only to the spatial distribution of radioactivity. It does not account for absorption or scattering in the medium or the source. It describes the dose dependence in free space. For a point source, $G(r,\theta) = 1/r^2$. For a line source, $G(r,\theta)$ can be derived from the Sievert integral.

The anisotropy function $F(r,\theta)$ describes the anisotropy around the source due to the effects of absorption and scattering in the source. This quantity has no units.

The radial dose function $g(r)$ describes absorption and scattering in the medium along the transverse axis. It includes the effects of filtration on the energy spectrum due to the encapsulation and the source itself. This quantity has no units.

Putting all these terms together, we write the TG-43 expression for the total dose rate at a point:

$$\dot{D}(r,\theta) = S_k \Lambda \left[\frac{G(r,\theta)}{G(1\,\text{cm}, 90°)} \right] g(r) F(r,\theta). \qquad (16.5)$$

Example 16.4

Calculate the dose for one of the I-125 seeds in Example 16.3 at the point $r = 2.8$ cm and $\theta = 0$. Assume that the seed is a model 6711 (see Table 16.2) and that the 3 mCi apparent activity corresponds to an air kerma strength of 3.81 U. The distance is large compared to the size of the seed (approximately 3 mm) and therefore $G(r,\theta) \approx 1/r^2$. For this seed model $g(2.8) = 0.672$ and $F(2.8, 0°) = 0.449$.

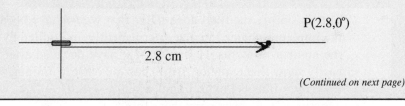

2.8 cm

P(2.8,0°)

(Continued on next page)

Example 16.4 (continued)

The geometry factor is: $\dfrac{G(r,\theta)}{G(1\,\text{cm},90°)} = \left(\dfrac{1.0}{2.8}\right)^2 = 0.128.$

The dose rate is given by:

$$\dot{D}(r,\theta) = S_k \qquad \Lambda \qquad \left[\dfrac{G(r,\theta)}{G(1\,\text{cm},90°)}\right] g(r) F(r,\theta)$$

$$= 3.81\,\text{U} \times 0.88\,\text{cGy}\,\text{h}^{-1}\text{U}^{-1} \times \quad 0.128 \quad \times \quad 0.672 \times 0.449$$

$$= 0.129\,\text{cGy}\,\text{h}^{-1}.$$

This is considerably less than the dose rate computed in Example 16.3 (0.52 cGy h^{-1}). That example did not take account of absorption and scattering or the anisotropy of the source. Absorption and scattering are very significant effects at a distance of 3.0 cm as shown in Figure 16.11. In addition, the calculation point is at a position where the anisotropy is expected to have its maximum effect.

16.9 Accumulated Dose from Temporary and Permanent Implants

We need to be able to calculate the total cumulative dose received at a particular point in a patient from a permanent implant, given the initial dose rate $\dot{D}_0$. The total dose is proportional to the total number of atoms undergoing radioactive decay: $D \propto N_0 = A_0\tau$, where A_0 is the initial activity. We can turn this into an equality by inserting a constant of proportionality k: $D = k A_0\tau$. The initial dose rate is proportional to the initial activity: $\dot{D}_0 = k A_0$ (we have assumed that the constant of proportionality is the same—this may not be obvious) and therefore:

$$D = \dot{D}_0\tau. \tag{16.6}$$

For a temporary implant the total accumulated dose after a time t is:

$$D = \dot{D}_0\tau\left(1 - e^{-t/\tau}\right). \tag{16.7}$$

This is simply the total dose, $\dot{D}_0\tau$, that would have been delivered had the implant remained in place permanently, multiplied by the fraction of the number of atoms, $(1 - e^{-t/\tau})$, that have decayed after time t. We can easily show that equation (16.7) has the correct limiting behavior. When $t = 0$, $D = 0$ as we expect, and when $t \to \infty$, $D \to \dot{D}_0\tau$, which is simply equation (16.6) for a permanent implant.

Example 16.5

The initial dose rate from an I-125 prostate implant is 5.0 cGy/h at a specified location. What total dose will that location receive?

$$\tau = 1.44\,(59.5\,\text{d}) = 2056\,\text{h}, \quad D = \dot{D}_0\tau = 5.0\,\text{cGy/h} \times 2056\,\text{h} = 10{,}300\,\text{cGy}$$

16.10 Systems of Implant Dosimetry

The required distribution and strength of sources necessary to accomplish a clinical goal clearly depends on the anatomical site that is to be treated. Rather than consider each site separately, it makes sense to consider various categories of source distribution and then to discuss those sites that are treated using such distributions.

Detailed calculations of the location of sources, their strength and the necessary treatment time are now carried out by digital computers. The simplest source distribution is a single point source. The next most complicated distribution is a linear array of sources. After this comes sources distributed on a plane surface. Finally, we could have sources distributed throughout a three-dimensional volume.

16.10.1 A Point Source

We can imagine a variety of increasingly complex source arrangements. The most elementary arrangement is a simple point source. A point source is of course an idealization. Any real source has a non-zero size. If however the distance from the source is large compared to the size of the source, then the source will effectively be a point source. In such a case, the dose on the surface of any sphere with the source at the center will be a constant (assuming no anisotropy) because every point on the surface of the sphere is an equal distance from the source. Therefore, surfaces of constant dose (isodose surfaces) are spheres centered on the source. The dose will decrease with distance according to the inverse square law [neglecting absorption, see equation (16.3) for a point source). Note that an inverse square decline with distance is *only* valid for a point source. At a sufficient distance from an implant of any shape, the isodose surfaces are spherical. This can be seen in a single plane for the source displayed in Figure 16.2.

It might be surprising to learn that a point source does have application in radiation therapy. A single source is sometimes used to treat the lumpectomy cavity for breast cancer patients. The surgeon places an inflatable balloon in the lumpectomy cavity. A catheter runs along a principal diameter of the balloon and out through the skin surface. This catheter allows an HDR source to be fed into the balloon, where it dwells in the center. After surgery the balloon is inflated with saline until it completely fills the cavity and the surrounding tissue conforms to the surface of the balloon. The balloon is spherical in shape. In this case, the isodose surfaces are spheres concentric with the balloon (neglecting anisotrophy). Typical diameters are 4 to 5 cm and the prescription point is 1.0 cm from the surface of the balloon. The HDR source size is roughly 0.5 cm, and therefore the prescription point is at a distance that is moderately large compared to the size of the source.

16.10.2   A Linear Array

The next most complex form of source arrangement is a linear array. This may be a single physical source or a series of sources arrayed along a straight line. It is possible that there may be spaces between the sources. A linear array can be characterized by the length and distribution of activity. The distance over which activity is distributed is called the active length.

A single linear array of sources is often encountered in endobronchial treatment and in treatment using a vaginal cylinder. The dose is prescribed at a certain distance from the linear array of sources, usually 1.0 cm for endobronchial treatment and 0.5 cm from the surface of a vaginal cylinder (in which the sources are arrayed along the central axis of the cylinder).

As an illustration, let us consider the case of an endobronchial treatment in which the desired treatment length is 10 cm. Activity is to be distributed over the length to be treated. We desire a uniform dose on the surface of an imaginary cylinder with a radius of 1 cm and a length of 10 cm. We will normalize the dose to 100% at a point 1 cm away from the linear array of sources and halfway between the endpoints. Let us suppose that we use 21 sources spaced 0.5 cm apart. If the activity of all of the sources is the same, then the dose distribution will be as shown on the left hand side of Figure 16.14. Note that the 100% isodose line is "pinched" in at the ends and therefore the ends are underdosed. The active length could be extended to provide better dose coverage, but the consequence of this would be to deliver more dose to healthy tissue. We can improve the dose distribution without extending the active length by using higher activity sources at the ends. The right hand side of Figure 16.14 shows the dose distribution from a non-uniform activity array. The activities have been chosen by treatment planning software to provide an optimum dose distribution. The relative activity of the sources at the center is given a weight of 1.00 and the activity of the sources near the ends is more heavily weighted. Figure 16.15 shows a graph of the weights as a function of position.

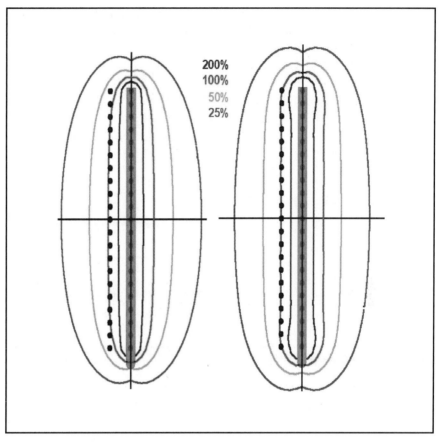

Figure 16.14: The dose distribution around a linear array of sources. The vertical shaded tube is a catheter containing the sources. There are 21 sources in each catheter, spaced 0.5 cm apart. The total active source length is therefore 10 cm. Next to each catheter is a series of dots arranged vertically. The dots are at a distance of 1.0 cm from the catheters and serve as reference markers. The dose has been normalized to 100% at a distance of 1.0 cm from the center of the active length of the catheters. The goal is to treat to 100% at all of the marker points. The sources in the catheter on the left all have equal activity. The sources in the catheter on the right do not have equal activity; the activity is higher at the ends than in the middle. Note that the 100% line on the left is "pinched" in near the ends of the catheter, whereas the 100% line on the right uniformly covers the desired treatment length. See COLOR PLATE 11.

It is not feasible to obtain a set of seeds with just the activity distribution shown in Figure 16.15. With an HDR afterloader, however, it is easy to deliver this treatment. The afterloader is programmed so that the source dwells at each of the 21 source positions for an amount of time that is proportional to the weightings shown in Figure 16.15. As a specific example, suppose that we wish to deliver 500 cGy, with a 10 Ci HDR source. The source will need to dwell for 10.8 seconds at the center (weight = 1.00) and 24.9 seconds at the ends (weight 2.3) The total treatment time is the sum of all the dwell times and, in this case, it is 266 seconds.

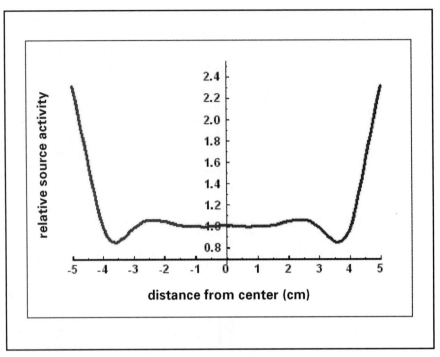

Figure 16.15: The relative weight of the sources used in the linear array shown on the right-hand side in Figure 16.14. The source weight at the center (distance = 0 cm) has been set to 1.00. The sources at the ends have a relative weight of 2.3. The optimized weights displayed here have been calculated using brachytherapy treatment planning software.

Dose distributions from brachytherapy implants are now calculated by computerized treatment planning systems. It is still useful, however, to know how to make manual calculations. Manual calculations can be used to interpret, understand, and check computer output. Rules for placement of sources remain valid. Geometry dominates implants because the inverse square effect is the predominant determinant of dose distribution. This implies that placement of sources is crucial. Poor source placement will lead to a poor dose distribution. Manual systems provide rules for how the sources should be distributed, what activity should be chosen, and how the dose is specified. Tables are used which specify the required amount of radium multiplied by the time (in mg h) for delivery of 1000 cGy.

16.10.3 Planar and Volume Implants

Over the years a large variety of systems have been introduced to deal with planar and volume implants. There are three major systems for planar and volume implants: Paterson-Parker (also known as Manchester), Quimby, and Paris. There are other systems that will not be discussed here, such as the Memorial system, etc. In the Paterson-Parker system, a non-uniform source distribution is used to obtain a uniform dose distribution. In the Quimby system, the source distribution is uniform, but this leads to a non-uniform dose distribution. Neither of these systems accounts for oblique filtration in the dose distribution nor do they account for photon attenuation and scattering (effectively $T(r) = 1$). These implant systems should therefore not be used for low-energy sources (<200 keV) such as I-125 or Pd-103.

Implant systems provide rules for the distribution of sources to treat a volume of tissue. Along with these rules are tables, graphs, nomograms, etc., which are used to determine the amount of activity necessary to deliver a desired dose. As we have already mentioned, such systems are no longer used to plan brachytherapy implants—digital computers generally do a more accurate and effective job of this. This is augmented with modern imaging modalities such as CT, ultrasound, and MRI. Nevertheless, it is still useful to study these old systems of implant dosimetry to understand how the sources should be distributed.

Quimby System

In 1932 Edith Quimby published the first paper on the system that became known as the Quimby system. This was followed in 1934 by the first paper describing the Manchester (Paterson-Parker) system. In the 1930s the isotope used for brachytherapy was Ra-226. The first article on the Paris system was published by Pierquin in 1960. This system was developed for the use of Ir-192.

In the Quimby system, source activity is distributed uniformly over the implant and the resulting dose distribution is non-uniform. The procedure for planning an implant involves determination of the area or volume to be treated. One then consults a table of the cumulated source strength in units of milligram hours (mg h) to deliver a specified dose of 1000 cGy. A multiplier is then used to determine the cumulated activity for the prescribed dose.

Paterson-Parker System

The Paterson-Parker system was designed to deliver a dose that is uniform to within ±10% to a plane or a volume. Planar implants are designed so that the dose is uniform to within ±10% over a plane within ±0.5 cm of the plane of the implant. The treated volume is therefore a slab of tissue 1.0 cm thick for a planar implant. A fraction of the radium is arranged around the periphery and the remainder is spread as evenly as possible over the interior. The rules for these implants were developed for radium needles. Even though radium needles are no longer used, these rules are still useful to know because they provide guidance on the placement and source strength for interstitial implants. The rules for these implants are described in terms of radium in the form of needles, ribbons, or catheters.

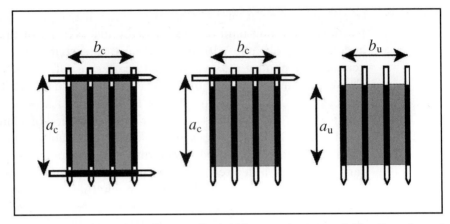

Figure 16.16: Various arrangements for radium needles (which are no longer used). The dimensions of the treated area are shaded. The dimensions are determined by the boundaries of the activity. The diagram on the left shows two crossed ends ("c" and "u" subscripts are for "crossed" and "uncrossed" dimensions, respectively). The active region of the crossing needles should overlap the active region of the interior needles if possible. This is not shown for clarity. (Adapted from Figure 15.11, p. 549 in Bentel, G. C. *Radiation Therapy Planning*, Second Edition. New York: © 1995 McGraw-Hill Professional.)

The source needles should be placed 1 cm apart. The dimensions of the implant are determined by where the activity is. See Figure 16.16.

Rules to follow:

I.   The ratio of activity on the periphery to the amount over the interior area depends on the area of the implant and should follow Table 16.3.

II. The spacing of the source needles or ribbons in the plane should not be more than 1 cm from one another.

III. If the ends of the implant are uncrossed, the effective area of dose uniformity must be reduced by 10% for each uncrossed end.

Crossing needles should cross the active ends. Tables are usually given in terms of the number of mg h/1000 cGy for radium with 0.5 mm platinum filtration (see Table 16.4). These tables can be used for other sources (e.g., Cs-137, Ir-192) provided the source strength is given in radium equivalents.

Table 16.3: Paterson-Parker Source Distribution for Planar Implants

Area (cm²)	Periphery fraction	Area fraction
<25	2/3	1/3
25–100	1/2	1/2
>100	1/3	2/3

Table 16.4: Paterson-Parker Planar Implant Tables
Cumulated Source Strength for 1000 cGy in Water @ 0.5 cm from Plane

Area (cm²)	Milligram hours (mg h)	Area (cm²)	Milligram hours (mg h)
0	31	52	757
2	101	54	777
4	147	56	796
6	185	60	835
8	215	64	874
10	245	68	911
12	272	72	948
14	301	76	987
16	329	80	1024
18	357	84	1061
20	384	88	1098
22	410	92	1135
24	435	96	1171
26	461	100	1206
28	487	120	1365
30	512	140	1527
32	536	160	1679
34	561	180	1823
36	583	200	1963
38	607	220	2096
40	630	240	2226
42	651	260	2355
44	672	280	2476
46	694	300	2605
48	715	320	2737
50	736	340	2858

(Adapted from Table 2, p. 305 in Anderson, L. L., and J. L. Presser, "Classical Systems I for Temporary Interstitial Implants: Manchester and Quimby Systems" in *Brachytherapy Physics,* J. F. Williamson, B. R. Thomadsen, and R. Nath (eds.), © 1995 American Association of Physicists in Medicine (AAPM), with permission from Medical Physics Publishing.)

Figure 16.17 shows the dose distribution for a source distribution like that of Example 16.6.

Example 16.6

A single plane interstitial implant is to be designed to deliver a dose of 6000 cGy to an area of 3 cm × 5 cm at a distance from the implant plane of 0.5 cm. The crossing needles cross the active ends of the other needles. The implant is shown in the diagram below.

a.   Are the Paterson-Parker distribution rules obeyed?

The total peripheral activity is 2.6 × 2 + 2.0 × 2 = 9.2 mg. The total activity is 9.2 + 4.6 = 13.8 mg. The peripheral fraction is therefore 9.2/13.8 = 0.67. This meets the distribution requirements outlined in Table 16.3. For implants with area less than 25 cm^2, the Paterson Parker rules require two-thirds of the activity on the periphery.

b.   What is the dose rate at 0.5 cm from the plane of the implant?

Interpolation in Table 16.4 shows that a 15 cm^2 implant with 315 mg h delivers 1000 cGy. Another way to state this is to say that 315 mgRaEq delivers a dose rate of 1000 cGy/h. The total activity of this implant is 13.8 mgRaEq; therefore the dose rate at 0.5 cm from the plane is (13.8/315) × 1000 cGy/h = 43.8 cGy/h.

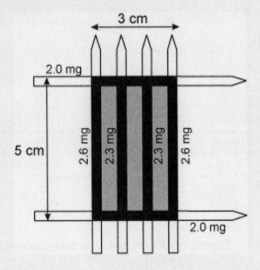

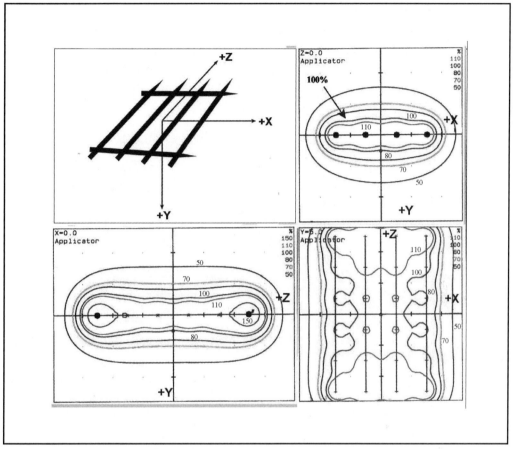

Figure 16.17: The interstitial 3 × 5 cm² planar implant discussed in Example 16.6. The interior needles are parallel to the Z axis and the crossing needles are parallel to the X axis. The activity is distributed according to Paterson-Parker rules. The dose distribution is shown in three planes. The distance between tick marks is 1.0 cm. In the $Z = 0$ plane, the 100% isodose line can be seen to be about 1 cm thick in the Y direction and to extend about 0.5 cm beyond the peripheral needles for a total width of about 4 cm. In the $X = 0$ plane, the 100% line is seen to bulge where the crossing needles intersect this plane. The $Y = 5$ plane shows the dose distribution in a plane 5 mm above the plane of the needles. It seems plausible that the dose in this plane is constant over the 3 × 5 cm² area to within ±10%. See COLOR PLATE 12.

16.11 Intracavitary Treatment of Cervical Cancer

Cervical cancer is routinely and successfully treated with brachytherapy. These treatments can be done at low dose rate (LDR) with Cs-137 or with an HDR afterloader. For LDR the patients are kept in the hospital. HDR treatments are given on an outpatient basis. HDR treatment for cervical cancer has now almost completely replaced LDR treatment.

The sources are placed into an applicator, which is inserted into the vagina and uterus. One of the most common types of applicators is the Fletcher-Suit applicator. This applicator consists of two parts: the tandem and the ovoids. The tandem is a 12 in. long stainless steel tube with

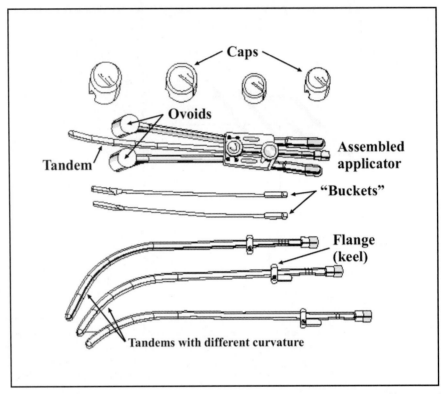

Figure 16.18: A Fletcher-Suit applicator set. Tandems come with different curvatures. The flange (keel) is normally closer to the tip of the tandem. The flange is positioned at the cervical os. The tandem extends up into the uterus and usually holds three sources. The "Buckets" are loaded with one source each. These are inserted into the ovoids and hold the source in position in the ovoids. The caps reduce the dose to the vaginal mucosa. (Courtesy of Best Medical, Springfield, VA, www.TeamBest.com)

outer diameter of ¼ in. The tube has a bend in it near the tip. Most patients have a uterus that is tipped toward the anterior. See Figure 16.18.

Different curvatures for the tandem are available (15°, 30°, and 45°). The tandems are loaded with sources such as those shown in Figures 16.1 and 16.4.

The ovoids or colpostats are cylinders about 3 cm long and 2 cm in diameter. They are each loaded with a single source, and have tungsten shielding built into the medial aspects at the ends of the ovoids to reduce the dose to the rectum and bladder by 10% to 20%.[8] Plastic caps are available which can be placed on the ovoids to increase the distance from the source to the vaginal mucosa. The caps are 2.5 to 3.0 cm in diameter. The caps reduce the dose to the mucosa and improve the dose distribution. The dose distribution is dominated by inverse square—move further away and the variation in dose becomes smaller, just like for percent

---

[8] Meli, J.A. "Dosimetry of Some Interstitial and Intracavitary Sources and their Applicators" in *Brachytherapy Physics,* J.F. Williamson, B.R. Thomadsen, R. Nath (editors), AAPM 1994 Summer School Proceedings, Madison, WI: Medical Physics Publishing, pp. 185–207, 1994.

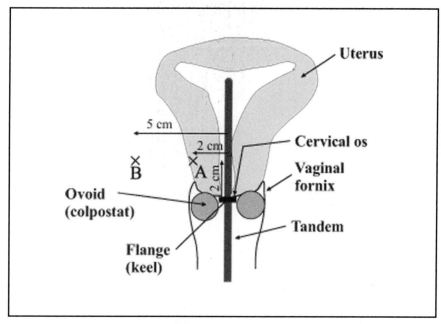

Figure 16.19: The position of the tandem and ovoids after insertion. The tandem extends up into the uterus. The ovoids are positioned at the vaginal fornix. The flange is at the position of the cervical os. Point **A** of the Manchester system is 2 cm superior to the cervical os (along the tandem) and 2 cm lateral. Point **B** is 2 cm superior to the cervical os and 5 cm lateral to the tandem.

depth dose. Before inserting the tandem into the uterus, the uterus is "sounded." The purpose of this is to determine the length of the uterus (usually 6 to 7 cm). The tandem has a "keel" or flange that is placed on it at a distance from the tip equal to the sounded depth of the uterus. This prevents the tandem from being pushed in too far and perforating the uterus. It is necessary to dilate the cervical os to allow passage of the tandem into the uterus. After insertion of the tandem and ovoids, the vagina is packed with sterile gauze to prevent shifting of the applicator. This also reduces the dose to surrounding sensitive structures.

The classical system of dosimetry for intracavitary cervix treatment is the Manchester system (Paterson-Parker). In this system the dose is prescribed to a point that is 2 cm superior to the top of the flange (at the cervical os) along the tandem and 2 cm lateral to the tandem. This point is called point **A**. Point **B** is 2 cm superior to the flange along the axis of the patient (or in some definitions of point **B**, along the tandem) and 5 cm lateral to the axis (see Figure 16.19). The dose is prescribed to point **A**. The dose at point **B** should be calculated and charted. Point **B** is at the approximate position of the obturator lymph nodes. Note that there are actually two point **A** locations, one to the left of the tandem and one to the right (see Figure 16.19). These are often designated A_L (left) and A_R (right). Likewise for point **B**. Only for an ideal implant will the dose be the same at A_L and A_R. It is customary to average the dose at these points, that is: dose at point **A** = (dose at A_L + dose at A_R)/2.

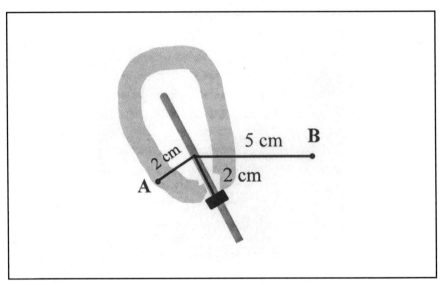

Figure 16.20: An anterior view. If the uterus is tipped, then point **A** tips with the uterus but not point **B**.

If the patient's uterus is tipped, then point **A** tips with the uterus but not point **B** (see Figure 16.20). The logic is that point **A** is supposed to represent a point in the uterine wall, whereas point **B** corresponds to lymph nodes. The location of the reference points **A** and **B** is usually determined from a set of isocentric orthogonal films of the patient that are taken on a simulator with the Fletcher-Suit applicator in place. These films are usually AP and lateral (see Figure 16.21). Orthogonal films allow anatomical points of interest to be uniquely located in three-dimensional space.

Critical normal structures are the vagina, bladder, and rectum. The maximum dose to the bladder and rectum should be approximately 80% or less than the dose to point **A**. The bladder point is determined as follows: a Foley catheter is inserted into the bladder and filled with 7 cc of contrast medium. The Foley is pulled down snug against the urethra. The bladder point is located by marking the center point of the filled Foley on the AP film and the most posterior point on the lateral film. The rectal point is located first on the lateral film at 0.5 cm from the most posterior face of the ovoid. On the AP film the rectal point is at the midpoint between the ovoids along the tandem.

The usual prescribed dose for LDR is 7500 cGy to point **A**.[9] This is delivered in two fractions of about 3 days each, with a week between fractions. The standard dose rate at point **A** is about 55 cGy/hr. The dose delivered to point **B** is usually about one-third the dose to point **A**.

The length of the uterine canal is usually 6 to 7 cm long. Cs-137 sources are 2 cm long (see Figure 16.1) and therefore there are usually

---

[9] This is only for very early stage disease when the entire treatment is brachytherapy.

three sources in the tandem. Only the part of the tandem inside the uterus should be loaded. A typical loading pattern in units of mgRaEq is shown in Figure 16.22. Each patient receives a custom plan. As a result, the loading for a particular patient may be different from that shown in Figure 16.22.

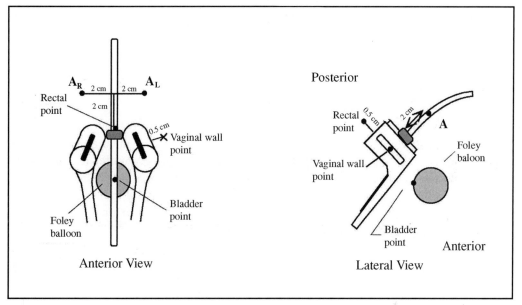

Figure 16.21: An anterior and a lateral view of a tandem and ovoid implant, showing the location of important reference points.

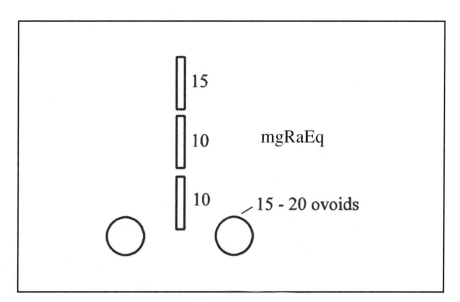

Figure 16.22: A typical loading pattern for tandem and ovoids.

Criticisms of the Manchester System

1. Point **A** relates to the position of the sources and not to a specific anatomic structure.
2. The dose to point **A** is very sensitive to the position of the ovoid sources relative to the tandem sources and this should not be a determining factor in implant duration.
3. Point **A** may lie inside or outside the uterus, depending on the size of the uterus. The dose distribution is pear shaped in the coronal plane (projected AP).

16.12 Along and Away Tables

Dose distributions are calculated by computerized treatment planning systems. It is useful however to be able to make manual calculations for a few points. This is valuable for checking computer output. Manual calculations also serve a pedagogical purpose. Tables are available (see Table 16.5) which allow the user to manually calculate the dose rate in cGy/h per mgRaEq for tubular sources of various designs (e.g., see Figure 16.1, principally Cs-137 sources).

The calculation point is located by specifying the distance from the center of the tube along the length of the tube and the distance away from the tube in a direction perpendicular to the long axis of the tube. This is illustrated in Figure 16.23. See Example 16.7.

Table 16.5: Dose Rates (cGy/h) per mgRaEq for Cs-137 Source*
(Active length 1.4 cm; wall thickness 1.0 mm stainless steel)

Distance from center along length of source (cm) ↓	Tranverse distance (away) from center of the source (cm)									
	0.5	1.0	1.5	2.0	2.5	3.0	3.5	4.0	4.5	5.0
0.0	21.052	6.808	3.241	1.866	1.204	0.837	0.614	0.468	0.368	0.295
0.5	17.445	5.997	2.996	1.773	1.162	0.816	0.602	0.461	0.364	0.293
1.0	8.404	4.177	2.409	1.536	1.051	0.758	0.569	0.441	0.351	0.285
1.5	3.663	2.597	1.777	1.245	0.902	0.676	0.521	0.411	0.331	0.271
2.0	1.943	1.639	1.275	0.975	0.750	0.585	0.464	0.375	0.307	0.255
2.5	1.187	1.093	0.925	0.757	0.613	0.498	0.407	0.336	0.280	0.236
3.0	0.794	0.768	0.686	0.591	0.500	0.420	0.353	0.298	0.259	0.216
3.5	0.566	0.564	0.522	0.466	0.408	0.353	0.304	0.262	0.226	0.196
4.0	0.422	0.429	0.407	0.374	0.336	0.298	0.262	0.230	0.202	0.177
4.5	0.326	0.335	0.325	0.304	0.279	0.252	0.226	0.201	0.179	0.159
5.0	0.258	0.268	0.263	0.250	0.233	0.214	0.195	0.177	0.159	0.143

*Data from Krishnaswamy, V. (1972). "Dose distributions about Cs-137 sources in tissue." *Radiology* 105:181–184.

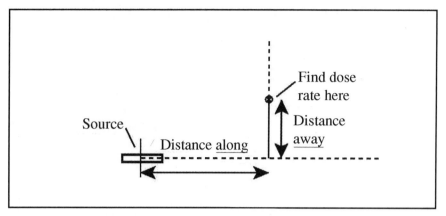

Figure 16.23: Geometry for "along and away" calculations.

Example 16.7

Two views are shown of the geometry and loading for a tandem and ovoid using 2.0 cm long Cs-137 tubes which have an active length of 1.4 cm and a wall thickness of 1.0 mm of stainless steel. The sources are numbered in the diagram. Use the along and away tables for this source design to compute the dose rate at point A_L.

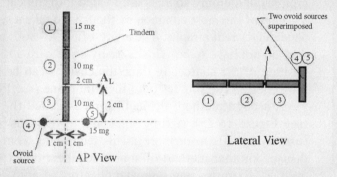

Point **A** Dose Rate Calculation

Source #	Distance along (cm)	Distance away (cm)	cGy/h/ mgRaEq	"Strength" mgRaEq	Dose rate at A (cGy/h)
1	3.0	2.0	0.59	15	8.9
2	1.0	2.0	1.54	10	15.4
3	1.0	2.0	1.54	10	15.4
4	0.0	3.6	0.58	15	8.7
5	0.0	2.2	1.60	15	24
				Total	72.4

Source #4 is a distance $\sqrt{2^2 + 3^2} = \sqrt{13} = 3.6$ cm away and source #5 is a distance of $\sqrt{1^2 + 2^2} = \sqrt{5} = 2.2$ cm. Which one contributes most of the dose? What is the dose rate for A_R?

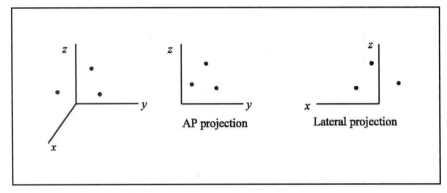

Figure 16.24: Two isocentric orthogonal films will uniquely locate objects in three-dimensional space. A three-dimensional perspective view is shown on the left. An AP projection gives y and z coordinates. A lateral projection gives x and z coordinates. It is necessary to know the magnification factor.

16.13   Localization of Sources

To compute the dose distribution for a brachytherapy implant, it is necessary to know the location of the sources in three dimensions. There are three main methods that are used to "localize" the sources. All of these methods rely on radiography. Prior to radiographic exposure radiopaque dummy sources are loaded into the catheter, applicator, etc.

One of the most common methods is to take a set of orthogonal (perpendicular) radiographs. These are often AP and lateral films although they do not have to be. This is easily done with a therapy simulator. The position of the sources in three dimensions can be ascertained from the projection of the sources onto the film plane (see Figure 16.24).

A second method of localization is called the stereo shift method (see Figure 16.25). A film is taken and then the x-ray tube is shifted (usually by 20 cm or more). This technique seems to have fallen into disuse. Another method of source localization exploits CT. CT can be used if the sources and source applicators (if any) do not produce severe artifacts. Conventional gynecological applicators are not CT compatible for this reason.

16.14   High Dose Rate Remote Afterloaders

A high dose rate (HDR) remote afterloader is a treatment machine that can deliver brachytherapy treatment at high dose rates and which can be operated remotely to reduce radiation exposure to health care workers. An HDR system consists of three components: the afterloader, the control console, and the treatment planning workstation. High dose rate is defined as dose rate >0.2 Gy/min.

The afterloader contains the radioactive source and delivers the treatment to the patient. See Figures 16.26 and 16.27. The afterloader is

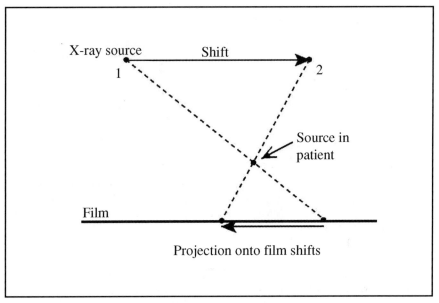

Figure 16.25: Illustration of the stereo shift method of source localization. An exposure is made with the x-ray tube at position 1 and then the tube is shifted a known distance to position 2 and another exposure is made. The projection of the source position on the film shifts as a result of the shift in the tube position. The position of the source can be determined by measuring the shift in the projection.

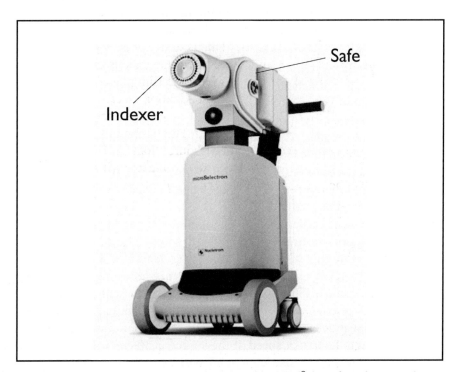

Figure 16.26: An HDR afterloader; the Nucletron microSelectron Digital®. Transfer tubes or catheters are connected to the indexer face where the source exits. The source resides in a shielded safe between treatments. (Courtesy of Nucletron B.V., Veenendaal, The Netherlands)

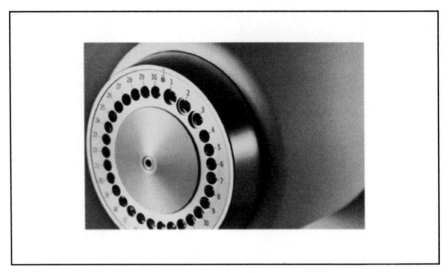

Figure 16.27: A close-up of the indexer face of the microSelectron Digital. Transfer tubes or catheters are attached to one or more of the 30 output channels. The source will exit through each channel in turn throughout the treatment. (Courtesy of Nucletron B.V., Veenendaal, The Netherlands)

in a shielded room with the patient. The control console is outside the treatment room. The control console enables the operator to deliver a treatment from the afterloader remotely. The control console consists of a computer that controls the afterloader and displays all the treatment parameters. The planning workstation consists of a digitizer, a computer, and a printer. Patient treatments are planned on this system. All HDR systems in the United States use a single Ir-192 source, which is either attached to or embedded in the end of a wire about 1.0 to 2.0 m long. When a fresh source is installed, the activity is typically 10 Ci. In between treatments the source resides in a shielded "safe" inside the afterloader. The safe is usually made of tungsten. One characteristic of Ir-192 that makes it ideal for an HDR afterloader is its high specific activity of 450 Ci/g. Iridium also has a very high density of 22.4 g/cm^3 and therefore a 10 Ci source can be made very small. One manufacturer has a source wire that is 0.6 mm in diameter (see Figure 16.28). The wire is made of a nickel-titanium "superelastic" alloy that enables it to negotiate highly curved pathways. The Ir-192 source is embedded inside this wire and has an active length of 5 mm.

HDR units employ stepper motors to advance the source by fixed increments in distance. The source can be sent out through one of 15 to 30 different channels (depending on the manufacturer), and dwell at various locations and for various times. Dwell times as small as 0.1 s are possible and the transit speed of the source is 50 cm/s. This is sufficiently fast that the transit dose deposited between dwell positions is negligible. The accuracy of source position placement is ±1 mm. The half-life of Ir-192 is only 73.8 days and this generally necessitates four source changes per year at a total cost of approximately $50,000.

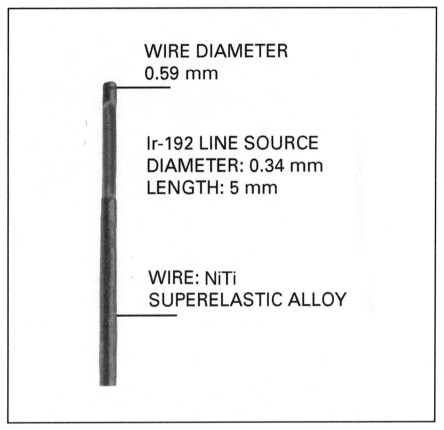

WIRE DIAMETER
0.59 mm

Ir-192 LINE SOURCE
DIAMETER: 0.34 mm
LENGTH: 5 mm

WIRE: NiTi
SUPERELASTIC ALLOY

Figure 16.28: HDR Ir-192 source embedded in wire. (Courtesy of Varian Medical Systems, Inc. Copyright © 2010, all rights reserved.) See COLOR PLATE 13.

HDR afterloader systems have numerous redundant safety features built in, particularly after an accident that occurred in 1992 (see chapter 18, section 18.7.2). They have a backup power supply for use in the event of a power outage. They have a battery which powers an emergency retract motor if the backup power fails. A hand crank on the afterloader can be used to attempt to pull the source back into the safe if the retract motors fail (see Figure 16.29). There is a maximum time that the source can dwell. If this time is exceeded, then the source is withdrawn. Some HDR units have a source park verification, which uses an internal GM (Geiger-Müller) counter. If the GM counter does not detect the source after it is parked, then an alert is issued. Optical encoders on the drive wheels are used to monitor the length of the extended wire. This informs the system of the position of the source. Before the actual source is driven out of the afterloader, a check cable with identical mechanical properties is driven to the same extension that the actual source will go. If the check cable encounters a constriction, it retracts and notifies the operator of the position of the constriction.

The U.S. Nuclear Regulatory Commission (or an Agreement State, see chapter 17) regulates the use of HDR afterloaders. A closed-circuit

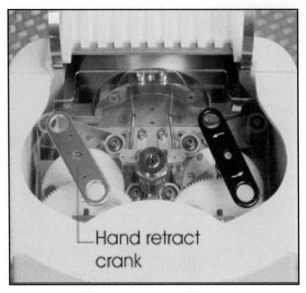

Figure 16.29: Inside the Nucletron microSelectron Digital®, as seen from the rear with the cover opened. If the retract motor fails to withdraw the source into the safe, the user can try the hand retract crank. (Courtesy of Nucletron B.V., Veenendaal, The Netherlands)

TV (CCTV) and intercom are required so that audiovisual communication is maintained with the patient at all times. The door to the treatment room has an interlock that prevents initiation of treatment when the door is open and interrupts treatment if the door is opened during treatment.

Treatment planning is based on source localization as described in section 16.13. The locations of the dummy sources in three dimensions are determined. One must then decide on the dwell positions and the dwell times at each of these positions. Treatment planning software is available to assist the user in adjusting the dwell positions and times to optimize the dose distribution.

Advantages of Remote Afterloading

1. Radiation protection; reduces personnel exposure.
2. No hospitalization for extended treatment; can treat as outpatient; fractionate.
3. Dose distribution optimization.

Disadvantages of Remote Afterloading

1. Expense of unit—about $350,000 circa 2004.
2. Requires shielded room.
3. Stiff regulatory requirements.

Chapter Summary

- **Sealed sources,** usually doubly encapsulated; HDR > 20 cGy/min, LDR 40–80 cGy/h.

- 1 mCi = 37 MBq

- **Specific activity** = (activity/total mass of element present).

- **Exposure rate:** $\dot{X} = \Gamma \dfrac{A}{r^2}$, where A is the activity, r is the distance from the source, and Γ is a proportionality constant having a different value for different isotopes. Typical units of Γ: R cm^2 h^{-1} mCi^{-1} (crazy mix—be careful to make sure you know what units you have).

- **Ra-226:** Originally used for brachytherapy; techniques based on this; $T_{1/2}$ = 1600 years; $^{226}_{88}\text{Ra} \to {}^{222}_{86}\text{Rn} + {}^{4}_{2}\text{He}$, α particles filtered out by encapsulation, $\overline{E}_\gamma = 0.83$ MeV, but $(E_\gamma)_{max} = 2.45$ MeV; shielding problem;
  —Disadvantages of radium: (1) hard to shield, (2) radon gas leakage, (3) helium gas pressure
  —1 mg of Ra has $A \approx 1$ mCi. $\Gamma = 8.25$ R cm^2 h^{-1} mg^{-1}. Specific activity is approximately 1 Ci/g.

- **Cs-137:** Replaced radium; byproduct material; comes in stainless steel tubes 2 cm long, predominantly for LDR gynecological applications; $T_{1/2}$ = 30 years, E_γ = 0.622 MeV, HVL = 5.5 mm-lead.
  —Advantages: (1) less shielding, (2) no radon hazard, (3) dose distribution almost identical to Ra within 10 cm of source—inverse square law dominates distribution nearby, $\Gamma = 3.3$ R cm^2 h^{-1} mCi^{-1} (standard filtration).

- **Ir-192:** Byproduct material; used for HDR and interstitial implants; has high specific activity (about 450 Ci/g) and density (small source has high activity); $T_{1/2}$ = 73.8 days, $\overline{E}_\gamma = 0.38$ MeV (complicated γ spectrum). HVL = 2.5 mm-lead, $\Gamma = 4.7$ R cm^2 h^{-1} mCi^{-1}.

- **I-125:** Often used for permanent implants (brain and prostate), $T_{1/2}$ = 59.5 days, E_γ = 0.028 to 0.035 MeV, HVL = 0.025 mm-lead; decays by electron capture → characteristic x-ray emission 27 to 35 keV; dose distribution around these seeds is highly anisotropic; $\Gamma = 1.5$ R cm^2 h^{-1} mCi^{-1}.

- **Pd-103:** Reactor produced; $T_{1/2}$ = 17 days; decays by electron capture; characteristic x-rays 20 to 23 keV, permanent implants.

- **Sr-90:** Eye applicator; long-lived fission fragment; $^{90}\text{Sr} \rightarrow {}^{90}\text{Y} \rightarrow \beta^-$ + ...; beta has 2.27 MeV max energy, $T_{1/2} = 28.0$ years.

- **Equivalent Mass of Radium:** mgRaEq = the number of milligrams of radium that will produce the same exposure rate as the given radioisotope:

$$M_{Ra} = \frac{\Gamma_x}{\Gamma_{Ra}} A_x, \text{ where } M_{Ra} \text{ is the mgRaEq.}$$

Rule of thumb: 2.5 mCi of Cs-137 is equivalent to 1 mg of Ra-226 (i.e., 1 mgRaEq).

- **Dose from Permanent Implant:** $D = \dot{D}_0 \tau$, where D is the total dose, and $\dot{D}_0$ is the initial dose rate, and τ is the mean life (1.44 $T_{1/2}$).

- **Systems of Implant Dosimetry:**
  —Planar and Volume
  (1) Paterson-Parker/Manchester: Non-uniform source distribution to get uniform dose (±10%) distribution, rules for planar and volume implants, tables.
  (2) Quimby: Uniform source distribution; non-uniform dose distribution.

  Neither accounts for photon attenuation and scattering: DO NOT use for low-energy sources <200 keV (e.g., I-125, Pd-103).

  —Intracavitary: Manchester System
  – Doses to points A, B, bladder and rectum.
  – Point A is tipped with the uterus but point B is not tipped.
  – LDR dose 7500 cGy to point A in two weeks, 2 fractions of about 3 days each, standard dose rate at point A is about 55 cGy/h, $D_B \sim 1/3\ D_A$.
  – Typical source loading shown in diagram to the right.

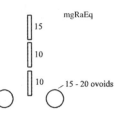

- **Fletcher-Suit Applicator**
  —Tandem: Usually stainless steel, ~12 in. long, outer diameter about ¼ in.; different curvatures available (e.g., 15°, 30°, 45° angle).
  —Ovoids = colpostats: Shielded with tungsten at medial aspect at end of ovoids; reduce dose to bladder and rectum by 10% to 20%; loading: length of uterine canal is typically 6 to 7 cm: 3 Cs-137 tubes.
  —Calculate point doses by hand: use Krishnaswamy "along and away tables" (see Table 16.5).

- **Localization of Sources:** (1) orthogonal films, (2) stereo shift, (3) CT.

- **HDR Units:** Definition of high dose rate >20 cGy/min; single Ir-192 source at end of wire 1.0–2.0 m long and 0.6 mm in diameter; source size is typically 5 mm long and 0.3 mm in diameter; fresh source is 10 Ci, 15 to 30 different channels; dwell times as small as 0.1 s— optimize dose distribution by using variable dwell time.

Problems

1. Approximately how much of a reduction in exposure will a 0.25 mm thick lead sheet make for I-125 radiation?

2. Ignoring attenuation in the patient, estimate the exposure rate (in units of mR/h) at a distance of 1.0 m from a patient with a 65 mgRaEq Cs-137 implant.

3. Under what circumstances is the effect of anisotropy on the dose distribution surrounding a single seed or tubular source expected to be a maximum?

4. A breast cancer patient is treated with a 4.0 cm diameter balloon implant using an HDR afterloader. The 7.0 Ci Ir-192 source dwells at the center of the balloon. A dose of 3.4 Gy per fraction is prescribed to a distance of 1 cm from the surface of the balloon. Assume that $T(r) = 1.0$ and neglect anisotropy.
    a. Calculate the dose rate at the prescription location using equation (16.3).
    b. Calculate the total dwell time for the source in units of minutes and seconds.

5. Repeat the calculation of problem 4 using the TG-43 formalism. Assume that the angle $\theta = 0°$. The air kerma strength is 2.86×10^4 U, $\Lambda = 1.108$ cGy h^{-1} U^{-1}, $g(3.0) = 1.008$, $F(3.0, 0°) = 0.660$, and assume that $G(r, \theta) = 1/r^2$.

6. a. What is the dose rate in tissue (in cGy/h) at a distance of 2.0 cm from a 20 mCi point source of Cs-137. (You may ignore scattering and anisotropy effects).
    b. For a 20 mCi tube source with an active length of 14 mm, what is the dose rate in tissue at a distance of 2.0 cm away from the source on the transverse axis (see Table 16.5).
    c. Explain the *major* reason for the difference in the dose rates.

7. A permanent I-125 implant delivers 100 Gy to a reference point. Calculate the initial dose rate at this point in units of cGy/h.

8. Compare the features of the Paterson-Parker and Quimby systems of implant dosimetry.

9. a. What is the typical dose rate at point **A** for an LDR cervical treatment?

   b. In Example 16.7 calculate the dose rate at point **B**$_L$ and compare with the dose rate at point **A**. Hint: For source #4 (which is off the table), use an inverse square ratio to estimate the dose rate at point **B**$_L$ from the dose rate at the nearest entry in the table.

10. Why isn't apparent activity a good measure of source strength?

Bibliography

AAPM TG-43. (1995). Nath, R., L. L. Anderson, G. Luxton, K. A. Weaver, J. F. Williamson, and A. S. Meigooni. "Dosimetry of interstitial brachytherapy sources: Recommendations of the AAPM Radiation Therapy Committee Task Group No. 43." *Med Phys* 22:209–234. Also available as AAPM Report No. 51.

AAPM TG-56. (1997). Nath, R., L. L. Anderson, J. A. Meli, A. J. Olch, J. A. Stitt, J. F. Williamson. "Code of practice for brachytherapy physics: Report of the AAPM Radiation Therapy Committee Task Group No. 56." *Med Phys* 24:1557–1598. Also available as AAPM Report No. 59.

AAPM TG-59. (1998). "High dose-rate brachytherapy treatment delivery: Report of the AAPM Radiation Therapy Committee Task Group No. 59." *Med Phys* 25:375–403. Also available as AAPM Report No. 61.

Anderson, L. L., and J. L. Presser, "Classical Systems I for Temporary Interstitial Implants: Manchester and Quimby Systems" in *Brachytherapy Physics*, J. F. Williamson, B. R. Thomadsen, and R. Nath (eds.). Madison, WI: Medical Physics Publishing, pp. 301–321, 1995.

Bentel, G. C. *Radiation Therapy Planning*, Second Edition. New York: McGraw-Hill Professional, 1995.

Glasgow, G. P. "Isodose Planning: Brachytherapy" in *Treatment Planning in Radiation Oncology*. F. M. Khan and R. A. Potish (eds.). Baltimore, MD: Williams & Wilkins, 1998.

Grove, Andy. "Taking on Prostate Cancer." *Fortune* magazine. May 13, 1996.

Khan, F. M. *The Physics of Radiation Therapy*, Fourth Edition. Philadelphia: Lippincott Williams & Wilkins, 2009.

Krishnaswamy, V. (1972). "Dose distributions about Cs-137 sources in tissue." *Radiology* 105:181–184.

Meigooni, A. S., J. F. Williamson, and R. Nath. "Single-Source Dosimetry for Interstitial Brachytherapy" in *Brachytherapy Physics*. J. F. Williamson, B. R. Thomadsen, and R. Nath (eds.). Proceedings of the AAPM 1994 Summer School. Madison, WI: Medical Physics Publishing, 1995.

Meli, J. A. "Dosimetry of Some Interstitial and Intracavitary Sources and their Applicators" in *Brachytherapy Physics*. J.F. Williamson, B.R. Thomadsen, R. Nath (editors). AAPM 1994 Summer School Proceedings. Madison, WI: Medical Physics Publishing, pp. 185–207, 1994.

Nag, S. (ed.). *High Dose Rate Brachytherapy: A Textbook.* Armonk, NY: Futura Publishing Company, 1994.

Paterson, R., and Parker, H.M. (1934). "A dosage system for gamma ray therapy." *Br J Radiol* 7:592–632.

Pierquin, B., A. Dutreix, and C. Paine. (1978). "The Paris system of interstitial radiation therapy." *Acta Radiol Oncol* 17:33.

Quimby, E. H. (1932). "The grouping of radium tubes in packs and plaques to produce the desired distribution of radiation." *AJR Am J Roentgenol* 27:18.

Thomadsen, B. R., M. J. Rivard, and W. M. Butler (eds.). *Brachytherapy Physics, Second Edition.* Proceedings of the 2005 Joint AAPM/American Brachytherapy Society (ABS) Summer School. AAPM Medical Physics Monograph No. 31. Madison, WI: Medical Physics Publishing, 2005.

Williamson, J.F., B. R. Thomadsen, and R. Nath (eds.). *Brachytherapy Physics.* Proceedings of the AAPM 1994 Summer School. Madison, WI: Medical Physics Publishing, 1995.

17 Radiation Protection

Various advisory and regulatory agencies are concerned with the protection of the public and protection of occupational workers from radiation. In the United States there is the National Council on Radiation Protection (NCRP), a non-profit corporation chartered by Congress in 1964 to: (1) make recommendations about radiation protection and (2) advise regarding radiation measurements and quantities particularly with respect to radiation protection. On the international level there is the International Commission on Radiation Protection (ICRP). Both the NCRP and the ICRP publish reports and make recommendations for radiation exposure standards.[1]

In the United States there are both federal and state regulatory agencies. On the federal level there is a patchwork of agencies involved in radiation regulation. This quirky arrangement has arisen through historical happenstance. The U.S. Nuclear Regulatory Commission (NRC) regulates: (1) "source material" (uranium or thorium) and (2) "byproduct" material. Byproduct materials are reactor-produced radioisotopes such as Ir-192 (HDR units), Co-60 (Co-60 units), Cs-137, etc. See Table 17.1 for

---

[1] For more information on the NCRP and ICRP and to order publications, access their web sites: http://www.ncrponline.org and http://www.icrp.org, respectively.

Table 17.1: Selected Isotopes Regulated by the NRC or Agreement States

Isotope	Applications
Cf-252	Neutron brachytherapy: temporary implants
Co-60	External beam therapy (including gamma stereotactic)
Cs-137	Intracavitary brachytherapy
Au-198	Brachytherapy: permanent implants
I-125	Permanent implants (prostate, brain)
I-131	Thyroid ablation (unsealed beta source)
Ir-192	Brachytherapy: HDR, temporary implants
Mo-99	Diagnostic nuclear medicine (produces Tc-99m)
Pd-103	Permanent implants
P-32	Intracavitary (unsealed beta source)
Sr-89	Metastatic bone pain
Sr-90	Eye applicators
Y-90	Microspheres for liver cancer

a more extensive list. The Energy Policy Act of 2005[2] expanded NRC regulatory authority to include: (1) naturally occurring radioisotopes, such as radium, and (2) accelerator-produced radionuclides. This became effective August 2009.[3] The NRC does not regulate the use of medical linear accelerators. NRC regulations can be found in Title 10 of the *Code of Federal Regulations* (*CFR*). Especially pertinent are: 10 CFR Part 19, Part 20, and Part 35 (Medical Use of Byproduct Material). Part 35 was extensively modified effective October 2002. Another useful NRC reference is NUREG-1556, Vol. 9, Revision 1 "Program Specific Guidance About Medical Use Licenses." A very useful online reference is the Medical Uses Licensee Toolkit.[4]

The Center for Devices and Radiological Health (CDRH) is a part of the U.S. Food and Drug Administration (FDA). The FDA regulates the manufacture and sale of radiation-producing machines including linacs and treatment planning systems. Such devices must be approved for sale in the United States by obtaining what is called 510(k) clearance.[5]

The U.S. Department of Transportation (DOT) oversees rules for the safe transport of radioactive materials, including packaging, labeling, etc. Individuals who (1) prepare radioactive material for shipment, (2) transport radioactive material, or (3) sign in or receive radioactive material are required to be trained, tested, and certified every 2 years.

---

[2] Section 651(e) of the Energy Policy Act of 2005 (EPAct) on "Treatment of Accelerator Produced and Other Radioactive Material as Byproduct Material."

[3] *Federal Register*, vol. 72, no. 202: Notification of the Plan for Transition of Regulatory Authority Resulting from Expanded Definition of Byproduct Material.

[4] http://www.nrc.gov/materials/miau/med-use-toolkit.html.

[5] The web site for the CDRH is http://www.fda.gov/AboutFDA/CentersOffices/CDRH/default.htm.

In 1959, the Atomic Energy Act was enacted, which authorized states to assume regulatory control for non-byproduct material and the use of diagnostic and therapeutic x-rays. Provided the state had an adequate program to protect the public health and safety, it could enter into an agreement with the NRC and assume control of byproduct material as well. There are currently 36 Agreement States that have a written agreement with the NRC, which includes stipulations that the state program must be compatible with NRC regulations. State governments generally regulate the use of x-ray–generating machines, such as simulators and linear accelerators, and all isotopes not regulated by the NRC. State oversight includes review of shielding plans for linac and simulator rooms. These devices must be registered with the state, and the states perform periodic inspections to ensure compliance with all regulations.

17.1 Dosimetric Quantities Used for Radiation Protection

One of the primary biological effects of concern for radiation protection is cancer induction. Different types of radiation have different biological effects for the same dose (see chapter 7, section 7.11). The quantity *equivalent dose* is introduced to account for these differences. The equivalent dose is defined as

$$H_T = D_T \times w_R, \tag{17.1}$$

where D_T is the average absorbed dose in a tissue or organ and w_R is the radiation weighting factor.[6] The radiation weighting factor depends on the type and energy of the radiation. The quantities H_T and w_R are only intended to be used for low doses of radiation for the purposes of radiation protection and not for large doses, such as those that might be administered for therapeutic purposes or those received in a serious radiation accident. The biological effects of ionizing radiation depend on the length of time over which the dose is delivered and on the type of effect considered. Values of w_R are listed in Table 17.2. This table shows that high-LET radiation, such as the alpha particles emitted by radon, is far more dangerous (for the same dose) than low-LET radiation such as from x-rays or electrons. The quantity w_R has no units and therefore H_T has units of J/kg in the SI system. In this context, this combination of units is given a name different from absorbed dose. The SI unit of H_T is sievert; 1 sievert = 1 Sv = 1 J/kg. Therefore H in sievert equals dose in gray times w_R. The old unit of equivalent dose is the rem,

---

[6] Unfortunately, there is also an older quantity called the *dose equivalent* (also symbolized by H). Do not confuse this with the equivalent dose. The dose equivalent $H = D \times Q$, where Q is the quality factor. The NRC still uses *dose equivalent,* as does NCRP Report No. 151.

Table 17.2: Radiation Weighting Factor w_R*

Radiation		w_R
X-rays, γ-rays, electrons, positrons, and muons		1
Neutrons	<10 keV	5
	10 keV to 100 keV	10
	>100 keV to 2 MeV	20
	>2 MeV to 20 MeV	10
	>20 MeV	5
Protons (other than recoil protons and energy >2 MeV)		2
Alpha particles, fission fragments		20

*Data from ICRP Publication 60, 1990 Recommendations of the International Commission on Radiological Protection, 1990.

which is still in widespread use. The equivalent dose in rem is equal to the absorbed dose in rads (or cGy) times w_R. Therefore 100 rem = 1 sievert.

Most exposures to radiation are non-uniform to the body. For example, when handling radioisotopes the hands may receive an exposure far higher than the rest of the body. Different organs and tissues also differ in their response to radiation. The quantity *effective dose, H_E,* is introduced to account for these differences.[7] It takes into account the radiation sensitivities for various organs and tissues. It is associated with the same probability of cancer and genetic effects for a non-uniform irradiation as for a uniform irradiation of the entire body. The effective dose equivalent is calculated as follows:

$$H_E = w_{T1}H_{T1} + w_{T2}H_{T2} + ..., \qquad (17.2)$$

where H_{Tn} is the mean equivalent dose received by tissue n and w_{Tn} is a weighting factor based on the relative detriment to each organ and tissue from cancer and hereditary effects in that tissue. The sum of all the weighting factors is equal to 1.00. Table 17.3 contains values of the weighting factors. If the dose is uniform, then $H_{T1} = H_{T2} = ... = H_{Tn} = H_T$ and therefore $H_E = H_T (w_{T1} + w_{T2} + ... + w_{Tn}) = H_T$, as expected.

There are several additional quantities which are used in personnel occupational radiation exposure reports. NRC radiation exposure limits are expressed in terms of these quantities. The *deep dose equivalent* for external whole body exposure is the dose equivalent at a tissue depth of 1.0 cm. Radioisotopes that are not sealed can potentially be absorbed, inhaled or ingested by the body. These isotopes will be eliminated from the body by two mechanisms: (1) physical radioactive decay and (2) biological elimination (excretion, exhalation, etc.). The *committed dose equivalent* is the dose equivalent to organs or tissues received from intake of radioactive materials by an individual during a 50-year period

---

[7] The NRC uses the older quantity *effective dose equivalent* for regulatory exposure limits.

Table 17.3: Tissue Weighting Factors w_T*

0.01	0.05	0.12	0.20
Bone surface	Bladder	Bone marrow	Gonads
Skin	Breast	Colon	
	Liver	Lung	
	Esophagus	Stomach	
	Thyroid		
	Remainder		

*Data from NCRP Report No. 116, Limitation of Exposure to Ionizing Radiation, 1993.

following the intake. The *shallow dose equivalent* applies to external exposure of the skin. It is the dose equivalent at a depth of 0.007 cm averaged over an area of 1 cm². The *eye dose equivalent* applies to the lens of the eye. It is the dose equivalent at a tissue depth of 0.3 cm. The *total effective dose equivalent* is the sum of the deep dose equivalent (for external exposure) and the committed effective dose equivalent (for internal exposures).

17.2 Exposure of Individuals to Radiation

There are two major sources of radiation exposure: natural and man-made. Natural sources are those sources that we would be exposed to even in the absence of human activity. Man-made sources are those that result from human activity. Table 17.4 contains a summary of the levels of radiation exposure listed in NCRP Report No. 160 (the reference of

Table 17.4: Annual Effective Dose for U.S. Population (2006)*

Source			Average Annual Effective Dose (mSv/y)
NATURAL	Cosmic rays		0.33
	Terrestrial		0.21
	Internal		0.29
	Radon		2.30
		Average subtotal	**3.13**
MAN MADE	Medical		3.0
	Consumer products		0.13
	Industrial, security, medical, educational, and research		0.003
		Average subtotal	**3.13**
		TOTAL	**6.26**

*Data from NCRP Report No. 160, Ionizing Radiation Exposure of the Population of the United States, 2009.

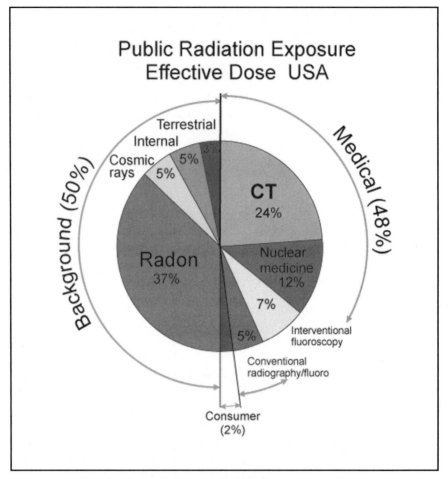

Figure 17.1: The relative contribution of various sources of radiation exposure in the United States as of 2006 (data from NCRP Report No. 160). Approximately half of the total exposure is from medical procedures (mostly CT). The remaining half is from background.

record), and Figure 17.1 shows a pie chart of the contribution from various sources. We are, on average, exposed to about 6.2 mSv/year (620 mrem/year) or about 0.017 mSv/day (there are 1000 mSv per sievert).

 Rule of thumb: The average effective daily dose equivalent to individual members of the public is about 0.017 mSv (1.7 mrem). This provides a context within which occupational exposure may be evaluated.

We are all continually exposed to naturally occurring radiation, which is present in the environment. Background radiation refers to naturally occurring radiation—from cosmic rays or radioisotopes found in nature. Background radiation levels as measured with a survey meter are typically 0.2 μSv/h, depending on locale. Cosmic rays are high-energy particles (mostly protons) from outer space, incident upon the upper atmosphere. Cosmic rays interact with the atmosphere and produce a shower of secondary particles such as electrons, photons, some neutrons, and particles called muons. Radiation levels from cosmic rays are much higher at elevation (in the mountains or on airline flights).

Terrestrial exposure results from the gamma rays emitted by natural radioactive materials in the earth such as potassium-40 (K-40), thorium-232, uranium-238, and the decay products of the latter two isotopes (see chapter 3, section 3.7).

Internal sources of radiation are found in food, water, and air. These include K-40 and carbon-14 in food. The single biggest contribution to natural radiation exposure is radon. This gas is continuously produced by natural radioactive decay of radium in soil and rocks. It seeps into houses, particularly lower levels such as basements. Radon is an alpha emitter. Alpha particles cannot penetrate the skin; however when radon is inhaled, the alpha particles ($w_R = 20$) damage the bronchial endothelium. The amount of radon in a residential basement depends on the amount of radium in the soil and on the rate of "turnover" of air in the basement. The concentration of radon in the air can vary greatly from neighborhood to neighborhood and even from house to house. The U.S. Environmental Protection Agency (EPA) recommends that the occupants consider remedial action if the concentration of radon in a living area exceeds 4.0 pCi per liter of air. It is possible to reduce the radon levels in a home by changing the ventilation in the house. The U.S. Surgeon General has said that radon is now the second leading cause of lung cancer in the United States. Radon levels can be measured using inexpensive activated charcoal kits available commercially and from state and local public health facilities.

The predominant source of man-made radiation exposure is from medical procedures. Medical radiation exposure is due to conventional radiography and fluoroscopy, nuclear medicine diagnostic procedures, and computed tomography (CT). Approximately half of the total annual exposure contribution is from medical procedures. This represents a substantial change over the previously reported value of 0.53 mSv/y from the early 1980s (NCRP Report No. 94). The increase is due mainly to a sharp rise in the use of CT and nuclear medicine procedures. CT now makes up approximately a quarter of the total annual exposure. A typical CT exam delivers an effective dose of about 10 mSv. There were about 67 million CT scans performed in the United States in 2006 alone.[8] Table 17.5 lists some nominal values of the effective dose for common radiographic medical exams. Many of these exams involve multiple projections (exposures).

---

[8] NCRP Report No. 160, Ionizing Radiation Exposure of the Population of the United States, 2009.

Table 17.5: Effective Dose for Radiographic Medical Exams*

Exam Type	Effective Dose (mSv)
Chest x-ray	0.1
Mammography	0.18
Lumbar spine x-ray	1.5
Barium enema	8.0
Dental bite wing (per image)	0.005
Computed tomography (CT)	10

*Data from NCRP Report No. 160, Ionizing Radiation Exposure of the Population of the United States, 2009.

Exposure from consumer products and activities includes building materials, cigarette smoking, and commercial air travel among others. (Refer to NCRP Report No. 160). According to NCRP Report No. 160, the average effective dose rate for domestic airline flights is 3.3 µSv/h. Thus for a 5-hour cross-country flight the effective dose is about 0.017 mSv, which is about the average amount of radiation received in a single day.

17.3 Biological Effects of Radiation

References of record are the BEIR V (Biological Effects of Ionizing Radiation committee) report from the National Academies of Science: "Health Effects of Exposure to Ionizing Radiation" and the BEIR VII report: "Health Effects from Exposure to Low Levels of Ionizing Radiation, Phase II".

The acute whole-body dose of radiation which is lethal to 50% of those humans exposed (LD_{50}) is approximately 400 cGy.[9] This is in the absence of any medical intervention.

Radiation injury to a cell can have one of three outcomes:

1. Cell death.
2. Failure to reproduce, which leads to eventual cell death.
3. Mutation, which is of primary concern in radiation protection.

Numbers 1 and 2 above are associated with the therapeutic effect of radiation or serious radiation accidents.

---

[9] Hall, E. J., *Radiobiology for the Radiologist,* 5th edition. Lippincott Williams & Wilkins, Philadelphia, PA, 2000.

The biological effects of radiation can be broadly classified into two categories:

I. **Deterministic Effects:** These are effects that increase in severity with increasing dose above a threshold dose; require high doses:
   - *Acute, early effects:* skin erythema (reddening), epilation (hair loss)
   - *Late effects:* cataracts, fibrosis, organ atrophy.

On a cellular level these are associated with numbers 1 and 2 above. The threshold dose for transient skin erythema is 2000 mSv.

II. **Stochastic Effects:** Probability of an effect increases with dose, but severity is independent of dose. It is an all or nothing phenomenon, e.g., cancer, genetic effects. This is associated with number 3 above.
   - *Threshold:* It has been suggested that below a certain level radiation has no harmful stochastic effects. Current data cannot rule out a threshold at 100 mrem (1 mSv) or below.
   - *Hormesis:* The hypothesis that small amounts of radiation may be beneficial to health due to an adaptive response. This is highly controversial.

17.3.1 Carcinogenesis

It is not possible to distinguish radiation-induced cancers from those due to any other causes. About 20% of the population will die of cancer due to all causes. Human data on radiation carcinogenesis is based on:

1. Atomic bomb survivors: About 120,000 persons have been carefully followed. About 90,000 of these were exposed to significant levels of radiation. As of 1990 about 6000 had died of cancer. Of these 6000, about 400 are considered to be excess deaths due to radiation.
2. Patients exposed to medical irradiation.
3. Early occupational radiation exposures.

Latency is the time interval between irradiation and the appearance of malignancy. The latency period for leukemia is 5 to 7 years, whereas it is a minimum of 10 years for solid tumors.

To estimate the risk of fatal cancer from low doses of radiation requires assumptions and extrapolation. All evidence of radiation-induced cancer is based on doses of 200 to 500 mSv and higher. It is assumed that since high doses of radiation increase the risk of cancer

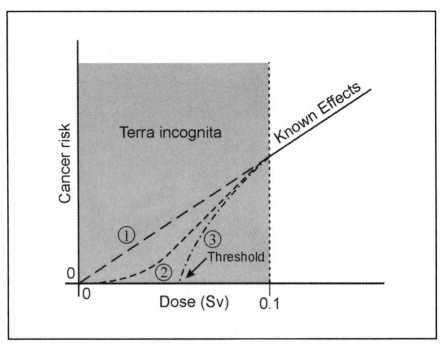

Figure 17.2: Models for cancer risk associated with exposure to low levels of radiation. Number ① is the linear no threshold model, number ② is the linear quadratic model, and number ③ is a model that exhibits a threshold. (Adapted from NRC Regulatory Guide 8.29, Instructions Concerning Risks from Occupational Radiation Exposure, 1996.)

that low doses will also increase the risk. Risk estimates for low doses of concern to occupational workers are based on extrapolations from high-dose data points. These extrapolations are educated guesses and are very contentious. The conservative approach to radiation protection regulations is based on the linear no threshold model (see Figure 17.2). The known risk of radiation exposure at higher levels is extrapolated linearly backward to lower dose equivalents assuming no threshold level below which there is no risk. This is a cautious approach that assumes that any radiation exposure is detrimental.

Based on the linear, no threshold dose response model adopted by the NRC: for occupational workers subjected to low doses and low dose rate, the *excess lifetime risk of developing a fatal cancer due to radiation exposure is 4 in 100 per sievert* (4×10^{-2}/Sv; equivalent whole body) of radiation exposure.[10]

It is very difficult to determine the effects of low dose and low dose rate. Most of the data for risk of carcinogenesis is based on high doses and often on high dose rates (acute exposure). Consider a numerical illustration: begin with a population of 10,000 radiation workers. Of

---

[10] ICRP No. 60, 1990 Recommendations of the International Commission on Radiological Protection, 1991; NCRP No. 115, Risk Estimation for Radiation Protection, 1993.

these, 2,000 would be expected to die of cancer without *any* occupational exposure. This number varies by about 80.[11] So it is quite probable that the number of deaths due to cancer will be anywhere in the range between 1,920 and 2,080 out of the original 10,000. The average career dose of workers at NRC licensed facilities is 0.015 Sv. Of our 10,000 workers a total of 6 would be expected to die from radiation-induced cancer (4×10^{-2} Sv^{-1} $\times$ 0.015 Sv $\times$ 10,000 = 6). We thus expect a total of 2,006 cancer deaths in an exposed population versus 2,000 in a non-exposed group. Now suppose we actually observe 2,006 fatal cancers. Are the extra six just part of the normal variation that could easily occur with high probability, or do they represent a real (statistically significant) increase? It is impossible to tell without studying a much larger group of workers. This is why it is so difficult to study radiation carcinogenesis at low doses—it is a bit like trying to hear a whisper in a hurricane!

17.3.2 Risk to Fetus/Embryo

Cells are most sensitive to radiation damage when they are undifferentiated (or stem cells) or rapidly dividing.[12] This explains why embryonic cells are more sensitive than mature adult cells.

It is a common misconception that radiation produces bizarre mutants and monsters. This is false, it only happens in cartoons or movies (see Figure 17.3). The normal incidence of "malformed" infants at birth is about 6%.

Effects of Radiation
1. Growth retardation
2. Pre-natal or neonatal death
3. Congenital malformation
4. Mental retardation
5. Childhood cancer (primarily leukemia)

For the purpose of studying the effects of radiation, gestation is divided into three periods:

1. *Pre-implantation:* Fertilization → embryo attaches to uterine wall; 0 to 9 days, radiation usually causes all or nothing effect → death of embryo (spontaneous abortion).

---

[11] Based on a binomial distribution and all of the assumptions implied by this. The standard deviation is approximately $\sigma = 40$.

[12] The law of Bergonie and Tribondeau.

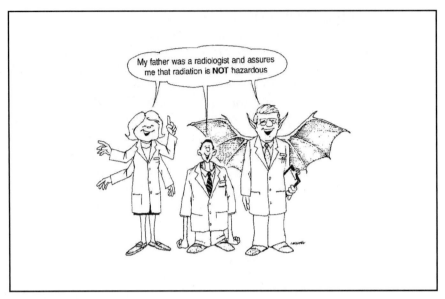

Figure 17.3: (Reproduced from Hall, E. J. *Radiobiology for the Radiobiologist,* 5th ed., Fig. 11.1, p. 169, © 2000, with permission from Lippincott Williams and Wilkins.)

2. *Organogenesis:* Period of rapid cellular differentiation and organ development; critical period; 10 days to 6 weeks; abnormalities, neonatal death.
3. *Fetal:* 6 weeks to term; permanent growth retardation, cancer.

The effects of irradiation of the embryo/fetus of mice is shown in Figure 17.4. The mice received an exposure of 200 R (or 2 Sv) at various times after fertilization. The outcomes studied were prenatal death, neonatal death, and "abnormalities." The graph shows the incidence of these outcomes as a function of days post conception. The equivalent time scale for humans is shown at the bottom. Assuming that these data are applicable to humans, the following conclusions may be drawn. Prior to implantation the result of this level of irradiation is almost always pre-natal death, presumably followed by spontaneous abortion. The woman may never know that she was pregnant. The period of organogenesis, roughly from day 10 to day 40 post conception for humans, is the phase during which the developing fetus is most sensitive to radiation. Differentiation of cells to form particular organs begins on specific days, resulting in specific abnormalities. During this phase a woman is unlikely to know that she is pregnant. Following this period the fetus is relatively insensitive to radiation. The incidence of abnormalities falls off rapidly as organogenesis progresses. One exception is the risk of severe mental retardation that peaks 8 to 15 weeks post conception, according to studies of individuals who were exposed as fetuses to atomic bomb radiation in Japan. The risk of severe mental retardation is estimated to be about 40% per Sv, with a threshold of about 15 Sv. Occupational workers are unlikely to be exposed to such large doses. Below

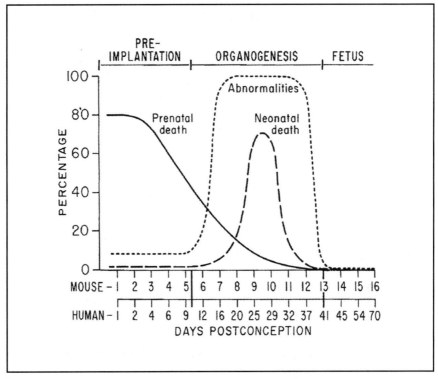

Figure 17.4: The effects of a 200 R irradiation of the embryo/fetus of mice at various times after conception. The human equivalent post conception time appears at the bottom. (Reproduced from Hall, E. J. *Radiobiology for the Radiobiologist,* 5th ed., Fig 12.1, p. 179, © 2000, with permission from Lippincott Williams and Wilkins.)

50 mSv the risk of congenital malformations is essentially nonexistent (1 in 800) compared to the risk of spontaneous congenital malformations (1 in 20) for all pregnant women. The developing embryo/fetus is most sensitive to radiation effects in the first trimester, less so in the second trimester, and significantly less so in the third trimester.

The crucial interval is before a woman is aware that she is pregnant. If you are a radiation worker and you are attempting to become pregnant, you may wish to take whatever steps you can to reduce your exposure to a minimum.

It has been reported that a few obstetric diagnostic x-ray images may increase the natural or spontaneous childhood cancer incidence by a factor of 1.5 to 2.0. An exposure of 1 to 2 cGy in utero increases the risk of leukemia (up to age 10) by a factor of 1.5 to 2.0 over the natural incidence. The natural incidence is about 4/10,000. The BEIR VII report indicates that exposures as low as 10 mSv in utero have been shown to result in excess cancers.[13]

---

[13] BEIR VII report: Health Effects from Exposure to Low Levels of Ionizing Radiation, Phase II, 2006.

17.3.3 Genetic Effects

Genetic effects are any abnormalities which can be inherited and therefore involve radiation exposure to reproductive organs. A large genetic study of the offspring of A-bomb survivors has failed to show any statistically significant genetic effects.[13] Genetic effects have been shown in animal studies and it seems likely that they do exist in humans also. According to the BEIR VII report, the mutation doubling dose is at least 1 Sv. Mutation induction resulting in damage to the human gene pool is not the primary concern for those who administer, receive or work with medical radiation. Nonetheless to minimize the radiation risk for genetic effects, gonadal doses should be kept to the practical minimum.

17.4 Radiation Protection Principles

The philosophy recommended is to assume maximum risk consistent with scientific data. To establish limits, it seems sensible to compare the risks of radiation with the risks in other industries that are considered safe. One can then set radiation exposure limits so that the risks are similar. ALARA: strive for exposure levels *As Low As Reasonably Achievable* taking into account social, technical, and economic factors. This can be basically summarized by saying that if there are easy steps that can be taken to reduce exposure, then these steps should be taken.

Exposure to radiation can come from external sources that deliver a radiation dose from outside the body. When radioactive material is introduced into the body, this is a source of internal exposure. Personnel exposure to external radiation can be minimized by considering three factors:

1. Time.
2. Distance.
3. Shielding.

Time: Reduce the time of exposure to a minimum. The amount of exposure is directly proportional to the time interval during which the exposure occurs.

Distance: Take advantage of the inverse square law, doubling the distance to a point source of radiation causes a four-fold decrease in radiation level.

Shielding: Adequate barriers can reduce radiation levels enormously. The thickness of the shielding required will depend on the material used, its distance from the source of radiation, and the energy and type of radiation to be shielded against. This is discussed further in section 17.8.

Some basic rules for avoiding internal radiation doses include restrictions on eating and drinking, use of protective clothing, hand washing, and avoidance of airborne radioactivity.

17.5 NRC Regulations

Important documents are 10 CFR Part 20, Standards for Protection Against Radiation and 10 CFR Part 35, Medical Use of Byproduct Material. NRC regulations pertaining directly to mandatory quality assurance (QA) procedures are discussed in chapter 18. We confine our attention to sealed sources; that is, the sources are encapsulated in some way and are not in the form of an open liquid or powder. This is a summary only; one must consult the full, detailed wording of the regulations to ensure full compliance.

The NRC formulates regulations, enforces those regulations, and conducts inspections. Inspections are performance based rather than a strict review of records and always include interviews with employees. Failure to comply with NRC rules and regulations can result in NRC press releases, fines, license revocation, and possibly criminal penalties. Leniency is usually shown for self-identified rule violations that are clearly disclosed and for which appropriate corrective action has been taken.

All radiation safety procedures must be carefully documented. If you didn't document it, you didn't do it! All of the records documenting compliance with the rules and regulations in Part 35 must be retained for various lengths of time depending on the nature of the document. For record keeping requirements, see Part 35, Subpart L.

17.5.1 Annual Dose Limits

The dose limits stated in 10 CFR Part 20 are based on general recommendations from the NCRP and the ICRP. It is useful to study these recommendations and in particular the rationale behind them. In this section, however, we will concentrate on NRC regulatory *requirements*. Permitted radiation exposure levels differ for occupational workers and members of the general public. Occupational workers are not permitted to exceed the occupational dose limits. Industrial and medical radiation facilities must take appropriate precautions so that they do not expose the public to levels in excess of the allowed levels for individual members of the public. Dose limits to the embryo/fetus apply to "declared" pregnant occupational workers. A declared pregnant woman is an occupational worker who has voluntarily informed her employer, in writing, of her pregnancy and the estimated date of conception.

I. Occupational Dose Limits for Adults
    Do not include:
    1. Background
    2. Medical exposure received as a patient
    3. Dose as a member of the general public

    Annual Limit; whichever is the more limiting of:
    1. Total effective dose equivalent of less than 50 mSv (5000 mrem)
    2. Deep dose equivalent + committed dose equivalent to any organ or tissue (except eye) less than 500 mSv (50 rems)
    3. Lens of the eye less than 150 mSv (15 rem)
    4. Shallow dose less than 500 mSv to skin or extremities

II. Individual Members of the Public
    1. Total effective dose equivalent less than 1.0 mSv (100 mrem)
    2. Dose equivalent in any unrestricted area cannot exceed 0.02 mSv in any one hour

III. Dose to Embryo/Fetus
    1. Must not exceed 5 mSv during the entire pregnancy
    2. It is recommended that the fetus receive no more than 0.5 mSv per month

IV. Occupational Dose Limits for Minors
    Must not exceed 10% of the annual dose limit for adult workers

V. ALARA
    To the extent practical, controls based on sound radiation protection principles are required to achieve occupational doses and doses to the general public that are as low as reasonably achievable (ALARA). Typically 10% of the dose limit is set as the guideline for investigations of the use of additional shielding or changes in the work environment so that lower exposure can be achieved.[14]

VI. Negligible Individual Risk Level (NIRL)
    The NCRP defines the NIRL as the "level of average annual excess risk of fatal health effects attributable to radiation below which efforts to reduce radiation exposure to the individual is unwarranted." It is considered a trivial risk compared to normal risk and is currently an annual effective dose of 0.01 mSv per source or practice.

---

[14] NRC Regulatory Guides 8.10, Operating Philosophy for Maintaining Occupational Exposures as Low as Reasonably Achievable; and 8.18, Information Relevant to Ensuring that Occupational Exposure at Medical Institutions will be as Low as Reasonably Achievable.

17.5.2 Medical License and General Requirements

Medical use of byproduct material requires a license from the NRC or Agreement State Radiation Control Agency and physician users must be authorized to use such materials. The term "authorized user" is a technical term. You are not an authorized user unless your name appears on an NRC (or Agreement State) license for the approved category of use (i.e. brachytherapy HDR, gamma stereotactic radiosurgery, etc.). The requirements to become an authorized user have become increasingly strict. To be an authorized user, a physician must be either board certified (in diagnostic, nuclear medicine, or therapeutic radiology) by an NRC-recognized medical board or possess specific educational training and experience as outlined in Part 35. Other physicians may be involved in the medical use of byproduct material if they work under the direct supervision of an authorized user (this covers, for example, medical residents). An authorized medical physicist is an individual who is named on a license. This individual is authorized to perform medical physics duties as specified on the license.

In addition to compliance with general NRC regulations, facilities must ensure that they abide by any special conditions appearing in their license. If you have any radiation safety responsibilities, you should carefully read the specific conditions of your clinic's license.

Medical licensee facilities are required to appoint a Radiation Safety Officer (RSO) who is charged with the task of oversight of the institution's radiation safety program. NCRP 105 (Radiation Protection for Medical and Allied Health Personnel) recommends that the RSO be a medical or health physicist. Medical institutions licensed for two or more types of use are required to have a radiation safety committee. This committee must include an authorized user for each type of use permitted by the license, the RSO, a representative from nursing, and a representative of management. The committee usually oversees all radiation safety policies and procedures including those under state and local jurisdiction, such as diagnostic x-ray units and linacs. The committee should meet as often as needed to ensure the radiation safety program is operating in compliance with the license, established procedures, and regulations. For most large programs, quarterly radiation safety committee meetings are necessary.

It is necessary for licensees to possess a survey meter. The survey meter must be calibrated before first use, annually, and after repair.

A semiannual inventory of all sealed sources (except gamma stereotactic) is required. This is to ensure that no sources are missing. Certain sealed sources must be tested for leakage before first use and at intervals not to exceed 6 months. This is to ensure that no radioactive material is leaking out of the encapsulated source. This is often referred to as a wipe test. Each source is wiped with a cotton swab or alcohol pad. An unused wipe is held in reserve as a control for background evaluation. The wipes are assayed in a well counter. The well counter must be shown to be capable of detecting a minimum of 0.005 μCi (185 Bq). If the assay reveals an amount of removable activity in excess of 0.005 μCi, then the source must be removed from use and a report must be sent to the NRC.

Only service personnel specifically licensed by the NRC or an Agreement State can "install, maintain, adjust or repair a remote afterloader unit, teletherapy unit or gamma stereotactic radiosurgery unit that involves work on the source(s), shielding, the source(s) driving unit, or other electronic or mechanical component that could expose the source(s), reduce the shielding around the source(s), or compromise the radiation safety of the unit or the source(s)."

Brachytherapy sources must be calibrated before first use, and positioning accuracy must be verified within applicators. The user must mathematically correct for source decay at intervals corresponding to not more than 1% change in activity. For Co-60 this means that the activity should be updated monthly. For Ir-192 the activity should be updated daily. HDR unit computers update the source activity at least twice daily.

17.5.3 Written Directives and Medical Events

The NRC requires a *written directive* prior to the administration of radiation treatment using any sealed radioisotope regulated by the NRC. In essence, this is a prescription that must meet the requirements spelled out below. The written directive must include the patient's name and must be dated and signed by an authorized user prior to administration. Additional requirements for various types of therapy are as follows:

1. Teletherapy (Co-60)
   a. total dose
   b. dose per fraction
   c. number of fractions
   d. treatment site
2. HDR brachytherapy
   a. radioisotope
   b. treatment site
   c. total dose
   d. dose per fraction
   e. number of fractions
3. Other brachytherapy
   a. prior to implantation
      i.   radioisotope
      ii. treatment site
      iii. total dose

    b. after implantation, but prior to completion
      i. radioisotope
      ii. treatment site
      iii. number of sources
      iv. total source strength and exposure time (or total dose)
4. Gamma or stereotactic radiosurgery
    a. total dose
    b. treatment site
    c. target coordinates

The "licensee shall develop, implement and maintain written procedures to" ensure that the patient's identity is verified prior to treatment and that each treatment is in accordance with the written directive. The reason for the first of these is to avoid treating the wrong patient. For example there may be two Mr. Smiths in the waiting room. Many clinics require two modes of identification. An example might be to ask the patient's name and to examine a photograph of the patient in the chart. Both manual and computer-generated dose calculations must be checked. Many clinics require a manual check for each patient.

The old term "misadministration" has been discarded by the NRC and the new term "medical event" has been introduced. A medical event is considered a serious deviation from the written directive. The NRC must be notified no later than the next calendar day of the discovery of a medical event and a written report must be submitted within 15 days. The patient and the referring physician must be notified within 24 hours.

One of the criticisms of the definition of the old term "misadministration" is that it included treatment of the wrong anatomical site. This resulted in endless debate about the meaning of this. If a treatment field is displaced by a few millimeters does this constitute treatment of the wrong anatomical site? The new term medical event attempts to remedy this, but unfortunately it results in a complicated and convoluted definition.

A **medical event** for sealed sources is defined as any treatment with a byproduct material in which:

1. A dose that differs from what would have been delivered following the written directive by more than 50 mSv effective dose equivalent, 0.5 Sv to an organ or tissue or a shallow dose equivalent of 0.5 Sv to the skin AND
    i. The total dose delivered *differs* from the prescribed dose by 20% or more;
    ii. The total dosage delivered *differs* from the prescribed dosage by 20% or more or falls outside the prescribed dosage range; or
    iii. The fractionated dose delivered *differs* from the prescribed dose, for a single fraction, by 50% or more.

2. A dose that exceeds 50 mSv effective dose equivalent, 0.5 Sv to an organ or tissue or a shallow dose equivalent of 0.5 Sv to the skin from any of the following:
   i.   administration of the wrong radioactive drug;
   ii. administration of dose to the wrong individual;
   iii. administration of dose by the wrong mode of treatment;
   iv. a leaking sealed source.
3. A dose to the skin or an organ or tissue other than the treatment site that exceeds by 0.5 Sv and 50% or more of the dose expected from the administration defined in the written directive. This does not apply to permanent seed implants in which the seeds were implanted at the correct location but have migrated outside the treatment site.[15]

The first part of the provision in 3 above appears to be designed to address the previous problem about "wrong anatomical site." Note that the criteria of this section are the same as occupational dose limits. If a treatment to the wrong anatomical site is delivered, it must exceed this threshold before it is defined as a medical event. Notice in 1, items i–iii, the word "differs". This means that an underdose can constitute a medical event. The allowed deviation for a single fraction (50%) is relatively large because a single fraction is only a portion of the total treatment and because compensation by adjusting the succeeding dose per fraction (presuming that there are any) is possible.

17.5.4   Examples of Events Reported to the NRC

This is a collection of events reported to the NRC. The descriptions are taken almost verbatim from the NRC web site.[16]

> A clinic delivered a 7 Gy dose to an unintended site using a HDR remote afterloader. The planned treatment site was a tumor in the bronchial area. The licensee measured and tested the patient's catheter using the dummy source. After the test, the catheter was placed in a box and sent for sterilization. On February 6, 2003, the licensee used what they thought was the correct catheter during one fraction. "When the patient returned on February 13, 2003, for the second fraction, a medical physicist discovered that the catheter was 30 centimeters too short." The

---

[15] Note that there is proposed rulemaking (preliminary draft rule changes to 10 CFR Part 35.40) that adds a unique category for permanent implants and specifies requirements for the written directive. It also specifically defines a reportable medical event for permanent implants, such as source implanted beyond 3 cm from the boundary of the treatment site.

[16] www.nrc.gov.

dose was delivered to the skin in the nasal passages rather than the bronchial area. The patient elected to continue treatment to the correct site.

This constitutes a medical event under the criterion 3 in section 17.5.3.

In the course of treating a breast cancer, a saline-filled balloon was used to aid in positioning the Ir-192 HDR source (approximately 9.6 Ci). A series of 10 fractionated treatments was prescribed. An ultrasound image was made to assure the continued proper placement of the source between each fraction. The ultrasound technician indicated all was okay for all treatments. After the series was completed, the balloon was deflated for removal and the physician then noted that the balloon had ruptured. A review of the retained ultrasound images indicated that starting with treatment 7, the balloon was deflated. The doses were recalculated and the tissue dose was 40% higher than prescribed. The adjacent skin dose was calculated to be 266 cGy rather than the 175 cGy as originally calculated. The licensee has proposed corrective measures to prevent a recurrence of this event. The balloon manufacturer has been informed of this event. The medical review indicates some additional fat necrosis and possible inflammation may occur. It will be reviewed as a part of the patient follow up.

This qualifies as a medical event under the criterion 1.i in section 17.5.3.

An HDR afterloader Ir-192 source (4.6 Ci) failed to retract following a patient treatment. The source became stuck in the transfer tube. The physicist started his stopwatch, entered the room and attempted to manually retract the source. Manual retract failed. The physicist called the physician, who was waiting outside the room. The physician entered the room and disconnected the apparatus from the patient and dropped the transfer tube into a lead pig (see Figure 17.5). The physicist and physician moved the patient out of the room. The physicist stopped the watch and it showed that 2 minutes had elapsed. The physicist surveyed the patient and obtained no measurement above background. The physicist re-entered the room and performed a radiation survey, and found the hot spot along the transfer tube to be in the pig. The pig measured 10 mR/h at 3 feet. The room was locked and posted until arrival of the manufacturer's representative, who also was unable to make the source retract. The manufacturer's representative placed the transfer tube into a shipping container and shipped it back to the manufacturer for further investigation. Doses to the patient, physicist, and physician were estimated as follows: patient skin dose (10 cm from

source for 2 minutes) = 9 rem; physicist for 2 minutes = 45 mrem; physician 125 mrem whole body and 15 rem extremity.
This is probably a medical event under criteria 1 of section 17.5.3.

It was discovered that 42 I-125 seeds were implanted into the bulb of a patient's urethra instead of his prostate. The urologist had misinterpreted the ultrasound scan. The total activity of the Iodine-125 seeds was 14.2 mCi. Each seed was 0.338 mCi. The patient and his referring physician have been notified of the error.
This requires dosimetric evaluation. It is likely to be a medical event under the criteria in 1 and 3 of section 17.5.3.

It was discovered that a patient receiving brachytherapy to the right lung using a HDR remote afterloader, received an actual dose less than the prescribed dose. The source was 5.2 Ci of Ir-192 and the prescribed dose was 2000 cGy, which was to be administered in four 500 cGy increments. The computer was programmed for the four fractions, but the total prescribed dose was set for 500 cGy, resulting in an actual dose delivered of 125 cGy during the first fraction. The patient was informed that the dose received was lower than intended and they would be receiving the total prescribed dose in the remaining three fractions.
This is a medical event under the criterion of 1.iii of section 17.5.3. The dose delivered during a single fraction was less than the prescribed dose per fraction by more than 50%.

A patient received a single-fraction HDR treatment for cervical cancer with a tandem and ovoid applicator. The written directive called for a dose of 500 cGy. Instead, the patient received a dose of 800 cGy. The dwell positions were incorrect because they had been entered in reverse order. The error was not detected until after treatment. This shows that the second check procedures were inadequate to detect the error.
This is a medical event. The total dose delivered differs from the prescribed dose by more than 20%.

17.5.5   Radiation Protection for Brachytherapy Procedures

Manual Brachytherapy Procedures

Manual brachytherapy procedures are those in which an afterloader is not employed. The sources are actually loaded by hand. Examples are

I-125 prostate permanent implants and temporary Cs-137 implants with tandem and ovoids for cervical treatment.

After implanting sources, a survey of the area must be conducted to account for all sources that have not been implanted. This is to prevent the loss of a source, which could expose personnel to unnecessary radiation. Immediately after a temporary implant is removed, the patient shall be surveyed. This is to ensure that no sources have been left inside the patient.

Temporary implants usually require the patient to remain in the hospital until the sources are removed. The door to the room must be posted with a "Radioactive Materials" sign. The patient should not be quartered in the same room as another patient who is not receiving brachytherapy.

For "in-patient" facilities, instruction must be given to care givers (usually nurses) initially and at least annually thereafter. The instruction must include a description of the size and appearance of the sources. Dummy sources or photographs (see Figure 16.4) can be used to accomplish this. Caregivers must be able to recognize a dislodged source. Instruction must be given in techniques of source handling and shielding. This may involve a set of tongs to pick up a dislodged source and a lead "pig" to place it in. A "pig" is a shielded container (see Figure 17.5). Such containers are routinely used for transporting sources around a hospital. Nurses are instructed to never pick up a source directly with their hands.

Caregivers must be aware of any restrictions on the patient. This may involve movement, bathroom privileges, etc. The nursing staff must be

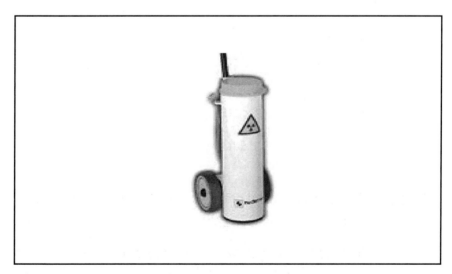

Figure 17.5: An emergency container, sometimes referred to as a "pig." (Courtesy of Nucletron B.V., Veenendaal, The Netherlands)

aware of restrictions on visitors. Usually no one under 18 and no one who is pregnant are allowed in the room. Visitors over 18 may not be permitted to sit closer than a certain distance and may be restricted on the amount of time that they may stay in the patient's room each day. Clear instructions must be posted and placed in the patient's chart about where and for how long visitors may stay in the patient's room.

A written log must be kept which accounts for the location and use of all brachytherapy temporary implant sources. This record must include the number and activity of sources removed from storage, the location of use, the date and time of removal, and the name of the individual who removed them from storage. When the sources are returned to storage, they must be logged back in.

Patients with permanent implants cannot be released from the hospital if they pose a radiation safety hazard to others. A patient may not be released unless the total effective dose equivalent to any other individual is not likely to exceed 5 mSv. To make this determination easier, the NRC has released practical guidelines for specific isotopes. For I-125 implants, if the total implanted activity is 9 mCi (0.33 GBq) or less the patient may be released. The patient may still be released, even if the implanted activity is higher than this, provided that the dose rate is less than or equal to 0.01 mSv/h at a distance of 1 m.

Source accounting is necessary for permanent implants as well as for temporary implants. The record must indicate the number and activity of sources removed from storage, the date they were removed and the individual who removed them. The disposition of all sources must be accounted for including the number and activity of sources not implanted, the name of the person returning them to storage and the number and activity of sources permanently implanted.

17.5.6   NRC Safety Precautions for Therapy Units

This covers afterloaders (HDR), teletherapy units (Co-60), and gamma stereotactic units (Gamma Knife®). Gamma Knife units are available in only a limited number of cancer centers and therefore we refer the reader to 10 CFR Part 35 for further details.

A radiation survey must be performed after initial installation and following certain repairs.

The treatment room must have a door with an interlock system. The interlock must prevent initiation of treatment if the door is open. The door interlock must also cause the source to be returned to the safe position if the door is opened while the source is exposed. The treatment unit must be secured when not in use. The keys must be removed from the console. The door to the room should be kept closed. This is to prevent any accidental irradiation. Any individual entering the room must

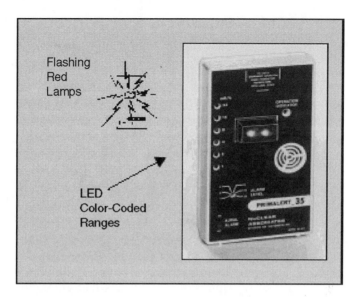

Flashing
Red
Lamps

LED
Color-Coded
Ranges

Figure 17.6: A fixed, wall-mounted radiation monitor. This unit can be placed in the entryway of a treatment room to indicate when a radioactive source is exposed.

verify that the source(s) have returned to the shielded position. This is usually accomplished by placement of a wall-mounted radiation monitor in the entryway (see Figure 17.6). These monitors are designed so that a red light blinks when the source(s) is(are) exposed. In the absence of such a monitor, a survey meter could be utilized.

The licensee must "develop, implement and maintain" written procedures to respond to an abnormal situation in which the operator is unable to place the source in the shielded position. These instructions must include a detailed description of how to respond when the source cannot be "turned off." A list must be available to the operator of the names and contact information for the RSO, authorized user(s), and authorized medical physicist(s).

Licensees must provide instruction to operators initially and at least annually on emergency and normal operating procedures for the unit. This must include drills of the emergency procedures. Licensees are required to have emergency response equipment to deal with a situation in which the source remains in the unshielded position, or lodged within the patient. For an HDR unit, emergency response equipment should include a shielded container (lead "pig") in which a dislodged source can be placed.

An intercom and viewing system must be available which allow continuous observation of the patient from the console during irradiation. The viewing system is frequently a closed circuit television system (CCTV).

NRC Safety Precautions for HDR Units

Each facility needs to develop local procedures depending on the model of HDR unit and the details of the particular installation. The discussion that follows is an overview for a typical installation. For a discussion of NRC-mandated HDR quality assurance procedures see *Specific Requirements for Remote Afterloading Units (HDR)* in chapter 18, section 18.2.2.

After treatment and before a patient is released the licensee shall perform a radiation survey of the patient and the afterloader to confirm that the source has been removed from the patient and returned to the afterloader safe. Occasionally, patients may arrive for HDR treatment who have had nuclear medicine imaging studies. These patients may be mildly radioactive and it is therefore useful to survey all patients both before and after HDR treatment.

At the beginning of any patient treatment both the authorized medical physicist and authorized user must be physically present. An authorized user or a physician (who has had emergency training) under the supervision of an authorized user (this could be a resident physician) and the authorized medical physicist must be physically present throughout the entire patient treatment.

Licensees are enjoined to only give treatments for which a stuck or dislodged source may be rapidly removed from the patient's body. The operator must know the signs of a stuck source. If the source fails to retract to the safe position, the console may show error messages and radiation warning lights may continue to be illuminated. The usual procedure is to first try the emergency off button at the console. If this fails, the operator or the physicist must go into the room and attempt to manually retract the source by turning a crank (see Figure 16.28). If this also fails, then the source (which will be attached to the cable) plus applicator/catheters must be removed from the patient. This may require physician assistance. The source is then to be placed in a shielded container ("pig", see Figure 17.5). The patient should then be removed from the room. The patient should be surveyed to ensure that no radioactive material is left inside the patient. The door to the treatment room should be secured and the HDR manufacturer should be notified.

NRC Safety Precautions for Co-60 Units

Licensees must have Co-60 units (and Gamma Knife units) fully inspected and serviced at the time of source change or at intervals not to exceed five years to "assure proper functioning of the source exposure mechanism."

The operator must know the signs that the source is stuck. An error message may appear on the console. The timer may indicate that the source has not returned to the shielded position even though the time "set" has been exceeded. The beam-on light at the console may continue to be illuminated. If there is a door light, it may continue to be illuminated. If there is any doubt, a survey meter should be used when entering the room. Many Co-60 units have a rod that protrudes from the end of the head when the source is exposed. The primary concern is to see to the safety of the patient. If the patient is ambulatory, the patient can be asked to get up and come out of the room. If the patient is not ambulatory, the therapists must go into the room and get the patient out. After the patient is safely out of the room, an attempt can be made to return the source to the "off" position. For most Co-60 units a "T-bar" can be used to attempt to manually push the rod that extends from the head of the machine (see Figure 9.25) back into the machine. This pushes the source back into the shielded position.

17.6 Personnel Monitoring

The NRC requires that personnel likely to receive 10% or more of the annual occupational limit and individuals entering a high radiation area must be monitored with a personal radiation detector. The NRC requires that personnel monitoring must include the deep-dose equivalent to the whole body, the eye dose equivalent, the shallow-dose equivalent to the skin, and shallow-dose equivalent to the extremities. There are several commercial firms that supply personal radiation detectors by mail. These detectors are in the form of a clip on badge (worn on the chest or at waist level, see Figure 17.7) or a ring, which measures exposure of the hands. Badges are usually worn for one month or for a calendar quarter. After this period the badges are returned to the vendor for evaluation. The vendor then sends the user a dosimetry report.

Originally, radiation badges used film to assess exposure. Today, whole-body badges contain a thin layer of aluminum oxide sandwiched between filters (see Figure 17.8) made out of aluminum, copper, or tin of varying thicknesses. When exposed to certain frequencies of laser light, aluminum oxide becomes luminescent in proportion to the radiation exposure. These badges can record exposures as low as 1 mrem. The amount of penetration through the filters enables some determination of the energy and type of radiation.

Things that can go wrong with badges:

- badge left in treatment room
- badge worn by individual during a medical procedure with radiation.

Badges are often worn on lab coats. It is not an uncommon occurrence to have a worker take off his lab coat and then leave it in the treatment room. If you know that your badge has inadvertently been exposed to radiation, inform the person in charge of the badge program or the RSO.

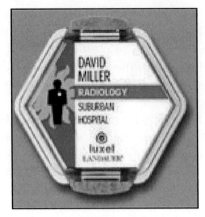

Figure 17.7: Personal radiation badge. (Courtesy of Landauer, Inc., Glenwood, IL)

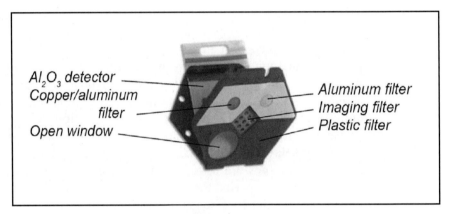

Figure 17.8: Inside of a badge showing the detector and the various filters which are used to determine the type of radiation exposure. (Courtesy of Landauer, Inc., Glenwood, IL)

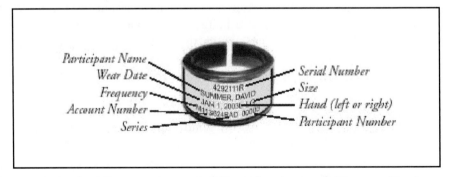

Figure 17.9: A ring badge should be worn whenever handling radioactive sources. (Courtesy of Landauer, Inc., Glenwood, IL)

Ring badges (see Figure 17.9) often have TLDs embedded in them. The readings are reported as shallow dose. A ring badge should be worn whenever handling radioactive sources.

A control dosimeter is shipped with badges. It is used to subtract the background radiation including dose received in transit. The control dosimeter must be kept shielded from stray radiation.

When you start a new job involving occupational radiation exposure, your employer should attempt to determine your exposure history from previous employers (if any) so that your total, cumulative radiation exposure can be followed. Your employer must maintain records of your exposure history.

A sample generic exposure report appears in Figure 17.10. Much of this report is self-explanatory. The first row shows the dose equivalent received by the control dosimeter. The "M" indicates that the dose equivalent is below the minimum threshold. The type of dosimeter depends on the monitoring needs and includes P for photon and beta; J for photon, beta, and fast neutron; T for photon, beta, fast/intermediate/ thermal neutron; and U for ring badges. The Use column indicates where the badge is to be worn. The radiation quality column specifies the type and energies of radiation contributing to the whole-body dose equivalent (PH: photon high energy > 200 keV; PM: photon medium energy 40 keV to 200 keV; PL: photon low energy < 40 keV). In succeeding columns the dose equivalent is listed for deep dose, eye dose, and shallow dose for the current dosimeter. These numbers are also given for the quarter to date because some states have quarterly limit criteria. The total lifetime deep dose equivalent is given in the next to last column.

RADIATION EXPOSURE REPORT

Dr RSO
Radiation Therapy Department
NoOaks Hospital
Rangaroon, MK

DATE BADGES RECEIVED	5/4/09
REPORT DATE	5/9/09
PAGE	1 OF 1

Badge Wearer Number	NAME (Last, first)	BIRTH DATE	SEX	DOSIMETER	USE	RADIATION QUALITY	MONITORING PERIOD		DOSE EQUIVALENT (MREM)										INCEPTION DATE (MM/YY)
									CURRENT			QUARTER TO DATE			YEAR TO DATE			LIFETIME TO DATE	
							BEGIN	END	DEEP	EYE	SHALL	DEEP	EYE	SHALL	DEEP	EYE	SHALL	DEEP	
	CONTROL				CNTRL				M	M	M								
12345	STACEY, MONICA	10/29/66	F	P	WH BODY	PH	09/01/08	09/30/08	23	23	23	23	23	23	254	248	248	1296	03/98
98765	PHILLIP, SEAN	6/27/89	M	P	COLLAR	PL	09/01/08	09/30/08	44	44	44	66	66	66	92	94	95	363	01/08
67891	ROSE, SHAYLA	10/20/77	F	P	WAIST	PL	09/01/08	09/30/08	37	38	38	37	38	38	307	306	303	2405	01/03
				U	FNGR						40			40			140		
54321	ATEN, RUDY	5/6/70	M	P	WH BODY		09/01/08	09/30/08	ABSENT										

NVLAP Accredited Laboratory

Figure 17.10: Sample radiation exposure report.

17.7 Shipment and Receipt of Radioactive Packages

The U.S. Department of Transportation (DOT) regulates the shipment of radioactive materials. The NRC regulates handling of packages once they are received. Radioactive materials must be in approved packaging that is appropriately labeled. The transport index (TI) is the highest radiation level (in mrem/h) that can be received by a person who is at 1.0 m from the external surface of the package.

Package labeling depends on the dose equivalent rate at the surface of the package.

17.7.1 Package Labels

Radioactive White I: All white background color, no special handling required, levels low, level at package surface ≤ 0.5 mrem/h (TI = background radiation).

Radioactive Yellow II: Label has upper half yellow (see Figure 17.11). At package surface radiation level is greater than 0.5 mrem/h but less than or equal to 50 mrem/h (TI ≤ 1.0).

Radioactive Yellow III: Yellow label with three stripes, transport vehicle must be placarded "Radioactive." Radiation level at the surface > 50 mrem/h but less than 200 mR/h (1 < TI < 10).

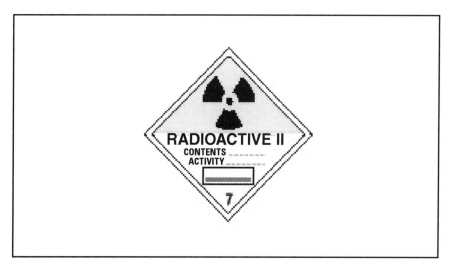

Figure 17.11: Radioactive package label "Yellow II".

17.7.2 Receipt of Radioactive Packages (NRC Regulations)

1. Monitor package surface as soon as possible after delivery, but not later than 3 hours after receipt if received during normal working hours—not later than 3 hours after beginning of next working day if received after working hours.
2. If radiation levels exceed 200 mrem/h at surface of package or 10 mrem/h at 1 m, immediately notify carrier and NRC.

17.8 Shielding Design for Linear Accelerators

In this chapter we will only discuss shielding of megavoltage external photon beam radiation. Other radiation-producing devices commonly found in radiation therapy departments are conventional simulators, CT simulators, HDR units, and superficial therapy units. Shielding considerations are somewhat different for these other devices. The details of shielding design for a linear accelerator room are complex. Here we shall discuss some of the main conceptual issues. The reference of record is NCRP Report 151, Structural Shielding Design and Evaluation for Megavoltage X- and Gamma-Ray Radiotherapy Facilities. Shielding calculations should be performed by a board-certified medical physicist or health physicist who is familiar with state and federal regulations and who represents the interests of the clinic.

In a radiation therapy facility, areas are classified as either controlled or uncontrolled. A controlled area is where personnel occupancy and activity are subject to control and supervision for the purpose of radiation protection. It is an area where the public is not allowed free access. An uncontrolled area is one in which the public has free access.

For multiple photon energy linear accelerators the shielding is generally designed for the highest beam energy. Linear accelerator beams with energies above 10 MV have a neutron contaminant that must be shielded against. Radiation shielding calculations are often based on "worst-case scenario" assumptions. In other words, estimates are always made to err on the side of extra shielding.

For radiation protection purposes, radiation is characterized in three different ways:

1. **Primary radiation:** This is radiation that comes directly from the source, it is the "useful" beam which is used to treat patients.
2. **Scatter:** This is radiation that is scattered out of the useful beam by the patient, treatment couch, etc.
3. **Leakage:** This is radiation that leaks out of the head of the treatment machine. The amount of leakage permitted is regulated to no more than 0.1% of the useful dose rate at 1 meter for linear

accelerators. The energy of the leakage radiation is usually somewhat less than the energy of the useful beam. In the absence of specific information to the contrary, a conservative assumption is that the energy of the leakage radiation is the same as for the useful beam.

The walls of a treatment room (or vault as it is sometimes referred to) must be shielded against each of these types of radiation. The point at which radiation levels are either calculated or measured is usually taken as 1 ft beyond the outside surface of a shielded wall. The reasoning is that this is about as close as an individual can come to a wall.

There are two types of shielding barriers. A primary barrier shields against the primary beam. The primary beam can point directly at this barrier. As the gantry is rotated through its range of angles, it may point at different primary barriers, usually the floor ceiling and two walls. A primary barrier may only be the section of a wall, floor, or ceiling that the primary beam strikes when the collimator jaws are open to their maximum setting. A secondary barrier shields against leakage and scatter. The primary beam cannot point at a secondary barrier for any gantry angle. See Figure 17.12 for an illustration.

Radiation protection levels quoted for shielding purposes are based on the allowable weekly dose equivalent in sievert. This quantity is given the symbol P and its units are $[P]$ = Sv/week or mSv/wk. In a controlled area the value of P that is consistent with NRC regulations (radiation workers, 50 mSv/50 weeks) is 1.0 mSv/wk. NCRP 151 recommends a value of 0.1 mSv/wk, which is one-tenth of the NRC regulatory limit. In an uncontrolled area (NRC public, 1.0 mSv/50 weeks) the value of P is 0.02 mSv/wk. This is also the value recommended by NCRP 151.

The shielding requirements of a treatment room depend on the amount of time that the beam is on. This is described by the workload, W, which is defined as the number of patients treated per week multiplied by the dose equivalent delivered per patient at a distance of 1 meter from the source of radiation. A busy treatment machine may treat 50 patients per day. If each of these patients receives 2 Gy then the workload will be W = 50 patients/day $\times$ 2 Sv/patient $\times$ 5 days/week = 5×10^2 Sv/week at 1 meter. Note that with the advent of IMRT, traditional estimates of the workload for secondary barriers may need to be revised upward to reflect the large increase in MU per treatment, which is sometimes associated with IMRT. As the beam is on longer for IMRT treatments, the cumulative amount of leakage is proportionately higher (see chapter 20).

The necessary thickness of a primary barrier will depend on the fraction of the time that the beam is pointed at this barrier. The use factor U for a primary barrier is the fraction of the time that the beam is pointed at that particular barrier. Recommended general values of the

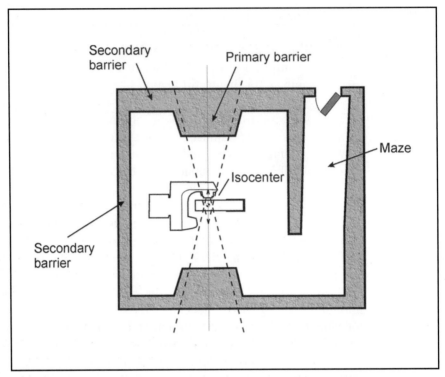

Figure 17.12: A "plan" view of a linear accelerator treatment room (vault). A primary barrier is any barrier that can potentially intercept the direct beam. Secondary barriers are all other barriers. Most treatment rooms have a maze, which is intended to reduce the amount of radiation that can reach the entryway. There is usually a door at the entryway.

use factor are shown in Table 17.6. The use factor for a secondary barrier is always 1.00, as leakage radiation is always present whenever the beam is on.

The areas adjacent to a treatment room may be offices, nursing stations, exam rooms, corridors, lavatories, etc. The exposure received by individuals depends on the fraction of the time that the area is occupied. The occupancy, T, is the fraction of the treatment day during which the area of interest is occupied by individuals. Some recommended occupancy values from NCRP 151 are:

> $T = 1$ (full occupancy): work areas, offices, treatment control rooms, nurses' station, etc.
> $T = 1/5$ (partial occupancy): corridors, staff rest rooms, employee lounge, etc.
> $T = 1/20$ (occasional occupancy): public lavatories, waiting rooms, storage areas, etc.
> $T = 1/40$ (transient occupancy): stairways, elevators, etc.

Some treatment machines are equipped with a beam stopper (see Figure 9.24). A beam stopper may be necessary if a treatment machine

Table 17.6: Use Factors*

Barrier	Use Factor U
Floor	0.31
Walls	0.21
Ceiling	0.26

*Data from NCRP Report No. 151: Structural Shielding Design and Evaluation for Megavoltage X- and Gamma-Ray Radiotherapy Facilities, 2005.

is to be housed in an existing room that is insufficiently shielded or in a new room where space is limited. A beam stop is inconvenient because it restricts accessibility to the patient couch. The mechanical tolerances of a linac gantry with a beam stop are generally not as good.

The basic procedure used to perform a shielding calculation for a specific barrier is to first determine the barrier transmission factor, B. This is the multiplicative factor by which the radiation level must be reduced so that it equals the design limit, P. The second step is to select the composition and required thickness of the barrier material. The barrier material selected depends on space and cost. Commonly used materials are concrete, lead, steel, and combinations thereof. Concrete is probably the most widely used material; it is effective for photons and for the neutron contaminate in high-energy linac beams.

In chapter 5 we discussed the half-value layer (HVL). Radiation shielding frequently requires a reduction in radiation levels by orders of magnitude. For this reason the thickness of shielding material is usually described in terms of tenth-value layers (TVLs). TVL = 1.0 corresponds to $B = 0.1$, TVL = 2.0 to $B = 0.01$, etc. Given the transmission desired, the number of TVLs needed is $10^{-\text{TVL}} = B$ and therefore:

$$\text{TVL} = -\log(B). \qquad (17.3)$$

An example of this is the case where $B = 0.1$, TVL $= -\log(B) = -\log(0.1) = 1$ as expected. The actual physical thickness of the material, in, say, centimeters, that corresponds to 1 TVL depends on the specific material and the radiation energy. For example, the TVL ($=1.0$) of concrete for an 18 MV beam is approximately 48 cm.

17.8.1 Primary Barriers

We can construct an equation for the necessary primary barrier transmission B_p in terms of the quantities W, U, and T that we have previously introduced and the distance d from the source of the radiation to the point protected, measured in meters. The radiation is attenuated by both geometric effects (inverse square) and absorption/scattering in the barrier material. The inverse square attenuation is governed by equation (5.5): $I_2/I_1 = (d_1/d_2)^2$. In this case $d_1 = 1$ meter (isocenter) and therefore $I_1 = W$. Let $d_2 = d$, the distance from the linac target (in meters) to the point protected. In this instance: $I_2 = P = W (1/d)^2$. If we add a barrier in the path of the radiation, then we must multiply by the barrier transmission B_p. We also multiply by the usage, U, and the occupancy, T. The weekly dose equivalent (in Sv) is then equal to:

$$P = \frac{WUT}{d^2} B_p, \qquad (17.4)$$

where d must be measured in meters. Given a limiting value of P, say 1.0 mSv/week, this equation can then be solved for the required barrier transmission B_p:

$$B_p = \frac{Pd^2}{WUT}. \qquad (17.5)$$

A typical value for the thickness of concrete necessary for a primary barrier is roughly 2 meters for a beam of 15–18 MV.

Example 17.1

A treatment room houses a linac with a 6 MV and 10 MV beam and no beam stopper. The distance from the radiation source to the inside of the primary barrier wall (+1 foot) of an adjacent room is 5 m. This room is a nurses station. The TVL of concrete for a 10 MV beam is 0.40 m. Assume a workload of 10^3 Sv/week. What is the total thickness of concrete needed to reduce P to 0.1 mSv/week (controlled, ALARA)?

$$B = \frac{Pd^2}{WUT} = \frac{10^{-4}(5)^2}{10^3(0.21)(1)} = 1.2 \times 10^{-5} \qquad (17.6)$$

TVL $= -\log(B) = -\log(1.2 \times 10^{-5}) = 4.9$ and therefore the required thickness of concrete is $= 4.9 \times 0.4$ m $= 2.0$ m.

17.8.2 Secondary Barriers

Leakage Radiation

This is radiation that escapes from the head of the treatment unit. Linear accelerators are designed so that the leakage radiation at 1.0 meter from the source is no more than 0.1% of the "useful beam." The use factor for secondary barriers is always assumed to be 1 since these barriers are always exposed to leakage whenever the beam is on. The weekly dose equivalent P for leakage radiation is given by

$$P = \frac{0.001 \, WT}{d_L^2} B_L, \qquad (17.7)$$

where the 0.001 represents the 0.1% leakage and B_L is the barrier transmission necessary to reduce the dose equivalent due to leakage and d_L is the distance from the isocenter to the point protected. This is a modified version of equation (17.4) where we have multiplied W by 0.001 and set $U = 1$. Given a regulatory limit for P, this equation can be solved for B_L:

$$B_L = \frac{Pd_L^2}{0.001 \, WT}, \qquad (17.8)$$

where d_L is in units of meters. The most conservative assumption is to assume that the energy of the leakage radiation is the same as the energy of the primary beam. Leakage barrier requirements are usually more important than scatter for megavoltage beams because leakage radiation is more penetrating, as we shall see.

Scatter Radiation

When a patient is irradiated, some of the radiation is scattered out of the patient. The amount of scattering depends on the dose rate, the beam energy, the area of the beam at the scatterer, and the scattering angle (see Figure 17.13). The quantity a is the ratio of scattered dose to incident dose. The value depends on the angle of scattering, the beam energy, and the field size. Tables for a as a function of scattering angle and beam energy are given in NCRP 151. For scattering at 90°, $a \approx 4 \times 10^{-4}$ for a 6 MV, 20 × 20 cm^2 beam. For the purpose of scatter to secondary barriers, the angle of scattering is approximately 90°. Recall from the discussion of Compton scattering in chapter 6 that the maximum energy of a photon scattered at 90° is 0.5 MeV. This radiation is much less penetrating than leakage radiation, which has roughly the

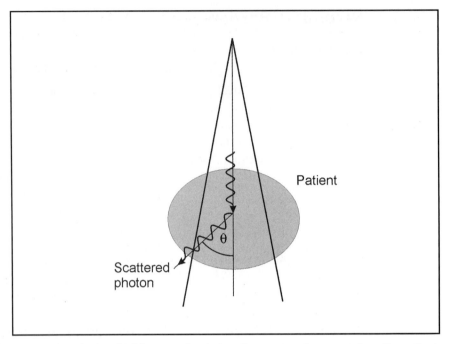

Figure 17.13: In general, radiation shielding must be designed to account for scatter from the patient. The scattering angle is θ.

same energy as the useful beam. For this reason, the scatter component of the radiation is generally less important than the leakage.

For a scatterer at a distance of 1 meter from the source,

$$P = \frac{aWT}{d_s^2}\frac{F}{400}B_s,\qquad(17.9)$$

where d_s is the distance from the scatterer to the point protected (in meters), F is the field size in units of cm^2, and B_s is the barrier transmission factor for the scattered radiation energy. The factor of 400 cm^2 corresponds to a 20 × 20 cm^2 field size. One usually assumes the maximum field size available for F. For most linacs this would be $F = 40$ cm × 40 cm = 1600 cm^2.

Given a limiting value of P, equation (17.9) can be solved for B_s:

$$B_s = \frac{P}{aWT}\frac{400}{F}d_s^2.\qquad(17.10)$$

Note that when looking up the TVL for B_s one must use the energy of the scattered radiation. For secondary barriers, B_L and B_s are calculated separately. One obtains a necessary barrier thickness for the leakage and a barrier thickness for the scatter. If the thickness of the barriers differs by 3 HVL, use the thicker barrier. If not, add 1 HVL to the larger one.

A nominal value of the thickness of a secondary concrete barrier for an 18 MV linac is about 1 m.

17.8.3 Neutrons

For linacs with beam energies above 10 MV, neutron contamination must be considered. Some neutrons are produced when high-energy photons and electrons are incident upon the target, flattening filter, and collimators. The neutrons are produced via photonuclear (γ, n) reactions, which are described briefly in chapter 6. These reactions are especially likely to occur for high-Z materials, such as the lead and tungsten in the head of a treatment machine. The neutrons produced by the (γ, n) reaction have energies ranging from 1 to 2 MeV. In the 16 to 25 MV range, the neutron contamination is roughly 0.05% neutron rem per cGy of photons. Note that the w_R value of the neutrons is already folded into this. The neutron contamination dose is clearly insignificant for patients, but it may not be insignificant in shielding considerations. If concrete is used for the primary and secondary barrier photon shielding, then the walls will be thick enough to absorb the neutrons. Concrete has a high hydrogen content and it absorbs neutrons efficiently. If lead or steel is used however, additional shielding may be necessary to absorb the neutrons. Barriers made of lead or steel may also be a source of neutrons as a result of (γ, n) reactions in the barrier material itself. This must be taken into account whenever using such materials.

17.8.4 The Entryway

Many treatment rooms have a "maze" (Figure 17.12). The purpose of the maze is to reduce the radiation level at the door. There are two sources of radiation at the doorway: primary x-rays (and neutrons) scattered off the walls and leakage/scatter transmitted through the inner wall of the maze. The maze is designed so that primary radiation must be scattered at least once to reach the door. If a room does not have a maze, then the door must be extra thick, particularly if the treatment machine has a high-energy beam (say, above 10 MV). In this case, the door may be so massive that it cannot be mounted on hinges and sliding doors may be necessary. Important considerations are the time it takes to open and close the door, whether the door can be opened manually in the event of a power failure, and safety features to prevent the door from closing if anyone gets caught in it. Evaluating the shielding necessary for a door in a room with a maze requires a method for determining the radiation levels at the end of the maze (doorway). A method for doing this is described in NCRP 151.

For linacs with beam energies above 10 MV neutron production is important. Some of these neutrons will diffuse down the maze and reach the door to the treatment room. By the time the neutrons reach the door some of the neutrons are thermal. These neutrons (thermal and fast) must be absorbed by the door. It is common to use borated polyethylene (5% boron by weight). The polyethylene has a high hydrogen content and is therefore very effective in slowing down the neutrons (see chapter 6, section 6.3). The boron absorbs neutrons. When the neutrons are captured by nuclei, the nuclei are left in an excited state and they emit γ-rays. The door must be shielded for the scattered x-rays, fast neutrons, thermal neutrons, and neutron capture γ-rays. For beam energies up to 20 MV, the typical treatment room door may have 4 to 5 in. of borated polyethylene, up to 1 in. of lead and ¼ in. of steel on the inside and outside face of the door. The lead must be on the *outside* of the door to attenuate the neutron capture γ-rays. A typical therapy room door for an 18 MV accelerator weighs approximately 3500 pounds and has a closing time of up to 19 seconds.

In addition to the door, provisions must be made for other room "penetrations," such as those needed for HVAC (heating, ventilation, and air conditioning).

17.8.5   Radiation Protection Survey of a Linear Accelerator

As soon as the first beam is generated during the installation of a linac, the "physicist of record" must perform at least a preliminary radiation survey to ensure that it is safe to continue to operate the linac.

Once the linac is completely operational and an initial calibration has been completed, a detailed radiation survey must be conducted. All occupiable areas near the linac must be surveyed to ensure that exposure limits are not exceeded. A Geiger-Müller counter may be used for locating hot spots, but this should be followed with measurements using an ion chamber survey meter (which is presumably more accurate, see chapter 8). For primary barriers the beam must be pointed at the barrier and the field must be set to the maximum size. Secondary barriers should be surveyed with a phantom in the beam and with the maximum field size. Door interlocks should be checked at this time (see chapter 9, section 9.2.4). A warning light, which is activated when the beam is on, should be located near the entrance to the room. The operation of this light should be checked during the survey. Some states may also require warning signs posted on the door to the room. In addition to measurements of high-energy photons, linacs operating above 10 MV should be assessed with a portable neutron survey meter to determine the neutron dose equivalent.

Chapter Summary

- **Equivalent Dose:** $H_T = D_T \times w_R$, where w_R is the radiation weighting factor, $[H_T]$ = sievert (Sv), 100 rem = 1 Sv. The value of w_R is 1.0 for x-rays and electrons. For neutrons the value of w_R depends on the energy and can be as high as 20. For alpha particles $w_R = 20$.

- **Effective Dose:** Effective whole body detriment (risk of fatal cancer and severe hereditary effects)

  $H_E = w_{T1}H_{1T} + w_{2T}H_{2T} + ... + $, where H_{Tn} is the equivalent dose to tissue/organ and w_{Tn} is the weighting factor for various tissues. The most sensitive tissues are gonads ($w = 0.2$) and bone marrow, lung, colon and stomach (all with $w = 0.12$).

- **Background Radiation:** Naturally occurring radiation from cosmic rays and radioisotopes found in nature.

- **Annual effective dose** for U.S. population is 6.2 mSv/y. Natural radiation contributes about half of this; medical exposure also contributes about half.

 Rule of thumb: The average daily effective dose equivalent to individual members of the public is about 0.017 mSv (1.7 mrem). This provides a context within which occupational exposure may be evaluated.

- **ALARA Principle:** *As low as reasonably achievable;* given social and economic factors

- **Basic Principles of Radiation Protection:**
  —Time
  —Distance
  —Shielding

Biological Effects of Radiation

- **$LD_{50} \sim 4$ Gy:** Acute whole body dose that is lethal to 50% of those humans exposed.

- **Deterministic Effects:** Increase in severity with increasing dose above a threshold, e.g., skin erythema, epilation, and cataracts.

- **Stochastic Effects:** Probability increases with dose, but severity is independent of dose. It is an all or nothing phenomenon, e.g., cancer, genetic effects.

- **Carcinogenesis:**
  —Latency: Time interval between exposure and appearance of malignancy (leukemia: 5 to 7 y; solid tumors: >10 y)
  —Lifetime risk of fatal cancer due to radiation exposure: 4×10^{-2}/Sv.

- **Risk to Fetus/Embryo:** Greatest during period of organogenesis (10 days to 6 weeks); rapid cellular differentiation and development.

Who Regulates What?

NRC: Regulates the use of "byproduct" material: Ir-192, Co-60, Cs-137, I-125, I-131, Pd-103, Sr-90; among others; naturally occurring isotopes or accelerator produced isotopes. See 10 CFR Part 20 and Part 35 (Medical Use of Byproduct Material, revised Oct 2002). Does not regulate linacs. Does regulate HDR units, Co-60 units. and Gamma Knife® because they use byproduct material.

FDA: Regulates manufacture and sale of radiation-producing machines (includes linacs); also treatment planning systems.

DOT: Regulates shipment of radioactive materials.

States: Regulate operation of x-ray machines and linear accelerators. If an "Agreement State," then takes over regulatory functions from NRC.

- **NRC Exposure Limits**
  I. Occupational Dose Limits
      Do not include:
      1. background
      2. medical exposure received as a patient
      3. dose as a member of the general public.
      Annual Limit; whichever is the more limiting of
      1. total effective dose equivalent of <50 mSv (5 rem)
      2. deep dose equivalent + committed dose equivalent to any organ or tissue (except eye): <0.5 Sv (500 mSv)
      3. lens of the eye: <150 mSv
      4. shallow dose: <0.5 Sv (500 mSv) to skin or extremities
  II. Individual Members of the Public
      1. total effective dose equivalent: <1 mSv (100 mrem or 1 mSv)
      2. dose equivalent in any unrestricted area cannot exceed 0.02 mSv in any one hour.

NRC Medical Event

Serious deviation from the written directive; NRC must be notified within 24 hours of discovery; written report must be submitted within 15 days. The patient and the referring physician must be notified within 24 hours.

1. A dose that differs from what would have been delivered following the written directive by more than 50 mSv effective dose equivalent, 500 mSv to an organ or tissue, or a shallow dose equivalent of 500 mSv to the skin AND
   i. The total dose delivered *differs* from the prescribed dose by 20% or more;
   ii. The total dose delivered *differs* from the prescribed dose by 20% or more or falls outside the prescribed dose range; or
   iii. The fractionated dose delivered *differs* from the prescribed dose, for a single fraction, by 50% or more.
2. A dose that exceeds 50 mSv effective dose equivalent, 500 mSv to an organ or tissue, or a shallow dose equivalent of 500 mSv to the skin from any of the following:
   i. administration of dose to the wrong individual;
   ii. administration of dose by the wrong mode of treatment;
   iii. a leaking sealed source.
3. A dose to the skin or an organ or tissue other than the treatment site that exceeds by 500 mSv and 50% or more of the dose expected from the administration defined in the written directive. This does not apply to permanent seed implants in which the seeds were implanted at the correct location but have migrated outside the treatment site.

Shielding Design

- **Controlled Area:** Where personnel occupancy and activity are subject to control and supervision for the purpose of radiation protection.

- **Uncontrolled Area:** Public has free access.

- **Radiation Categories for Shielding Design:**
  1. *Primary:* This is the "useful beam" used to treat patients.
  2. *Scatter:* Radiation scattered by a patient in the beam.
     a = ratio of scatter dose to incident dose ($a \sim 10^{-4}$); for 90° Compton scatter the maximum energy is 0.5 MeV.
  3. *Leakage:* Leakage from head of machine, regulated to be no more than 0.1% of useful beam at 1 meter.

- Barriers:
  1. *Primary:* Any barrier which useful beam can point toward; typical thickness is 2 m concrete for 15–18 MV beam room.
  2. *Secondary:* All barriers which are not primary, only need shielding for scatter and leakage; typical thickness is 1 m concrete for a 15–18 MV beam energy

  P = permissible radiation level in Sv/wk; depends on controlled or uncontrolled; NCRP 151 recommends 0.1 mSv/wk for controlled areas and 0.02 mSv/wk for uncontrolled areas.

  W = workload; dose equivalent delivered per week; typical value is 10^3 Sv/wk.

  U = use factor; fraction of the time beam is pointed at barrier ($U = 1$ for secondary barriers).

  T = occupancy; fraction of time area is occupied; $T = 1$ for work areas.

  B = barrier transmission factor.

  d = distance from target to point protected.

  d_L = distance from isocenter to point protected

  TVL = tenth-value layer; thickness necessary to reduce radiation level by a factor of 10; depends on beam energy and barrier composition: $10^{-\text{TVL}} = B$,   TVL $= -\log B$.

- **Primary Barrier:** $B_p = \dfrac{Pd^2}{WUT}$.

- **Secondary Barrier:**
  1. Leakage (usually dominates scatter) $B_L = \dfrac{Pd_L^2}{0.001\,WT}$.

  2. Scatter $B_s = \dfrac{P}{aWT}\dfrac{400}{F}d_s^2$.

- **Neutrons:** Neutron contamination important if beam energy >10 MV; if barriers designed for photons are concrete, they will be adequate for neutrons.

- **Entryway:** Maze reduces dose equivalent at door. Typical door: 4 to 5 in. borated polyethylene; 1 in. of lead outside poly to absorb neutron capture γ-rays; ¼ in. steel on inside and outside face of door.

Problems

1. Convert 1 mrem to mSv.

2. If the annual effective dose from radon exposure is 200 mrem,
   a. what is the equivalent dose to the bronchial endothelium?
   b. what is the absorbed dose in this tissue?

3. A chest x-ray delivers an absorbed dose of 10 mrad to the lungs (assume that only the lungs are irradiated).
   a. What is the value of the effective dose?
   b. What is the risk of developing a fatal cancer as a result of this x-ray exam?

4. Cancer caused by radiation can be distinguished from cancer caused by other factors. *True* or *False*.

5. Exposure to radiation has been shown to cause hereditary genetic effects in humans. *True* or *False*.

6. Of the 120,000 atomic bomb survivors that have been followed, the total number of excess cancer deaths as of 1990 has been _____ .

7. The effective dose from an average CT scan is approximately _____ times the average annual effective dose.

8. What is the single biggest natural source of radiation exposure for the average person?

9. There is some evidence that a few abdominal x-ray images of a pregnant patient can double the likelihood of childhood cancer. *True* or *False*.

10. Which personnel must wear radiation badges?

11. What is the purpose of the use of filters in radiation badges?

12. An 18 MV linac treats 40 patients per day, 5 days per week. If the average number of fields per patient is 2 and the average dose per field is 100 cGy, what is the workload?

13. What is the numerical value of the use factor in a secondary barrier calculation? Why?

14. a. What materials are used to shield against neutrons in radiation therapy room doors?

    b. What types of linacs require such shielding?

15. The control room of an 18 MV linear accelerator is shielded by the primary concrete barrier of the treatment room. When the beam is pointed toward the control room, the distance from the linac target to a point of protection (1 ft beyond the wall) is 6.6 m.

    a. Assuming a workload of 10^3 Sv/wk, what barrier transmission is necessary to reduce the exposure to 0.1 mSv/wk?

    b. How many TVL are necessary?

    c. If the TVL for an 18 MV beam is 48 cm in concrete, what is the required thickness of this primary barrier?

16. Three therapists work at the treatment console of a linear accelerator. What value should be used for the occupancy factor? Justify your answer.

17. What is the current NRC total effective dose limit for (a) radiation workers and (b) members of the general public?

18. Who must be on a radiation safety committee?

19. What information is required as part of the written directive for a high dose rate brachytherapy treatment?

20. Under what conditions can a patient with a radioactive implant be released from the hospital?

Bibliography

American Association of Physicists in Medicine (AAPM) Report No. 53, Radiation Information for Hospital Personnel. Woodbury, NY: American Institute of Physics, 1995.

Biological Effects of Ionizing Radiation (BEIR V). Health Effects of Exposure to Ionizing Radiation. Washington, DC: National Academies Press, 1990.

Biological Effects of Ionizing Radiation (BEIR VII). Health Effects from Exposure to Low Levels of Ionizing Radiation, Phase II. BEIR VII. Washington, DC: National Academies Press, 2006.

Code of Federal Regulations, Title 10, Part 20: Standards of Protection Against Radiation, October 2007.

Code of Federal Regulations, Title 10, Part 35: Medical Use of Byproduct Material. April 24, 2002.

Gottfried, K-L. D., and G. Penn (eds.) *Radiation in Medicine: A Need for Regulatory Reform.* Committee for Review and Evaluation of the Medical Use Program of the Nuclear Regulatory Commission. Washington, DC: National Academies Press, 1996.

Hall, E. J. *Radiobiology for the Radiologist,* 5th Edition. Philadelphia: Lippincott Williams & Wilkins, 2000.

International Commission on Radiological Protection (ICRP) Publication 60: 1990 Recommendations of the International Commission on Radiological Protection. Annals of the ICRP 21/1–3, 1990.

McGinley, P. H. *Shielding Techniques for Radiation Oncology Facilities,* Second Edition. Madison, WI: Medical Physics Publishing, 2002.

National Council on Radiation Protection (NCRP) Report No. 94: Exposure of the Population in the United States and Canada for Natural Radiation. (Supercedes NCRP Report No. 45). Bethesda, MD: NCRP, 1987.

National Council on Radiation Protection (NCRP) Report No. 105: Radiation Protection for Medical and Allied Health Personnel. (Supercedes NCRP Report No. 48). Bethesda, MD: NCRP, 1989.

National Council on Radiation Protection (NCRP) Report No. 115: Risk Estimates for Radiation. Bethesda, MD: NCRP, 1993.

National Council on Radiation Protection (NCRP) Report No. 116: Limitation of Exposure to Ionizing Radiation. (Supercedes NCRP Report No. 91). Bethesda, MD: NCRP, 1993.

National Council on Radiation Protection (NCRP) Report No. 151: Structural Shielding Design and Evaluation for Megavoltage X- and Gamma-Ray Radiotherapy Facilities. Bethesda, MD: NCRP, 2005.

National Council on Radiation Protection (NCRP) Report No. 160: Ionizing Radiation Exposure of the Population of the United States. Bethesda, MD: NCRP, 2009.

Nuclear Regulatory Commission (NRC) Guide 8.29: Instructions Concerning Risks from Occupational Radiation Exposure. Washington, DE: NRC, 1996.

Shapiro, J. *Radiation Protection: A Guide for Scientists, Regulators and Physicians,* Fourth Edition. Cambridge, MA: Harvard University Press, 2002.

18 Physical Quality Assurance and Patient Safety

18.1 Introduction

It is important to follow the recommendations of official organizations with respect to quality assurance (QA) tests, the frequency of these tests, and tolerance values. Generally such recommendations are becoming more voluminous with time and tolerances are becoming more stringent. Regulators and accrediting bodies are mandating more and more QA procedures. At the same time, with the advent of managed care, it is becoming increasingly difficult to afford costly QA programs. It has been estimated that the total cost of a comprehensive QA program in radiotherapy is approximately 3% of the annual billing for combined technical and professional charges. The impetus for QA hopefully stems from a desire to practice good radiotherapy. Perhaps a secondary consideration is the wish to avoid litigation. The International Commission on Radiation Units and Measurements (ICRU) has called for a dose delivery accuracy of ±5% based on the steep dose response curves for tumor control and for normal tissue complications (see ICRU reports 24 and 42).

This is a very stringent requirement. This implies that all of the uncertainties in the radiotherapy "chain" of treatment from simulation to treatment delivery must have an accuracy of better than 5%. The spatial accuracy required for dose delivery is generally 5 to 10 mm although in some cases (stereotactic radiosurgery) it is clearly smaller than this.

Recommendations pertaining to radiation oncology have been published by a bewildering "alphabet soup" of bodies, organizations, regulatory agencies, etc. These are the American College of Radiology (ACR), the American Association of Physicists in Medicine (AAPM), the American College of Medical Physics (ACMP), the International Commission on Radiation Units and Measurements (ICRU), the Joint Commission on Accreditation of Health Care Organizations (JCAHO), and the U.S. Nuclear Regulatory Commission (NRC). It would be unwise and perhaps legally indefensible to deviate from the recommendations of relevant advisory bodies. Medical professionals are generally expected to follow "standard and customary practice" in their specialty. The AAPM has published a comprehensive guide for quality assurance in radiation therapy: "Comprehensive QA for radiation oncology: Report of AAPM Radiation Therapy Task Group 40."[1] This "TG-40" document is the *de facto* standard among physicists and much of this chapter will be based on it. The TG-40 report has recently been updated for medical accelerators by Task Group 142.[2]

We will only address the physical aspects of QA here because it is this that is generally under the purview of the physicist, and even at that we will only cover some of the major aspects of QA. This is a huge subject on which large monographs have been written. There are many nuances and subtleties that are beyond the scope of this discussion. The reader is referred to the bibliography for more detail. In this text we distinguish between equipment QA and patient QA. Equipment QA consists of tests carried out on equipment or software whereas patient QA consists of various checks, tests, or measurements to ensure that a specific patient receives the correct treatment.

18.2 Equipment Quality Assurance

In this book the term "tolerance" will be used to indicate the maximum allowable difference between the measured value of a parameter and the expected value. *If the difference exceeds the tolerance value, then some action must be taken.* An example is provided by beam output measurements. Suppose a linear accelerator (linac) is calibrated to produce an output of 1.000 cGy/MU in phantom under some standardized conditions. The tolerance for daily checks of photon beam output is given by AAPM TG-40 as ±3%. Suppose on a certain day, the output is measured

---

[1]*Medical Physics*, vol. 2, issue 4, April 1994, page 581 (AAPM Report No. 46).
[2]*Medical Physics*, vol. 36, issue 9, September 2009, pages 4197–4212 (AAPM Report No. 142).

under standard conditions and the value is 1.05 cGy/MU. In this instance, the output exceeds tolerance and some action must be taken. Every radiation therapy department must establish policies and procedures for dealing with situations like this.

When new equipment is acquired, it is generally subjected to acceptance testing. Examples are linear accelerators, simulators, HDR units, and treatment planning systems. Acceptance testing consists of those tests and measurements designed to verify that a new piece of equipment or software meets the specifications given by the manufacturer. Generally these are the generic specifications listed by the manufacturer, although in some cases custom specifications may be stated during the purchase negotiation. Usually the acceptance testing protocol is specified by the manufacturer; that is, the manufacturer specifies measurement techniques. These procedures are usually carried out jointly by the installation technician and the physicist. Once the physicist is satisfied that the machine has been installed properly and that it meets all specifications, he or she will sign a document formally accepting the machine. The machine is then turned over to the customer and the unpaid balance of the purchase price is remitted.

Once acceptance testing is complete, the process of commissioning begins. This process consists of all those procedures necessary to put the device or machine into routine clinical use. For a linear accelerator with two photon energies and a variety of electron energies, the AAPM (TG-45 report[3]) has estimated that this process is expected to take "6–8 weeks of intensive effort (requiring 16 hour shifts)". The commissioning process for a linear accelerator begins with a careful radiation survey of all contiguous occupiable areas (see chapter 17, section 17.8.5). All beams must have an absolute calibration following the AAPM TG-51 protocol (see chapter 10). Depth dose data must be collected for the full range of field sizes for every beam energy. Both cross-plane and in-plane beam profiles are measured at a range of depths for every beam energy for open beams and for all wedges. These are just some of the measurements that must be made. It is then necessary to enter all of this data into the treatment planning system.

Acceptance testing and commissioning establish the baseline performance of the product.

Regular and on-going QA testing is necessary for linear accelerators, conventional simulators, CT simulators, HDR units, and treatment planning systems. An equipment quality control program must specify these elements:

1. Parameters to be tested or the tests to be performed.
2. Instruments to be used to perform the tests.
3. Test set up (geometry, etc.).
4. Frequency of the tests.

---

[3]*Medical Physics,* vol. 2, issue 7, July 1994, page 1093 (AAPM Report No. 7).

5. Individuals responsible for testing.
6. Expected results or values.
7. Tolerance level.
8. Action to be taken when tolerances are exceeded.

These elements should be in the form of written policies and procedures.

18.2.1 Linear Accelerators

There are now over 4000 medical linear accelerators in the United States. An essential reference for linac QA is the TG-45 report "AAPM code of practice for radiotherapy accelerators: Report of AAPM Radiation Therapy Task Group No. 45."[3]

QA procedures for linear accelerators can be divided into three major categories:

1. Mechanical.
2. Dosimetric.
3. Safety.

Most mechanical tolerances for linear measures, such as laser position, optical distance indicator, etc., are ±2 mm. Angular tolerances, such as gantry angle readout, are 1.0 degree; dosimetric tolerance for beam output is 2% for the monthly check.

QA procedures for linear accelerators are carried out on a daily, monthly, and annual basis. At most centers the daily QA is performed by the therapists as part of the machine warm-up process. The monthly check is generally much more extensive and is performed by a physicist. A monthly QA check of a dual-energy linac with electron beams may take as long as 5 to 7 hours, with perhaps many hours of later follow-up work. The annual QA is a very extensive set of checks and measurements that may take several days of machine time and many subsequent days for data analysis and report writing. The order in which some tests are done is crucial because they depend on previous tests.

Daily Checks

A summary of the TG-40 recommendations for daily checks is given in Table 18.1.

Mechanical Checks

Localizing lasers are used for patient setup (see Figure 18.1). Lasers help to level, align, and orient the patient and to ensure that the patient is in the same position for every treatment. Some of these lasers pro-

Table 18.1: Daily Quality Assurance Procedures for Linear Accelerators

	Procedure	Tolerance
Mechanical	Localizing Lasers	±2 mm
	Distance Indicator (ODI)	±2 mm
Dosimetry	X-ray Output	±3%
	Electron Output	±3%
Safety	Door Interlock	Functional
	Audiovisual communication	Functional

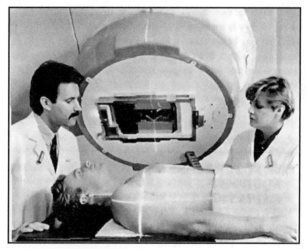

Figure 18.1: Side laser fan beams as they appear on a patient's skin. (Reprinted from Karzmark et al., *Medical Electron Accelerators,* Fig. 1-26b, p. 28, © 1993, with permission from McGraw-Hill.)

duce fan beams (see Figure 18.2). Side lasers are mounted on the walls to the left and right of the gantry, as seen when facing the gantry. These are generally set up to produce a fan beam in a vertical plane and a fan beam in a horizontal plane with perhaps a spot in the center of the fan beam that points toward the isocenter. The side lasers are used to ensure that the patient is leveled properly before treatment. The table must be at the correct height and the patient must lie flat with no rotation about the inferior-superior axis. The sagittal laser is mounted on the wall opposite the gantry stand and produces a fan beam in a vertical plane. This laser is used to ensure that the patient is lined up along the long axis of the table. The ceiling laser is mounted in the ceiling and points vertically downward toward the position of the isocenter. This is sometimes just a spot laser. Lasers must be firmly mounted. They should be anchored in concrete or metal support beams and not in drywall. Lasers

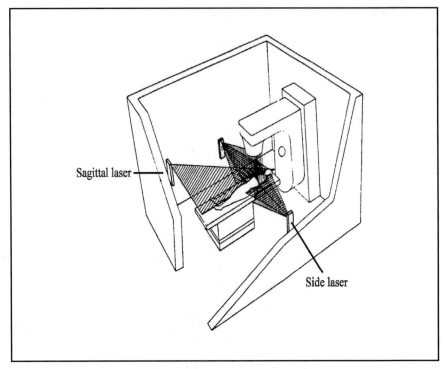

Figure 18.2: Side and sagittal fan beam lasers. Note that for the side laser there are both horizontal and vertical fan beams. (Courtesy of Gammex, Inc., Middleton, WI)

are frequently placed in a recess in the wall to prevent them from being bumped. They must be relatively insensitive to mechanical shock from carts, etc., bumping up against the walls. Most radiation therapy lasers are solid-state diode lasers with 0.05 mW power (although some helium-neon gas lasers are still around). They are similar to lasers used as grocery store scanners. They are relatively safe for the eyes for *very brief* exposures.

Laser beams must be checked on a daily basis. Lasers beams must point to the isocenter and they must be collinear. This is illustrated in the diagram in Figure 18.3. The tolerance for laser positioning is ±2 mm. The side lasers can be checked by positioning the treatment tabletop at the gantry isocenter using the distance indicator (or optical distance indicator, ODI). For most linacs the tabletop would be set at 100 cm SSD. The lasers should then just skim the tabletop on both sides. This presumes that the ODI is correct. The side lasers can be checked for collinearity by taking a semitransparent card and moving it back and forth in the cross-plane direction. Your hand can be used to block one beam and then the other beam. The two beams should overlap one another. Lack of collinearity, if severe, should be corrected. Another method of checking side lasers is with the use of wall marks. When the lasers are first installed and adjusted, marks can be made on the opposite walls where the beam strikes (see Figure 18.4). These marks can

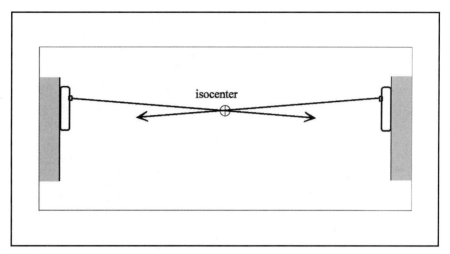

Figure 18.3: Side laser beams that point properly toward the isocenter but are not collinear; that is, they do not overlap except at the isocenter. Adjustment is needed to make these collinear.

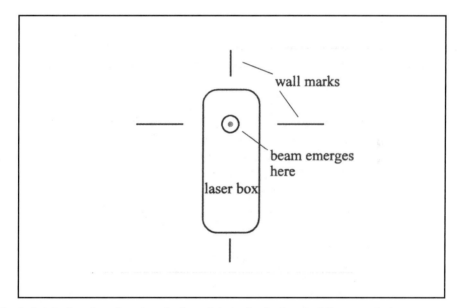

Figure 18.4: A sketch of wall marks set up for laser "aiming" adjustment of the opposite laser.

then be used in the future as reference fiducials to check the "aim" of the laser. The aim point of a laser can change as a result of mechanical shock (a cart bumping into the wall), temperature changes in the room, etc. There are usually knobs (or sometimes hex or Allen head screws) that can be used to adjust the aim point of the fan beam (either horizontally or vertically). There are now some positioning lasers available that feature remote control steering.

The field light of a linac projects down from the collimator onto the patient's skin and shows the region that will be irradiated when the beam is turned on (see Figure 9.20). There is usually a reticule in the beam that has a cross hair on it. The center of the cross hair indicates the axis of rotation of the collimator (i.e., the central axis). The sagittal laser can be checked by noting whether the fan beam line on the table runs through the center of the cross hair of the field light. The ceiling laser can be checked by positioning the gantry upright, marking the location of the cross hair on a piece of tape attached to the table, and then rotating the gantry out of the way to verify that the spot from the laser coincides with the mark on the piece of tape.

The distance indicator, range finder, or optical distance indicator (ODI) is a scale that is optically projected downward and shows the distance to the surface. The ODI must be checked daily; the ODI tolerance is ±2 mm. The ODI can be checked against the lasers by positioning the tabletop to the SAD (100 cm for most linacs) and then verifying that the lasers just skim the tabletop. For daily checks it is often the case that both the ODI and the side lasers are checked simultaneously in this way. If a discrepancy is found, it may not be immediately obvious whether the problem lies with the ODI or lasers. In this case, further tests are necessary.

The ODI can also be checked with the use of a front pointer. A front pointer is a long rod that can be inserted into the collimator (see Figure 18.5). The rod extends downward along the axis of rotation of the collimator. The rod can slide up and down. The rod is ruled so that the distance from the radiation source to the end of the rod can be read. During installation the technician will carefully adjust the reading of this rod so that its tip corresponds to the position of the gantry isocenter when the rod reads 100 cm. As front pointers are adjusted specifically for each individual linac, they should not be "swapped" between machines. The front pointer can be used to check the ODI by raising the table until the tip of the front pointer just touches the tabletop. The ODI should then read the same as the front pointer. If it is out of tolerance, the ODI can be adjusted by a service technician or a physicist.

Dosimetry Check

The "output" of a linac should be checked daily for all beams. The tolerance for the daily check is ±3% for both electron and x-ray beams. There are a variety of devices that can be used to perform this test. There are dedicated specialized devices, sometimes called "beam analyzers," that are designed for this purpose. These often consist of an array of ion chambers or diodes. An example is shown in Figure 18.6. There is a central detector that is used to check output and off axis

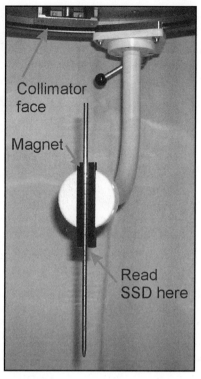

Figure 18.5: A front pointer for an Elekta linac. The front pointer assembly is clamped to the collimator face. The pointer itself extends along the central axis and is held in place by a magnet. The front pointer rod can slide up and down. When the tip of the pointer is in contact with a surface, the SSD can be read from the scale as shown. This can be used as a check against the optical distance indicator.

detectors to check beam flatness and symmetry.[4] For ion chamber beam analyzers, corrections must be made for temperature and pressure variations if the ion chambers are not sealed. On some devices this is done automatically by the beam analyzer. It is permissible to use a single diode for output checks provided that it can be shown that the reading is accurate enough that discrimination on the 3% level is possible. The diode might be the same one used for patient in vivo dosimetry measurements. Another possibility is to use a single ion chamber, such as a Farmer chamber, and a plastic phantom. For any one of these devices it is the responsibility of the physicist to calibrate the check device and to establish tolerance readings.

---

[4] TG-40 does not require that beam flatness and symmetry be checked on a daily basis.

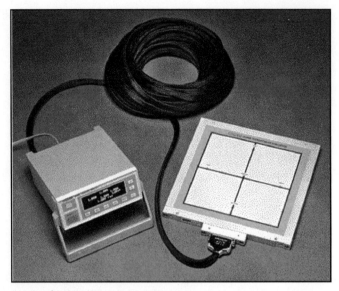

Figure 18.6: A radiation beam daily output check device. The detector, shown on the right, has five built-in ion chambers. The central ion chamber is used to check output, and the four outlying chambers can be used to evaluate flatness and symmetry. The display, shown on the left, is usually placed at the linac console. (Courtesy of Fluke Biomedical, Everett, WA)

Safety Checks

An intercom providing two-way communication with patients must be in working order. A closed-circuit television (CCTV) monitor that provides for continuous observation must be operational. All treatment rooms must have door interlocks that prevent the beam from turning on if the door is open and that interrupt the beam if the door is opened while the beam is on. Door interlocks must be checked daily. Warning lights on the console and at the room entry must illuminate when the beam is on. On the console of some linacs the buttons may be illuminated indicating the status of the linac. On older linacs there may be a lamp test button to check that all buttons can be illuminated when necessary. This should be checked daily.

Monthly Linac QA

We will describe here some of the main checks that are done on a monthly basis.

Mechanical

The light field on an external beam treatment unit is used to show where radiation will go. It is presumed that outside the light field there will be no primary radiation and that inside the light field there will be. The light field and the radiation field should be congruent or coincident with one another. That is, they should correspond in both size and position. One way to test this is with the use of "ready pack" film. This is a single sheet of film that is enclosed in an opaque paper wrapper. The ready pack film is taped to the tabletop, which is set to the height of the isocenter. The collimator is set for a nominal field size such as 20×20 cm^2. The light field is turned on and the edges of the light field are traced onto the paper-covered film with a ball-point pen and a ruler. The pen marks should be made with "heavy" pressure on the pen tip so that some of the emulsion on the film inside the wrapper will be scratched off. The marks will then clearly show up when the film is processed. Square plates of phantom material such as polystyrene, "virtual water," or acrylic are then placed over the film. The thickness of the stack of plates should be at least as great as the d_m value for that beam. The reason for this is to prevent any electron contamination from reaching the film. The film is then irradiated. On the processed film, the lines drawn to delineate the light field should correspond to the sides of the irradiated field. The tolerance for the mismatch between the light and radiation field is 2 mm. The position of the light field can be adjusted by changing the angle of tilt of the mirror in the treatment head (see Figure 9.20).

The gantry angle is displayed by both a digital and mechanical indicator. Both of these must be checked for accuracy. The gantry angle can be checked with the use of a bubble level. A level with a magnet is useful for magnetic surfaces. Most linacs have a machined surface somewhere on the treatment head. When the gantry is upright, this surface is perfectly horizontal. The level is attached to this surface, the gantry is rotated until the bubble is centered, and then the digital and mechanical readouts are read. They should both read 0° (IEC scale). A gantry angle of 180° can be checked in a similar fashion. Gantry angles of 90° and 270° can also be checked with most bubble levels since they generally also have a bubble that indicates when a surface (the collimator face) is perfectly vertical. The tolerance for either the gantry or the collimator angle is 1°. The digital and the mechanical readout can be adjusted to give the correct value.

The field size indicator displays the size of the field as measured at the isocenter. If the coincidence of light and radiation field has already been checked, then the field size can be evaluated by measuring the size of the light field projected onto the treatment table with the table surface at the SAD of the unit. A range of field sizes are set from 5×5 to 35×35 cm^2. These field sizes can be measured directly with a ruler and compared with the field displayed. The field size tolerance is 2 mm. If there is a disagreement between the measured field size and the displayed field size, then the value of the displayed field size is adjusted by a service technician so that it agrees with the measured value.

The central axis of a teletherapy treatment beam corresponds to the rotation axis of the collimator. The shadow of the cross hair that is visible on the treatment table when the light field is turned on should correspond to the location where the central axis "pierces" the table. It is very important that the cross hair be centered in this way, because the cross hair is used to locate the central axis on the patient's skin. The cross hair centering can be checked by placing a piece of masking tape on the treatment table so that the shadow of the cross hair falls on it. The position of the cross hair is marked with a small dot of ink from a pen. The collimator is then rotated through its full range. If the cross hair remains centered on the original dot of ink, then the cross hair is truly centered on the collimator rotation axis. If collimator rotation results in movement of the cross hair with respect to the original dot, then new dots can be placed at the location of the cross hair for various collimator angles. The result will be a partial circle of dots as shown in Figure 18.7. This is sometimes called "run out." We do not see a full circle because the collimator cannot rotate through 360°. The diameter of this circle should not be more than 2 mm. If it is, then the cross hair needs to be moved in an attempt to eliminate the "run out." It may not be possible to completely eliminate the run out because the collimator may not rotate about a single fixed axis (it may wobble a bit) as a result of worn bearings, etc.

Dosimetry

At the time of absolute calibration, a monthly check system must be established for the purpose of evaluating changes in output (see chapter 11, section 11.8). This may need to be a more accurate system than the daily

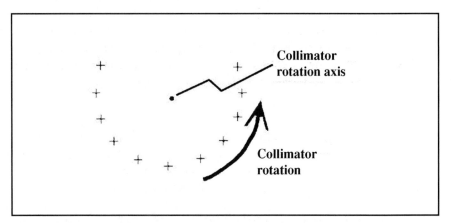

Figure 18.7: In this view the collimator rotation axis is into the page. When the cross hair (+) is not on the rotation axis (central axis) of the collimator, a circular pattern is traced out by the position of the cross hair as the collimator is rotated. This "run out" must be minimized by adjusting the location of the cross hair.

check device provides since the tolerance for the monthly output check is only ±2% for both x-rays and electrons. Most centers use an ion chamber of some type along with a solid phantom such as square sheets (typically 25×25 or 30×30 cm^2) of polystyrene or "virtual water" of various thicknesses (see chapter 8, Figure 8.1). A large square block of the phantom material can be machined with a hole to accept the ion chamber so that the chamber can effectively be embedded in it. Then additional blocks or sheets can be used for build-up material or backscatter material.

When the absolute calibration is performed, the monthly check procedure is established immediately afterward. This consists of a 10×10 cm^2 field size with an ion chamber at a depth of at least d_m for the given beam. The build-up material is necessary to filter out the electron contamination of the beam. The chamber can be placed at the SAD, or the SSD to the top of the phantom can be set to 100 cm. Once the system is set up, it is irradiated (100 MU is common). The charge measured by the electrometer is then known to correspond to the absolute dose that was just measured. The electrometer signal should be corrected to standard dosimetry temperature and pressure conditions: 295 K and 760 mm-Hg. This setup can then be used in subsequent months to evaluate whether the output has changed. If the output changes by more than 2%, then the output must be adjusted.

Beam energy can be checked by making measurements at two different depths (for example d_m and 10 cm) in phantom. The ratio of these measurements is a parameter that should remain constant over time.

The intensity of a therapy radiation beam should be uniform throughout the cross section of the beam. Ideally, the intensity of the beam would be the same at the edges as it is at the central axis. Without the flattening filter the x-ray beam of a linac would be much more intense at the center than at the edges. This was discussed in chapter 9. Recall that this is due to the properties of the bremsstrahlung x-ray emission process. For electrons it is the scattering foil that provides for a uniform beam. The uniformity of the beam is measured by two quantities called the *flatness* and *symmetry*. Unfortunately there are no universal definitions of these quantities (see chapter 9).

Safety

The following safety items should be checked on a monthly basis: emergency off switches, touchguard (on the linac head, if any, and for electron applicators), wedge and electron applicator interlocks.

18.2.2 NRC Regulations Pertaining to QA

NRC regulations were discussed at length in chapter 17. We have deferred a discussion of NRC QA requirements to this chapter. The NRC has specific QA requirements for Co-60 teletherapy units, HDR units, and gamma stereotactic units. We concentrate on HDR units here as Co-60 teletherapy units are now rare and gamma stereotactic units are only found at a relatively small number of centers.[5]

Licensees are required to have a calibrated dosimetry system. One way to comply with the requirement is that the system be calibrated by an Accredited Dosimetry Calibration Laboratory (ADCL) (see chapter 11) within the previous 2 years. All units require a calibrated electrometer. For a Co-60 unit a Farmer ionization chamber is used. For an HDR unit a well ionization chamber is used (see Figure 8.8 in chapter 8).

Specific Requirements for Remote Afterloading Units (HDR)

A full calibration of source strength (to within ±5%) is required before first use and following source replacement. Full calibration (and mathematical decay calculations) must be performed by the authorized medical physicist. Full calibration must be accompanied by the following tests.

1. A check of source positioning accuracy. The tolerance is ±1 mm. This can be accomplished with a CCTV system (the same one used for patient viewing) and a source positioning check device.
2. The source retracts under backup battery power upon power failure. This is tested by interrupting the power to the unit.
3. Timer accuracy and linearity
4. Check length of transfer tubes and applicators
5. Function of the source transfer tubes, applicators, and transfer tube–applicator interfaces.

A number of spot checks are required before first use each day and after a source change.

1. Door interlocks must be functional.
2. All source exposure indicator lights must be functional.
3. The viewing and intercom systems must be functional.
4. Emergency response equipment must be present.
5. Radiation monitors must be operable.
6. Timer accuracy must be checked.
7. The date and time in the console computer must be correct. The date in the console computer is used by the console to correct for source decay; therefore it is very important that the clock be accurate.
8. The current source activity in the computer must match independent source decay calculations.

---

[5] For a sample Gamma Knife™ QA program, see AAPM Report No. 54, page 71.

If the HDR unit fails any of these checks, then it must not be used for patient treatment. There are additional requirements for mobile remote afterloader units, which will not be discussed here.

Treatment Planning Systems

The NRC requires acceptance testing of treatment planning systems. At a minimum this testing must include verification of:

1. Source-specific input parameters required by the dose calculation algorithm. An example of this might be the value of the dose rate constant Λ for a particular source.
2. Accuracy of dose, dwell time, and treatment time calculations at representative points.
3. Accuracy of isodose plots.
4. Accuracy of source localization software.
5. Accuracy of manual or electronic data transfer from the treatment planning system to the treatment console.

18.2.3 Dosimetry Instrumentation

A variety of equipment is used for dosimetry measurements. Measurements made with this equipment are only as reliable as the equipment itself. QA tests carried out on a regular basis are necessary for this instrumentation. A list of this equipment is lengthy: ionization chambers, electrometers, triaxial cable, thermometers, barometers, computer-controlled water phantom scanning systems, thermoluminescent dosimeters (TLDs), and TLD readers.

18.3 Patient Quality Assurance

Patient QA consists of all those procedures that are designed to ensure that each individual patient receives the specific intended treatment.

18.3.1 Physics Chart Checks

Chart checks should be performed by a physicist for all new or modified patient ports. Some facilities require this check before delivery of the third fraction or before delivery of 20% of the total dose, whichever comes first. Some of the items to be checked follow: Has the patient had previous radiation therapy? If so, is there any overlap between the prior treatment volume and the new treatment volume? Does the patient have a pacemaker or ICD (implanted cardioverter-defibrillator device)? (See section 18.6.)

Prescription review should address the following:

1. Anatomical site description clear?
2. Signed and dated by attending physician?
3. Beam arrangement, modality and energy.
4. Dose per fraction.
5. Total dose.
6. Location of dose delivery. Dose delivery can be specified to isocenter, to a specific isodose line (e.g., 95% line), to a specific depth (e.g., 3 cm, or mid-depth) or volumetrically as for IMRT (e.g., 95% of planning target volume (PTV) should receive prescription dose).
7. Bolus or other beam modifiers.
8. Critical organs specified.

Treatment plan review should include the following: Is the anatomical site correct? Have the dose distribution and DVH been signed by the physician? Does the dose distribution correspond to the prescription goals in terms of total dose, modality, beam arrangement, etc.?

Most linear accelerator facilities have record and verify (R&V) software. The R&V software accepts information from the treatment planning system and then communicates that information to the linac control system. The R&V software also records the daily treatment received by individual patients. and is used to set the linac parameters for daily patient treatment. It is therefore crucial that the information in the R&V software for a particular patient be correct. The data in the R&V software must be checked against the original treatment plan. Some of the information to be checked includes the port numbering; beam modality and energy; monitor units; presence and orientation of a wedge; the dose for each port; gantry, collimator, and pedestal angles.

An independent check of the MU for each port is necessary. This can be accomplished either by using software that is separate from the main treatment planning software or by carrying out manual calculations using the methods described in chapters 12 through 14.

18.3.2 Weekly Physics Chart Checks

The purpose of a weekly chart check is to ensure that treatment delivery is as intended. The patient setup instructions should be clear and unambiguous. The charted treatment should correspond to the prescription in the following particulars:

1. Beam modality and energy.
2. Field arrangement.
3. Number of fractions.

4. Dose for all ports should add to prescribed dose per fraction.
5. Cumulative dose delivered to date is correct.
6. Measured SSDs are within some tolerance of expected values.
7. In vivo dosimetry performed if prescribed and results within tolerance.
8. Bolus (if prescribed) is being applied.

The R&V software can be overridden if necessary and linac parameters can be entered manually by the radiation therapist. The R&V software should be checked for overrides. The reason for any override should be explained.

18.3.3 Portal Imaging

Portal imaging utilizes the treatment radiation beam to form an image of the treatment aperture and the patient's anatomy. This is discussed in more detail in chapter 19, section 19.9. Portal imaging should be performed at the beginning of any new or modified treatment and then on a regular basis (perhaps weekly) thereafter. There are two purposes: (1) To verify the field placement: is the isocenter in the correct location? (2) To verify that the beam aperture is correct: Is the blocked field the correct size and shape?

18.3.4 In Vivo Dosimetry

In vivo dosimetry can be used to verify the dose actually received by a patient. While portal imaging verifies targeting, in vivo dosimetry verifies that the correct dose is delivered to the target. In vivo dosimetry can also be used to measure skin dose. It is difficult to predict or calculate skin dose accurately (see chapter 14, section 14.9). Another application of in vivo dosimetry is to measure peripheral dose. This is the dose outside the region that intercepts the direct beam. Peripheral dose is deposited by scatter and leakage radiation. An example of this is the measurement of the dose to a pacemaker (see section 18.6). Dosimeters used for in vivo dosimetry include diodes, TLDs, and MOSFETs. These devices were described in chapter 8, section 8.4. You may wish to review that section.

Most routine patient dosimetry verification programs use diodes. These are small solid-state devices that come with (or without) build-up material (see Figure 8.27). A cable attached to the diode leads to a dedicated electrometer. The electrometer readout is calibrated to read directly in units of cGy (see Figure 8.26). The build-up material is non–tissue-equivalent. Non–tissue-equivalent build-up material is used so that the diodes can be made reasonably compact in size. The amount and composition of the buildup is designed for the energy range of intended use. As an example, a diode for use in the energy range from 6 to 12 MV might use molybdenum or brass (1.6 g/cm^2), whereas a diode designed for the 15 to 25 MV range might use tungsten (2.6 g/cm^2).

It is common to make diode measurements for each new radiation field that is accessible. The skin surface is not easily accessible for some fields, such as for a PA field in a supine patient. Diodes are generally not used for IMRT treatments because of the possibility of high-dose gradients and secondarily due to the difficulty in calculating expected readings. They are also not usually used for peripheral dose measurements or to measure skin dose (although diodes are available with minimal buildup). Skin dose is usually measured either with TLDs or MOSFETs. MOSFETs have only a small amount of buildup on them.

Diodes are placed on the patient skin surface where the beam enters the patient. They are usually placed on the central axis unless the field edge is closer than 1 to 2 cm from the central axis. Diodes should be placed firmly on the patient skin surface with no gaps underneath. If it is necessary to position the diode off the central axis, the graticule should be used for placement (a graticule is an accessory which projects a grid down onto the patient skin surface). A ruler should not be used for placement because of the possibility of a sloping skin surface and because distances off axis usually refer to a plane through the isocenter. Careful diode positioning is particularly crucial in the presence of a wedge. It is also advisable to orient a cylindrical diode so that the long axis of the diode is perpendicular to the direction of the wedge gradient. Problems are more likely for anatomical sites with steep skin slopes and wedged fields; e.g., especially breast tangents.

Diodes are usually calibrated to measure the entrance dose in the patient at a depth of d_m. Exit dosimetry is possible, although much more complicated, by placing the diode on the skin at the location of the beam exit, if accessible.

Diodes are calibrated for entrance dosimetry by placing them on the surface of a geometric phantom (at least 5 cm thick for backscatter) at the beam central axis and at some specified SSD (usually 90 or 100 cm). The field size is usually set to 10×10 cm^2. The readout of the diode is adjusted so that it corresponds to the known dose (as measured with an ion chamber) delivered to a depth of d_m in the phantom.

Diodes need periodic calibration. Sensitivity changes slowly with accumulated dose. The sensitivity decreases at the rate of roughly 0.1% per 10,000 Gy for photons. The gain of the electrometer used to read the diodes can also drift over time. Generally the calibration is checked monthly as part of the monthly linac QA.

The "gold standard" for clinical dose measurement is an ionization chamber. Diodes do not respond to changes in measurement conditions in the same way that ion chambers do. Diodes exhibit an anomalous response (a response different than an ion chamber) to changes in field size, SSD, and the presence of a wedge. In principle, therefore, the predicted diode reading should be corrected for these effects. The corrections actually applied in practice in a given clinic depend on the accuracy desired. If no corrections are applied, then the tolerance needs to be made larger to avoid needless investigation. Diodes also exhibit some angular dependence; the reading may depend on the angle at which the beam enters the diode.

The expected diode reading is calculated by computing the dose at depth d_m in the patient modified by correction factors (if desired). This calculation is based on the patient's beam parameters such as MU, SSD, field size, etc. The measured value is compared to this value. Each clinic must establish a tolerance range. If the measured value falls outside the tolerance range, some action must be taken. A tolerance range of ±7% is common. This means that if the expected calculated value is 100 cGy, then the measured value should fall in the range 93 to 107 cGy. If the measurement should fall outside this range, then an investigation is necessary.

What sort of problems can diodes catch? The ±7% tolerance can catch incorrect delivered MUs, presence or absence of a wedge or other beam modifier (e.g., compensator), incorrect beam energy, confusion of SAD and SSD setups. This tolerance will not catch small errors (e.g., missing tray factor in an MU calculation or small errors in SSD).

What action should be taken when a diode reading is out of range? The parameters that were used to calculate the expected diode reading should be checked. These should be double-checked prior to the first reading anyway as part of the physics chart check. The patient treatment plan and setup should be checked carefully. Is there anything about the geometry or placement of the diode that would help to explain an anomalous reading? Are readings for other patients out of tolerance, either all low or high? If so, then the diode calibration should be checked. If no error can be found in the expected value, then the diode reading should be repeated as soon as possible. It is useful to measure the SSDs to the diode placement position on the same day as the diode reading to verify that they correspond to the treatment plan (and to the expected reading calculation). It may be helpful to take a portal image at the same time. Diodes can be seen on portal images and this may allow verification of placement position.[6] It may be useful to have a physicist observe the diode placement. If no explanation for an out of tolerance measurement is evident, it may be necessary to measure the diode reading in a phantom using the patient's beam parameters.

---

[6] The fact that a diode can be seen on a portal image indicates that the diode does "shadow" tissue underneath it. The magnitude of the dose shadow is on the order of 5% if a diode is used which is within its stated energy range.

18.4 Starting New Treatment Programs

Examples of new treatment programs are Gamma Knife® or stereotactic radiosurgery, IMRT, HDR, TBI (total body irradiation), and total skin electron irradiation (TSEI). Each one of these treatment modalities represents a complex *program*. Before beginning a new treatment program it is necessary to ensure that the required resources will be in place. These programs are usually not "turnkey" systems, despite vendor claims to the contrary. They have to be adapted to local conditions relating to the clinic and the regulatory environment.

Establishing such programs involves more than simply acquiring the hardware and turning it on. As an example, a new treatment planning system is not just "a toaster" that you plug in and turn on.

Careful acceptance testing and commissioning is required that may take many full-time equivalent weeks in the case of a treatment planning system and perhaps many months in the case of IMRT or HDR. In addition to hardware and software, extra staff may be needed. Policies and procedures must be developed and checklists and forms must be generated. Equipment QA and patient QA procedures must be established. Treatment procedures and techniques must be developed for specific anatomical sites. The staff must receive on site (and possibly off site) training. Careful rehearsal and planning for contingencies is also necessary. Shortcuts are an invitation to disaster.

18.5 Mold Room Safety[7]

The main concern is exposure to toxic heavy metals; lead and especially cadmium (see chapter 13 for a discussion of cast block fabrication). The use of cast blocks for field shaping has declined significantly in favor of MLC field shaping. Despite this, a small number of cast blocks are still utilized even in departments that have been using MLC for years. In addition, electron cutouts are still fabricated from low-melting-temperature alloys. To avoid heavy metal exposure, workers should wear protective clothing: an apron, a lab coat, or a smock and eye protection. Personnel should wear gloves and wash their hands after handling blocks or cutouts. There should absolutely be no eating, drinking, or smoking in the mold room. The door to the room should be kept closed and a "tacky" mat should be placed at the entrance to trap particulates on footwear. A fume hood is desirable; otherwise a respirator may be necessary. The melting pot should be kept under the fume hood. Toxic fumes appear not to be an issue provided that

---

[7] The material in this section is drawn from the Civco Medical Solutions publication: *Radiation Therapy Mold Room Safety.* For more information, refer to http://www.civco.com/customer_support/ customer_tools/oncology/.

the molten alloy is maintained at a low temperature. The higher the temperature, the greater the toxic fume concentration. The temperature of molten Lipowitz metal should be no more than 85 °C. The major concern is from alloy dust, which may be produced when filing or sanding occur. Cleanup should be with a vacuum cleaner, preferably one with a HEPA filter.

18.6 Patient Safety

Pacemakers and Implantable Cardioverter-Defibrillators[8]

An increasing number of radiation therapy patients have pacemakers or implanted cardioverter-defibrillator devices (ICDs). Pacemakers are used to maintain normal heart rhythm. ICDs provide an electrical shock to the heart to restore normal rhythm in the event of ventricular tachycardia or fibrillation. Failure of these devices can lead to potentially life threatening consequences. The solid-state electronics in these devices may be damaged by exposure to ionizing radiation. The operation of these devices may be adversely affected by the presence of the strong radiofrequency electromagnetic fields present in linear accelerator rooms. Every radiotherapy department must have a mechanism for identifying such patients prior to treatment. There are two categories of possible malfunction: transient and permanent. *Transient effects* can potentially occur during treatment. *Permanent effects* are due to radiation damage to solid-state electronics. To avoid transient effects, it is sometimes recommended that the device be turned off during beam delivery, if possible. If the device is in the direct planned radiation field, it should be moved. It is necessary to estimate the cumulative dose to the device from scatter and leakage. The absorbed dose to a pacemaker should be less than 2 Gy unless otherwise specified by the manufacturer. ICDs are more sensitive and the dose to these devices should be limited to 1 Gy (unless otherwise specified by the manufacturer). A cardiologist should assess the status of the patient and the device to provide a baseline prior to initiation of radiation therapy. In vivo dosimetry measurements should be made at the first treatment to verify dose estimates. The patient should be monitored carefully during treatment and weekly by a cardiologist. At the conclusion of treatment there should be a full assessment of the function of the device by a cardiologist.

---

[8] The recommendations outlined here are taken from: "Treatment of patients with cardiac pacemakers and implantable cardioverter-defibrillators during radiotherapy," Solan, A.N., et al. *Int J Radiat Oncol Biol Phys* 59(3):897–904, 2004. Also see "Implanted cardiac defibrillator care in radiation oncology patient population," Gelblum, D.Y., and H. Amols, *Int J Radiat Oncol Biol Phys* 73(5):1525–1531, 2009.

18.7   Radiation Therapy Accidents

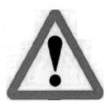

It is difficult to obtain information about radiation therapy accidents within the United States because of the medico-legal climate. Naturally, radiation therapy facilities and equipment vendors are not eager to see any publicity about mistakes or accidents. NRC-regulated activities result in information about medical events because of the reporting requirements.

Equipment instruction manuals include more and more legal disclaimers and warnings to the point of attention overload. There may be up to a half dozen warnings per page. There are so many warnings that there is a risk that no one will pay attention to any of them.

Accidents can involve an underdose as well as an overdose. An underdose puts the patient at risk for disease progression or recurrence. Some accidents are insidious because they may take months or years to discover. During this period large numbers of patients may be treated incorrectly. Many current NRC regulations originated as a result of specific accidents.

18.7.1   A Linear Accelerator Calibration Error

In 2005 a cancer center in Florida delivered an overdose of approximately 50% to 77 patients. The overdose was the result of an error in calibration of a linear accelerator used for cranial stereotactic radiosurgery. The error was discovered through the mailed TLD program of the Radiological Physics Center (RPC) (see chapter 11, section 11.8). It has been reported that the error occurred upon calibration of the linac. The AAPM TG-51 protocol requires calibration measurement of the dose rate at a depth of 10 cm followed by mathematical calculation of the dose rate at depth d_m. It appears as if there was an error in a computer spreadsheet and that the last step was not performed. If we assume a 6 MV beam, the percent depth dose at a depth of 10 cm (for a 10×10 cm^2 field size) is approximately 67% and $1/0.67 = 1.49$, leading to an error of approximately 50%.

18.7.2   An HDR Accident

On November 16, 1992, in Indiana, PA, an HDR error occurred that resulted in the death of a patient. The patient was an 82-year-old female who was treated for anal carcinoma using a 4.3 Ci Ir-192 source inserted using an afterloader. The room monitor indicated high radiation levels after the treatment; but the monitor had been malfunctioning, so it was disregarded. A survey meter was available, but it was not used to survey the patient. The control console indicated that the source had returned to the HDR unit safe. In reality, the source had broken off the end of the wire and was in one of the catheters inside the patient. After treatment, the patient was transferred to a nursing home. On November 20, the catheter came loose and nursing home personnel placed it in a biohazards bag and put it into storage for later disposal. The patient died the next day. It was later estimated that the patient received a dose (at 1 cm from the source) of 1.6×10^6 cGy. The coroner listed the cause of death as "acute radiation exposure and consequences thereof." From November 16 through November 25, numerous residents, employees, and visitors to the nursing home were unknowingly irradiated. On November 25, the biohazards bag was collected by a waste disposal company. On November 27, it was taken to a waste disposal facility where fixed radiation monitors at the gate identified radiation emanating from the truck. The source was found and eventually traced back to the nursing home.

On December 2, 1992, a second source wire from the same model afterloader broke in Pittsburgh, PA. The wire broke at the same location as the first incident. The physicist was aware of the first incident and safely retrieved the source.

The cause of the break in the wire is uncertain. The following scenario has been offered as a likely explanation. Prior to installation the source was stored in a Teflon™-lined container. The purpose of the Teflon was to reduce friction and to make it easier to insert the source cable into the container. When Teflon is exposed to radiation, it emits hydrogen fluoride. If moisture is present, the hydrogen fluoride becomes hydrofluoric acid, which is extremely corrosive. Presumably the acid weakened the weld between the wire and the source, allowing the source to break free.

The afterloader equipment manufacturer has since gone out of business and the licensee of the Pennsylvania clinic was fined $360,000 by the NRC. The fine has been appealed. This incident was the impetus for many NRC requirements for HDR treatments. The NRC now requires that patients be checked with a survey meter after treatment.

18.7.3 Malfunction 54

This is probably one of the most serious linear accelerator accidents in history. Details of this incident are somewhat sketchy, because there was never any official investigation.

On March 21, 1986, in Tyler, TX, a 33-year-old patient was receiving the 9th electron treatment with a Therac 25 linear accelerator for a tumor on his back. From prior fractions the patient knew the treatment to be painless and uneventful. When the beam came on the patient felt an electric shock like pain. He said that it felt as if someone had poured hot coffee on his back. The patient began to get off the table when he again felt a sensation like an electric shock. The control console showed that only 20 MU had been delivered. The physicist at the facility ran tests, found nothing wrong with the linac, and patient treatment was resumed. The next day this patient presented with a mass over the left deltoid muscle. Engineers from the manufacturer came to test the machine but could find no apparent problem. The Therac 25 was put back into service.

On April 11, 1986, a patient was treated with electrons at the same facility for a superficial cancer near the right ear. While programming the console the therapist inadvertently selected x-ray mode. Realizing her mistake, she quickly changed to electron mode and turned the beam on. Within 1 second the message "MALFUNCTION 54" appeared on the display console. The only time she had seen this message before was when the March 21 patient was treated. In the meantime, the patient was moaning for help and complaining that his face felt like it was on fire. The patient said that it felt like something had hit him in the face, that he saw a flash of light, and that he heard a sizzling sound like frying eggs.

The physicist at the facility was later able to reproduce "MAL-FUNCTION 54." The physicist discovered that under these circumstances the linac was delivering 25,000 cGy in less than a second! It was later learned that the buttons were pushed so fast that the linac was somehow able to remain in "x-ray mode" during electron treatments even though the target and flattening filter were moved out of the way of the beam. In x-ray mode the beam current is 100 to 1000 times higher than in electron mode. As a result, the patients were exposed to a very high intensity electron beam. The problem was later traced to an error in the software that controls the linac.

The second patient died 3 weeks after the accident. An autopsy showed an acute radiation injury to the right temporal lobe and brainstem. The first patient was eventually hospitalized for radiation-induced myelitis of the cervical cord and numerous other complications from the overdose. He died 5 months after the accident.

18.7.4 Co-60 Overdose

During the period March 1975 through January 1976, almost 400 patients treated with Co-60 external beam radiation at a hospital in Columbus, OH, received an overdose of up to 40%.[9] The overdose was due to an incorrect calibration and not a machine malfunction. At the time the incident was reported to NRC, two patients had already died as a "direct result of the miscalibration." Over the ensuing months eight more patients died of suspected radiation overdose. This incident prompted the NRC to eventually require full annual calibration, monthly spot checks, and detailed record keeping.

---

[9] *Radiation in Medicine: A Need for Regulatory Reform*, Institute of Medicine, National Academies Press, 1996.

Chapter Summary

- **Equipment Quality Assurance:** Tests on treatment equipment/software (linacs, HDR, simulators, etc.).

- **Patient Quality Assurance:** Quality assurance procedures to ensure that patients receive the specific, correct treatment.

Equipment Quality Assurance

- **Acceptance Testing:** Consists of those tests and measurements designed to verify that a new piece of equipment meets the specifications given by the manufacturer.

- **Commissioning:** Consists of all those procedures necessary to put the device or machine into routine clinical use. For a linac this includes the process of acquiring all the data that must be put into the computer treatment planning system.

- QA procedures for treatment machines are performed on an annual, monthly, and daily basis. QA procedures for linacs/Co-60 units fall into three categories: mechanical, dosimetric, and safety.

- **Selected Linac QA Tests**

Category	Test	Frequency[a]	Tolerance
Mechanical	Laser position	D, M, A	±2 mm
	Distance indicator (ODI)	D, M, A	±2 mm
	Congruence of light/radiation field	M, A	±2 mm
	Gantry/collimator angle accuracy	M, A	1°
	Field size indicator	M, A	±2 mm
	Cross hair centering	M, A	2 mm
Dosimetry	X-ray/Electron beam "output"[b]	D, M, A	±3% (D), ±2% (M)
	Flatness & symmetry	M, A	(See AAPM TG-45)
Safety	Door interlock	D, M, A	Functional
	Audiovisual monitoring	D, M, A	Functional
	Emergency off switches	M	Functional

[a] D = daily,   M = monthly,   A = annually

[b] All beams should be calibrated annually following the AAPM TG-51 protocol; monthly and daily checks are for constancy.

NRC HDR QA Requirements

- Must possess calibrated dosimetry system (ADCL calibration every 2 years)

Following Source Replacement:

- Full calibration

- Check of source position accuracy (±1 mm)

- Source retracts under battery backup

- Timer accuracy & linearity

- Transfer tubes, applicators (length, function)

Daily Checks:

- Door interlocks

- Viewing/intercom

- Emergency response equipment present

- Radiation monitors operating

- Timer accuracy

- Date/time on console

- Current source activity in computer

Patient QA

Physics Chart Checks: Each radiation port, usually before 3rd fraction or before delivery of 20% of total dose

- Review of prescription

- Review of treatment plan

- Independent MU calculation

Weekly Physics Chart Check: Ensure that treatment is delivered as intended.

- Pacemaker/ICDs
  —Possible malfunction due to linac radiofrequency (RF) fields or radiation
  —Transient/permanent effects

- Pacemakers: Limit dose to 2 Gy unless otherwise specified by manufacturer

- ICD: Limit dose to 1 Gy unless otherwise specified by manufacturer

Radiation Therapy Accidents

- Linac delivers 25,000 cGy in less than a second in 1986 when beam current remains in x-ray mode during planned electron treatments. Two patients die. Cause is a software error.

- HDR source breaks off from end of wire in 1992, remains in patient, unknown to treating clinic. Patient dies later in nursing home; numerous people exposed to radiation before source is found at waste site.

Problems

1. What document is an important reference for general standards regarding physical quality assurance in radiation therapy?

2. What is the difference between acceptance testing and commissioning?

3. Name the three major categories of QA tests for linear accelerators and give an example of each.

4. What are the tolerances for daily and monthly output checks for x-ray beams?

5. What is a front pointer and what is it used for?

6. How is gantry angle checked and what is the tolerance?

7. If you have access to a linear accelerator, ask a physicist to assist you in performing a light field/radiation field congruence test for one x-ray beam. Does the unit meet the tolerance for this test?

8. If you have access to a linear accelerator, perform the daily QA with the therapist assigned that task. For each test, record the following: a description of the test, the instruments used to perform the test (type, make, and model), the setup, the result of the test, and the tolerance.

Bibliography

AAPM Report No. 13. Physical Aspects of Quality Assurance in Radiation Therapy. Report of AAPM Radiation Therapy Committee Task Group 24 with contribution by AAPM Radiation Therapy Committee Task Group 22. New York, NY: American Institute of Physics, 1984.

AAPM Report No. 46. Reprinted from Kutcher, G. J., L. Coia, M. Gillin, W. F. Hanson, S. Leibel, R. J. Morton, J. R. Palta, J. A. Purdy, L. E. Reinstein, G. K. Svensson, M. Weller, and L. Wingfield. "Comprehensive QA for radiation oncology: Report of Task Group 40 of the Radiation Therapy Committee." *Med Phys* 21(4):581–618, 1994.

AAPM Report No. 47. Reprinted from Nath, R., P. J. Biggs, F. J. Bova, C. C. Ling, J. A. Purdy, J. van de Geijn, and M. S. Weinhous. "AAPM code of practice for radiotherapy accelerators: Report of AAPM Radiation Therapy Task Group No. 45. *Med Phys* 21(7):1093–1121, 1994.

AAPM Report No. 54. Stereotactic Radiosurgery. Report of Task Group 42 of the Radiation Therapy Committee. New York, NY: American Institute of Physics, 1995.

AAPM Report No. 56. Reprinted from Purdy, J. A., P. J. Biggs, C. Bowers, E. Dally, W. Downs, B. E. Fraass, C. J. Karzmark, F. Khan, P. Morgan, R. Morton, J. Palta, I. I. Rosen, T. Thorson, G. Svensson, and J. Ting. "Medical accelerator safety considerations: Report of AAPM Radiation Therapy Committee Task Group No. 35." *Med Phys* 20(4):1261–1275, 1996.

AAPM Report No. 67. Reprinted from Almond, P. R., P. J. Biggs, B. M. Coursey, W. F. Hanson, M. S. Huq, and R. Nath. "AAPM's TG-51 protocol for clinical reference dosimetry of high-energy photon and electron beams." *Med Phys* 26(9):1847–1870, 1999.

AAPM Report No. 87. Diode In Vivo Dosimetry for Patients Receiving External Beam Radiation Therapy. Report of Task Group 62 of the AAPM Radiation Therapy Committee. Madison, WI: Medical Physics Publishing, 2005.

AAPM Report No. 142. Reprinted from Klein, E. E., J. Hanley, J. Bayouth, F. F. Yin, W. Simon, S. Dresser, C. Serago, F. Aguirre, L. Ma, B. Arjomandy, C. Liu, C. Sandin, T. Holmes. "Task Group 142 report: Quality assurance of medical accelerators." *Med Phys* 36(9):4197–4212, 2009.

Committee for Review and Evaluation of the Medical Use Program of the Nuclear Regulatory Commission, Institute of Medicine, K.-L. D. Gottfried (ed.), and G. Penn (ed.). *Radiation in Medicine: A Need for Regulatory Reform.* Washington, DC: National Academies Press, 1996.

Constantinou, C. *Protocol and Procedures for Quality Assurance of Linear Accelerators.* Brockton, MA: Brockton Hospital, 1993.

Gelblum, D. Y., and H. Amols. (2009). "Implanted cardiac defibrillator care in radiation oncology patient population." *Int J Radiat Oncol Biol Phys* 73(5):1525–1531.

ICRU Report No. 24. Determination of Absorbed Dose in a Patient Irradiated by Beams of X or Gamma Rays in Radiotherapy. Bethesda, MD: International Commission on Radiation Units and Measurements (ICRU), 1976.

ICRU Report No. 42. Use of Computers in External Beam Radiotherapy Procedures with High Energy Photons and Electrons. Bethesda, MD: International Commission on Radiation Units and Measurements (ICRU), 1976.

International Commission on Radiological Protection (ICRP). Publication 86. *Prevention of Accidents to Patients Undergoing Radiation Therapy.* Amsterdam: Elsevier, 2002.

Karzmark, C. J., C. S. Nunan, and E. Tanabe. *Medical Electron Accelerators.* New York: McGraw-Hill, 1993.

Khan, F. M. *The Physics of Radiation Therapy.* Fourth Edition. Baltimore: Lippincott Williams & Wilkins, 2009.

Lessons Learned from Accidental Exposures in Radiotherapy: Safety Reports Series No. 17. Vienna, Austria: International Atomic Energy Agency (IAEA) (available on-line).

Leveson, N. "Medical Devices: The Therac 25," chapter in *Safeware: System Safety and Computers*. Reading, MA: Addison Wesley, 1995.

Podgorsak, E.B. (ed.). *Radiation Oncology Physics: A Handbook for Teachers and Students*. Vienna, Austria: International Atomic Energy Agency (IAEA) (available on-line).

Radiation Therapy Mold Room Safety. Publication OF-M0095131-EN Rev NR. Orange City, IA: Civco Medical Solutions. www.civcomedical.com. No date given.

Solan, A. N., M. J. Solan, G. Bednarz, and M. B. Goodkin. (2004). "Treatment of patients with cardiac pacemakers and implantable cardioverter-defibrillators during radiotherapy." *Int J Radiat Oncol Biol Phys* 59(3):897–904.

Starkschall, G., (ed.). *Quality Assurance in Radiotherapy Physics*. Madison, WI: Medical Physics Publishing, 1991.

19 Imaging in Radiation Therapy

19.1 Introduction

The improvement in non-invasive imaging of the human body over the last 35 years has been nothing short of astonishing.[1] The imaging needs of radiation therapy are often quite different from those of diagnostic radiology and can be divided into two broad categories: imaging for treatment planning and imaging for treatment verification. Both of these categories are complex and we can only address the main features here.

Imaging for treatment planning is used to define the gross tumor volume and organs at risk and to select geometric parameters such as the location of the isocenter and treatment beam angles. The imaging modalities used for treatment planning can be divided into two categories: conventional and three-dimensional. Conventional imaging

---

[1] See *Naked to the Bone: Medical Imaging in the Twentieth Century* by B. Kevles, 1997.

includes general radiography and fluoroscopy. Conventional treatment simulators (see section 19.3) provide these capabilities. Conventional imaging can be thought of as two-dimensional imaging in which three-dimensional anatomy is projected onto a plane. Plane film radiographs are "shadow pictures" or projection images. Three-dimensional imaging modalities include CT (computed tomography), MRI (magnetic resonance imaging), ultrasound, SPECT (single photon emission computed tomography), and PET (positron emission tomography). These modalities provide true three-dimensional anatomical information and in the case of SPECT and PET, metabolic information.

Plane film, fluoroscopy, and CT are based on x-rays as the imaging agent. MRI is based on nuclear magnetic resonance (NMR). It involves "interrogating" the magnetic properties of atomic nuclei in a magnetic field. Radio frequency electromagnetic waves are used to accomplish this. *No ionizing radiation is employed in MRI.* There is an "urban legend" regarding the name "magnetic resonance imaging." The original name for this technique was nuclear magnetic resonance. As the public is so averse to anything with the word "nuclear" in it, the name was changed to MRI. Ultrasound (US) imaging is based on the propagation and reflection properties of sound at tissue interfaces. PET imaging is based on the administration of a positron emitter and the differential uptake of the radiopharmaceutical in different organs and tissues.

For treatment planning purposes it is often necessary to be able to discriminate between various types of soft tissue. Ordinary or "plane" radiographs can distinguish between soft tissue and bone and between soft tissue and air, but not between different types of soft tissue. Generally you cannot see tumors on plane films.

The three most widely used modalities for soft tissue imaging are CT, MRI, and ultrasound. For high spatial resolution and soft tissue discrimination MRI is unsurpassed (see Figure 19.1).

The imaging that we have described so far is *anatomical imaging*. *Functional imaging* such as PET and fMRI (functional MRI) display physiological activity such as glucose metabolism. This promises to play an increasingly important role in the future of radiation therapy.

Traditionally, megavoltage imaging using the treatment beam has been employed for treatment verification using either film or electronic portal imaging devices (EPIDs). EPIDs have now replaced film in most clinics. A new development is image-guided radiation therapy (IGRT). In IGRT the patient is imaged on the treatment machine just prior to treatment. The location of the target is compared with the expected location and the patient is moved to bring the target into alignment with its expected location. A variety of imaging modalities are in use for IGRT including on-board kVp imagers and ultrasound.

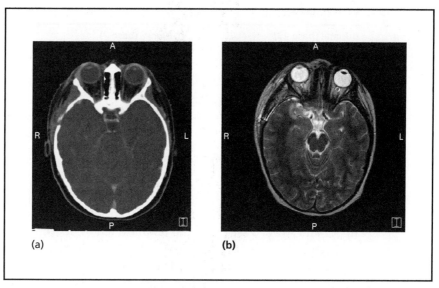

Figure 19.1: Side-by-side images of the same axial section made with CT (a) and MRI (b). The superior soft-tissue discrimination of MRI is evident. CT shows bone better than MRI. Note that it is conventional to always display the patient's right on the left-hand side (patients are viewed from inferior to superior direction).

19.2 Digital Images

Digital images are images that can be stored in a computer in numerical form. CT and MRI produce digital images directly. Ordinary radiographic film produces analog images. Film images can be "digitized" by scanning them with a film scanner such as the one shown in Figure 8.24 in chapter 8.

Electronic computers are fundamentally based on a large number of switches. Physically these switches are transistors that reside on integrated circuits ("chips"). A switch may be either "on" or "off." There is no in-between state. An on or off state is like a "yes" or a "no" or like a 1 or 0. For this reason the natural number system for electronic digital computers consists of the digits 0 and 1 only. This system of numbers consisting of only two digits is called base 2 or binary. Our commonly used number system, the decimal system, is base 10. It consists of the digits 0, 1, 2, . . . , 9. The term "bit" is shorthand nomenclature for a binary digit. It is either a 1 or a 0; it is the most elementary unit of information.

Any base 10 number can be expressed as a binary number. Table 19.1 shows the conversion from decimal to binary for the decimal numbers 0 through 5.

A byte is 8 bits of information. An example is the 8-bit number 11000010.

Table 19.1: Binary Numbers

Decimal (base 10)	Binary (base 2)
0	0
1	1
2	$10 = \underline{1} \times 2^1 + \underline{0} \times 2^0$
3	$11 = \underline{1} \times 2^1 + \underline{1} \times 2^0$
4	$100 = \underline{1} \times 2^2 + \underline{0} \times 2^1 + \underline{0} \times 2^0$
5	$101 = \underline{1} \times 2^2 + \underline{0} \times 2^1 + \underline{1} \times 2^0$

Alphanumeric characters are the 26 letters of the alphabet (both upper and lower case) plus the ten base ten digits 0, 1, . . . , 9 and special symbols such as \$, #, etc. A byte can be used to represent a particular alphanumeric character. There are 2^8 different ways to represent a string of 8 ones and zeroes. Therefore there are $2^8 = 256$ possible characters a byte can represent. This is the reason that the original PC character set contains 256 characters.

There are some useful prefixes in computer science that are a little different (we won't make a bad pun and say "a bit different") than defined in Table 2.2. A kilobyte is $2^{10} = 1024$ bytes. A megabyte (MB) is $2^{20} = 1,048,576$ bytes. A gigabyte is 2^{30} bytes, etc. As an example, a 100 GB storage disk will hold approximately 1.074×10^{11} bytes of data.

There is a standard binary coding scheme for alphanumeric characters, the *A*merican *S*tandard *C*ode for *I*nformation *I*nterchange, known as *ASCII* (pronounced ass-key) for short. There are 128 standard characters and each character is represented by an 8-bit (one byte) number. For example a "W" is represented as the 8-bit binary number 01010111. ASCII is the *lingua franca* of the computer world. Most computers recognize ASCII. A page of ASCII text is about 2 kbytes. A more recent industry standard is Unicode, which is used to represent about 100,000 different text characters in use throughout the world.

Digital images are divided up into an array or grid of *pic*ture *el*ements called *pixels*. The pixel size influences the spatial resolution of an image. The larger the pixel size the poorer the resolution (see Figure 19.2). For a specific image, smaller pixel size means that more pixels are necessary to depict the entire image. More pixels provide higher spatial resolution. There is a cost however; more pixels mean more storage space required. Radiological images are generally either 512×512 pixels or 1024×1024 pixels. This is crude compared to the resolution available in consumer digital cameras.[2]

---

[2] At the time of this writing, 10 megapixel cameras are common. This corresponds to an image of 3888×2592 pixels.

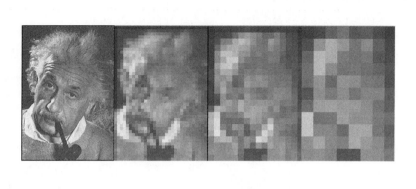

Figure 19.2: A series of four images with different numbers of pixels. The first image on the left has 345×487 pixels. The second image is approximately 30×45 pixels. The third is approximately 16×22 and the fourth is 8×11. The larger the number of pixels, the greater the spatial resolution.

Example 19.1

The field of view of a fluoroscopic unit is 9 in. (23 cm) across. Images are acquired in a 512×512 pixel format.

What is the pixel size and what is the size of the smallest object that can be resolved?

The pixel size is 23 cm/512 = 0.45 mm per pixel. Any object that is about 0.5 mm or smaller will be difficult to discern.

Images that we might normally describe as "black and white" (such as in old movies) actually have many shades of gray. In a "gray scale" image, each pixel is assigned a number that represents a shade of gray or a gray level. This is called the gray scale. In a color image each pixel is assigned a number that represents a color. The numerical values assigned to a pixel are binary. An example is an 8-bit gray scale which has $2^8 = 256$ shades of gray. The number of shades of gray in an image affects the *contrast* resolution of the image. This is illustrated in Figure 19.3.

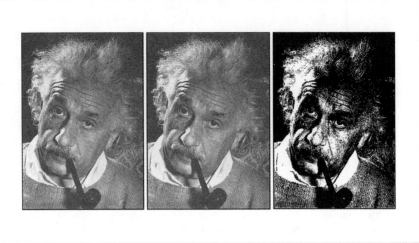

Figure 19.3: Three images having different gray-scale levels. The image on the left has an 8-bit gray scale. The middle image has a 4-bit gray scale. The image on the right is a 2-bit image: there are only two shades—black and white. This image is true black and white.

Example 19.2

A CT image is 512×512 pixels and has 16-bit pixel values (only 12 bits are used for the gray scale). How many bytes are required to store this image?

The total number of bits = 512×512×16 = 4,194,304 bits. The number of bytes = 4,194,304/8 = 524,288 and 524,288/1024 = 512 kbytes. The file will be slightly larger because of the presence of an image "header" containing information about the image (patient name, date, etc.).

For three-dimensional imaging purposes the region of interest in a patient is divided up into a large number of small volume elements or voxels. The goal of three-dimensional imaging is to determine the value of some quantity characterizing the tissue in each one of the voxels. This value is presumed to be constant within each of the small voxels. The image can only be displayed however in two dimensions as either a sectional image or a projection image.[3] A sectional image is often described as a "slice." A slice may be as little as one voxel thick. There are three principal types of sectional images. An axial or transverse slice divides a patient into two halves, a superior half and inferior half.

---

[3] This paragraph follows the discussion in *Radiation Oncology: A Physicist's Eye View* by M. Goitein, 2008.

A coronal section divides a patient into an anterior half and a posterior half and a sagittal section divides a patient into left and right halves. A projection image is one in which each pixel represents a transmission value through all tissue traversed between the source and image plane. The prime example is an ordinary radiograph.

Standardization of image data files is a very critical issue. It is important to be able to seamlessly transfer images between imaging devices, treatment planning systems, record and verify systems, etc. Most manufacturers now comply with the DICOM (Digital Imaging and Communication in Medicine) standard. An extension of this standard is called DICOM-RT and includes specific provisions for radiation therapy. Radiological images are often stored and transferred within a *Picture Archiving and Communication System (PACS)*. This replaces hardcopy film and allows remote access. A PACS consists of servers for image storage that are connected to client viewing stations via a network system. A PACS enables easy access to radiological images anywhere throughout a hospital or hospital system.

19.3 Conventional Simulators

There are two types of simulators used for radiation therapy: conventional and CT. Both types of simulator are intended to provide information necessary for the planning and treatment of patients. A conventional simulator is a device which mechanically simulates the behavior of a linac or Co-60 unit (see Figure 19.4). There is a gantry, which can rotate, and a couch, which may be identical to a linac or Co-60 treatment couch. All of the motions that are possible on a linac are duplicated in a conventional simulator. In addition, the source-axis distance (SAD) can be set on a simulator. Simulators also have a block tray holder. The tray slot must be at the same distance from the x-ray source as the tray on the linac. In addition, a conventional simulator is capable of kV (diagnostic quality) imaging including fluoroscopy. This is needed to assist in planning patient treatments. Linear accelerators are not capable of diagnostic quality images or fluoroscopy. This is the major reason a simulator is used rather than a linac to plan a patient's treatment. Fluoroscopy allows adjustment of the beam position under real time conditions. Conventional simulators are likely to disappear over the next ten years in favor of CT simulators.

A simulator room is divided into two areas: a control console area and an area containing the simulator. The simulator consists of a console, a gantry, a gantry stand, and an x-ray generator. The simulator room is the place where most of the information necessary to plan and to treat a patient is gathered. Once simulation data are collected (films, gantry angles, etc.), it will be passed along to a dosimetrist for treatment planning on a treatment planning computer system. The simulator room has wall-mounted lasers for patient positioning just like a treatment

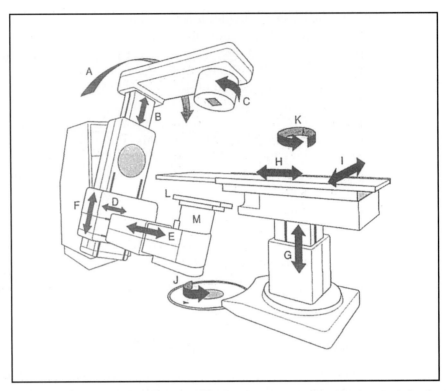

Figure 19.4: A conventional simulator is designed to be mechanically like a linac in that it mimics the motion of a linac. The exception is that the SAD can be changed (B). The head houses a diagnostic x-ray tube and at the other end of the gantry there is a grid, film cassette holder (L), and an image intensifier (M) for fluoroscopy. The image intensifier can be moved laterally (D and E) and up and down (F). (Reproduced from *Radiotherapy Physics in Practice*, J. R. Williams and D. I. Thwaites (eds.), Fig. 7.3, p. 125, © 2000 by permission of Oxford University Press.)

room (see Figure 18.2 in chapter 18). Treatment aids, such as immobilizing devices, are usually fabricated during a patient's simulation appointment. The patient is usually marked or tattooed in the simulator room.

The simulator has a diagnostic x-ray tube in the head, which is used for fluoroscopy and plane film imaging. Focal spot sizes range from 0.4 to 0.6 mm for the small spot and 1.0 to 1.2 mm for the large spot. The simulator has a grid, a film cassette holder, and an image intensifier (II) for fluoroscopic imaging. Newer simulators have digital flat-panel, solid-state detectors instead of an II. Fluoroscopy is activated with the use of a foot pedal. The II can be moved up and down, from side to side, and in and out. The presence of the II constrains gantry and table motion. A collision avoidance system is built into the II so that it cannot hit the treatment couch.

The II is a large, evacuated tube with a cesium iodide fluorescent screen at one end that converts x-rays to light (see Figure 19.5). The light from this screen strikes a photocathode, which in turn emits low-

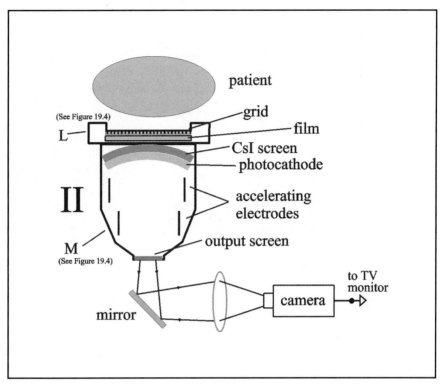

Figure 19.5: An image intensifier (see L and M in Figure 19.4) is a large evacuated tube that contains a fluorescent cesium iodide input screen. The CsI input screen converts x-rays to visible light, which in turn strikes the photocathode and generates electrons. The electrons are accelerated and focused. When the electrons strike the output screen, they produce a smaller and much brighter image.

energy photoelectrons. In this way the x-ray image is converted to an electronic image. The electrons are accelerated and focused by a high voltage (up to 30 kV) between the ends of the tube. At the end of the tube the electrons strike a small output fluorescent screen, producing a visible light image of high brightness. The brightness gain is due to two factors: the energy acquired by the accelerated electrons and the reduction in the diameter (minification) of the image. The image is directed into a camera through a mirror tilted at a 45° angle. The image is viewed on a TV monitor in the control console area. Many simulators have "last image hold," which enables continued viewing of an image after the x-ray beam turns off. The brightness level is set by the automatic brightness control (ABC). A photocell located between the II and the camera sends a signal back to the generator to adjust the kVp or mA. As the patient is moved with respect to the II, the ABC maintains the proper brightness level.

When planning patient treatment it is necessary to select gantry, collimator, and couch (pedestal) angles for each beam or treatment field. In addition, the location of the isocenter must be chosen with respect to

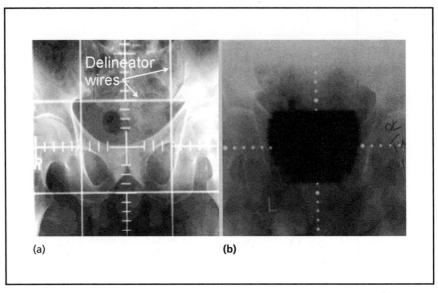

Figure 19.6: A simulation film of a patient's pelvis (a) next to a 6 MV localization film (b). The quality of the simulation film is far superior to the localization film. The delineator wires are shown on the "sim" film. A graticule on the sim film shows lateral distance as measured at isocenter. The wires are set for a 10×10 cm² field. The dark central area on the localization film is the treatment field.

the patient. Simulators have four independent delineator wires which take the place of linac independent jaws and cast a shadow which shows where the jaws will be positioned on the linac. This allows the physician to view adjacent anatomical structures. Radiographic contrast agents may be used in the bladder, etc. A graticule scale projected onto the film shows the beam central axis and graduated scale (see Figure 19.6).

The control console is used to set the radiographic technique: kVp, mA, and time. Modern generators produce high-frequency dc with low ripple (see chapter 5, section 5.2). The control console is behind a barrier which is shielded against kV scatter x-rays. There may be an interlock on the exterior door so that the x-ray beam is shut off if the door is opened. The simulator and patient can be viewed from the control console, usually through a leaded glass window. The control console can also be used to remotely set the gantry angle, collimator angle, delineator wires, and position of the II. The control area also has the video display monitor for fluoroscopy.

19.4 Computed Tomography

Computed tomography (CT) was developed by G. N. Hounsfield and A. M. Cormack. The first commercially available unit was introduced by EMI Ltd., in 1970. This company is perhaps best known for first recording the Beatles! Hounsfield and Cormack won the Nobel Prize for

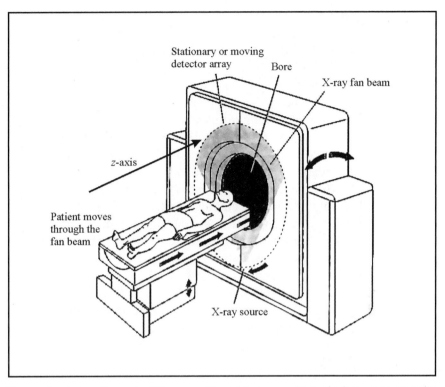

Figure 19.7: The mechanical motions of a CT scanner. The table is moved into the bore. An x-ray tube inside the gantry rotates around the patient. A detector array registers the x-ray intensity passing through the patient. The detector signals are fed to a computer, which then "reconstructs" a series of axial images ("slices") of the patient. (Reproduced from *Radiotherapy Physics in Practice*, J. R. Williams and D. I. Thwaites (eds.), Fig. 7.8, p. 135, © 2000 by permission of Oxford University Press.)

Medicine in 1979. CT was one of the most significant developments in medical imaging in the twentieth century. What's the breakthrough?

(1) Three-dimensional imaging.
(2) Soft tissue discrimination.

Herein lies the power of CT.

As shown in Figure 19.7 the patient lies on a table, which can move up and into the aperture (sometimes called the bore). The inferior and superior scan limits are selected first by performing a transmission scan (also called a topogram, scout, or surview). For this purpose the patient is moved through the bore while the x-ray tube is on but stationary (not rotating). Based on the image formed by this procedure, the operator then selects the inferior and superior limits of the scan. During the scan itself the x-ray tube rotates around the patient. The x-rays pass through the patient and are detected by a detector array opposite the tube and converted into electrical signals. The signals from the array are fed into a computer, which then "reconstructs" an axial slice or tomogram (see Figure 19.1) of the patient. This is quite different from the "shadow" picture formed by plane radiography. As the table moves further into the bore, successive slices in the inferior direction are reconstructed. These slices can be stacked to form a three-dimensional image of the patient. This provides a digital model of the patient, including both geometric data (location of skin surface, tumor, and organs at risk) and composition data (linear attenuation coefficient). This digital model is exported to a treatment planning system.

CT images are the primary imaging modality used for radiation therapy treatment planning purposes. There are three reasons for this: CT images are spatially accurate. They are not subject to spatial or geometric distortions. An accurate model of the patient is necessary for accurate dose calculations, both spatially and in terms of composition (i.e., electron density). The second reason is that the spatial resolution of CT is relatively high (compared to PET, for example). The third reason is that electron density data can be derived from the CT number (CT#), provided that a calibration curve is available (see section 19.4.3). MRI can suffer from spatial distortion, and it does not provide electron density data.

CT images represent a "virtual" patient. CT units are either diagnostic scanners or speciality scanners, called CT simulators, sold specifically for radiation therapy treatment planning. The advent of CT simulators and the use of "virtual simulation" may signal the end of conventional simulators. Virtual simulation involves the use of CT images along with software to "virtually" simulate and plan treatment. The role that CT plays in treatment planning is twofold:

(1) *Contour data:* provides true 3-D data on spatial location of skin, tumor, normal organs and tissues.
(2) *Electron density:* recall that Compton scattering is the dominant photon interaction at megavoltage therapy energies—depends primarily on the electron density (electrons/cm^3) $\Rightarrow$ inhomogeneity corrections depending on electron density.

19.4.1 Development of CT scanners

Early model CT scanners acquired a single axial slice at one time with the table immobile during tube rotation. The x-ray tube generates a fan beam of x-rays that rotates around the patient. The table is then advanced to acquire the next slice. In this way contiguous axial slices are generated. In the early 1990s spiral scanners were developed in which the table moves continuously while the x-ray beam remains on, tracing out a helical path around the patient. At about the same time, multi-slice scanners were introduced. These scanners are capable of acquiring multiple slices simultaneously. We will discuss each of these important developments below.

We begin with a discussion of the development of axial (non-spiral), single slice scanners. These scanners have evolved through four generations as shown in Figure 19.8. The first generation scanners used a pencil beam (Figure 19.8a) and a single detector. Both the x-ray tube and the detector first moved horizontally (translate) through 180 positions and then the x-ray tube and detector rotated 1°. This translate-rotate process was repeated until sufficient projections were obtained to form an image. It is not surprising that scan times were long, about 5 minutes for a single axial slice. Second-generation scanners (Figure 19.8b) used an x-ray fan beam and a multiple linear detector array. These scanners also operated in a translate-rotate mode. The multiple detectors increased speed considerably, but it still took as long as 20 seconds to image a single slice. Third-generation scanners use a fan beam and a detector array containing at least 30 elements (Figure 19.8c). Translation is no longer necessary, and both the tube and detector rotate. Scan times are as low as 1 second for an axial slice. In a third-generation scanner, each detector element images a particular annulus of the patient's anatomy. If an element is not functioning properly, a "ring" artifact may result. In a fourth-generation scanner (Figure 19.8d) the detectors form a ring completely surrounding the patient and therefore only the x-ray tube rotates. Most scanners sold today are actually third-generation scanners.

The x-ray detectors are either xenon gas ionization detectors, used in some third-generation scanners, or solid-state scintillation crystals used in third- and fourth-generation scanners. The thinnest slice thickness is determined by detector collimation and reconstruction parameters. Various slice thickness settings are possible: 1, 2, 5, and 10 mm are common. Spatial resolution can be as good as 0.6 mm in the axial plane.

Single-slice scanners have two major disadvantages. First, they are very slow, and second they suffer from poor resolution in the longitudinal direction. A non-spiral set of single-slice CT scans for treatment planning using a third- or fourth-generation scanner can take as long as 45 minutes. This is time-consuming for staff, and it is difficult for some patients to remain in immobilization devices this long. Practical values of the slice thickness are relatively large. The resolution in the axial plane of a CT image is typically about 1 mm. It is not uncommon with old scanners to use a slice thickness of 5 mm or even 10 mm. The slices are then stacked to form what could be described as a "pseudo 3-D" image. Because the resolution in the longitudinal direction is considerably poorer than in the axial plane, any object or boundary within a given slice will be imaged, but its location within the slice will be

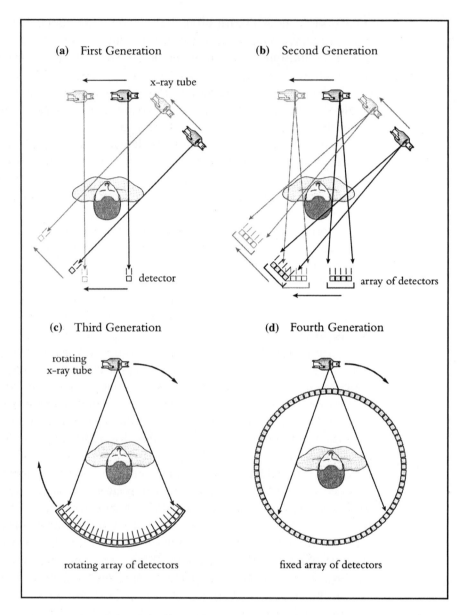

Figure 19.8: The four generations of CT units described in the text. (a) is a first generation unit, (b) is second generation; (c) and (d) are third and fourth generations. Most CT units sold today are third generation. (Reproduced from "CT Basics" by D. Cody in *The Physics and Applications of PET/CT Imaging,* Figs. 1 and 2, pp. 30, 32. © 2008, with permission from American Association of Physicists in Medicine (AAPM); previously printed in "Computed Tomography" by T. G. Flohr, D. D. Cody, and C. H. McCullough in *Advances in Medical Physics: 2006,* A. B. Wolbarst, R. G. Zamenhof, and W. R. Hendee (eds.), Figs. 3-4a/b, p. 63, © 2006, Medical Physics Publishing.)

unknown. This is sometimes called "volume averaging." This implies that the location of anatomical boundaries is uncertain by an amount approximately equal to the slice width. A 10-mm uncertainty in the superior/inferior direction may be unacceptable for highly conformal radiation therapy. In addition, digitally reconstructed radiographs (DRRs, see section 19.4.4) suffer from poor quality when the slice thickness is large.

New CT scanners are now helical (sometimes called spiral) scanners. These were introduced in the early 1990s. A non-spiral scan will be referred to as an axial or sequential scan. Modern CT scanners can acquire images in either axial or spiral mode. Spiral scanners are third generation and as such both the tube and detector rotate. Electrical cables run both to and from the tube and the detector, carrying power and data. In an axial scan the x-ray tube rotates as much as 360° around the patient.

If rotation in an axial scanner were to continue in the same direction past 360°, the cables would become increasingly wound or twisted. Therefore tube rotation must stop to avoid winding up cables. During this time interval, the table is moved (indexed) further into the bore by an amount that is usually equal to the slice thickness and then the next slice is acquired. Spiral CT is based on a continuous rotation of the x-ray tube as the patient is translated through the scanning aperture. Spiral scans eliminate the dead time associated with table motion. In this way it is possible to obtain up to 40 slices in a single breath hold. This reduces motion artifacts. Spiral CT has become possible through the introduction of "slip-ring" technology, which avoids the problem of cable winding. The faster the tube can rotate, the more rapidly a scan can be completed. CT units are now available in which the tube can rotate through 360° in as little as 0.3 seconds. This places severe cooling demands on the x-ray tube and housing. These tubes must be capable of handling a heavy heat load. They are therefore expensive, over $100,000. Oil is pumped through the tube housing and circulated through a radiator. The rapid rotation requires the gantry to be spin balanced like an automobile tire.

Newer CT units are capable of multiple-slice scanning (see Figure 19.9). These units can acquire more than a single slice simultaneously. There are units that can acquire up to 64 slices at one time. These use multiple rows of detectors extending along the longitudinal direction (z-axis, see Figures 19.7 and 19.9). The signals can be combined from adjacent elements to form slice thicknesses that are multiples of the size of a single detector element. The detector elements often have varying width—smaller near $z = 0$. The total scan thickness in a single rotation is related to the entire detector. The x-ray beam is now a cone beam instead of a fan beam. Multi-slice units are third-generation scanners. The advantages of multi-slice scanning are faster acquisition time, reduced tube loading, the option of respiratory gating or sorting,

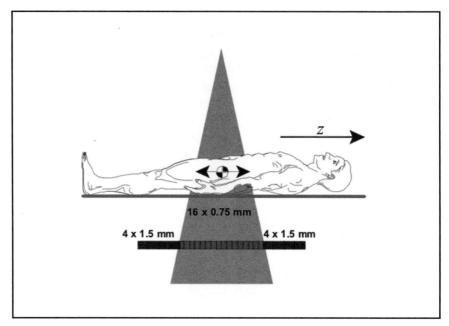

Figure 19.9: A multi-slice CT scanner showing the detector array and the cone beam diverging in the longitudinal direction. A single-slice scanner would have a very narrow (in the longitudinal direction) fan beam whereas a multi-slice scanner has a cone beam. In this illustration the collimator has been set to produce a 16-slice scan; each slice is 0.75 mm thick (all dimensions measured at the isocenter). The largest total scan thickness for this scanner is 16×0.75 + 8×1.5 = 24 mm.

thinner slices, and greater volume coverage on a single tube rotation. Slice thicknesses of as little as 0.5 mm are feasible. This is true 3-D imaging—the resolution in the z-direction is as good as the resolution in the axial plane. Multi-planar reconstruction becomes a useful option; the resolution in coronal and sagittal planes is as good as in an axial plane.

There are some disadvantages of multiple slice scanning. The use of a cone beam as opposed to a fan beam leads to increased scatter in the patient and to the detector. To maintain image quality, scattered photons are partially eliminated by using radiopaque separators (septa) between detector elements in the z-direction. This arrangement acts like a grid in a film cassette to eliminate image degradation due to scatter radiation (see chapter 4, section 4.4). The dose is higher for a multi-slice scan compared to an axial scan of like quality. This is due in part to increased scatter in the patient from the large cone beam and decreased efficiency because of the presence of the septa between detector rows.

Each patient may have hundreds or up to perhaps one thousand images (4D CT). As an example of data storage requirements, suppose 100 patients are under treatment at a given time. Let us assume that there are 150 images per patient and each image is 512×512 pixels. Each pixel is 2 bytes (actual gray scale is 12 or 14 bits, they do not use the full 16 bits). This requires $512 \times 512 \times 2 \times 150 \times 100 = 7.3$ GB storage just for current patients.

Reconstruction of images from a spiral scan is affected by the distance that the table moves in one revolution of the x-ray tube and by the beam thickness. The quantity pitch has been defined to describe this. With the introduction of multi-slice scanners the definition of pitch has been refined so that it is relevant to both axial and multi-slice scans:

$$P = \frac{\text{Table travel per rotation} \left(\text{mm}\right)}{T'} \qquad (19.1)$$

For a single slice axial scanner T' is the beam thickness as determined by the x-ray collimator in millimeters. For a multi-slice scanner T' is the total length of the tissue irradiated in millimeters (the length covered by the beam in Figure 19.9).

The pitch has a direct impact on patient dose and image quality. When $P < 1$ (see Figure 19.10) there is an improvement in image quality, but the dose is increased because of overlapping helical slices. When $P > 1$, less time is required for the scan, but not all regions are fully sampled; some z interpolation may be necessary resulting in a loss of resolution along the z-axis. The pitch values for one commercially available CT simulator range from 0.07 to 1.7 (for 4D CT, see section 19.4.6).

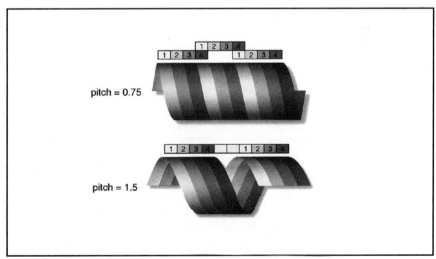

Figure 19.10: A side view of a four-slice scan. In the top diagram the pitch is 0.75. This means that the table travels 3/4 of the beam width (i.e., three channels) in one rotation. This causes detectors 1 and 4 to overlap. When the pitch = 1.5 (bottom diagram), there is an underlap and there is a gap in the coverage. [Reprinted from *The Modern Technology of Radiation Oncology*, vol. 2, J. Van Dyk (ed.), Fig 2.4, p. 38, © 2005; previously adapted and printed in "McCullough, C. H., and F. E. Zink, "Performance evaluation of a multi-slice CT system," *Med Phys* 26:2223–2230, © 1999 with permission from American Association of Physicists in Medicine (AAPM).]

Some radiation therapy departments do not have a dedicated CT unit. There are special considerations when using a diagnostic radiology department CT unit for RT planning. The size of the bore is an important factor. Diagnostic CT scanners generally have a bore diameter of 70 cm. This can be too small for RT for two reasons. The first reason has to do with patient immobilization and positioning devices; the second has to do with the size of the "scanned field of view." The prime example of the first reason is breast treatment where the patient is often lying on a breast board with her arm extended (see Figure 19.11). In this case, the patient may not fit through the bore. It is important that patients be scanned in the same position in which they will receive treatment so that there is no distortion in patient geometry. For accurate treatment planning, patient position must be identical during CT scan and treatment. Immobilization devices such as breast boards, alpha cradles, etc., may not fit through the bore. CT units cannot image over the entire bore aperture. The imaging size is specified by the scanned field of view. This must be large enough to encompass a patient's skin surface completely. The treatment planning system needs complete information about the location of the patient's skin surface to calculate treatment depths accurately. CT scanners with bore sizes up to 90 cm are now on the market for radiation therapy planning purposes.

The couch top of diagnostic CT units is concave. For RT purposes the couch top must be flat like the treatment couch, otherwise patient anatomy will be distorted. Couch inserts are available to make the couch top flat. In fact, a simple board will suffice provided that it is placed level, does not flex, and does not interfere with imaging.

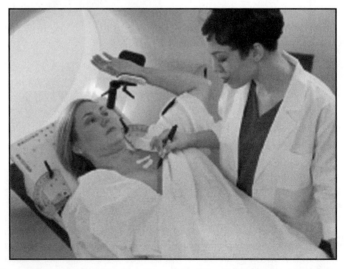

Figure 19.11: A patient undergoing simulation for a breast treatment. The patient is lying on a breast board. Note the position of her arm. This requires a large bore size for CT imaging. (Courtesy of Philips Healthcare, Andover, MA)

For radiation therapy, external lasers are needed for patient positioning and marking. Diagnostic CT units only have internal gantry lasers. The internal lasers show the location of the scan plane. The external lasers are mounted outside the gantry. A set of lateral lasers is mounted either on the floor or on the walls. These project perpendicular lines defining coronal and axial planes, usually 50 cm inferior to the scanning plane (assuming patient goes in head first). An overhead laser projects a sagittal fan beam perpendicular to the scan plane. This laser is sometimes mobile, as it is not possible to move the CT couch laterally.

19.4.2 CT Image Reconstruction

The goal of image reconstruction is to use transmitted x-ray intensity information to determine the μ value for each volume element (called a voxel). The value of μ is then used to construct a gray-scale map, which can be portrayed as an image. The process is described in this and the following section. A simple heuristic explanation follows.

In Figure 19.12 we consider the most elementary "patient" possible, one consisting of a single voxel of known side length x. A single x-ray projection is used. A known intensity, I_0, is incident on the voxel. The transmitted intensity, I, is measured by the detector (see Figure 19.8A). The relationship between the incident intensity and the transmitted intensity is $I = I_0 e^{-\mu x}$ (see chapter 5, section 5.5). In this equation the known quantities are I_0, I, and x. Therefore we can solve for the one unknown μ.

Now let us consider a slightly more realistic example: a patient consisting of two voxels, as shown in Figure 19.13. We again use a single x-ray projection. The relationship between the transmitted intensity and the incident intensity is $I = I_0 e^{-(\mu_1 + \mu_2)x}$, where I_0, I, and x are known and μ_1 and μ_2 are unknown. In this case, we have a single equation in two unknowns and we cannot solve for μ_1 and μ_2 without more projections.

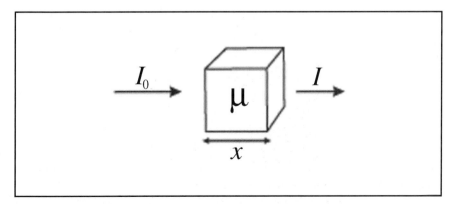

Figure 19.12: A "patient" consisting of a single voxel.

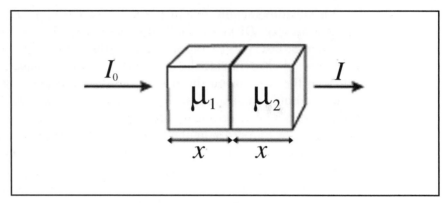

Figure 19.13: A "patient" consisting of two voxels.

Let us now consider a patient consisting of four voxels. We will use four x-ray projections, as shown in Figure 19.14. We have the following relationships between the incident and transmitted intensities:

$$I_1 = I_0 e^{-(\mu_1 + \mu_2)x}$$
$$I_2 = I_0 e^{-(\mu_3 + \mu_4)x}$$
$$I_3 = I_0 e^{-(\mu_2 + \mu_4)x}$$
$$I_4 = I_0 e^{-(\mu_1 + \mu_3)x}.$$

(19.2)

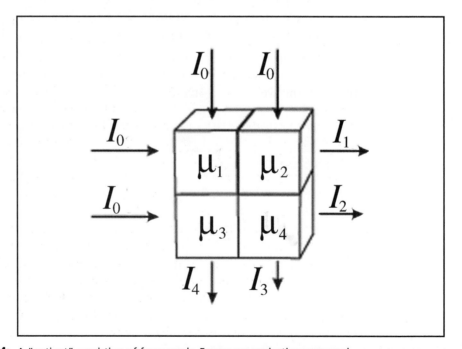

Figure 19.14: A "patient" consisting of four voxels. Four x-ray projections are used.

We have four equations in the four unknowns μ_1, μ_2, μ_3, and μ_4. These equations can be solved for the unknowns.

In general, a patient consists of a large number of voxels n. The illustration above has shown that provided there are enough projections, it is possible to solve for μ_1, μ_2, . . ., μ_n; that is, to find the μ value for each voxel. In practice, we are faced with the mathematical task of solving n equations in n unknowns where the value of n may be quite large. Sophisticated methods are used such as: 2-D Fourier transforms or "filtered backprojection." In this way one obtains three-dimensional information about the object imaged. This is called *image reconstruction* (recon). The calculations are carried out on a specialized computer in almost "real time." In the next section we discuss the problem of using the μ values to form an image.

19.4.3   CT Numbers and Hounsfield Units

Each pixel in a CT image requires a numerical gray-scale value for display. The values of μ are converted to CT# or CT pixel value. These are sometimes known as Hounsfield units:

$$CT\# = 1000 \frac{\mu_t - \mu_w}{\mu_w}, \tag{19.3}$$

where μ_t is the linear attenuation coefficient of the tissue in a particular voxel (for a given beam quality) and μ_w is the linear attenuation coefficient for water. Hounsfield units have no dimensions. For air $\mu_t \simeq 0 \text{ cm}^{-1}$ and therefore CT# = -1000 HU. For water $\mu_t = \mu_w$ and therefore CT# = 0 HU. The value of the CT# for dense bone depends on the kVp of the CT. At 100 kVp, $\mu_w = 0.206 \text{ cm}^{-1}$ and $\mu_{bone} = 0.528 \text{ cm}^{-1}$, therefore CT# = $1000(0.528 - 0.206)/0.206 = +1560$ HU. Most CT units have a CT# number range between -1000 HU and $+3000$ HU. High-density metal clips or prosthetic devices may have CT# approaching $+3000$ HU.

One HU represents a difference of 0.1% in attenuation coefficient with respect to water. Most CT units have a noise error of ± 5 HU. This allows discrimination at the level of $\pm 0.5\%$ in μ_t, enabling good contrast resolution. This sensitivity is what makes CT useful for soft tissue imaging.

CT images are usually 512×512 pixels. CT numbers may span the range from -1000 HU to $+3000$ HU. There are therefore 4000 possible values associated with each pixel. A 2-byte number associated with each pixel can accommodate this as $2^{16} = 6.6 \times 10^4$. Storage requirements are therefore 512×512×2 bytes = 0.5 MB for each slice. CT numbers must be converted into a gray level for display. The number of shades of gray that can be perceived by the human eye is at most 256.

One could assign $4000/256 \approx 16$ HU to the same shade of gray, but this would compress the scale and we would lose information. Instead, one should only throw away information that is not needed. This is accomplished by the use of a "window" and "leveling" system. A CT# is chosen that corresponds roughly with the average CT# in the region of interest. This value is called the "level" or center. A "window" width is chosen: for example, 128 shades below the center and 128 shades above the center. Pixels within the window are assigned gray-scale values between 0 and 255. Pixels below the window are set to black and pixels above the window are set to white. The window and level are chosen to obtain the required brightness and contrast for the type of tissue to be examined. Reducing the size of the window increases contrast. Changing the level allows inspection of a different range of CT numbers within the window. As an example of this process, suppose that the level chosen is 200 HU and the window is 500. In this case CT numbers less than $200 - 500/2 = -50$ are displayed as black and CT numbers above $200 + 500/2 = 450$ are displayed as white. One can adjust the window and level to obtain the desired brightness and contrast. This procedure is followed whenever CT images are examined.

For treatment planning with inhomogeneity corrections (see chapter 14, section 14.13), it is necessary to convert Hounsfield units to electron density (electrons/cm^3) by using a calibration curve. These curves are "bilinear" (see Figure 19.15). Calibration curves may be particular to the scanner and the kVp used. They are obtained by scanning a special

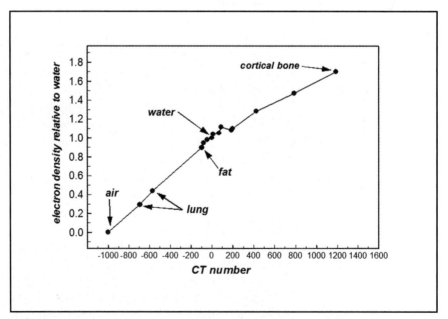

Figure 19.15: The relative electron density as a function of CT# for a representative CT scanner. Some tissues are heterogeneous and it is therefore not possible to assign a single unique CT#. This curve displays a typical bilinear character.

phantom containing about a dozen inserts with various known electron densities. An average CT number is measured for each insert and the electron density can then be plotted versus CT number as in Figure 19.15. The calibration curve is used by the treatment planning system to make inhomogeneity corrections.

High-density materials such as metal prosthetic implants, dental fillings, etc., may lead to streak artifacts. These streaks may have very high CT numbers. These high CT numbers are translated into high electron densities. Such images must be used with care if inhomogeneity corrections are turned "on" in the treatment planning system.

19.4.4   Digitally Reconstructed Radiographs

A plane film radiograph such as produced with a conventional simulator provides a beam's-eye view but not 3-D information. CT provides axial slices but not a beam's-eye view. The data contained in the CT record have information on the linear attenuation coefficient of each voxel. From these data it is possible to mathematically reconstruct a beam's-eye view image for any treatment port. This is known as a *d*igitally *r*econstructed *r*adiograph (*DRR*) because it is constructed from the digital CT data. A DRR is like a simulated radiograph and can be used like an ordinary simulation film for comparison with port films. An example is shown in Figure 19.16. The DRR is constructed by considering ray lines that emanate or diverge from the presumed source (e.g., the target of a linac) and strike an imaging plane a chosen distance away. The

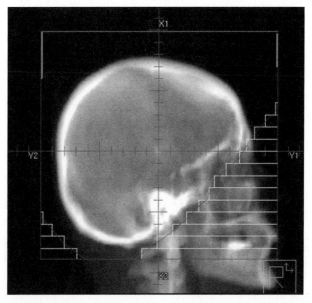

Figure 19.16: A beam's-eye view DRR for a lateral whole-brain irradiation field. The MLC leaf positions for blocking are superimposed.

value of any image pixel is related to the transmission of the associated ray line through the patient. The magnification of a DRR can be specified and various other image parameters can be easily manipulated because of the digital nature of these images. For example, it is possible to emphasize bone. DRR spatial resolution is improved by smaller slice thickness for the CT scan.

19.4.5 Virtual Simulation

The images acquired during a CT examination contain three-dimensional information about the patient's anatomy. These images can be used in conjunction with computer software to perform a virtual patient simulation immediately following CT image acquisition. The virtual simulation software mimics the mechanical motion of the linac. This allows beam's-eye view display for various gantry, collimator, and pedestal angles. The virtual simulation is used to define the treatment isocenter. The patient can then be marked with tattoos before getting off the CT couch. This often involves a set of lateral marks and an anterior or posterior mark. A system is necessary to ensure that the patient is in the same position on the treatment table as during the CT scan. Lasers are used to locate the spot where the skin marks are placed. The simulation software indicates the necessary couch position for laser marking. Radiopaque BBs are sometimes placed over the marks. These will be visible in the CT images and can be used to establish a coordinate system. As CT couches cannot be moved laterally, CT simulators have a moveable overhead sagittal laser. The sagittal fan beam is moved laterally to indicate the correct position of the isocenter on the patient's skin.

19.4.6 4D CT

The term "4D CT" refers to three spatial dimensions plus a time dimension. This is used to track respiratory motion. Let us first consider the effects of motion on CT images.

Refer to Figure 19.17. We imagine a spherical object in a patient's lung. This object is moving up and down sinusoidally with the patient's respiration. This object is shown in the figure (coronal view) at various times throughout two respiratory cycles. These snapshots in time are labeled with numbers 1 through 11. For simplicity we assume pure axial scans (no helical scan). The first axial scan shows the very top of the sphere. A side view of the axial scan slice is shown on the left in Figure 19.17. The top of the sphere is evident in this slice. The table is then indexed for the second axial scan, but by this time the sphere has moved out of the scan plane and does not show up on the axial slice labeled 2. The couch con-

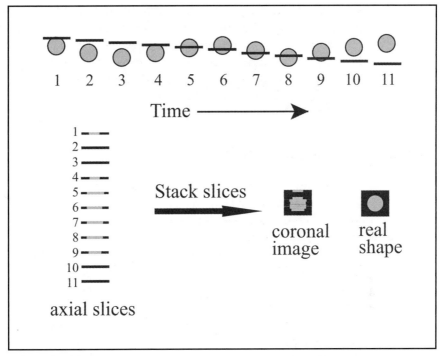

Figure 19.17: Illustration of the effects of motion on CT imaging. The region of interest is a sphere that is oscillating up and down as a result of respiratory motion. See the text for details. (Adapted from *The Modern Technology of Radiation Oncology,* vol. 2, J. Van Dyk (ed.), Fig. 2.5, p. 40, © 2005; previously printed in *International Journal of Radiation Oncology Biology and Physics,* "Can PET provide the 3D extent of tumor motion for individualized internal target volumes?" C. B. Caldwell, K. Mah, M. Skinner, and C. E. Danjoux, vol. 55, pp. 1381–1393, © 2003 with permission from Elsevier.)

tinues to move inward acquiring successive scans. A side view of each axial scan is shown at the bottom left. These can be stacked up to show a coronal image of the object (bottom right). The shape of the image of the object is clearly distorted. Figure 19.18 shows the respiratory motion distortion of a patient's lung tumor.

There are two types of 4-D imaging: prospective gated imaging and retrospective correlation imaging. In both types of imaging a device that monitors respiratory motion is attached to the patient's chest.

Prospective gated imaging is illustrated in Figure 19.19. During axial scans patients hold their breaths at either maximum inspiration or maximum expiration. The patient then resumes breathing while the couch is moved in. The patient then holds his breath again until the next axial scan is completed. The process continues until the entire scan is acquired. A disadvantage of this technique is that it requires patient cooperation and training.

In retrospective correlation (Figure 19.20) the patient breathes freely during a helical ultra low pitch scan. The pitch is made low

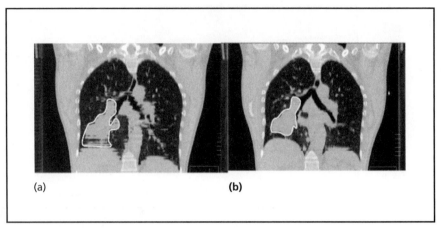

Figure 19.18: (a) A coronal reconstruction of a free breathing spiral CT. The jagged motion artifacts illustrated in Figure 19.17 can be seen in the diaphragm. The outline of a tumor is shown. (b) An expiration-correlated image. The motion artifacts are considerably reduced although not completely eliminated (examine the diaphragm). The shape of the tumor is now significantly different. (Courtesy of Rafael Vaello, TomoTherapy® Inc.)

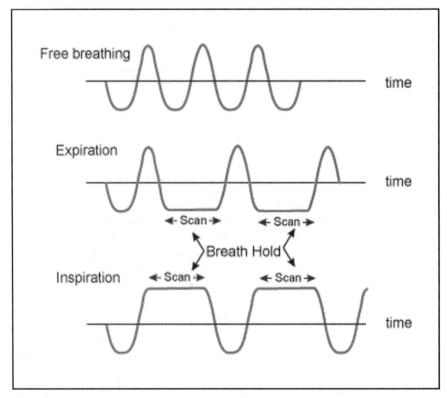

Figure 19.19: Gated prospective 4D CT. The top line shows the patient's free breathing pattern. The middle line shows 4D CT gated on full expiration. The patient is asked to hold his or her breath at full expiration while scanning is underway. This is repeated until the entire volume of interest is scanned. The bottom line shows 4D CT gated on inspiration.

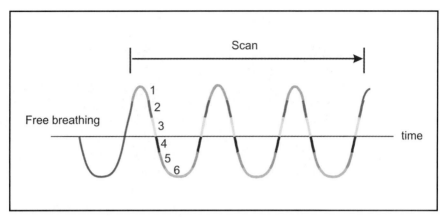

Figure 19.20: Retrospective 4D CT. The patient breathes freely while a very low pitch scan is acquired. Every portion of the relevant anatomy is imaged through a minimum of one respiratory cycle. The breathing cycle is divided into phases. In this figure there are a total of six phases. Eight to ten phases are common. All axial images acquired during a particular phase are grouped together into sets. See COLOR PLATE 14.

enough so that all portions of the anatomy are imaged through several respiratory cycles. The couch should not move more than one detector length in the time it takes to complete one breathing cycle. For a tube rotation time of about 0.5 s and a breathing rate of 12 breaths/min, the pitch should be about 0.1. The respiratory cycle is divided into phases. The operator can choose the number of phases. A typical number is 10. The slices are then arranged in groups according to the phase of the respiratory cycle in which they were acquired. One then has 10 groups of CT scans of the patient's entire chest at 10 moments in time. This can result in over 1000 axial slices. These data can then be used to study the three-dimensional motion of lung tumors in detail. This allows an assessment of the internal target volume (ITV) (see chapter 14, section 14.6).

19.5 Magnetic Resonance Imaging

Magnetic resonance imaging is capable of superb soft-tissue discrimination. MRI is used to diagnose diseases of the central nervous system and musculoskeletal disorders. Breast MRI is used to evaluate lesions discovered with mammography. MRI is widely used as an adjunct to CT in localizing treatment volumes, particularly in the brain. MRI is also capable of direct multi-planar imaging. A CT unit acquires images directly in an axial plane. Images in any other plane, such as the coronal or sagittal, require additional computer processing whereas MR images can be acquired directly in any desired plane. The 2003 Nobel Prize in "Physiology or Medicine" was awarded to Paul Lauterbur and Peter Mansfield "for their discoveries concerning magnetic resonance imaging." This Nobel Prize was somewhat controversial because another important contributor to the development of MRI, Raymond Damadian, was excluded.

An MRI imager appears much the same as a CT imaging unit (Figure 19.7), although the bore is deeper. Some patients experience claustrophobia when in the bore. It may take as long as 10 to 15 minutes to acquire a series of MRI images. A very uniform high-intensity magnetic field is established inside the bore (see chapter 2, section 2.3.6). The field strengths can range from 1 to 3 T and are generally produced with superconducting electromagnets (see chapter 2, section 2.3.4). These magnets require cooling with liquid helium. Higher field strengths allow shorter imaging time and higher signal to noise ratio. MRI units cannot be situated near linear accelerators because the strong magnetic fields would interfere with the motion of the electrons in the linac. Patients with any ferromagnetic implants may not be eligible for an MRI scan. This includes patients with pacemakers or aneurism clips, etc. Exposure to magnetic fields of the strength used for MRI are not known to cause any significant side effects. MRI units are now available with an "open" magnet configuration. These units do not have a donut and thus eliminate claustrophobia.

Nuclear magnetic resonance is based on a fundamentally quantum mechanical effect. A classical physics description of this is simply not possible. We will do our best to explain by drawing classical analogies and "waving our hands." Do not be distressed if you feel that you do not have a detailed or fundamental understanding of this topic. Our task here is to simply provide some flavor of the basic science of MRI. Magnetic resonance imaging is complex and requires years of study to understand fully.

Elementary particles possess an intrinsic angular momentum or "spin." The comic book depiction of this is a small spinning top (like most comic book depictions, this is not reality). A small magnetic field is associated with this spin. The particle acts like a tiny bar magnet (see Figure 19.21) or a "dipole." In an atomic nucleus protons tend to pair up with spins in opposite directions. The same is true for neutrons. When nucleons pair up, their magnetic fields cancel. A nucleus with an odd number of neutrons, protons, or both, however, will have a residual magnetic field. Hydrogen, with a single proton, is one such nucleus. Hydrogen is abundant in tissue and is therefore used for most MR imaging.

In the absence of an externally applied magnetic field, the magnetic fields of the individual nuclei will point in random directions and thus, over the bulk of the material, they will cancel out. If an external magnetic field is applied however, the magnetic nuclei will tend to line up with this field, like iron filings on a piece of paper subjected to a magnetic field. The aligned nuclei will contribute to the external field, reinforcing it. The magnetic field associated with the aligned nuclei is called the "magnetization" and the symbol for this quantity is $\vec{M}$.

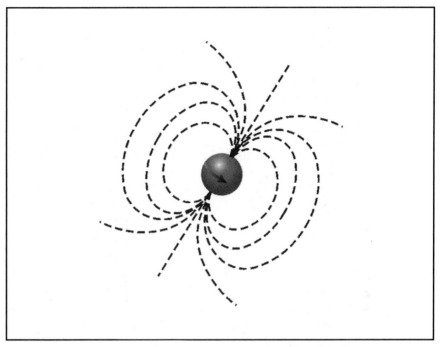

Figure 19.21: Elementary particles such as neutrons and protons possess a property called "spin." A small magnetic field is associated with this. Elementary particles act like small bar magnets.

When the nuclei, which act like little bar magnets, are subjected to an external magnetic field, they behave like a spinning top or a gyroscope in a gravitational field. A top that is spinning will "precess" under the action of gravity (see Figure 19.22). The rotation axis of the top slowly rotates around a vertical axis. In an analogous fashion, nuclei precess in an externally applied magnetic field. The frequency of precession is called the Larmor frequency, ν, and it is directly proportional to the strength of the external magnetic field:

$$\nu = \frac{\gamma B_0}{2\pi}, \qquad (19.4)$$

where γ is a quantity that depends on the particular atomic nucleus and is called the gyromagnetic ratio. The value of $\gamma/2\pi$ for protons is 43 MHz/T. For a magnetic field strength of $B_0 = 1.5$ T, the precession frequency is 64 MHz. This is in the radio region of the electromagnetic spectrum just below FM radio in frequency (see chapter 2, section 2.4).

After the external magnetic field is applied to the patient, there are three stages in the process of MR imaging: excitation, relaxation, and detection. *Excitation* involves tipping or rotating the magnetic moment away from the axis defined by $\vec{B}_0$ using the addition of a briefly applied weak

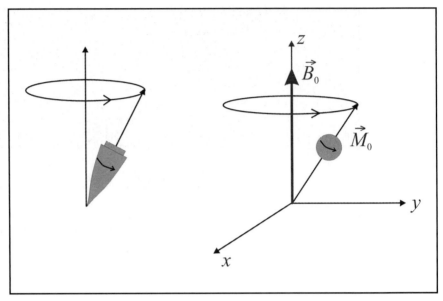

Figure 19.22: A spinning top precesses in a gravitational field; that is, the spin axis itself rotates around a vertical axis. In a similar way, the magnetic moment of a proton precesses around the direction of an externally applied magnetic field. The direction of the magnetic field is taken to be along the z-axis.

magnetic field in the form of a radio frequency (RF) pulse. The angle through which $\vec{M}$ is tipped can range from 0° through 180°, depending on the duration of the pulse. If $\vec{M}$ is tipped 90°, this is called a 90° pulse. After the RF pulse, $\vec{M}$ "wants" to return to its undisturbed direction along $\vec{B}_0$. This is *relaxation*.

After excitation, the amplitude of the component of $\vec{M}$ in the x-y plane will decrease at a rate 1/T2 and the z-component will increase at a rate of 1/T1. The values T1 and T2 depend on the external field strength B_0 and on the characteristics of different types of tissue. As the nuclei return to their equilibrium state, they emit an RF signal which can be detected by an RF coil. This is *detection*. The closer the receiving coil to the patient, the better. A number of different types of RF coils are available: head coils, body coils, and coils for other body parts.

The precession frequency depends on the applied magnetic field [see equation (19.4)]. If small gradients are deliberately introduced into this field, then the precession frequency will vary with position in the patient. In this way spatial information can be encoded in the data and this information can be used to reconstruct an image.

Typical images are one of three types: proton density or spin density, T1 weighted, or T2 weighted (see Figure 19.23). These are produced using different combinations of echo time (TE) and repetition time (TR). T2 weighted images have TE of 60 to 100 ms and TR of about 3000 ms. T1 weighted images have TE about 10 ms and a value of TR comparable to T1 for the tissue of interest (about 500 ms at

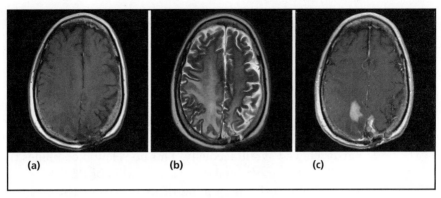

(a)   (b)   (c)

Figure 19.23: Three axial MRI images of a GBM tumor. (a) is a T1 weighted image. This image displays the tumor and edema as dark. (b) is T2 weighted. This image displays the tumor and edema as light. T2 images do not show fat and they highlight CSF and gray matter. The image in (c) was made with a gadolinium contrast agent. (Courtesy of Brigham and Women's Hospital, Boston, MA)

1.5 tesla).[4] Fluid attenuated inversion recovery (FLAIR) is a pulse sequence that creates images that have T2 weighted contrast for brain tissue but in which signals for CSF are suppressed.

FLASH stands for fast low angle shot, and about 70% of MRI is done this way. A contrast agent that is commonly used contains the paramagnetic element gadolinium.

MR images by themselves are generally not adequate for treatment planning purposes. They are more susceptible to spatial distortions than CT. It is important to have reliable geometric information about the patient. The determination of the location of a voxel in MRI is governed by the magnetic field gradients. Any irregularities in the magnetic field can therefore cause spatial distortion. In addition, MR imaging takes longer than CT and therefore there is an increased likelihood of distortion due to patient motion. Furthermore, MRI does not provide information about electron density, which is necessary for inhomogeneity corrections in dose calculations. The physical dimensions of the scanner and its accessories limit the use of immobilization devices. Dense bone contains very little hydrogen and therefore the bone signal is weak. For this reason useful DRRs cannot be generated for comparison with portal images. Instead of being used by themselves, MRI images are often used in conjunction with CT data for treatment planning. This requires image fusion, which is discussed in the next section.

---

[4] "MRI in Radiation Treatment Planning" by Y. Cao and L. Chen, pp. 401–424 in *Integrating New Technologies into the Clinic: Monte Carlo and Image-Guided Radiation Therapy,* AAPM 2006 Summer School Proceedings, AAPM Medical Physics Monograph No. 32, B. H. Curran, J. M. Balter, and I. J. Chetty, Program Directors, 2006.

19.6 Image Fusion/Registration

For the purpose of treatment planning it is very useful to be able to combine or correlate images from different modalities, in particular CT and MRI. Tumors frequently appear very different on MR images than on CT (if they show up at all). Image fusion (or registration, as it is sometimes called) is the process of placing two sets of images on the same coordinate system so that they can be superimposed like an overlay or viewed simultaneously. This correlation combines the advantages of CT with another modality such as MRI or PET. Most treatment planning systems offer the option of image fusion. Sometimes it is desired to register two sets of CT images obtained on different dates. The process of image-guided radiation therapy (IGRT; see section 19.10) depends on image registration.

We first consider the problem of registration for images of an object that is a rigid body. A rigid body is one that cannot change shape or be deformed. The two objects in the different image sets can be brought into coincidence by coordinate translations (shifts) and rotations. It is best if both sets of images are obtained at about the same time, ideally the same day. The patient should be in the same position for each imaging modality. Ideally any immobilization devices should be used for both sets of scans. We will discuss three methods for registration of a rigid body: point-to-point matching, surface to surface matching and voxel-to-voxel matching.[5]

In point-to-point matching, a set of corresponding reference points or fiducial markers is necessary in both sets of images. These can be externally placed markers positioned in key locations on the patient's skin. Adhesive markers are available commercially, which show up clearly in both CT and MRI images. A bare minimum of three points in each image, not all lying in the same plane, is required and more are preferred. Once the fiducial points are specified, the image fusion software shifts (translates) and rotates the images so that they correspond to one another. In the absence of externally placed markers, which are preferable, internal anatomical reference points may be used. It may not be easy to find anatomical points of reference that can be clearly seen in both image sets.

Anatomical surfaces may be easier to delineate in both image sets than discrete points. Surface matching involves matching anatomical surfaces in the two images. Voxel-to-voxel matching uses all of the information in the images. In this technique there is an attempt to correlate all of the voxels to one another. One shortcoming of this technique is that parts of the image may be unreliable. An example is the mandible, which may be in different positions with respect to the skull

---

[5] *Radiation Oncology: A Physicist's Eye View* by M. Goitein, 2008, p. 48.

in the two image sets. A method of image registration that has achieved some success involves the maximization of "mutual information."[6] Although the pixel intensities of tissues may differ in different modalities, there is a relationship between them. For example, bone is bright in CT images and dark in MRI images. Mutual information registration relies on the predictable relationship between corresponding tissue types in the two image sets.

If there are significant differences in the shape of the patient between the two image sets, then deformable image registration is desirable. Differences in shape may result from imaging on different days, in different positions, or with and without immobilization devices. Respiratory motion may cause deformation also. Deformable image registration is not yet commonly available in commercial treatment planning software.

For treatment planning, the primary set of images is the CT set. Dose calculations are done from this set. Once the software has performed the fusion, it is up to the user to examine the images to assess the quality of the result (see Figure 19.24). Do not take the quality of the fusion for granted. The correlation of the two image sets must be carefully examined. The radiation oncologist can draw tumor outlines (GTV, CTV, etc.) on the fused MR (or PET) images, which will then automatically be transferred to the CT images used for dose calculations. The reliability of this process depends critically on the quality of the registration.

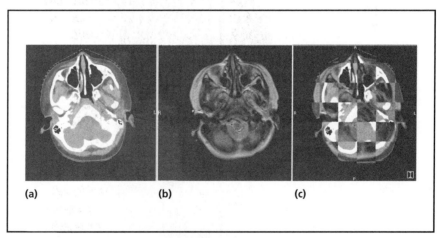

(a)   (b)   (c)

Figure 19.24: An example of image fusion between CT and MRI images. The image in (a) is the CT image. The image in (b) is the reconstructed (fused) MRI image that corresponds to this. The quality of the fusion (which is marginal) is assessed from the "checkerboard" image in (c). Alternating squares are either CT or MRI.

---

[6] Chen et al., in Chapter 2, Imaging in Radiotherapy in *Treatment Planning in Radiation Oncology,* 2nd edition (F. Khan, ed.).

19.7 Ultrasound Imaging

The use of ultrasound for diagnostic imaging is widespread in medicine. Ultrasound is one of the three means of imaging soft tissue. Ultrasound equipment is relatively inexpensive and there is no ionizing radiation exposure. An ultrasound system is shown in Figure 19.25. Ultrasound is frequently used as an adjunct to mammography for breast cancer detection. In radiation therapy ultrasound is used for treatment planning, particularly for prostate brachytherapy implants, and for treatment position verification, primarily for external beam prostate therapy (see section 19.10).

Sound waves are longitudinal waves—a small parcel of matter in the medium oscillates back and forth in the direction in which the wave moves (see Figure 19.26). This contrasts with transverse waves in which the motion of the medium is perpendicular to the direction of wave travel (as in Figure 2.12). Examples of transverse waves are waves on a string or (approximately) waves on the surface of water.

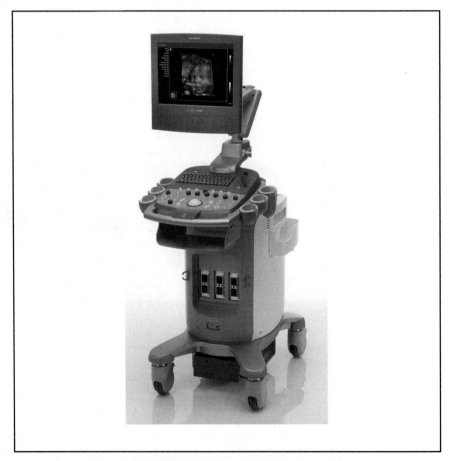

Figure 19.25: Ultrasound imaging cart. (Courtesy of Siemens Medical Solutions USA Inc., Concord, CA)

Sound can be thought of as a compressional wave. This is illustrated in Figure 19.26. This figure shows a snapshot at an instant in time of a compressional wave.

The speed of sound in a given medium depends on the elastic properties of that medium. The speed of sound in soft tissue is approximately 1540 m/s. Ultrasound imaging is dependent on differences in the sound speed of various tissues. When an ultrasound wave is incident upon an interface where the sound velocity changes, part of the wave will be reflected. It is these reflections that form the basis for conventional ultrasound imaging.

The frequencies of audible sound waves extend from about 20 Hz up through perhaps 20 kHz (if you are a child with excellent hearing). Ultrasound frequencies are approximately 5 MHz, well beyond the range of human hearing (hence the name ultrasound). As an example, we will calculate the wavelength of a 3.5 MHz sound wave in soft tissue. We use the equation $v\,\lambda = c_s$ [essentially equation (2.19)] where c_s is the sound speed: $\lambda = c_s/v = (1540 \text{ m s}^{-1})/(3.5\times10^6 \text{ s}^{-1}) = 4.4\times10^{-4}$ m or 0.44 mm. To achieve high spatial resolution, small wavelength is desirable. If the wavelength is comparable to, or larger than, the object to be imaged, then the wave will simply "bend" (diffract) around the object and no clear (specular) reflection will occur. It is apparent from the previous calculation that high frequencies are necessary to achieve small wavelength, and this is why ordinary audible sound would be inadequate for high-resolution imaging.

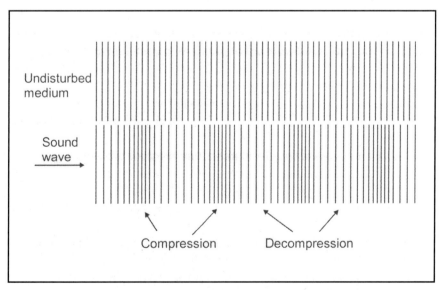

Figure 19.26: A longitudinal sound wave. The top portion of the figure shows an undisturbed medium (no sound wave). The bottom portion is a snapshot at a particular instant in time showing regions of compression and decompression. A small element in the medium moves back and forth horizontally as the wave passes by from left to right.

Ultrasound waves are produced and detected by a device called a transducer. A transducer is any device that converts one form of energy to another. The ultrasound transducer converts electrical energy to mechanical energy. An electrical signal fed into the transducer converts electrical energy to mechanical vibrational energy. The transducer is coupled to the patient surface (sometimes a coupling gel is used to get good mechanical contact) and sound is transmitted into the patient's body. A transducer also detects and converts the reflected sound waves into electrical energy—similar in function to a microphone. The reflected wave provides the basis for image formation. The longer it takes a wave reflected from an interface to return to the transducer, the further the interface is from the transducer.

19.8 Functional/Metabolic Imaging

Functional imaging shows the location and strength of physiological activity at the cellular and molecular levels.

The promise of functional imaging:

(1) *Improve disease detection:* functional imaging is capable of detecting microscopic disease.
(2) *Cancer staging:* functional imaging may reveal areas of disease not visible with anatomical imaging. For example, it may more readily reveal the existence of metastatic disease.
(3) *Treatment planning:* functional imaging may be of assistance in planning radiation therapy by providing more accurate localization of disease; radioresistance of tumor, tumor phenotype; identify areas of hypoxia that may require a higher dose. In the future it may become possible to identify a biological target rather than simply an anatomical target.
(4) *Response to therapy:* may allow a more rapid indication of cellular response to therapy.
(5) *Earlier detection of recurrence.*

Positron emission tomography (PET) provides metabolic information such as glucose metabolism rates. Cancer cells generally metabolize glucose at higher rates than normal cells. The patient is administered a pharmaceutical tagged with a positron emitter either by injection or inhalation. PET scans frequently employ F-18 (fluorodeoxyglucose, ^{18}F-FDG). This is a marker for glucose metabolism. The distribution of activity throughout the patient is imaged. FDG uptake is enhanced in most malignant tissues and in some benign structures as well. FDG uptake can be used to measure tumor response to treatment as well as for initial staging. New PET radiopharmaceuticals that are more specific markers of tumor activity are under development.

F-18 undergoes positron decay with a half-life of 110 minutes. The positron emitters used in PET imaging have a short lifetime and therefore the supply for these isotopes must be physically close at hand. Positron emitters are produced in cyclotrons. Therefore PET facilities must either have a cyclotron on site or a cyclotron must be located relatively nearby.

There is a waiting period of about an hour between injection of FDG and the scan to allow time for uptake. PET scan data acquisition takes on the order of 20 minutes. This is clearly a problem when significant respiratory motion is present. 4D PET scanning is on the horizon and is expected to be available soon.

The positrons travel only a short distance before annihilating and forming two 0.5 MeV photons that travel in almost completely opposite (180°) directions. These photons are detected by scintillation detectors made of bismuth germanate (BGO) or (LSO:ce).[7] The visible photons that emerge from the scintillator are detected by photomultiplier tubes.

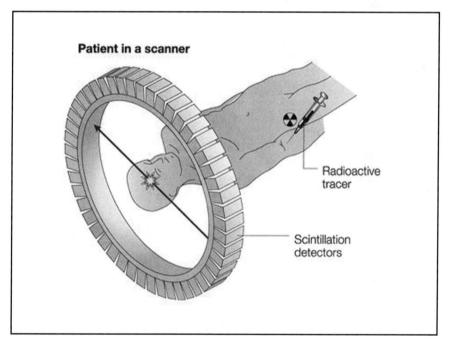

Figure 19.27: The detectors in a PET scanner form an axial ring around the patient. Event counting is based on annihilation coincidence. Events must occur nearly simultaneously in opposite detectors or they are rejected. Coincidence detection confirms that the annihilation must have occurred somewhere along the line joining the detectors. (Reprinted by permission from MacMillan Publishers Ltd: *Nature Reviews Cancer*, vol 4, pp. 457–469, "The potential of positron-emission tomography to study anticancer-drug resistance," C. M. L. West, T. Jones, and P. Price, © 2004.)

---

[7] Sasa Mutic in "Use of Imaging Systems for Patient Modeling PET and SPECT" by S. Mutic, pp. 375–400, in *Integrating New Technologies into the Clinic: Monte Carlo and Image-Guided Radiation Therapy*, AAPM 2006 Summer School Proceedings, AAPM Medical Physics Monograph No. 32, B. H. Curran, J. M. Balter, and I. J. Chetty, Program Directors, 2006.

PET uses annihilation coincidence detection to reconstruct axial images showing the activity distribution or uptake. There is a series of detectors in a ring around the gantry bore (see Figure 19.27). Each detector in the ring is paired with detectors on the opposing side of the ring. If a signal is detected in one of the detectors, a gating circuit "listens" for a signal in the paired detectors on the opposite side for a short interval of time called the coincidence window. If a signal is detected during this interval, it is assumed that the signal must represent a true annihilation photon corresponding to the detection on the opposite side. It is then known that the annihilation must have occurred somewhere along the line joining the two detectors. If no second signal is detected during the coincidence window, the original signal is discarded. The coincidence window is usually about 5 to 10 ns in duration, which corresponds roughly to a time $t = D/c$, where D is the maximum thickness of the patient and c is the speed of light.

Currently, 90% of PET scans are for oncology purposes. Combined PET/CT scanners now completely dominate the market. In a PET/CT unit the two gantries are combined in the same housing (see Figure 19.28). PET/CT machines have the advantage that fusion is more accurate because the patient is scanned on the same couch and almost at the same time as the CT scan. Therefore the patient is positioned identically in the two scans. Fusion of separate PET images and CT is more difficult because of the low spatial resolution of PET images (on the order

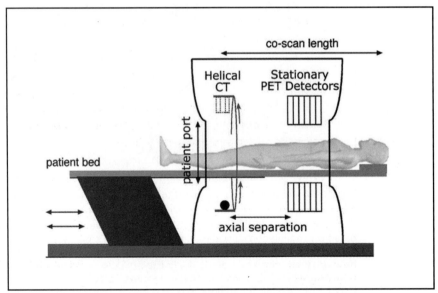

Figure 19.28: A PET/CT unit. This is a long bore design in which the housing covers both the PET and CT unit. (Reprinted from *The Modern Technology of Radiation Oncology*, vol. 2, J. Van Dyk (ed.), Fig. 2.14, p. 63, © 2005; previously printed in *Radiologic Clinics of North America*, vol. 42, issue 6, A. M. Alessio, P. E. Kinahan, P. M. Cheng, H. Vesselle, and J. S. Karp, "PET/CT scanner instrumentation, challenges, and solutions," pp. 1017–1032, © 2004 with permission from Elsevier.)

of 5 mm). The CT data allow for attenuation corrections of the PET image, resulting in sharper images and significantly shorter (by up to 40%) PET scan time.[7]

The uptake of FDG can be quantified by the use of the standard uptake value (SUV), which is defined as:

$$SUV = \frac{\text{Activity per unit volume} / \text{decay factor}}{\text{Injected activity} / \text{body mass}}, \qquad (19.5)$$

where the activity per unit volume is measured in units of MBq/ml, the decay factor is the fraction of decay between administration and the time of the scan, and the injected activity/body mass is in units of MBq/g. The SUV will vary throughout a tissue. The maximum SUV is a more useful parameter than average SUV.[8] SUV may not be useful in tissue that normally has a high SUV such as the brain (high glucose metabolism rate) and the kidneys (the kidneys clear FDG from the body). It is common to use an SUV threshold of 2.5 as an indicator of the presence of malignant tissue although SUV values have not been shown to be useful for defining GTV boundaries.[9]

19.9 Portal Imaging

How do we verify correct treatment delivery?

(1) *Positional accuracy:* Are we hitting the target?
    Portal imaging.
(2) *Dosimetric accuracy:* Are we delivering the right amount of dose to the target?
    In vivo dosimetry: TLDs, diodes, MOSFETs, etc., discussed in chapter 8 (see also chapter 18, section 18.3.4). In the future these two may be "married" with portal imagers that can simultaneously image and verify dose.

Portal images can be acquired with either film (rapidly disappearing) or electronic portal imaging devices (EPIDs). Portal images are used to verify both the shape of the aperture and the position of the central axis with respect to the patient's anatomy. It is common to superimpose an open field on the portal aperture field so that surrounding anatomy can be viewed for reference. This is sometimes referred to as a "double exposure."

---

[8] The SUV must be used with caution. Caldwell and Mah have pointed out that some researchers refer to SUV as standing for "silly, useless, value."

[9] C. B. Caldwell and K. Mah in chapter 2, *Imaging for Radiation Therapy Planning, The Modern Technology of Radiation Oncology,* Volume 2, J. Van Dyk (ed.), page 67.

19.9.1 Port Films

(1) *Localization film:* Exposure is short compared to the daily treatment time, need sensitive film.

(2) *Verification film:* Exposure is for the duration of the treatment delivery with that field, use slow film such as Kodak XV film.

These films are compared with films from the simulator or DRRs produced by the treatment planning system. The purpose is to verify targeting.

Why is portal image quality so poor compared to diagnostic images?

(1) *Poor contrast:* Predominant interaction is Compton, weak dependence on Z, very little differential absorption is seen compared to diagnostic films.

(2) *Scattered photons and secondary electrons:* Scattered photons are not easily removed, cannot use a grid.

(3) *Large penumbra:* Geometric + phantom scatter.

The quality of port images degrades with increasing beam energy and patient thickness (>20 cm). Portal images should be made using the lowest energy photon beam available.

For portal films, the film is placed in a special cassette. Compton recoil electrons form the image on the film, not the photons directly. The secondary electrons generated in the patient, treatment couch, etc., tend to smear out images because electrons are very easily deflected. We want to filter out these electrons. We would also like to have some build-up in front of the film. For these two reasons metal screens are used inside portal film cassettes. The screen is placed in close contact with the film. The screen is made of a high-density material such as lead or copper. It is common to use a copper screen about 1 mm thick. Port films are not made in real-time—they have to be developed. They are impractical to do before every treatment. This leads to a motivation to have real-time imaging.

19.9.2 Electronic Portal Imaging Devices[10]

There are three major types of electronic portal imaging devices (EPIDs):

(1) Screen camera systems.
(2) Matrix ion chamber.
(3) Flat-panel arrays.

This field is evolving rapidly. Linac manufacturers have now moved to flat-panel arrays.

---

[10] Much of the information in this section is taken from *The Modern Technology of Radiation Oncology*, J. Van Dyk (ed.), 1999.

Screen camera systems use a video camera and a mirror oriented at a 45° angle. A phosphor-coated metal plate produces visible light photons, which are imaged by the camera. Camera images are digitized at 30 frames/s, then averaged to produce a final image. They have good resolution, but they are bulky and tend to get in the way.

Matrix ion chamber EPIDs consist of an array of ionization chambers. One design uses a 256×256 array of ion chambers with an electrode separation of 0.8 mm and is filled with a volatile liquid. When the liquid is irradiated, ion pairs are formed which are collected when a bias is applied between the electrodes.

Flat-panel arrays have replaced camera-based and matrix ion chamber EPIDs. The image quality is superior to the older technology. The flat-panel arrays overcome the bulkiness of camera systems and the relatively long irradiation times for matrix ion chamber EPIDs. Flat-panel EPIDs are solid-state devices in which amorphous silicon (a-Si) is deposited on a thin substrate, usually 1 mm of glass. Amorphous silicon is highly resistant to radiation damage and can therefore be placed in the direct beam. Each pixel is a photodiode, which detects light generated by a screen/phosphor combination. The screen/phosphor combination consists of a metal plate and a phosphor screen. The metal plate removes secondary electrons generated in the patient as well as low-energy scattered photons. A commercial model is the Varian aS500 Portal Vision with an array size of 40×30 cm^2 and 512×384 pixels (see Figure 19.29). This model has a 1 mm copper plate and a gadolinium oxysulfide (Gd$_2$O$_2$S) screen. Each pixel value is represented by a 16-bit word.

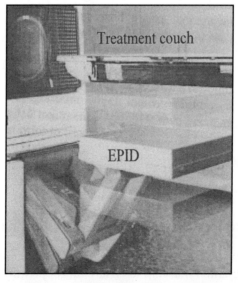

Figure 19.29: A portal imager on a robotic arm. The imager folds away at the base of the gantry when not in use. The arm can move the imager vertically and horizontally. (Courtesy of Varian Medical Systems, Inc. Copyright © 2010. All rights reserved.)

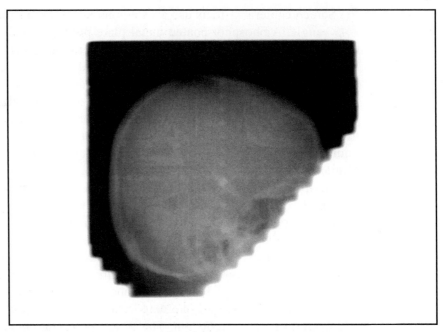

Figure 19.30: An electronic portal image made with a flat-panel array. This is a lateral skull image made with a 6 MV beam using 2 MU for a whole-brain irradiation field. The graticule is visible in the image. The faint outline of a diode placed on the patient's skin is visible at the center. Compare this image with the DRR for the same patient in Figure 19.16.

What are the differences between the use of EPIDs and film? One obvious difference is an immediate result without having to wait for processing. EPIDs are sensitive to the dose rate whereas film is sensitive to the total cumulative dose. For the EPID, one sets a specific number of MU regardless of the patient thickness. For film one must take into account the patient thickness. The digital format of EPID images allows image enhancement, window and leveling, and digital storage and dissemination. Both film and EPID images are available in hard copy. With film, what you see is what you are stuck with.

The ease of use of EPIDs makes more frequent imaging easily feasible (see Figure 19.30). It becomes feasible to image the patient daily and to use correction algorithms that indicate shifts (and possibly rotations) of the patient with respect to the intended treatment position. It then becomes possible to move the patient into the intended position just prior to treatment.

19.10 Image-Guided Radiation Therapy

Image-guided radiation therapy (IGRT) employs imaging of soft tissue or implanted markers to ensure target positioning prior to treatment. The location of key anatomical structures or markers is compared to the expected location (based on CT images used for treatment planning) and the patient is moved if necessary. The geometric accuracy of treatment delivery is limited by three factors: set up uncertainty, intrafraction target movement, and interfraction target movement. These issues have been discussed in chapter 14, section 14.6. The desire for highly conformal therapy is the motivation for IGRT. IGRT reduces the chance of a geometrical miss and allows a reduction in the size of the PTV with all the benefits that follow: fewer treatment complications and/or dose escalation.

There are quite a variety of commercially available systems for IGRT. Conventional linear accelerators can now be purchased with optional on-board kV imagers that are capable of cone beam CT (see Figures 19.31 and 19.32). The imager consists of an x-ray tube and a flat-panel detector. The axis of the x-ray beam is perpendicular to the MV beam axis. These are now widely available. Another option is a conventional linac and a CT scanner that share a common couch. A third option is CT images generated from the same MV beam that is used to treat the patient. This technique is used on an innovative treatment machine that delivers "tomotherapy." We defer a discussion of tomotherapy units to the next chapter. Ultrasound is used in some clinics to image the prostate prior to prostate radiotherapy. Yet another choice is implantable markers that are available from several vendors. These

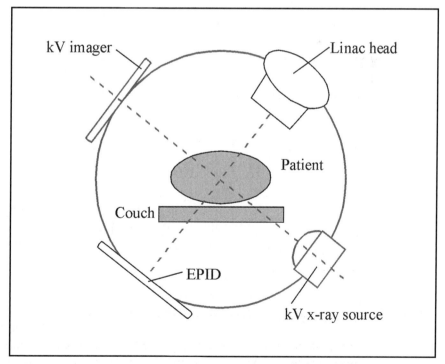

Figure 19.31: A conventional linac with on-board kV cone beam imaging. The gantry rotates around the patient with the MV beam off and the kV beam on. Given a sufficient number of projections, a set of axial CT images may be reconstructed.

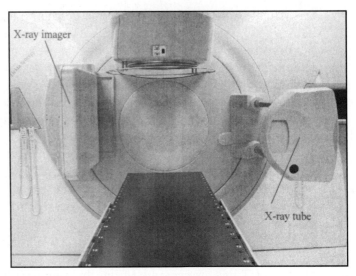

Figure 19.32: The Elekta Synergy® with on board kV imager. (Courtesy of Elekta, Norcross, GA)

markers can be observed in MV images. Provided that there are a sufficient number of these, the location and orientation of the organ in which they are embedded can be determined. Markers have been used widely for prostate treatments. A more exotic illustration of IGRT is provided by the imaging capabilities of a robotic linac (see the discussion of radiosurgery in chapter 20).

For kV cone beam CT the gantry rotates around the patient while the kV x-ray tube is on and the MV beam is off. During gantry rotation the kV imaging panel is acquiring numerous projections. The projection data can be reconstructed to provide a set of CT axial images. The shape of the kV x-ray beam is a cone and thus this modality is referred to as cone beam CT (CBCT). For IGRT purposes it is crucial that the MV beam and the kV beam share the same isocenter. During gantry rotation the x-ray tube and imager may sag or flex. It is necessary to correct for this by use of a "flexmap" which characterizes the flex with gantry angle.

CBCT images can be compared to the treatment planning CT. The CBCT software on the linac allows the operator to determine the shift in patient position that will best bring the two sets of images into alignment (see Figure 19.33). In general, this requires three shifts (translations), one in each of three perpendicular coordinate directions and rotations about three axes. Rotational correction is available on some specialized linacs. Linacs without this capability use the three translations that give the best fit. If the movements are small, the table can be moved automatically from the control console without having to enter the treatment room.

Ultrasound is used in some clinics to image a patient's prostate gland prior to delivery of radiation for prostate cancer (see Figure 19.34).

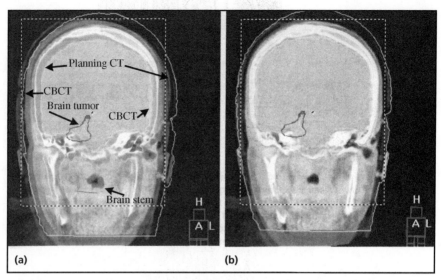

Figure 19.33: Cone-beam image-guided radiation therapy. (a) A patient's cranium as imaged with the Elekta XVI (x-ray volume imaging) system shown in Figure 19.32. Contours of a brain tumor (in red) have been imported from the treatment planning CT. This is the view prior to image registration. The planning CT image is in pink and the cone beam CT is in green. There is a clear mismatch between the two sets. (b) This is the same as (a) except that this is the image after registration. The patient is now positioned very accurately for treatment. (Courtesy of Elekta, Norcross, GA) See COLOR PLATE 15.

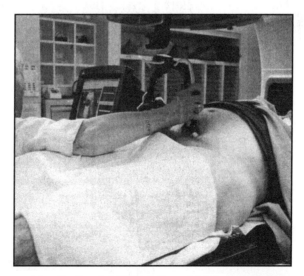

Figure 19.34: Prostate ultrasound localization for IGRT. A therapist is holding the transducer against the patient's skin. The head of the linac and the docking station can be seen at the top of the photo. (Courtesy of Best Medical, Springfield, VA, www.TeamBest.com)

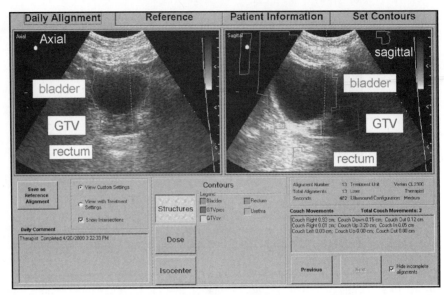

Figure 19.35: A screen capture from the NOMOS BAT (B-mode Acquisition and Targeting) ultrasound IGRT system. The image on the left is an axial image. A sagittal image is shown on the right. The operator has superimposed contours of the bladder, GTV, and rectum from the treatment plan. These contours have been aligned with the corresponding structures in the ultrasound images. The shift necessary to bring about this alignment on the computer is then used to calculate how the patient should be moved. This information is shown in the box on the lower right. (Courtesy of Best Medical, Springfield, VA, www.TeamBest.com) See COLOR PLATE 16.

The tricky part is to register the images with the planning CT (see Figure 19.35). The ultrasound transducer is at the end of an articulated arm. This arm is able to keep track of both the position and orientation of the transducer. Prior to imaging the transducer is docked at a docking station attached to the head of the linac. The position of the docking station is known with respect to the isocenter. Image information can be referenced in this way to the linac isocenter.

Chapter Summary

- **Imaging for Treatment Planning**
  - (i) Plane film
  - (ii) Fluoroscopy

  > Conventional

  - (iii) CT
  - (iv) MRI

  > 3-D & soft tissue discrimination

  - (v) Ultrasound

- **Digital images** are composed of picture elements called **pixels**; radiological images are usually 512×512 pixels.

- **Gray Scale:** The number of levels of gray assigned to a pixel; this determines the contrast resolution of the image; an 8-bit gray scale has $2^8 = 256$ shades of gray.

- **CT:** Provides three-dimensional reconstruction of patient anatomy and electron density data for inhomogeneity corrections.

  —*Image reconstruction:* Need a sufficient number of projections to calculate μ for each voxel.

  —*Image size* usually 512×512 pixels; requires about 0.5 MB/slice for storage

  — $CT\# = 1000 \dfrac{\mu_t - \mu_w}{\mu_w}$, where μ_t is linear attenuation coefficient for tissue in a particular voxel and μ_w is the linear attenuation coefficient for water.

  —CT# sometimes called Hounsfield units (HU). CT#'s range between -1000 and $+3000$. For air CT# $= -1000$, for water CT# $= 0$, for dense bone 1300–1600.

  —Window and level: Level is center value of CT# displayed and window is range.

  —Modern scanners are spiral multislice units.

  —Pitch = (table travel per tube rotation)/(total length of tissue irradiated by the cone beam).

  —*Pitch < 1:* improvement in image quality but increase in dose.

  —*Diagnostic CT scanners:* Bore diameter 70 cm; concave couch top.

—*CT simulators:* Bore diameter 80 to 90 cm; flat couch top; moveable external lasers

—*Relative electron density* for patient treatment planning derived from calibration curve plot of relative electron density vs. CT#.

- **DRR:** Digitally reconstructed radiograph; simulated radiograph mathematically calculated from CT data, usually beam's-eye view for each treatment port.

- **4D CT:** Adds time dimension to the three spatial dimensions to assess or manage motion
  (1) *Prospective gated imaging:* Breath hold at either inspiration or expiration while scanning
  (2) *Retrospective/correlation imaging:* Patient breathes freely and CT slices are binned according to phase of respiratory cycle during which they were acquired.

- **MRI:** Magnetic resonance imaging uses non-ionizing RF radiation, based on magnetic properties of protons in tissue

  —Magnetic field strengths of 1 to 3 T

  —Contraindicated for patients with ferromagnetic implants: pacemakers, aneurism clips, etc.

  —Proton precesses with Larmor frequency $v = \dfrac{\gamma B_0}{2\pi}$ (in the radio region of the spectrum), where γ is a constant called the *gyromagnetic ratio.*

  —*Magnetic field gradients* used so that Larmor frequency varies with position throughout patient

  —Three stages for imaging:
  (1) *Excitation:* tip direction of magnetic field of proton
  (2) *Relaxation:* magnetic field of proton returns to equilibrium with associated time scales T1 and T2
  (3) *Detection:* detect "echo" from relaxation images are weighted by spin density, T1 or T2

  —MRI images are usually not used directly for treatment planning because:
  (1) They are subject to geometric distortion.
  (2) They do not provide electron density information for inhomogeneity corrections.

(3) Bone signal is weak, hard to produce useful DRRs for treatment verification.

- **Ultrasound Imaging:** Uses high-frequency sound, sound reflects off boundaries between tissues having different sound speeds.

  —Speed of sound in soft tissue $c_s = 1540$ m/s; ultrasound frequency is approximately 5 MHz.

  —*Transducer:* Converts mechanical energy to electrical energy and vice versa; used to produce and detect ultrasound.

- **PET:** Positron emission tomography; images the distribution of positron-emitting radiopharmaceutical throughout the body; metabolic imaging.

  —*Coincidence detection:* Events are counted only if seen nearly simultaneously on opposite sides of ring.

  —*Common radioisotope* is ^{18}F ($T_{1/2} = 110$ min), incorporated in glucose analog FDG; malignant cells exhibit enhanced glucose uptake.

  —*Standard uptake volume (SUV):*

  $$SUV = \frac{\text{Activity per unit volume / decay factor}}{\text{Injected activity / body mass}}$$

  —High SUV is a sign of possible malignancy.

- **Imaging for Treatment Verification (Portal Imaging)**
  (i)   Film
  (ii) Electronic portal imaging devices (EPIDs)

  —A screen is used to filter out electron contamination and to provide some build-up.

  —Poor quality is due to:
  (1) *Poor contrast:* Predominant interaction is Compton, weak dependence on Z; very little differential absorption is seen compared to diagnostic films.
  (2) *Scattered photons and secondary electrons:* Scattered photons are not easily removed, cannot use a grid.
  (3) *Large penumbra:* Geometric + phantom scatter.

  —The quality of port images degrades with increasing beam energy and patient thickness (>20 cm).

- **IGRT:** Image-guided radiation therapy; large variety of methods are used to assure correct geometric targeting:
  (1) Cone beam CT (CBCT): X-ray tube and flat-panel detector attached to linac.
  (2) MV CT: Use megavoltage beam to produce CT image: tomotherapy unit.
  (3) Ultrasound image registration for prostate treatment.
  (4) Implanted markers.

Problems

1. An axial CT image has a field of view of 250 mm in width. The image is 512×512 pixels. What is the pixel size? What is the smallest object that you are likely to be able to perceive?

2. Estimate the computer storage requirements for 100 CT axial slice images used for treatment planning. Assume that the images are 512×512, 16-bit gray scale. Give the answer in MB.

3. Estimate the time necessary to transfer these 100 CT slices over a network with a speed of 10 Mbps (megabits per second).

4. At a particular kVp, $\mu_w = 0.267$ cm^{-1}, and for a particular sample of bone $\mu_{bone} = 0.511$ cm^{-1}. Calculate the CT# of this bone.

5. List the following tissues in order of increasing Hounsfield number: bone, muscle, fat, lung.

6. The window and level of a CT image are chosen as +300 and +100, respectively. What CT#'s are displayed as black? What CT#'s are displayed as white?

7. A CT scanner with a 24-mm wide detector is operated at a pitch of 0.06 for a 4-D respiratory scan. How far does the table move during one tube rotation?

8. How can the quality of DRRs be improved?

9. Briefly describe the three stages in the process of MR imaging.

10. What are the contraindications for MR imaging?

11. What are the relative advantages and disadvantages of CT and MRI for treatment planning?

12.   What contrast agent is frequently used in MR imaging?

13.   How is the quality of portal images affected by beam energy?

14.   Why do MV portal images show lower bone/soft tissue contrast than kV images?

Bibliography

Alessio, A. M., P. E. Kinahan, P. M. Cheng, H. Vesselle, and J. S. Karp. (2004). "PET/CT scanner instrumentation, challenges, and solutions." *Radiol Clin North Am* 42(6): 1017–1032.

American Association of Physicists in Medicine Report No. 24. Radiotherapy Portal Imaging Quality. Report of AAPM Task Group No. 28. New York: American Institute of Physics, 1988.

Bushong, S. C. *Radiologic Science for Technologists: Physics, Biology, and Protection,* 9th edition. St. Louis: Mosby, 2008.

Caldwell, C. B., and K. Mah. "Imaging for Radiation Therapy Planning." Chapter 2 in *The Modern Technology of Radiation Oncology,* Vol 2. J. Van Dyk (ed). Madison, WI: Medical Physics Publishing, pp. 31–89, 2005.

Caldwell, C. B., K. Mah, M. Skinner, and C. E. Danjoux. (2003). "Can PET provide the 3D extent of tumor motion for individualized internal target volumes? A phantom study of the limitations of CT and the promise of PET." *Int J Radiat Oncol Biol Phys* 55:1381–1393.

Chen, G. T. Y., C. A. Pellizzari, and E. R. M. Rietzel. "Imaging in Radotherapy." Chapter 2 in *Treatment Planning in Radiation Oncology,* 2nd edition. F. Khan (ed.), Philadelphia: Lippincott Williams and Wilkins, pp. 11–32, 2007.

Cody, D., and O. Mawlawi (Program Directors). *The Physics and Applications of PET/CT Imaging.* Proceedings of the AAPM 2008 Summer School. AAPM Medical Physics Monograph No. 33. Madison, WI: Medical Physics Publishing, 2008.

Coia, L., T. Schultheiss, and G, Hanks (eds.). *A Practical Guide to CT Simulation.* Madison, WI: Advanced Medical Publishing, 1995.

Curran, B.H., J. M. Balter, I. J. Chetty (Program Directors). *Integrating New Technologies into the Clinic: Monte Carlo and Image-Guided Radiation Therapy.* Proceedings of the AAPM 2006 Summer School. AAPM Medical Physics Monograph No. 32. Madison, WI: Medical Physics Publishing, 2006.

Goitein, M. *Radiation Oncology: A Physicist's-Eye View.* New York: Springer, 2008.

Hazle, J. D., and A. L. Boyer (eds.). *Imaging in Radiation Therapy.* Proceedings of the AAPM 1998 Summer School. AAPM Medical Physics Monograph #24. Madison, WI: Medical Physics Publishing, 1998.

Herman, M. G., J. M. Balter, D. A. Jaffray, K. P. McGee, P. Munro, S. Shalev, M. Van Herk, and J. W. Wong. (2001). "Clinical use of electronic portal imaging: report of AAPM Radiation Therapy Committee Task Group 58." *Med Phys* 28(5):712–738. Also available as AAPM Report No. 75.

Kevles, B. *Naked to the Bone: Medical Imaging in the Twentieth Century.* New York: Perseus Publishing, 1997.

McCullough, C. H., and F. E. Zink. (1999). "Performance evaluation of a multi-slice CT system." *Med Phys* 26:2223–2230.

Mutic, S. "Use of Imaging Systems for Patient Modeling PET and SPECT" in *Integrating New Technologies into the Clinic: Monte Carlo and Image-Guided Radiation Therapy.* AAPM 2006 Summer School Proceedings, AAPM Medical Physics Monograph No. 32. B. H. Curran, J. M. Balter, and I. J. Chetty, Program Directors, pp. 375–400, 2006.

Podoloff, D. A., R. H. Advani, C. Allred, A. B. Benson 3rd, E. Brown, H. J. Burstein, R. W. Carlson et al. (2007). "NCCN task force report: Positron emission tomography (PET)/computed tomography (CT) scanning in cancer." *J Compr Canc Netw* 5(Suppl. 1):S1–S23.

Van Dyk, J. (ed.). *The Modern Technology of Radiation Oncology.* Chapters 4, 5, 6, 7, and 13. Madison, WI: Medical Physics Publishing, 1999.

Van Dyk, J., and K. Mah. "Simulation and Imaging for Radiation Therapy Planning." Chapter 8 in *Radiotherapy Physics in Practice,* 2nd edition. J. R. Williams and D. I. Thwaites (eds.). Oxford, UK: Oxford University Press, 2000.

West, C. M. L., T. Jones, and P. Price. (2004). "The potential of positron-emission tomography to study anticancer-drug resistance." *Nat Rev Cancer* 4:457–469.

20 Special Modalities in Radiation Therapy

20.1 Introduction

This chapter contains a discussion of three specialized treatment modalities in radiation therapy: IMRT, stereotactic radiosurgery, and proton therapy. IMRT has now become quite mainstream and is commonly used in most clinics. Stereotactic radiosurgery is offered in most large clinics. Although the use of proton therapy has been growing, it is still only available in a small number of centers. Proton therapy is very costly in comparison to conventional photon therapy and the degree to which it represents an improvement over conventional therapy is still controversial. We have not included a discussion of total or whole-body photon irradiation. Anecdotal evidence (and experience in our clinics) indicates that this form of radiation therapy is waning in use. We have also not included coverage of total skin electron irradiation as this form of therapy is used only infrequently for rare skin conditions (e.g., mycosis fungoides).

20.2 Intensity Modulation in Radiation Therapy

Wedges and compensators are used in radiation therapy in an effort to improve the dose distribution. These devices modify or modulate the intensity of the beam. We can carry this idea further by asking about the benefit of being able to set the intensity at all points across the beam to any arbitrary value between 0 and 100%, independent of the intensity at adjacent points. This is the concept of intensity modulation. Treatment with such intensity-modulated beams is called _i_ntensity-_m_odulated _r_adiation _t_herapy, or IMRT for short. IMRT may be the most technically complex development in radiation therapy in the last 25 years. The use of this modality has expanded rapidly and is now quite routine. We will show that intensity-modulated beams, custom designed for each patient, can produce remarkably conformal dose distributions. The increase in dose conformality allows for the possibility of "dose escalation." In principle, it should be possible to raise the dose to the tumor without increasing the rate of complications associated with the irradiation of organs at risk.

It is not currently technically feasible to have the intensity vary continuously over the plane perpendicular to the central axis. Instead the beam cross section is usually divided up into an array of small beams called beamlets (or sometimes bixels). The intensity is constant within each beamlet. In addition the intensities may be restricted to discrete values. A common arrangement is to use 1 cm × 1 cm beamlets. In this case, a 10 × 10 cm^2 field would be divided up into 100 beamlets. The set of intensity values at each point in a plane perpendicular to the central axis is called the intensity map. Figures 20.1 and 20.2 show intensity maps.

Figure 20.3 shows how IMRT differs from conventional therapy. The top portion of the figure shows the conventional treatment of a target with an irregular shape using three beams. Each beam is shaped so

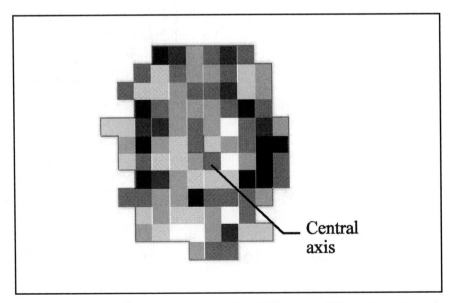

Figure 20.1: An intensity map showing 1 cm × 1 cm beamlets. There are ten different intensity levels (dark is more intense). See COLOR PLATE 17.

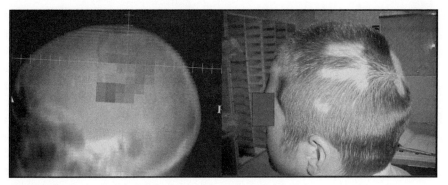

Figure 20.2: Intensity map for an IMRT beam superimposed on a patient DRR (left) and reflected in hair loss on the patient's scalp (right). See COLOR PLATE 18.

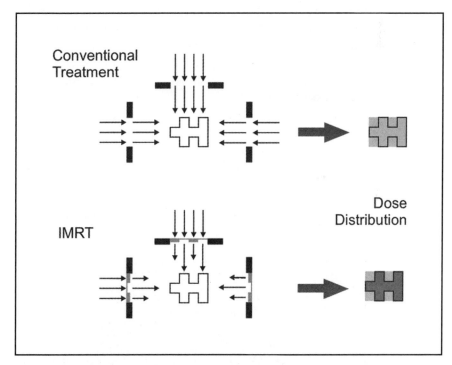

Figure 20.3: The difference between conventional radiation therapy and IMRT. Three beams are used to treat a target with an irregular shape. In the conventional treatment shown at the top, the jaws are used to shape the beams to correspond to the beams eye view shape of the target. The resulting dose distribution is shown as shading on the right. In the IMRT treatment the beam is modulated in an attempt to reduce the dose to the "nooks and crannies" that contain normal tissue. The resulting dose distribution shows a reduction in dose in these regions.

that the entire target is exposed to the full beam, but tissue outside the target region is blocked. The entire target receives full dose coverage but so does the normal tissue in the "nooks" and "crannies" near the target. In the intensity-modulated treatment, shown at the bottom of the figure, the same three beams are used, but this time they are intensity modulated. The resulting dose distribution still fully covers the target, but now the normal tissue receives reduced dose.

Figure 20.4 shows the dose distribution for the treatment of a hollow sphere (in a geometric phantom) with an organ-at-risk inside. The plan uses seven gantry angles and five intensity levels. The dose distribution is remarkably conformal. The 100% line wraps tightly around both the inside and the outside of the sphere (at least in the plane shown). The uniformity however is poor; the maximum dose inside the target is 148%. This is characteristic of IMRT. IMRT plans tend to be much more conformal than conventional plans, but the dose distribution in the target is usually less uniform. This may be acceptable, perhaps even desirable, provided that the hot spots are not near the periphery of the target, especially if the target is adjacent to a critical structure. Hot spots can occasionally appear outside the tumor volume!

Figure 20.5 shows a treatment plan for multiple targets using a single isocenter. The targets are cylinders. The long axes of the cylinders are perpendicular to the page. Seven gantry angles were used for this plan. Again the dose distribution is remarkably conformal, and it is amazing that this dose distribution can be delivered with only a single isocenter. The maximum dose is 115%.

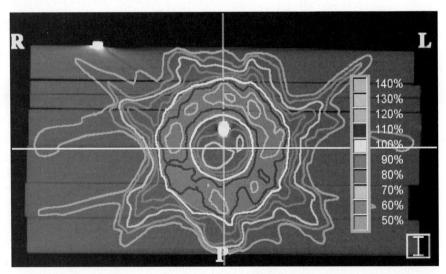

Figure 20.4: The dose distribution in a geometric phantom illustrates the power of IMRT. The target is the hollow sphere with an organ at risk inside (not shown). Seven gantry angles and five different intensity levels were used. The 100% isodose line wraps tightly around both the inside and outside of the sphere giving outstanding conformity. The uniformity of the dose distribution in the target however is relatively poor. The hot spot is 148%. The phantom is a stack of square slabs of virtual water. See COLOR PLATE 19.

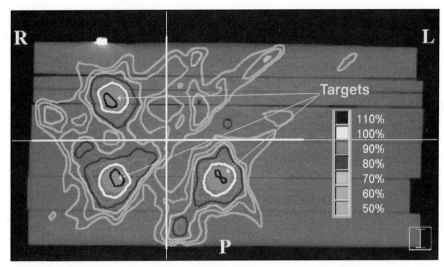

Figure 20.5: The dose distribution in a geometric phantom with three targets. The targets are cylinders with axes perpendicular to the page. The conformality is impressive considering that only a single isocenter was used. Seven gantry angles were used. The maximum dose in the targets is 115%. The intersection of the white lines shows the location of the isocenter. See COLOR PLATE 20.

IMRT should be considered for tumors where a lack of local control is a significant factor in disease progression and dose escalation is currently limited by the radiation tolerance of adjacent critical structures. IMRT is useful for tumors with concavities, particularly those wrapped around radiosensitive structures and for multiple isolated targets, such as brain metastases. IMRT is currently being used for brain tumors, head and neck tumors, mesothelioma, breast cancer, paraspinal tumors, and prostate cancer. IMRT is now being used for almost every anatomical site that has been traditionally treated with conventional radiation therapy.

There are disadvantages to IMRT. Treatment planning is much more labor intensive than for conventional therapy and the delivery time can be up to twice that for conventional treatment. There is a danger in being too conformal. The PTV must be realistically defined to account for issues of target definition, set up uncertainty, immobilization, and organ motion. Dose distributions resulting from IMRT treatment are usually more inhomogeneous than for conventional treatment. Finally, the whole-body dose received by the patient can be two to three times that of conventional therapy (see section 20.2.7).

The questions to be addressed are: how to determine the desired intensity map and once determined how can it be delivered? We will give the short answer to these questions now and elaborate later throughout this section. Delivery of intensity-modulated radiation beams almost always involves some sort of a computerized MLC. Determination of the intensity map usually entails some sort of "inverse treatment planning." For inverse treatment planning, one specifies treatment planning goals and the computer software is given the task of finding intensity maps that will meet these goals. It may not be physically possible to achieve the specified goals; therefore inverse treatment planning software calculates the intensity map which will most *closely* match those goals. This process is one of optimization.

20.2.1 IMRT Delivery Techniques

The use of a wedge is a crude type of intensity modulation. It is intensity modulation in one dimension—along the wedge gradient—and the beamlet intensities are not independent of one another. The use of a compensator is a more sophisticated implementation of intensity modulation (see chapter 14, section 14.12). This is two-dimensional intensity modulation. Compensators however have the limitation that they do not have a full 0 to 100% intensity range. Compensator material has a maximum thickness, which might correspond, for example, to a minimum 60% transmission. The maximum transmission is close to 100% (zero compensator thickness, which leaves just tray transmission). For a compensator, no location can have a transmission lower than the minimum value. True IMRT involves the use of a computerized MLC. This allows transmission that ranges from (close to) 0% to 100%. There are three major categories of MLC IMRT delivery systems: tomotherapy, cone beam, and intensity-(or volumetric-)modulated arc therapy (IMAT or VMAT). Each type of delivery requires a unique treatment planning system. We discuss each of these below.

Tomotherapy means literally "slice therapy." There are two methods by which tomotherapy can be delivered: serial (also called sequential) and helical. For both of these delivery methods the gantry rotates around the patient while the beam remains on, delivering a thin fan beam of radiation that is modulated as the gantry turns.

In serial tomotherapy a single axial slice of the patient is treated at a time. To deliver the next slice the patient couch must be moved very precisely (couch indexing). Any error in couch motion can lead to either an overdose due to an overlap or an underdose due to an "underlap." The NOMOS MIMiC® system is a commercial serial tomotherapy system (see Figure 20.6)[1]. The MIMiC device is mounted on the head of a conventional linac (which need not have an MLC). The slice width is 2 cm (measured at the isocenter). There are two rows of square leaves, each of which can be either open or closed. A pneumatic system opens and closes these rapidly as the gantry rotates through an arc. An advantage of this system is that it can be mounted on a "garden variety" linac. The linac does not have to have a built-in MLC. A disadvantage is that the MIMiC has to be mounted to treat IMRT and then removed for conventional treatments.

---

[1] This has now been replaced by the nomosSTAT system.

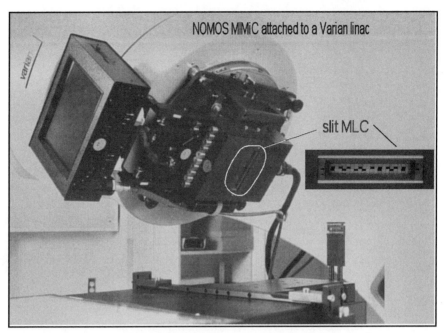

Figure 20.6: An add-on device that can be used to deliver serial tomotherapy using an ordinary linear accelerator without an MLC. A close-up of the slit MLC is shown on the right. (Courtesy of Best Medical, Springfield, VA, www.TeamBest.com)

The second type of tomotherapy is helical. Instead of delivering a single slice at a time, the fan beam is delivered in a helical fashion (just like a spiral CT, see chapter 19, section 19.4.1). The couch moves continuously while the source of radiation rotates around the patient. A commercial firm, TomoTherapy Inc., is now marketing a helical tomotherapy machine called the Hi-Art® system (see Figure 20.7). The machine has a "donut"-like gantry similar to a CT machine. Within this gantry there is a small in-line 6 MV linac with a fan beam MLC that rotates around the patient while the couch moves through the donut. The linac does not have a flattening filter. Recall that the purpose of a flattening filter is to produce a uniform beam profile (see chapter 9, section 9.4). The TomoTherapy linac does not need a flattening filter as the intensity is always modulated anyway. The linac can be used to construct tomographic images of the patient—just like a CT unit except using the 6 MV linac beam. This allows an adjustment in patient positioning prior to each treatment or adjustment in treatment delivery based on the position of the patient.

Cone beam IMRT uses a conventional linear accelerator and MLC. This is the most common type of IMRT delivery. A conventional MLC operating under computer control can deliver an intensity-modulated beam. The beam shape from a conventional linac is cone shaped because of beam divergence and hence the name "cone beam" IMRT. In cone beam IMRT the gantry is stationary while the beam is on. The treatment planner chooses a number of beam directions (typically 5 to 9).

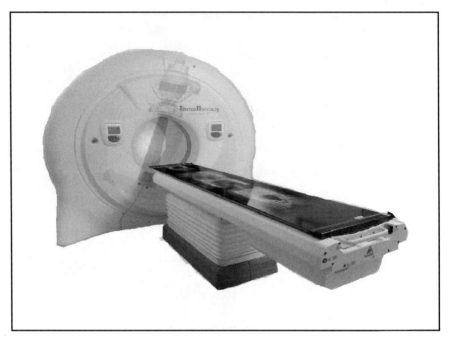

Figure 20.7: A helical TomoTherapy® unit. This drawing shows the linac inside the (semi-transparent) gantry cover. The linac rotates around the patient as the couch moves continuously inward. (Courtesy of TomoTherapy Inc., Madison, WI)

Each beam direction is specified by a couch angle and a gantry angle. Each one of these beams is modulated. The treatment planning system determines the optimum modulation of each beam so that the entire delivery of all the modulated beams chosen will result in the optimum dose distribution.

The beamlets are produced by MLC leaf motion. The dimensions of the beamlets are 0.2 to 1.0 cm along the direction of MLC leaf motion and equal to the leaf width in the other direction. The beamlets are established by performing a ray trace from the x-ray source to the patient target. Only those beamlets that traverse the target are turned on. Some additional beamlets may be turned on around the periphery to provide scatter to the edge of the target.

For conventional non-IMRT treatments the MLC (see chapter 13, section 13.2.3 for a discussion of MLC properties) is set to the desired shape and the leaf positions are fixed throughout the entire delivery of that beam. There are two methods of accomplishing cone beam IMRT. In dynamic MLC (DMLC, sometimes called "sliding window") the MLC leaves move throughout the entire time that the beam is on (see Figure 20.8). The dose rate (in MU/min) may vary while the leaves are moving. The leaves are computer programmed to move in such a way as to produce the desired intensity map. Opposing pairs of leaves sweep across the beam. The speed of the leaves, the dose rate, and the opening

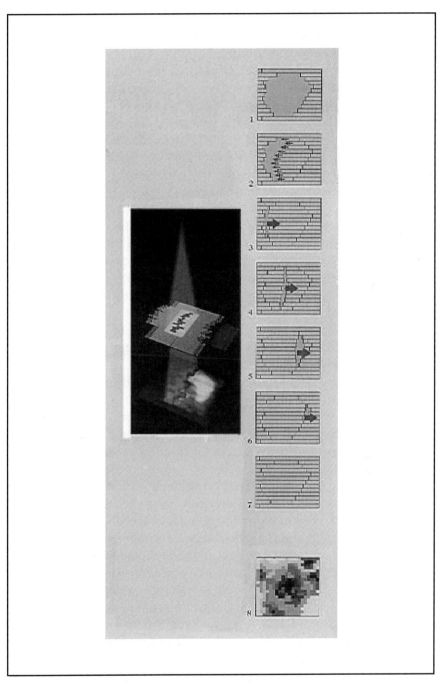

Figure 20.8: Illustration of DMLC IMRT delivery. The illustration on the left side of the figure shows the cone beam shaped by the MLC at some instant. The first frame at the top on the right shows an open field used for portal verification. The second frame shows the leaves closing down in preparation for treatment delivery. In frames 3 through 7 the beam is turned on and the "window" is shown sweeping across the field. The dose rate may vary during the sweep. The frame on the bottom right shows the resulting intensity map for this port. (Courtesy of Varian Medical Systems, Inc. Copyright © 2010. All rights reserved.) See COLOR PLATE 21.

between the leaves determines the final amount of radiation delivered at each location along the leaf motion.

In segmental multileaf IMRT (SMLC, sometimes called "static window, step-and-shoot, or stop & shoot") the leaves form a series of fixed aperture shapes to deliver the desired intensity map. This is the most widely used form of IMRT. The sequence of events for SMLC is as follows. The MLC leaves form an initial aperture. The beam is turned on and a certain number of MUs are delivered. The beam is then turned off, the leaves are moved to define a new aperture, and then the beam is turned on again, delivering (most likely) a different number of MUs. This process continues until the desired intensity map is delivered. The beam is turned on only when the leaves are stopped. Each MLC aperture is referred to as a "segment." The number of segments necessary may vary widely depending on the treatment plan and the hardware used to deliver the radiation. Thirty or forty segments are possible. The shape of the apertures and the number of MU delivered through each aperture are arranged to produce the desired intensity map. Sometimes the term "control point" is used to indicate a change in the stage of delivery, either the beam turning on or off and configuration of a new set of leaf positions (window). The number of control points is equal to two times the number of segments minus one.

Intensity-modulated arc therapy (IMAT) uses a conventional MLC to make a cone beam. The gantry rotates while the beam is on and while the MLC leaves are simultaneously in motion. Treatment extends over a range of gantry angles. Single or multiple arcs can be used. IMAT may be more efficient than other forms of cone beam IMRT.

After a desired intensity map is calculated by the treatment planning system, it is necessary to calculate a series of leaf positions that will deliver the intensity map as accurately as possible. There is no unique or exact solution to this problem. Algorithms created to accomplish this are called "leaf sequencing" algorithms, a number of which have been created for this purpose. For SMLC the leaf sequencing algorithm produces a series of static leaf configurations (segments) along with the fractional number of MU to be delivered for each segment. For DMLC the leaf sequencing algorithm produces a table of leaf positions as a function of MU. Leaf sequencing algorithms are not perfect and the resulting delivered intensity map may not be identical to the optimum map. For this reason, treatment planning systems usually perform a final dose calculation after leaf sequencing so that the user can see what will actually be delivered. It is possible, although more difficult, to avoid the intermediate leaf sequencing step by optimizing directly in terms of machine leaf positions and segment weights.[2]

---

[2] This is called Direct Machine Parameter Optimization (DMPO) in the Pinnacle (Philips) treatment planning system.

There are other considerations in determination of the leaf sequence. It is desirable to minimize the total number of MU and to exclude segments that are too small. As the total number of MU become larger, the delivery efficiency is reduced. In addition, a large number of MU leads to increased whole-body dose and shielding requirements (see section 20.2.7). Segments smaller than about 3 cm $\times$ 3 cm may not be delivered accurately because of uncertainties in output factors.

20.2.2 Inverse Treatment Planning

Specifying treatment planning goals is not as easy as it might at first seem. Ideally, we would like all of the dose to go to the PTV and none to normal tissues. This is, of course, physically impossible to achieve. Furthermore, it may not be convenient to specify the desired dose to be delivered to every single voxel inside the patient. A way of condensing the information about the dose distribution is to use cumulative dose volume histograms (DVHs, see chapter 14, section 14.7). A dose distribution can be summarized by giving the DVH for the target volume(s) and for normal tissues and organs.

Information about the desired dose distribution is usually provided by the user in the form of a DVH. A DVH is specified for the targets and all normal tissues and organs. One way to do this is to define three points (or more) on the DVH curve as shown in Figure 20.9. For the target, a

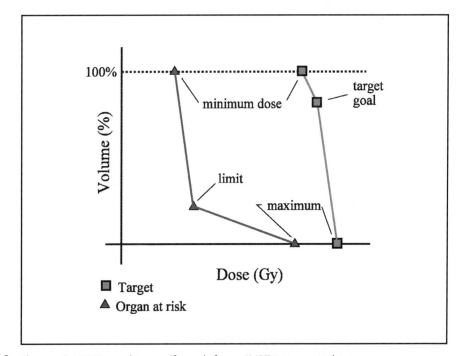

Figure 20.9: Three point DVHs used to specify goals for an IMRT treatment plan.

minimum dose is specified, a target goal (e.g., prescribed dose to 95% of the target), and a maximum dose. For organs at risk a maximum dose, a "limit" (e.g., no more than 33% of the kidney receives 30 Gy), and a minimum dose. For an organ at risk, it is tempting to set the minimum dose to zero. This may not be realistic and in fact may be an unreasonable constraint resulting in a poor plan. A more reasonable approach is to think of the minimum dose as the dose below which there is no known effect.

Inverse treatment planning software is used to calculate the intensity map that will provide the desired dose distribution. Conventional treatment planning is sometimes described as dose simulation. The treatment planner chooses (by making educated guesses) couch and gantry angles, beam modifiers (wedges or compensators), and relative beam weights. Once these parameters are chosen, the resulting dose distribution is calculated. The dose distribution is examined and the planner makes changes in the parameters and then iterates until an acceptable dose distribution is found. In inverse treatment planning, the planner specifies information about the desirable dose distribution (as in Figure 20.9). The computer then calculates the intensity maps, which will come as close as possible to delivering the desired dose distribution. This process is called "optimization." As of this writing, commercially available inverse treatment planning systems still require the planner to choose couch and gantry angles. The software then optimizes the dose distribution producing intensity maps for each beam portal.

The problem of finding optimum intensity maps is daunting, as the following example illustrates. Suppose that a patient's treatment consists of four 5×5 cm^2 fields. If each of the 5×5 cm^2 fields is divided up into 1×1 cm^2 beamlets, there will be 25 beamlets per field and a total of 100 beamlets for all the fields. Further suppose that we allow each beamlet to have one of ten discrete intensity levels. Consider the first portal and the first beamlet. There are ten choices of intensity. For the second beamlet there are ten more choices. For the first two beamlets there are a total of $10 \times 10 = 100$ possible choices of intensity maps. For the entire first portal there are thus 10^{25} possible combinations of beam intensity assignment. For all four portals there are 10^{100} possible combinations. That is a lot of combinations to check, even for a computer. Let us consider what would be involved. Each one of the 10^{100} possible combinations represents a different plan. Which one is the best choice? The brute force approach is to evaluate every one of these possibilities. Let us suppose that we use a computer with a processor having a 2 GHz "clock" speed. Let us be wildly optimistic and assume that we can evaluate one plan per clock cycle. Under these optimistic conditions it would take 10^{74} times the age of the universe to evaluate all of the possible combinations! Clearly the brute force approach fails and some finesse is called for. This leads us to the topic of optimization.

Let us suppose that our patient is divided up into I voxels and that there are a total of J beamlets for all of the beams combined. Any arbitrary beamlet will deposit some dose in every voxel. This is illustrated in Figure 20.10. Let a_{ij} be the dose deposited in the ith voxel by beamlet j for unit incident fluence. The total dose deposited in the ith voxel by all of the beamlets will be given by the sum over all the beamlets:

$$D_i = \sum_{j=1}^{J} a_{ij} w_j,$$

(20.1)

where w_j is the intensity of the jth beamlet. We see from equation (20.1) that the total dose in any voxel can be written as a linear combination of all of the beamlet intensities. Before starting the optimization process we compute the dose in every voxel, assuming unit intensity for all beamlets (i.e., all $w_j = 1$). The dose calculation is performed up front before the optimization process begins. Notice that the method of dose calculation is immaterial.

We would like the dose distribution to come as close as possible to the prescribed dose distribution. To achieve this goal, we introduce an objective or cost function, C, which describes how close a plan is to meeting the objectives. This function must be designed to quantify the

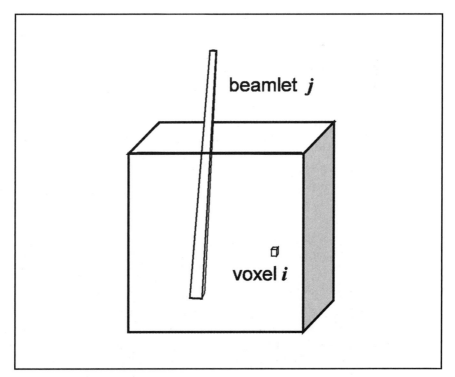

Figure 20.10: The patient is shaped like a cube for simplicity. Any arbitrary beamlet j will deposit some dose in every voxel, such as voxel i.

departure of the values of the dose from the prescribed values. The smaller the value of the objective function, the closer the candidate plan is to the desired plan. The objective function will depend on the beamlet intensities w_j:

$$C = C(w_1, w_2, ..., w_J).$$ (20.2)

We have not yet specified the specific form of the function in equation (20.2). There are many possible functions that we might "cook up" to accomplish the goal. The task is to find the set of values of w that minimize this function. Keep in mind that the number of beamlets, J, is of the order of 100.

An example of a very simple cost function follows. The cost is a sum of the costs for the target and the normal tissues:

$$C = TC + \sum_{m=1}^{M} NC_m,$$ (20.3)

where TC is the cost associated with the target and NC_m is the cost associated with the mth normal structure (organs at risk) and M is the number of normal structures. For the target, the cost can be related to the difference between the actual dose and the desired dose. A fairly simple way of doing this is to use the formula:

$$TC = \left\langle \frac{\left(D_t - D_p\right)^2}{D_p^2} \right\rangle,$$ (20.4)

where D_t is the actual dose in a target voxel and D_p is the prescribed dose to the target. The angular brackets in equation (20.4) indicate an average over all voxels in the target. Note that the square of the difference is used because $D_t - D_p$ may be positive in some voxels and negative in others. If we were to simply average $D_t - D_p$, some of the negative values would cancel some of the positive values, even if the values themselves were quite large in magnitude. To avoid this we square the difference in the doses. If all of the doses in all of the voxels in the target are equal to the prescription dose, the cost is zero.

For the normal tissues:

$$NC_m = NW_m \left\langle \frac{D_m^2}{D_{\lim,m}^2} \right\rangle,$$ (20.5)

where m is the mth normal structure, NW_m is a weighting factor for the importance of this structure compared to other normal structures, D_m is the dose in this structure, $D_{\lim,m}$ is the limiting dose specified for this structure. The quantity $D_{\lim,m}$ could be the largest dose for which there is no known effect. We do not want to make it zero, because this would be unrealistic. The ratio in the brackets of equation (20.5) is to be evaluated for every voxel in the normal structure and then averaged over all voxels. If the value of $D_m = 0$ for all voxels, then the value of the objective function (NC_m) is zero.

The doses D_m and D_t are a function of the beamlet intensities w_j; therefore C in equation (20.3) is a function of the w_j values. The optimization problem is to find a set of values w_j that makes C as small as possible. There are two broad categories of mathematical algorithms for accomplishing this: *deterministic* and *stochastic*. A stochastic method is one in which an element of probability or chance is built in and a deterministic method is one in which there is no chance or probability built in. We will discuss one example of each of these types of methods below.

The gradient method is a deterministic method. It has the advantage of being fast but the possible disadvantage of getting stuck in a "local minimum." This potential problem is illustrated in Figure 20.11. In this figure the cost function is a function of a single beamlet intensity. This

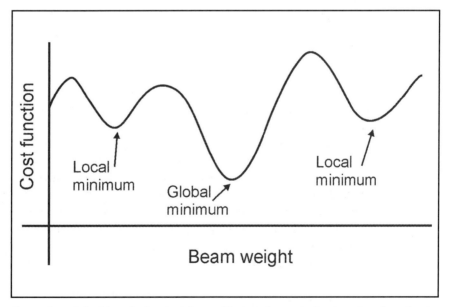

Figure 20.11: Illustration of the idea of a local minimum. The cost is assumed to be a function of a single beam weight. The optimum solution occurs where the cost is an absolute minimum value. This is labeled "global minimum." Gradient methods run the risk of getting stuck in a local minimum, which is not the best possible solution.

is a vast oversimplification, but it is illustrative nonetheless. This curve exhibits three minima. The minimum we seek is the absolute or global minimum. Gradient methods have the potential of finding one of the local minima rather than the global minimum.

There is a good analogy between the mathematical gradient algorithm and the problem faced by a hiker in the mountains who wishes to descend to the lowest valley. Let us imagine that it is foggy and that the hiker cannot see very far. The natural course of action for the hiker is to examine the ground nearby and take a few steps in the direction of steepest descent. The hiker would then pause and again take a few steps in the possibly new direction of steepest descent. This procedure is repeated (or iterated) until finding the lowest valley. In this process the hiker is attempting to find the latitude and longitude that will minimize the altitude. The altitude is like the objective function and the latitude and longitude are like beam weights. The dose optimization problem can be solved in a closely analogous fashion. Start with some arbitrary (but not ridiculous values) of the intensities w_j, for example, set all w_j = 1.00 (uniform intensity beams). Then proceed mathematically downhill in the direction of steepest descent.[3] In the dose optimization problem, negative values of w_j are prohibited. If the hiker always refuses to walk uphill, then the hiker could get stuck in a small dip or depression—a local minimum (see Figure 20.11). In the same way, the dose optimization algorithm can potentially get stuck in a local minimum. Furthermore, it may not be apparent that this has occurred.

There is also the issue of knowing when to stop taking steps. One can stop after a certain number of iterations or after the objective function drops below some small cutoff value or, more likely, whichever of these conditions is reached first. Thirty iterations is not uncommon. If the value of the cost function is changing very little from iteration to iteration, there is no point in continuing. The algorithm is said to have converged.

Stochastic methods make it possible to escape a local minimum. The stochastic method that we shall discuss is called "simulated annealing." As we shall see later, there is an analogy between this method and the annealing of metals. The algorithm begins by making an initial guess for the beamlet intensities (again perhaps all 1.00). Then the algorithm takes a step in a random direction (negative values of w prohibited). If the cost goes down as a result of the step, then the step is accepted. If the cost goes up, the step is not automatically rejected (because we could be in a local minimum) but is accepted based on a certain probability. The idea here is that if the system lands in a local minimum, we allow it some probability of jumping out. The probability is related to the change in the cost function:

$$P = e^{-\Delta C/kT}, \tag{20.6}$$

---

[3] For the mathematically minded, this can be accomplished by always moving in the direction of the negative of the gradient: $-\vec{\nabla}C$.

where ΔC is the change in the cost function associated with the step, k is a constant, and T is a parameter called the "temperature." The larger the value of the temperature, the more likely it is that the step will be accepted. The algorithm begins with a high value of the temperature and then as the steps proceed, the temperature is reduced according to some predefined schedule called the "annealing schedule." This means that early on, the algorithm is likely to jump out of a local minimum, but that as the iterations proceed, it settles down and becomes less likely to do so. If the system is "cooled" too quickly, it may not be able to escape local minima. If it is "cooled" too slowly, it may take excessively long to converge.

There is a close analogy between the methodology of this technique and the annealing of metals. If a liquid metal is cooled too fast, it may not reach the lowest energy crystalline state, instead reaching some amorphous state. If instead the metal is cooled slowly, crystalline order can be achieved over some long distance. This minimizes the internal energy of the metal.

All else being equal (it never is), simulated annealing is less efficient and consumes more CPU time than deterministic methods such as the gradient method.

The method of simulated annealing has been applied to a classic mathematics problem called the "traveling salesman problem." The problem is for a salesman to visit N cities in succession, following the shortest possible path and returning to the home city in the end. Consider the case in which there are 10 cities (not including the home city). There are 10 possible choices for the first city to visit. There are 9 possible choices for the second city, 8 possible choices for the third city, and so on. Therefore, there are a total of $10 \times 9 \times 8 \times ... \times 1 = 4 \times 10^6 = 10!$ possible routes. For N cities there are $N!$ total possible paths, a quantity that increases very rapidly as N increases. For the purpose of optimization, the objective function is the total distance traveled. Figure 20.12 shows the optimum path between 100 randomly positioned cities.

The traveling salesman problem is not just a curious academic puzzle. It is applied in the design of integrated circuits in which hundreds of thousands (or perhaps millions) of circuit elements have to be placed somewhere on the chip and interconnected. The United Parcel Service (UPS) uses optimization techniques for delivery of packages. If a driver has only three destinations, he can take six possible routes. If there are 25 deliveries, there are $25! = 1.6 \times 10^{25}$ possible routes. A typical UPS driver has about 150 drop off points per day.[4] There are additional constraints also, such as specified pick up and drop off times. Clearly the selection of an optimum route goes beyond casual thought.

---

[4] "Algorithms: Business by Numbers," *The Economist,* September 15, 2007.

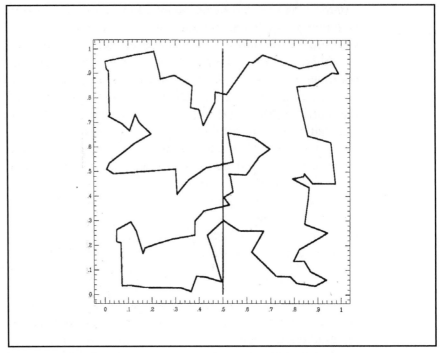

Figure 20.12: A solution to the traveling salesman problem for 100 randomly positioned cities. The number of possible routes is 100! $\approx 10^{158}$. (Reprinted from Press, W. H., S. A. Teukolsky, W. T. Vetterling, and B. P. Flannery. *Numerical Recipes: The Art of Scientific Computing*, 1st Edition, Fig. 10.9.1, p. 329. © 1986 Cambridge University Press. Printed with permission.)

20.2.3 Inverse Planning Issues

It is a misconception that inverse planning is less labor intensive or more automatic—in fact, it is quite the opposite. There are many parameters to be chosen before optimization, and the optimized plan will depend on these parameters. The search for the best plan often requires exploration of these parameters and therefore it can be very time consuming. IMRT is very labor intensive for the physician, the treatment planner, and the physicist. Because of the complexity of optimization, IMRT treatment planning can be counterintuitive.

It should now be clear that careful contouring of every structure entering the cost function is crucial. The optimization depends critically on the voxels contained in each structure in the cost function. Contours must be drawn carefully and accurately. Another issue relates to target volumes that extend toward the skin surface and into the build-up region. In the build-up region the dose would normally be low. In an attempt to raise the dose to the prescription level, the optimization algorithm may increase some beamlet intensities to compensate. The result may be hot spots elsewhere.

Furthermore, it may not be apparent to the planner that a better dose distribution is possible if the target volume is retracted from the skin surface. Most of the buildup occurs over the first several millimeters (see Figure 14.39). Some clinics will retract the PTV by 3 mm from the skin surface for 6 MV head and neck treatment. If the dose really needs to be high closer to the skin surface, bolus should be used. It is best if the bolus is placed on the patient prior to the planning CT. All contours should be checked carefully prior to optimization. This includes contours that are expanded by the treatment planning system such as GTV expansion to CTV and PTV.

Structures that are contiguous or overlap raise questions. One has to be careful when specifying doses for adjacent structures. As an example, it does not make sense to insist that a target receive a dose of 70 Gy and that an adjacent or contiguous organ at risk receive no more than 40 Gy. Poor plans can result from such unreasonable demands! If two structures overlap, which one takes priority upon optimization? An example is prostate treatment planning in which there is an overlap of the prostate PTV with the rectum. How does one state the dosimetric goals under this circumstance?

There are two ways that this can be handled, as described by Wu et al.[5] The first is to create non-overlapping structures, such as "PTV_without_overlap", "overlap", and "rectum_without_overlap", and to set dosimetric goals for each of these. This can get complicated if there are multiple overlapping structures. Another approach is to specify priorities. For example, if the PTV is to take precedence, then the priority is set in such a way that any overlap region of the PTV and another structure is treated as PTV.

It may be possible and desirable to place a limit on the size of small segments in an SMLC plan. It is difficult to accurately measure the output ($S_{c,p}$, see chapter 12, section 12.3) for fields with equivalent field sizes of 3 cm $\times$ 3 cm or 2 cm $\times$ 2 cm and smaller. Large uncertainties in the measurement of $S_{c,p}$ imply that the treatment planning software will be unable to calculate the dose for small apertures accurately. Some planning systems allow the planner to limit the area of the smallest segments. A choice of 5 cm^2 or 8 cm^2 might be reasonable. It may also be desirable to limit segments to some minimum number of monitor units. Some linacs (especially older linacs not designed for IMRT) do not deliver a small number of MU accurately. An example might be to limit segments to 2 MU or greater.

The number of beams used in IMRT plans is generally more than in conventional treatment planning. In principle, the more beams, the better the plan. For example, a nine-beam plan should, in principle, be at least as good, if not better, than a seven-beam plan, "provided that the nine beams include the original seven beams."[5] The worst that can happen is that the additional two beams get shut off (beamlet intensities set

---

[5] Wu, Q., L. Xing, G. Ezzell, and R. Mohan, "Inverse Treatment Planning," chapter 4 in *The Modern Technology of Radiation Oncology, Volume 2*, J. Van Dyk (ed.), pp. 133–183, 2005.

to zero). A seven-beam plan with different beams, however, may be better than the nine-beam plan because of optimal choice of beam angles. A larger number of beams spread out the dose more and allow for greater dose conformity with the target. Of course more beams require more time for delivery. One may reach a point of diminishing returns in which adding beams does not significantly improve the dose distribution. The use of five to nine beams is typical. Studies have shown that a larger number of beams is usually not helpful. Some planners feel that an odd number of beams is best. Parallel opposed beams should usually be avoided because these beam pairs produce a very uniform dose distribution along the common axis of the beams. This is not what we want from IMRT, but rather a very high dose in the target and little dose elsewhere. Non-coplanar beams can be useful to spread the dose out, but they require the therapists to enter the room to rotate the couch and therefore treatment time may become considerably longer. These beams also present the possibility of a collision of the gantry with the patient.

The choice of beam direction is important for IMRT. Whenever possible, it is advisable to choose beam directions in which the target is separated from organs at risk. This should result in less beam modulation, a more efficient plan, and a more homogeneous dose distribution. If it is possible, avoid beams that traverse critical structures. If no beam traverses a critical structure, then the only contribution to the dose in that structure is from scatter. For some standardized types of treatment (e.g., prostate) a "class solution" for beam angles may exist. This is a set of beam angles that usually gives the best plan for most patients.

We turn to the question of beam energy. There are reasons to favor lower energy beams even though higher energy beams may yield a somewhat better dose distribution for deep targets. Possible disadvantages of using higher energy beams are increased whole-body dose (see section 20.2.7) and non-equilibrium effects. Most clinics have both 6 MV and either 15 MV or 18 MV beams available. For relatively shallow targets (head and neck) 6 MV is adequate and perhaps preferred for its enhanced shallow dose. For deep targets in the pelvis, high-energy beams are usually preferred, especially when the number of beams is small. Low-energy beams will have a higher proximal dose, although they also have a more rapid falloff and thus a lower exit dose. When a small number of low-energy beams are used to treat a deep target, the proximal dose must be high to deliver the necessary dose at depth. As the number of beams is increased however the dose at d_{max} will tend to be diluted. The proximal dose will therefore go down. Studies have shown that for deep targets, such as the prostate, plan quality is relatively independent of energy for 6 MV and above, provided that the number of beams is at least nine.[6] The use of six beams or fewer with

---

[6] Pirzkall et al., (2002), "The effect of beam energy and number of fields on photon-based IMRT for deep-seated targets," *Int J Radiat Biol Phys* 53:434–442.

beam energy of 6 MV may result in significant hot spots far from the target (near the skin surface).[6] Arc therapy, such as tomotherapy, is equivalent to some large number of static beams at various gantry angles. This is why tomotherapy can achieve very good dose distributions even for deep targets using a 6 MV beam.

20.2.4 Case Study: Prostate Cancer

A prostate SMLC IMRT treatment plan is shown in Figure 20.13. The structures contoured are the PTV, bladder, bowel, rectum, and femoral heads (contour not shown). The PTV overlaps the bladder and rectum. For optimization calculations, the region of overlap with the rectum is called "overlap" and the region that does not overlap is called "no overlap." Other structures entering into the optimization are the bladder, small bowel, and femoral region (region around the femoral head and neck). Five coplanar 18 MV beams are used for this treatment plan. The beam angles, which are shown in Figure 20.13, are placed symmetrically. The prescription dose is 7740 cGy. The volume of the PTV receiving the prescription dose is 98.5%.

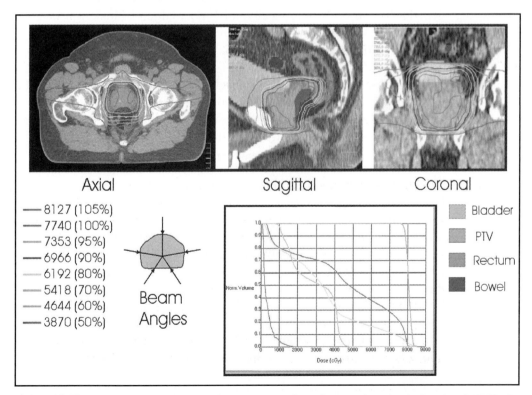

Figure 20.13: Prostate IMRT plan using five 18 MV co-planar beams. The prescription dose is 7740 cGy. See COLOR PLATE 22.

20.2.5 Aperture-Based Optimization

Generally the procedure followed in IMRT is to find the beamlet intensities and then to find the necessary apertures using a leaf sequencing algorithm. Aperture-based optimization (sometimes called "field within a field" or "multiple segment RT") is a different approach to IMRT. Aperture-based IMRT can be performed using a conventional 3D treatment planning system. In this type of IMRT (not everyone agrees that this actually *is* IMRT) a given port is created by adding beam segments that may only cover a portion of the target as seen in a beam's-eye view (BEV). Sensitive structures are blocked in some segments. The various segments are weighted in some way so as to produce a desirable dose distribution. This approach avoids leaf sequencing and the compromises that are sometimes associated with this method. This technique produces simple plans with only a few segments per beam and fewer MU than for inverse planning.

Aperture-based planning is now widely used for treating breast cancer. The conventional treatment technique is to use opposed tangents (see Figure 14.58) with wedges or compensators. The aperture-based IMRT technique can produce homogeneous dose distributions superior to wedge-based plans and reduce the dose to the lung. In addition, the absence of a beam modifier (wedge or compensator) reduces the scatter dose to the contralateral breast. The apertures are based on isodose curves generated from open field calculations (no wedge or blocking). Isodose lines from 120% to 100% are contoured in 5% increments. Segments are then added to conform to the BEV of these contours. Additional medial and lateral MLC segments are added for lung blocking.[7] This typically results in three to six segments for each of the two tangential beams. The segment weights are optimized to produce the final IMRT plan. The dose distribution for an aperture based breast treatment plan is shown in Figure 20.14. The lateral apertures used to produce this are shown Figure 20.15.

20.2.6 Physics Plan Validation

For conventional radiation therapy, individual ports can be checked by making manual MU calculations. This is not possible for IMRT. An alternative method to validate individual patient IMRT plans is needed. There are two aspects that need to be checked: the treatment planning system and the delivery system. Both must function properly. There are a number of validation methods in use at various clinics. We discuss two of these methods below.

One possibility is to take all of the beams computed for the patient and actually deliver them to a specified phantom. There are two steps in

---

[7] Shepard et al. "Aperture-Based Inverse Planning" in *Intensity Modulated Radiation Therapy: The State of the Art.* J. R. Palta and T. R. Mackie (eds.). AAPM 2003 Summer School Proceedings. Medical Physics Monograph No. 29, 2003.

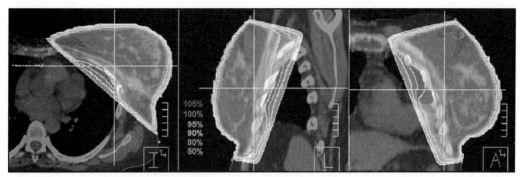

Figure 20.14: Breast aperture-based optimized treatment plan. From left to right: axial slice, sagittal slice, and coronal view. The white lines in the axial view show the location of the sagittal and coronal cut planes. The dose distribution is displayed as a "color wash." The red areas have doses between 100% and 105%. The color legend is shown in the middle (sagittal) frame. The beams are two 6 MV tangent beams matched at the posterior border as described in chapter 14, section 14.14. The segments for the lateral beam are shown in Figure 20.15. See COLOR PLATE 23.

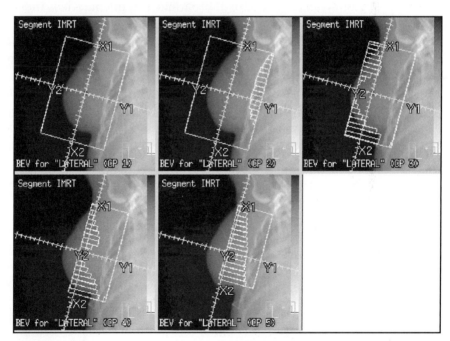

Figure 20.15: Apertures for the lateral beam of the dose distribution shown in Figure 20.14. The apertures for the medial beam are similar. The first aperture in the upper left corner is an open field (control point 1: CP1). The weighting of this aperture is 81.3%. In the second aperture (CP2, weighted 4.6%) some of the lung is blocked. In succeeding apertures (CP3, CP4, and CP5, weighted 5.4%, 3.5%, and 5.2%, respectively) anterior portions of the breast, which are thinner, are blocked to suppress hot spots there. See COLOR PLATE 24.

doing this. First, the beams must be applied to the phantom by the treatment planning system to compute the expected dose distribution in the phantom. The phantom can be somewhat arbitrary, provided that there is a CT representation of it stored in the treatment planning system. It is often a geometric phantom and may simply be a stack of virtual water plates (see chapter 8, Figure 8.1). The second step is to actually deliver the entire treatment to the phantom. The phantom will have dosimeters placed within to measure the dose and compare it to the expected dose. Often a small volume ion chamber is used in regions of both high-dose and low-dose gradient; film is used in regions of high-dose gradient. The ion chamber measurements are compared to the absolute dose expected at the location of the ion chamber and the film is used to check the relative dose distribution, particularly in regions where the dose gradient is high. Disadvantages of this technique are that patients are not shaped like geometric phantoms and, because all of the beams are evaluated as a whole, it is difficult to determine the source of discrepancies.

Another method is to check each beam individually. A number of check devices are sold to accomplish this purpose. These devices utilize embedded ionization chambers or diodes. Criticisms of this method are that each beam has to be analyzed individually and that each beam is usually (in practice) delivered with an upright gantry instead of the actual gantry angle used for the patient treatment. Also, these specialized devices do not have the spatial resolution that film has. One such device is called MapCHECK™ (Sun Nuclear, see Figure 20.16). It contains a grid of 445 diodes embedded in acrylic. The treatment planning system must first calculate the expected dose on a plane at a given depth and SSD for comparison with measurements. It is necessary to do this for every port. An example of the analysis for one port is shown in Figure 20.17.

The percent of the diodes passing is based on a comparison of the dose between corresponding points in the measured dose data versus the

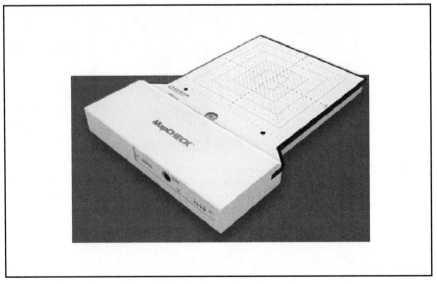

Figure 20.16: MapCHECK™ device that is used to validate IMRT treatment fields. This device contains an array of 445 diodes embedded in acrylic. The signal from the irradiated diodes provides a "map" of the dose distribution, which can be compared to an expected dose distribution calculated using the treatment planning system. (Courtesy of Sun Nuclear Corporation, Melbourne, FL)

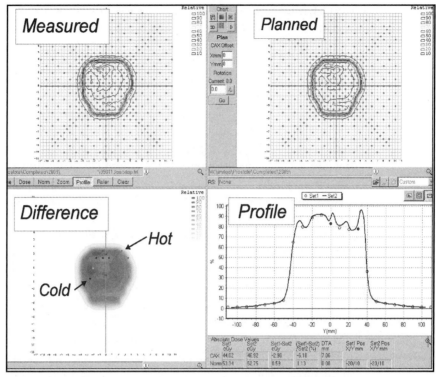

Figure 20.17: MapCHECK™ screen showing the comparison between measured IMRT field (ap prostate) labeled "Measured" and the dose distribution calculated by the treatment planning system (labeled "Planned"). The device shown in Figure 20.16 was used to acquire these data. The criteria for acceptance are that the percent difference is 3% or less and the distance to agreement is 3.0 mm or less. The diodes that fail to meet these criteria are shown as "hot" or "cold" dots in the "Difference" window on the lower left. In this example, 96% of the diodes pass and the difference between the measured and calculated dose at the norm point is 1.1%. A profile is shown in the lower right window. This is a profile along the gray vertical line shown in the "Difference" window. The solid line is the calculated profile and the dots are the measured values. See COLOR PLATE 25.

planned dose data. If the dose agrees within a certain percentage (usually taken to be 3%), then the point passes. If the dose does not agree within the tolerance, then the software searches the planned dose distribution to see if there is a point within some specified distance that is in agreement. This distance, called the "distance to agreement," is usually taken to be 3 mm. If the software finds such a point, then the point is considered to pass. With these criteria for passing, one would usually like to have about 95% of the diodes pass.

20.2.7 Whole-Body Dose and Shielding

The dose to the patient's entire body can be significantly larger for IMRT than for conventional therapy. In addition, the room shielding requirements are generally greater when IMRT is used. Both of these issues are discussed in this section.

The total number of MU necessary to deliver a given IMRT dose can be much higher than for conventional therapy. Let m be the ratio of the MU for an IMRT plan versus a conventional plan. The value of m is between 2 and 3 for an SMLC plan and up to 10 for serial tomotherapy. The reason for the latter is the inefficiency of serial tomotherapy delivery; only a small slice of tissue is being irradiated at any given time.

There are two contributions to whole-body dose: scatter and leakage. The scatter component of the dose is the same for IMRT as for conventional therapy because the dose delivered to the target is approximately the same. Whenever the beam is on, leakage radiation is present (see chapter 17, section 17.8). The leakage component comes from head leakage and leakage through the MLC. This radiation contributes dose to the patient's entire body. The leakage component for IMRT is larger because the beam is on longer. The IMRT whole-body dose from leakage is m times the whole-body dose from conventional therapy. In addition, for IMRT the dose absorbed by normal tissue is likely to extend over a larger volume of normal tissue because of the use of a larger number of beams, although this dose is likely to be lower.

Let us consider some numbers for a low-energy beam (less than 10 MV). For a conventional prostate treatment a patient might receive on the order of 7000 cGy. The delivery of this dose might require roughly 10,000 MU. The leakage radiation from the linac is restricted to no more than 0.1% (see chapter 17, section 17.8). We assume the leakage radiation has the same energy as the useful beam. At depth $d_{\max}$, 1 MU corresponds to roughly 1 cGy, and therefore the whole-body dose associated with 10,000 MU is 10,000 MU $\times$ 1 cGy/MU $\times$ 0.001 = 10 cGy or (for x-rays) 100 mSv. Recall that the annual occupational dose limit for radiation workers is 50 mSv. For SMLC dose delivery, the whole-body dose from leakage could be 300 mSv.

For high-energy beams, such as 18 MV, the situation is worse because of neutron contamination in the beam. Recall that the value of the radiation weighting factor w_R (see section 17.1) can be as high as 20 for neutrons. At 18 MV, serial tomotherapy could deliver a dose-equivalent as high as 3000 mSv. For this reason, IMRT is sometimes restricted to lower energy beams, particularly if the value of m is high, and especially when the patient is young.

For prostate patients the incidence of radiation-induced cancer is likely to double with the use of 6 MV IMRT, and increase by as much as a factor of 3 to 5 at energies of 15 MV and above.[8] The greatest concern must be for children. "Children are more sensitive to radiation induced cancer than adults by at least a factor of ten." In addition, as a child is smaller than an adult, the scatter and leakage dose may be higher because the sensitive tissues are closer to the central axis.

[8] Hall, E. J. (2006). "The inaugural Frank Ellis lecture—Iatrogenic cancer: The impact of intensity-modulated radiotherapy." *Clin Oncol* 18:277–282.

IMRT has implications for the design of room shielding, specifically for the workload (see section 17.8). In chapter 17 no distinction is made between the workload for primary radiation and leakage radiation. It becomes necessary to make this distinction for linacs that deliver a significant amount of IMRT, particularly if the value of m is large. The dose that is delivered to patients with IMRT is usually no different from the dose for non-IMRT (generally 180 cGy per fraction). Therefore, the workload for primary barriers is no different for IMRT than for non-IMRT. If the value of m is large, there may be a significant fraction of the treatment time during which little primary dose is delivered but during which there is leakage from the linac. For this reason, the workload for leakage radiation usually needs to be higher than for primary radiation. The leakage workload should be two to five times higher than for non-IMRT treatment.

20.3 Stereotactic Radiosurgery

20.3.1 Introduction

Stereotactic radiosurgery (SRS) is a form of single-fraction radiation therapy in which a stereotactic coordinate system is used for precise targeting. The term "stereotactic" refers to a method for locating points in the body by using an external three-dimensional reference frame or coordinate system. SRS can be thought of as a form of surgery in which radiation substitutes for a scalpel. High doses are used to cause "ablation," which destroys the ability of the target tissue to function or to grow. This is analogous to removal of the tissue by conventional surgery except that SRS is non-invasive. SRS treatments can be completed in a single day, on an outpatient basis. Single-fraction treatments do not provide for the normal tissue sparing associated with fractionated radiotherapy. The term "stereotactic radiotherapy" is usually reserved for multiple-fraction stereotactic treatments. Traditionally, SRS has been used for intracranial targets, although in the last few years some extracranial targets, such as the spine, have been treated using this technique. We will confine the discussion here to intracranial SRS.

Various forms of radiation have been used for SRS, including x-rays, gamma rays, and heavy particles such as protons. A number of treatment machines are used for SRS including conventional linacs and specialized treatment units such as the Gamma Knife® (Elekta) and CyberKnife® (Accuray). All of these units employ multiple non-coplanar beams to provide a highly conformal dose distribution with a very rapid falloff away from the target. There are a few clinics where stereotactic implants of radioactive sources (stereotactic brachytherapy) are performed.

There are three categories of diseases that are treated with SRS: functional disorders, arteriovenous malformations (AVMs), and tumors (benign and malignant). Functional disorders treated with SRS are primarily trigeminal neuralgia and to a lesser extent Parkinson's disease and epilepsy. Trigeminal neuralgia is a painful condition of the face involving the cranial trigeminal nerve. The dose prescription for a Gamma Knife treatment of trigeminal neuralgia is 40 Gy to the 50% line. This implies that the maximum dose in the target is 80 Gy!

An AVM is an abnormal tangle of blood vessels in the brain consisting of a "nidus" through which arteries connect directly to veins instead of through a capillary bed as normal. AVMs can bleed suddenly and without warning. The dose for AVMs is about 25 Gy. This results in a high obliteration rate, ranging "from 70 to 98%, depending on the nidus volume and the dose delivered."[9] It may take one to three years for ablation to become complete.

Benign tumors treated with SRS include acoustic neuromas (also called acoustic schwannomas), meningiomas, and pituitary adenomas. Local control for acoustic neuromas is 98%, with 50% to 70% of patients retaining their preexisting hearing levels.[9] Meningiomas are tumors in the dural lining of the brain. These tumors are often close to critical structures such as the brain stem or optic chiasm. Accurate targeting is therefore absolutely critical. The goal is to achieve tumor control while preserving existing function.

Malignant tumors fall into one of two categories: metastatic brain lesions or primary malignant brain tumors. Most metastatic tumors in the brain originate from the lungs or from melanoma primary (Flickinger 1994).[10] Sometimes SRS is used as a "boost" for conventional large or whole-brain irradiation. Metastatic tumors form the bulk of clinical practice for most clinics. It is possible to treat multiple "mets" in a single session. The prescribed dose ranges from 12 to 20 Gy, depending on the tumor size. Larger doses are given to smaller lesions. The local control rate is 85% to 90%.[11] SRS can significantly improve the quality of life for some of these patients.

SRS is usually restricted to target volumes of less than about 35 cm^3. Targets are generally less than 3 cm across. Larger target volumes imply more dose to a greater amount of normal tissue due to greater overlap of the incident beams. For larger volumes, the advantage of steep SRS dose gradients is lost, and one may revert to standard RT.

The dosimetric accuracy required for SRS is the same as for general radiotherapy (±5%). The geometric accuracy required is more stringent than for conventional radiotherapy. The mantra for SRS is *geometry,*

---

[9] Niranjan, A., and L. D. Lunsford, (2000), "Radiosurgery: Where we were, are, and may be in the third millennium." *Neurosurgery* 46:531–543.

[10] Flickinger et al. (1994), "A multi-institutional experience with stereotactic radiosurgery for solitary brain metastasis," *Int J Radiat Oncol Biol Phys* 28:797–802.

[11] Lippitz, B.E., "Treatment of Brain Metastases Using Gamma Knife Radiosurgery – The Gold Standard" at www.elekta.com/assets/Elekta-Oncology/Image-Guided-Radiation-Therapy/case-studies/lippitz.pdf. Accessed April 12, 2010.

geometry, geometry. Accurate targeting is absolutely essential; otherwise the wrong portion of the patient's brain will be ablated. For this reason, the positional accuracy required is ±1 mm. This stringent tolerance is affected by three factors: the accuracy of the established stereotactic coordinate system, the accuracy of delivery to the target, and motion of the target between the time of localization and treatment.

The stereotactic coordinate system is established with the use of a rigid coordinate frame that is attached to the patients skull (see Figure 20.18). A localization "box" is attached to the frame for imaging that has fiducial structures and can be used to establish the stereotactic coordinate system (see Figure 20.19). A CT scan and often an MRI are obtained with the localizer in place (see Figure 20.20). Specialized treatment planning software is used to analyze the CT/MRI images and to establish a coordinate system. The coordinates of any structure in the brain can then be ascertained. A common arrangement is for the fiducial markers on the side of the box to form the shape of a letter "N." On axial slices the outer marks always have the same separation, but the position of the central mark will depend on the location of the particular axial slice. For CT scans the fiducial markers are made of a high-Z material that will show up clearly in the images. For MRI, hollow plastic tubes are embedded in the localizer and filled with a solution of copper sulfate. It is possible to dispense with a frame provided that some method is available to locate the target in three-dimensional space. This is referred to as "frameless targeting." Among systems that are available to do this are

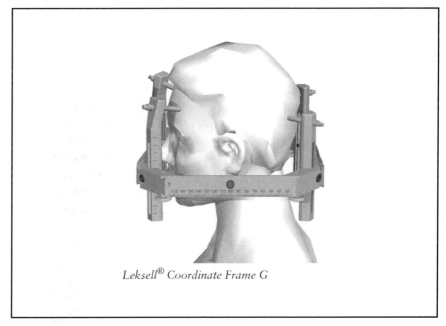

Leksell® Coordinate Frame G

Figure 20.18: Leksell Gamma Knife® stereotactic frame attached to the patient's skull with four pins. (Courtesy of Elekta, Norcross, GA)

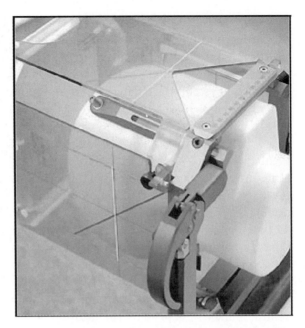

Figure 20.19: SRS head frame with localization box attached. (Courtesy of Elekta, Norcross, GA)

camera-based and x-ray–based systems. One camera-based system uses a reflector array attached to a patient bite block. The reflectors are illuminated by infrared light and a multiple camera imaging system detects the 3D position of each reflector with respect to the linac isocenter. The targeting system can calculate the shifts and rotations necessary to bring the reflectors into alignment with the expected treatment position. X-ray based frameless imaging systems are based on the position of the skull. These systems have the advantage that no reflectors or markers are needed.

20.3.2 Linac-Based Radiosurgery

Linac-based SRS was first developed in the 1980s. There are two approaches: the use of a temporarily modified general-purpose linac or specialized linacs such as the Accuray CyberKnife.

General-purpose linacs, which are temporarily modified, employ add-on tertiary collimators. There are two types of these: fixed-field circular apertures and a (mini- or micro-) MLC with small leaf width. The add-on collimator may be only a short distance from the patient, raising collision issues (see Figure 20.21). Typically, these systems are set up for SRS treatment at the end of the normal treatment day. The linac also requires table brackets or a floor-stand for immobilizing the SRS frame during treatment. The system used in Figure 20.21 uses a table bracket. The patient is set up by aligning markers on the stereotactic frame with

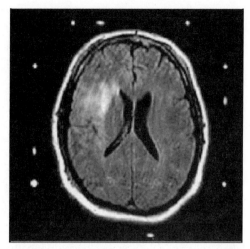

Figure 20.20: MRI localization for SRS. Fiducial markers attached to the head frame appear as bright spots around the periphery. The treatment planning software uses these markers to establish the stereotactic coordinate system. (Permission granted by Integra LifeSciences Corporation, Plainsboro, New Jersey, USA.)

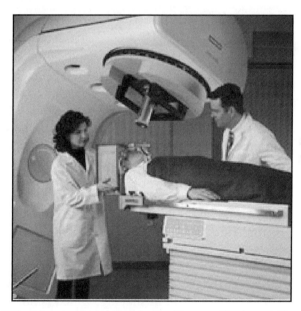

Figure 20.21: Linac-based SRS with a tertiary cylindrical collimator. The immobilization frame is mounted to the end of the table. (Permission granted by Integra LifeSciences Corporation, Plainsboro, New Jersey, USA.)

the room lasers. Mechanical specifications are more stringent than for routine therapy. Of particular importance is isocentricity with respect to gantry and couch rotation (see chapter 9, Figure 9.1). Ideally, the rotation axis of the gantry and of the couch intersect. Here we define the isocenter as this point of intersection. As the gantry or the couch is rotated, their rotation axes may wander. For SRS the total amount of wander must be less than 1 mm.

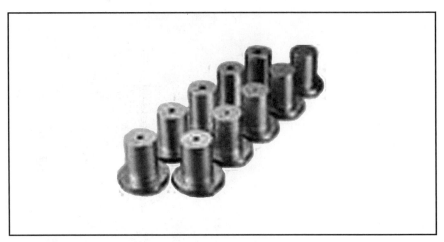

Figure 20.22: Cylindrical collimators with a range of circular aperture sizes for a linac-based SRS system. (Courtesy of BrainLAB, Feldkirchen, Germany)

Fixed-field circular cone apertures are defined by a cylindrical insert as shown in Figures 20.21 and 20.22. Aperture diameters range from about 5 to 40 mm. The cones are usually focused to reduce the penumbra (see chapter 13, Figure 13.4). The proximity of the cones to the patient helps to reduce the geometric penumbra (see chapter 9, section 9.4). Dynamic treatment involves the delivery of arcs. The technique of multiple non-coplanar converging arcs is probably the most commonly used. This is illustrated in Figure 20.23. Delivery is achieved by gantry rotations at fixed pedestal angles. For example, an arc in a sagittal plane is accomplished by gantry rotation at a pedestal angle of 90° or 270°. The arc angles are usually smaller than 180° to avoid parallel opposed beams in the plane of the arc. The number of arcs typically ranges from 4 to 11.[12]

Static treatment involves the use of a miniature or micro MLC with narrow leaf width for high precision in field shaping. Leaf widths are typically 3 to 4 mm. SRS MLCs are sold for mounting on a generic linac (see Figure 20.24). Multiple non-coplanar beams are employed. The MLC allows BEV field shaping, which is not possible with the circular collimators. The entire target volume is treated with a single isocenter rather than multiple isocenters or "shots" (Gamma Knife). Some of the advantages of this approach are: "improved dose homogeneity inside the target, sharper dose fall off outside the target, and less time consuming treatment planning."[12]

The CyberKnife (Accuray) is a miniature 6 MV linac mounted on a robotic arm (see Figure 20.25). The linac uses X-band microwaves with

---

[12] Podgorsak, E. B., and M. B. Podgorsak, IAEA Slide Set on Special Procedures and Techniques in Radiotherapy. http://www-naweb.iaea.org/nahu/dmrp/pdf_files/Chapter15.pdf.

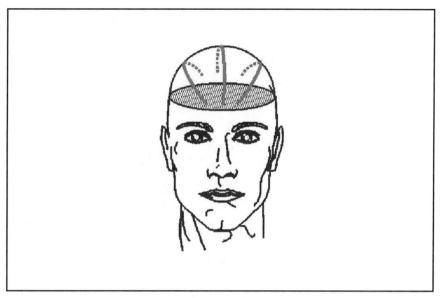

Figure 20.23: Dynamic stereotactic radiosurgery treatment technique using a linear accelerator to create multiple non-coplanar arcs. Each arc corresponds to gantry rotation at a separate couch angle. The beam is on while the gantry is rotating. If a jet of red ink were issuing from the collimator, it would trace the patterns shown on the patient's scalp (beam entry trace). Only three arcs are shown for clarity. Typically 4 to 11 arcs are used. See COLOR PLATE 26.

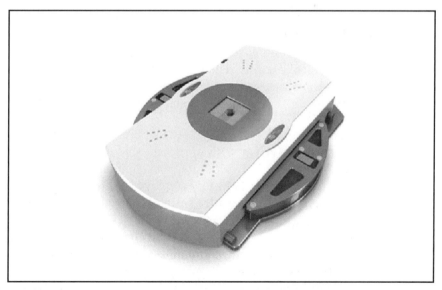

Figure 20.24: An MLC with small leaf size can be attached to a general-purpose linac for SRS. The MLC slides into the accessory mount. The leaf width of this MLC is 3 mm (projected to isocenter). The penumbra is small. (Courtesy of BrainLAB, Feldkirchen, Germany)

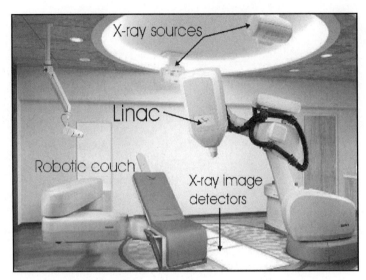

Figure 20.25: Robotic linac (CyberKnife®) used for SRS. The miniature X-band linac is mounted on a robotic arm. The system dispenses with the stereotactic frame. Target localization is accomplished with the use of two (diagnostic energy) x-ray sources producing orthogonal beams. The real time imaging detectors are located in the floor. The couch is also on a robotic arm. (Courtesy of Accuray, Sunnyvale, CA)

a frequency of about 10,000 MHz. This is to be compared with S-band microwaves used in conventional linacs that have a frequency of 3000 MHz (see chapter 9, section 9.2). The shorter wavelength of the X-band microwaves allows the waveguide to be shortened. The CyberKnife system provides frameless SRS. The system monitors patient position continuously with orthogonal x-ray beams and can track moving target volumes, thus compensating for intrafraction motion. Treatment is with multiple non-coplanar beams. There are very few constraints on beam direction. The geometrical accuracy is reported to be on the order of 1 mm. The CyberKnife is often used to treat extracranial targets.

20.3.3 Gamma Knife®

The Gamma Knife® was first employed in the late 1960s by neurosurgeon Lars Leksell. The basic idea has not changed since that time. Early models were the U, B, and B2. We will not discuss the details of those models. The current models are the 4C and the Perfexion™ (see Figure 20.26). There are approximately 250 units worldwide. As of 2008 approximately 500,000 patients have been treated worldwide.[13] Of these treatments, 44% were for malignant tumors, 35% for benign tumors, 13% for vascular disorders, and 8% for functional disorders.[13]

---

[13] Leksell Society Report. Indications Treated. December 2008. Available on-line at http://www .elekta.com/healthcare_international_leksell_gamma_knife_society.php.

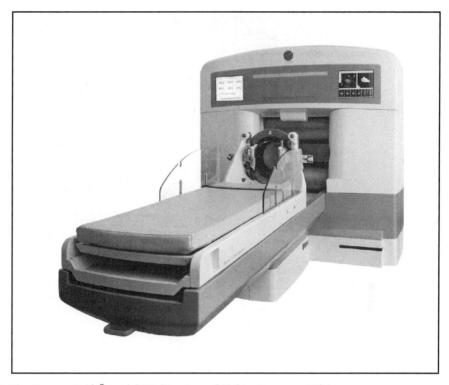

Figure 20.26: The Gamma Knife® model 4C. (Courtesy of Elekta, Norcross, GA)

The model 4C contains 201 Co-60 sources with a total activity of about 6000 Ci (220 TBq) when freshly loaded. This is a "quantity of concern" to the U.S. Nuclear Regulatory Commission and the U.S. Department of Homeland Security. Strict security precautions are now required in the United States. The properties of Co-60 are discussed in chapter 9, section 9.3. The sources are arranged in a hemispherical shell of radius approximately 40 cm around a point called the "unit center." Channels in the spherical shell direct 201 beams to a hemispherical helmet, which provides final collimation (see Figure 20.27). There are four helmets available with collimator apertures of 4 mm, 8 mm, 14 mm, and 18 mm diameter.

The treatment process proceeds as follows. The patient frame and a helmet are bolted to the end of the couch (see Figure 20.28). The staff leaves the room. When the start button is pressed, the shielding doors open and the couch moves in. The helmet "docks" with the beam channels (see Figure 20.29).

The dose distribution at the unit center is nearly spherical. To treat a nonspherical target, multiple "shots" are used. A shot is a portion of the treatment with a particular helmet aperture size and with the unit center set to a particular anatomical location. Multiple shots form a cluster of spherical high-dose regions, which combine to form a very

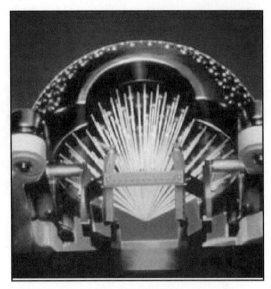

Figure 20.27: Light converging on the unit center as it traverses the collimator plugs in a Gamma Knife helmet. The head frame is in the foreground at the bottom. The patient target is positioned at the unit center. (Courtesy of Elekta, Norcross, GA). See COLOR PLATE 27.

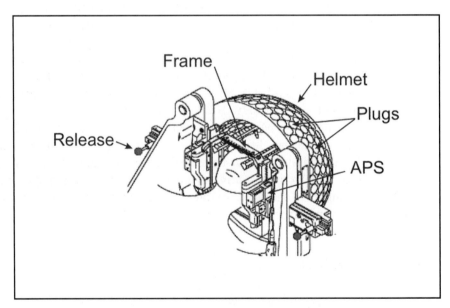

Figure 20.28: The Gamma Knife® frame and helmet are attached to the end of the couch. The 201 plugs in the helmet provide final collimation. Four helmets are available with plug aperture diameters of 4, 8, 14, and 18 mm. The automatic positioning system (APS) will move the patient with respect to the unit center. The patient is removed by pulling on the release knob shown. (Courtesy of Elekta, Norcross, GA). See COLOR PLATE 28.

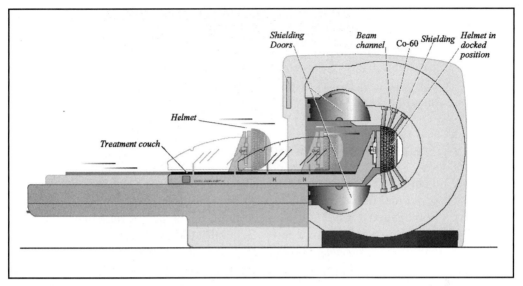

Figure 20.29: Schematic diagram of the model 4C Gamma Knife. The patient stereotactic frame and the helmet are attached to the end of the couch (as in Figure 20.28). After the staff have left the room, the shielding doors open and the couch moves in until the helmet is "docked" with the beam channels. (Courtesy of Elekta, Norcross, GA)

conformal dose distribution. Most treatments require multiple shots to produce dose distributions that conform to irregularly shaped targets and/or to treat multiple mets. The anatomical location of the unit center can be moved with the automatic positioning system (APS, see Figure 20.28). Multiple shots are easy to deliver with the APS in contrast to the difficulty of using multiple isocenters in linac-based SRS. It is not uncommon to use up to 10 shots.

The Perfexion™ is the latest model Gamma Knife. It has an expanded anatomical reach allowing treatments inferior to the limit of the Model 4C. This unit has 192 Co-60 sources and collimator sizes of 4, 8, and 16 cm. Collimator changes are made internally and are automatic. It is possible to deliver a "composite" shot which mixes collimator diameters in a single shot.

20.3.4 Imaging

The imaging requirements for SRS are similar to those for radiotherapy in general. The exceptions are discussed below.

MR imaging is almost always used along with CT imaging for SRS. As discussed in chapter 19, tumors are often not well visualized on CT. One must be cautious about the possibility of geometric distortion with MRI (see section 19.5). It is common to fuse CT and MR images (see section 19.6). The images must be examined very carefully for any signs of distortion, mirroring, etc.

AVMs are not very well visualized with either CT or MRI. Instead, digital subtraction angiography is used along with a special angiographic target localizer. The localizer is in the form of plastic plates with metal BBs (diameter 1 mm) or crosses embedded in them. The plates attach to the stereotactic head frame. Orthogonal images are taken (AP and lateral).

20.3.5 Treatment Planning

There are three factors to consider in planning SRS: conformity, volume of normal tissue irradiated by the prescription isodose surface, and dose homogeneity inside the target volume.[14] There is some tension between conformity and homogeneity. Generally the more conformal a dose distribution is, the less homogeneous it is. In conventional radiation therapy planning, dose homogeneity is a goal. The variation in dose over the target may be as little as ±5%. In SRS conformity is prized above all else to the point that homogeneity may be sacrificed. In SRS the dose is often prescribed to the lowest isodose surface encompassing the target. This implies that the dose distribution in the target may be very inhomogeneous. For the Gamma Knife it is customary to prescribe to the 50% isodose line (maximum dose 100%). The maximum target dose is therefore two times the prescribed dose. For linac-based SRS it may be possible to prescribe to the 80%–90% line. Targets that depart from spherical symmetry may require multiple isocenters (multiple shots on Gamma Knife) for adequate coverage. Critical structures are the optic chiasm, optic nerves, eyes, and brain stem. The SRS tolerance dose of these structures is different than for conventional fractionation.

Linac

The dose distribution for dynamic SRS is determined primarily by the location of the isocenter and the size of the collimators. Linac-based SRS usually uses a small number of isocenters. A change in isocenter requires a shift of the patient followed by whatever QA procedures are performed to verify targeting. This is time consuming. On a Gamma Knife the patient can be moved with respect to the unit center automatically using the APS. The collimator size is chosen according to the size of the target. Arcs which cross critical structures (eyes, optic chiasm, etc,) should be avoided. This may require restricted arcs. Arcs that are favorable can be preferentially weighted.

---

[14] Podgorsak, E.B., and M. B. Podgorsak, Special Procedures and Techniques in Radiotherapy (IAEA Slide Set based on Chapter 15 of *Radiation Oncology Physics: A Handbook for Teachers and Students*, IAEA, 2006).

Gamma Knife

The dose distribution at the unit center is approximately spherical. Planning proceeds by placing shots. A shot is characterized by the diameter of the 50% isodose spherical surface and the location of the center of the sphere. The diameter of the 50% isodose surface is determined by the helmet used. By placing shots of various diameters, locations, and weighting, it is possible to generate very conformal dose distributions (see Figure 20.30).

Evaluation of Dose Distributions

The tools used to evaluate and compare treatment plans are similar to those used for other forms of radiation therapy. The DVH is used to describe the dose distribution in the target and normal structures. The quantity PITV (prescription isodose to target volume) has been defined by the Radiation Therapy Oncology Group (RTOG) as the ratio of the volume encompassed by the prescription isodose surface divided by the target volume. This is a measure of the conformity of the prescription isodose surface to the target volume.[14] A range in PITV of $1.0 \leq \text{PITV} \leq 2$

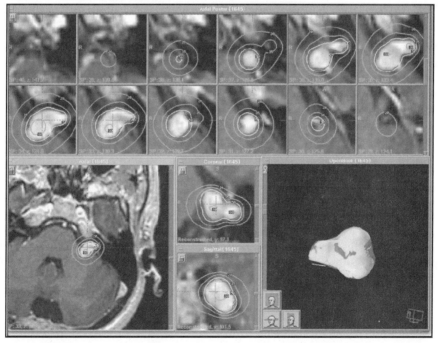

Figure 20.30: Gamma Knife treatment plan. The lower left-hand panel shows an axial image zoomed out. The upper panel shows various zoomed axial slices covering the inferior to superior extent of the target. The two middle frames on the bottom show a coronal and sagittal slice. The window on the lower right shows a 3-D rendering. The target contour is red. The yellow contour is the prescription isodose line (50%). The other two isodose lines are 35% and 20%. The 50% prescription isodose surface is highly conformal. (Courtesy of Elekta, Norcross, GA). See COLOR PLATE 29.

is considered to meet protocol. Values of the PITV in the range 2.0 < PITV < 2.5 or 0.9 < PITV < 1.0 are considered minor but acceptable deviations. A major and unacceptable deviation is PITV > 2.5.

20.3.6 Dosimetry

There are three different types of quantities which must be measured to establish an SRS linac dosimetry system: PDD or TMR, beam profiles and output factors ($S_{c,p}$). Measurements for the very small fields used in SRS present difficulties. Measurement of the profiles requires a detector with high spatial resolution. The detector must be considerably smaller than the field size and probably even smaller than the penumbra. Dose gradients are crucial in SRS, and it is therefore important to be able to measure the penumbra accurately so that the calculated dose distributions will be accurate. Film has high spatial resolution and is preferred for measuring beam profiles. PDD, TMR and $S_{c,p}$ should be measured with a small ion chamber (diameter less than 3 mm). Ion chambers are accurate and they have no energy dependence, but they are usually large. Very small micro or pinpoint ion chambers are available that have inner diameters as small as 2 mm. The Gamma Knife output is calibrated in a plastic spherical phantom provided by Elekta. The TG-21 calibration protocol is followed (recall that the TG-51 protocol requires water).

20.3.7 Quality Assurance

An "end to end" or "A to Z " test of the SRS treatment procedure is advisable. The Radiological Physics Center (RPC) provides an anthropomorphic head phantom, which is sent by mail. The phantom contains a dosimetric insert with radiochromic film (see chapter 8, section 8.4.2) and TLDs. The phantom is imaged, a treatment plan is made, and then the phantom is irradiated according to the plan. The phantom is then shipped back to the RPC for analysis. The RPC evaluates geometric and dosimetric accuracy. This provides independent confirmation of a clinic's ability to accurately deliver SRS. This should be performed prior to first patient treatment and perhaps once per year thereafter.

QA requirements for linac-based SRS are strict and demanding. This is in part because linacs are not dedicated SRS delivery units. Quality assurance procedures for SRS consist of equipment QA and patient QA (see chapter 18). Of chief concern is mechanical stability of the isocenter with couch and gantry rotation and laser alignment. As the lasers are used for patient alignment, they must be very accurately aimed—to better than 1 mm. Patient treatment QA should be meticulous. A treatment checklist is necessary. Items on the checklist might include: jaw setting, proper collimator inserted, target coordinates checked for each isocenter, couch position, arc angles programmed, etc.

20.4 Proton Radiotherapy

20.4.1 Introduction

Advocates of proton therapy have recently argued that within 10 to 15 years protons will likely replace photons as the most common type of radiation used for curative radiation therapy.[15] There are now five centers in the United States that routinely treat patients with protons. There are at least three additional centers that are planned to open within the next few years. At the time of this writing there are approximately 25 proton therapy facilities worldwide and over 60,000 patients have been treated. The major reason why there are so few facilities is cost: with current technology, acceleration of protons to the very high energies required for the treatment of deep-seated lesions (about 200 MeV) requires extremely large and heavy (over 100 tons) accelerators, which cost an order of magnitude more than the most sophisticated medical linear accelerators. However, considerable effort is being expended to develop smaller, lighter, and less expensive accelerators for proton therapy (see section 20.4.10), so the number of centers offering such treatments will likely increase significantly, especially if the clinical results obtained with current proton units prove to be better than for photons.

Physicists have been producing beams of accelerated protons since at least the early 1930s when Ernest Lawrence developed the cyclotron at UC Berkeley for research in nuclear physics.[16] The idea of using these particles for radiation therapy is hardly new. The physicist Robert Wilson (see Figure 20.31) made the first known suggestion that protons might have properties that are useful for radiation therapy in 1946. He was one of the founders and the director of Fermilab. When Wilson was called to appear before the Congressional Joint Committee on Atomic Energy, a senator asked him how a multimillion-dollar particle accelerator at Fermilab could improve the security of the country. He answered, "It has nothing to do directly with defending our country except to make it worth defending."

Patients were first treated with protons by C.A. Tobias and J. H. Lawrence (Ernest's physician brother!) on the 184 in. cyclotron at Lawrence Berkeley Laboratory beginning in 1954. They treated pituitary

---

[15] Maughan, R. L., F. Van den Heuvel, and C. G. Orton, (2008), "Point/Counterpoint. Within the next 10–15 years protons will likely replace photons as the most common type of radiation for curative radiotherapy." *Med Phys* 35(10):4285–4288.

[16] It is likely that protons were being accelerated at the Cavendish Laboratory in England prior to the development of the cyclotron.

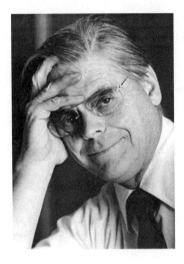

Figure 20.31: Robert Wilson (1914–2000) first suggested the use of protons for radiation therapy. (Courtesy of Fermi National Accelerator Laboratory, Batavia, IL)

tumors in approximately 30 patients. In the 1950s Larson and Leksell in Uppsala, Sweden, developed radiosurgical techniques for the treatment of brain tumors. They used a 180 MeV synchrocyclotron. They were the first to use range modulation and beam scanning to produce large treatment fields. They treated 73 patients. Lars Leksell later went on to develop the Gamma Knife. In 1961 Ray Kjellberg, a neurosurgeon at Massachusetts General Hospital began treating intracranial targets at the Harvard Cyclotron Laboratory. Although the use of protons in radiation therapy has a long history, the technology for beam delivery and field shaping is still evolving rapidly.

It is only recently that protons have begun to be used outside of a few research centers with accelerators that were not originally designed and built for physics research and housed in laboratories. The first hospital-based proton machine in the United States, built by Fermilab specifically for radiotherapy, was opened in 1990 at the Loma Linda University Cancer Center in California. As of 1998, 64% of the patients treated were prostate patients. The next highest percentage was 5.8% for head and neck patients.

20.4.2 Potential Advantages of Protons

The major rationale for proton therapy is the potential dose distribution benefit related to the Bragg peak (see chapter 6, section 6.2.5): as protons traverse matter such as tissue, they gradually lose energy and deposit dose more or less uniformly until they have almost come to rest at which point they lose energy precipitously. Consequently, the depth-dose curve is fairly flat after the protons enter the patient (the "plateau" region) until close to the end of their range when it rises suddenly (the

Bragg peak) and thereafter falls to zero (see Figure 6.12). The depth of the Bragg peak can be adjusted by changing the energy of the incoming protons: increasing the energy increases the depth. Figure 20.32 shows approximate depths of the Bragg peak as a function of proton beam energy. It is clear from this figure that to treat deep targets at a depth of, say 30 cm, requires a beam energy of between 200 and 250 MeV.

The width of the Bragg peak (distance from the proximal to distal depths) is only a few millimeters, so only small lesions can be treated with these "raw" proton beams. Fortunately it is possible to spread out the Bragg peak by combining beams of different energies. This is illustrated in Figure 6.12, which shows a number of depth dose curves for different energy proton beams (in this example, nine energies) adding together to produce the so-called "spread-out Bragg peak" (SOBP). If the intensities of the beams of each energy are selected appropriately, a flat SOBP can be obtained, as shown. The number of different energy beams can be adjusted to match the extent (in depth) of the target. Methods for production and selection of different energy beams will be presented in section 20.4.4.

Another advantage of protons is the increase in depth dose due to inverse-square law falloff of dose with distance. This falloff is significant with photons, for which typical SADs are about 100 cm, but is much reduced at the very long SADs used for proton therapy machines, which are usually greater than 200 cm.

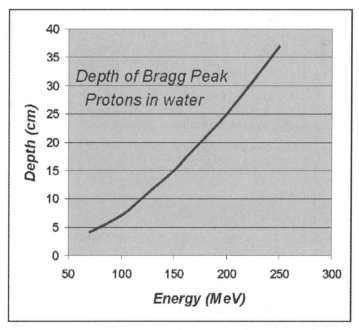

Figure 20.32: Depth of the Bragg peak for protons in water as a function of energy. These depths are considerably larger than those found with clinical machines because of attenuation in materials placed in the beams such as scatterers, range modulators, monitor chambers, compensating filters, etc., before they strike the patient.

The advantage of protons is due almost wholly to the improved dose distribution and not to any special radiobiological properties. Although the protons that deliver dose in the raw Bragg peak have a high LET, the LET in a SOBP is relatively low. The SOBP is a mixture of the radiations in the several low-LET plateau regions plus one high-LET Bragg peak. This significantly reduces the average LET of the clinical beam, and it turns out that any radiobiological benefit of proton therapy is likely to be minimal. For this reason, clinical proton beams do not exhibit the biological advantages claimed for high-LET radiotherapy, such as reduced effect of hypoxic cells in tumors. There is a small increase in biological effectiveness of the protons in the SOBP compared to photons, however, and this needs to be accounted for when prescribing dose and comparing clinical results. The ICRU Report No. 78 recommends that a generic Relative Biological Effectiveness (RBE) of 1.1 be used when comparing proton and photon radiotherapy doses i.e. that the radiation in the proton spread out Bragg peak is 10% more biologically effective than photons.[17] This is an oversimplification, however, since RBE depends on a number of factors, such as dose rate and fractionation, the energy spectrum of the protons at the point of interest, and the specific tissue being irradiated. Some references quote "cobalt gray equivalent" (CGE). This is the dose in gray multiplied by 1.1.

20.4.3 Proton Therapy Accelerators

There are five stages of proton acceleration common to all types of accelerators:

1. Ion source: produce protons for acceleration (use hydrogen gas)
2. Injection: get protons into the accelerator
3. Acceleration
4. Extraction: get protons out of accelerator
5. Beam transport/switchyard: direct beam to various treatment rooms

There are two main types of accelerators that are used to accelerate protons for radiation therapy:

1. Cyclotrons
   (a) isochronous
   (b) synchrocyclotron
2. Synchrotrons

Both of these types of accelerators are circular machines that use electric fields to accelerate the protons and magnetic fields to bend the

---

[17] ICRU Report 78: Prescribing, Recording, and Reporting Proton-Beam Therapy, 2007.

beams into circular paths. These accelerators can have superconducting or nonsuperconducting magnets.

Cyclotrons

Before the operating principles of the cyclotron are described, we must take a diversion to discuss the motion of a charged particle in a uniform magnetic field. A moving charged particle is deflected by a magnetic field (see chapter 2, section 2.3.6).[18] Figure 20.33 shows a region of uniform magnetic field. The magnetic field points perpendicular to, and into the page. A positively charged particle moving in the plane of the page will travel in a circle as shown in the figure.

The force on the charged particle is given by $F = QvB$, where Q is the charge of the particle, v is the speed of the particle, and B is the strength of the magnetic field. A particle in circular motion with constant speed experiences a centripetal acceleration: $a = v^2/R$ (see section 2.2). An expression for the radius of the circle can be found from Newton's second law:

$$F = ma$$

$$QvB = m\frac{v^2}{R},$$

(20.7)

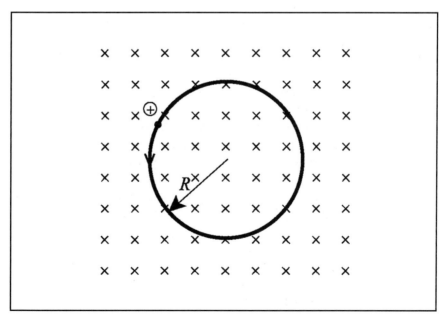

Figure 20.33: A charged particle moving perpendicular to a uniform magnetic field follows a circular path. In this illustration the magnetic field is directed into the page and the particle is positively charged.

---

[18] Unless the motion happens to be along the direction of the field.

where m is the mass of the particle. This can be solved for the radius of the circle:

$$R = \frac{mv}{QB}. \tag{20.8}$$

The time that it takes for a particle to travel once around the circle (the period) is given by:

$$P = \frac{2\pi R}{v} = \frac{2\pi m}{QB}. \tag{20.9}$$

Equation (20.9) shows that the period is independent of the speed (and thus energy) of the particle! A particle with greater speed will travel in a larger circle, but the time necessary to traverse the circle will remain constant. As we shall see, this is the crucial feature of a cyclotron.

The cyclotron was invented by Ernest Lawrence in the early 1930s for research in nuclear physics. Lawrence was awarded the Nobel Prize in Physics in 1939 for the development of the cyclotron. The cyclotron exploits a clever idea; instead of accelerating charged particles once through a large potential difference, accelerate them many times through a small potential difference. Lawrence's original cyclotron used two hollow electrodes in the shape of the letter "D" (see Figures 20.34 and 20.35).

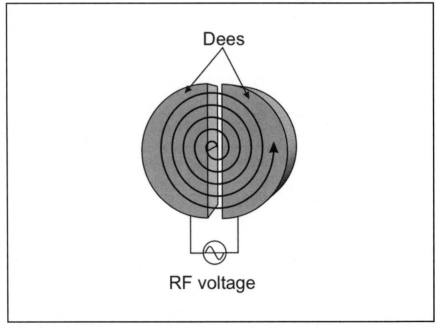

Figure 20.34: Schematic diagram of a cyclotron. The two electrodes are called "dees" because of their resemblance to the letter "D." There is a magnetic field directed into the page. The protons are initially injected at the center. Each time a proton passes between dees, it is accelerated. The protons travel inside the hollow dees, following a spiral path outward as they gain energy.

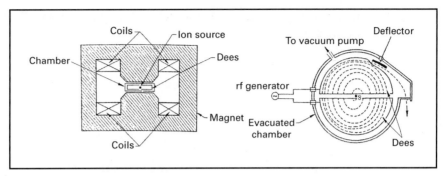

Figure 20.35: On the left is a side view of a classical cyclotron showing the massive magnet yoke and coils. On the right is an overhead view similar to Figure 20.34 but showing some additional detail such as the deflector used to extract the beam. (Modified from chapter 11, "Medical Accelerators," Fig 11-1b, p. 355, E. B. Podgorsak, P. Metcalfe, and J. Van Dyk, in *The Modern Technology of Radiation Oncology*, J. Van Dyk (ed.), © 1999 with permission.)

The particles are injected into the gap near the center and between the dees. They are then accelerated across the gap. The acceleration results in a gain in energy. If the polarity of the dees is changed in just the right way and at just the right rate, the particles will always be accelerated when they find themselves between the dees. This is illustrated in Figure 20.36.

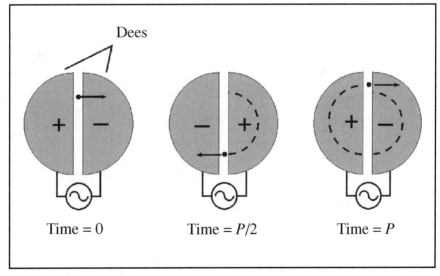

Figure 20.36: On the left, a proton is in the gap between the dees. If the dees have the polarity shown, the proton will be accelerated in a clockwise direction. Half a period later (middle diagram) the proton again finds itself between the dees. If the voltage polarity of the dees has now been reversed, the proton will again be accelerated in a clockwise direction. After one period elapses, the proton finds itself once more between the dees. If the polarity has now returned to the original configuration, then the proton will once again be accelerated in a clockwise direction.

The crucial feature of the cyclotron is that the period is independent of the speed (or energy) of the protons. Under these circumstances it is possible to have a constant frequency RF source tuned to the rotation frequency of the protons for a given magnetic field strength. In this way the protons can be repeatedly accelerated across the gap as they circulate around. As an example, suppose that the potential difference between the two dees is 10^5 volts. Each time a proton crosses the gap, it will acquire an additional 10^5 eV. A proton crosses the gap twice each time it makes a round trip (in time P). If the proton goes around 1000 times, it will gain an amount of kinetic energy equal to $2 \times 1000 \times 10^5$ eV = 200 MeV.

The protons are extracted from the cyclotron by using an electrostatic field applied by a deflector (see Figure 20.35). Modern cyclotrons used for medical therapy are considerably more complicated than the simple presentation given in Figure 20.35, although the basic idea remains the same. Figure 20.37 is a photograph of a proton therapy cyclotron.

The protons used for radiation therapy have kinetic energies up to 250 MeV. The rest mass energy of a proton is 950 MeV. The kinetic energy of therapy protons is a significant fraction of the rest mass. Under these circumstances, Newtonian mechanics begins to break down and we must consider the effects of special relativity (see chapter 2, section 2.5). In special relativity an object's mass increases when its speed becomes a significant fraction of the speed of light. When this occurs, equation (20.7) is no longer valid. This ruins the very basis for

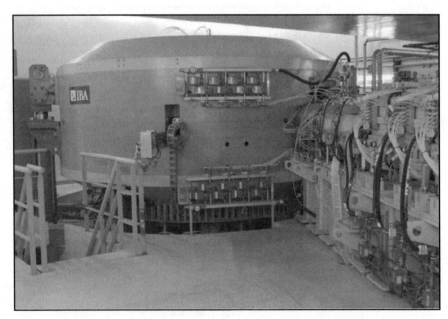

Figure 20.37: Photograph of an IBA isochronous cyclotron used for proton radiation therapy. The beam line is visible on the right. (Courtesy of Penn Medicine, Philadelphia, PA, and IBA, Louvain-la-Neuve, Belgium; www.iba-worldwide.com). See COLOR PLATE 30.

the classical cyclotron. For this reason a classical cyclotron is limited to a relatively low energy of roughly 10 MeV.

One method of overcoming relativistic behavior is to make the magnetic field stronger at larger distances from the center of the cyclotron. If the gradient in the magnetic field is just right, the protons will continue to circulate with the same period as they gain energy and move out toward the perimeter of the cyclotron. Such a cyclotron design is referred to as *isochronous*. An advantage of the isochronous cyclotron is that the radiofrequency can remain constant throughout acceleration. To satisfy requirements of particle stability and focusing, it is necessary to have spiral-shaped magnetic pole pieces, as illustrated in Figure 20.38, with "hills" and "valleys" in the magnetic field strength. Most proton therapy accelerators are isochronous cyclotrons.

Synchrotrons

The Loma Linda accelerator is a synchrotron built by Fermilab specifically for therapeutic use. Synchrotrons are not limited by relativistic behavior. A synchrotron is shown in Figure 20.39. The protons are injected into the "ring" and travel around in an orbit of constant radius due to the magnets in the curved sections of the structure in Figure 20.39. To maintain a constant orbital radius, the magnetic field strength is increased as the protons gain energy. The acceleration occurs in RF

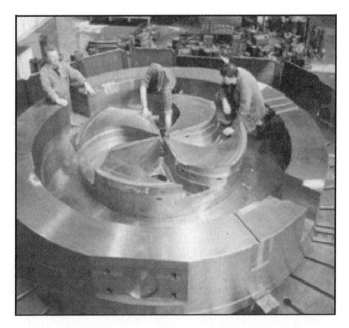

Figure 20.38: Magnet yoke for an isochronous cyclotron showing spiral shaped magnetic pole pieces. (Courtesy of IBA, Louvain-la-Neuve, Belgium; www.iba-worldwide.com). See COLOR PLATE 31.

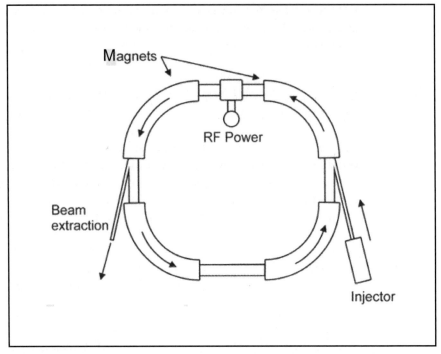

Figure 20.39: A proton synchrotron. The protons are accelerated in the RF cavity section of the ring. As they gain energy both the RF frequency and magnetic field strength must increase in synchrony. Synchrotrons are the only method currently in widespread use to accelerate protons to the highest energies (>1 TeV).

acceleration cavities spaced around the synchrotron. These are in the straight sections and the acceleration mechanism is basically the same as in the RF waveguide of a linac. The frequency of the RF must increase in synchrony with the magnetic field to stay in phase with the circulating protons (and hence the name synchrotron).

The steps in beam production are:

1. Inject protons from the ion source and the injector into the accelerator.
2. Accelerate the particles in the ring.
3. Extract the beam.
4. Return to step 1 and repeat.

Note that the final proton beam is pulsed and not continuous. This makes spot scanning difficult, which might limit some of the potential for intensity-modulated proton radiotherapy (see section 20.4.8).

Synchrotrons are the only method currently in widespread use to accelerate protons to very high energies (>1 TeV). The Large Hadron Collider (LHC) at CERN is a synchrotron. The energy of the protons in the LHC is about 9 TeV, about 5 orders of magnitude higher than the protons we use for therapy. Synchrotrons offer the advantage of variable energy. The beam current and hence the dose rate are lower for a synchrotron.

20.4.4 Production and Selection of Different Energy Beams

There are two ways to produce the different energy beams that combine to create the SOBP. They can be created either by the use of varying thickness filters placed between the source and the patient, or by changing the beam energy electronically. For the former, it is common to use a rotating variable thickness filter called a "ridge filter," "propeller," or "modulation wheel," such as the one shown in Figure 20.40. Most existing proton therapy machines use this method. Changing beam energies electronically is conceptually more elegant and versatile but technologically more difficult. It requires rapid energy selection changes in the

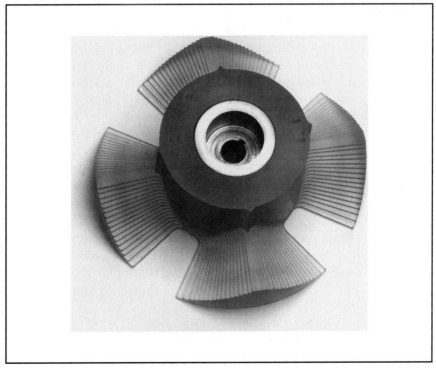

Figure 20.40: A range modulating "propellor" that can be inserted into the beam line to spread out the Bragg peak. The thickness of the propellor that is intercepted by the beam varies as the propellor rotates. This is for the Loma Linda eye beam line. It produces a uniform dose over 22 mm in depth. (Reprinted from chapter 20, "Proton Therapy," Michael F. Moyers, Fig. 20.16, p. 842, in *The Modern Technology of Radiation Oncology*, J. Van Dyk (ed.), © 1999 with permission.)

accelerator while the beam is "on." Many of the early difficulties have now been resolved, however, so most future proton therapy machines are likely to use this method of energy modulation.

20.4.5 Lateral Beam Spreading and Field Shaping with Protons

The beam produced by a proton accelerator is very small in cross section. When the beam emerges from the accelerator, it may be only a few millimeters in diameter, much like that of the electron beam in a linear accelerator. There are two main approaches to widening such beams: passive scattering and active scanning. With *passive scattering*, the beam is spread laterally by the use of a scattering foil positioned upstream of the collimation system. With *active scanning*, magnets are used to deflect the beam much like the raster scanning of electron beams in a cathode-ray television or cathode-ray oscilloscope tube. Until fairly recently, only the first technique had been used. It is technologically simpler but requires compromises in dose distribution.

Passive Scattering

This involves placing a scattering foil in the beam, just as we do in electron beam radiotherapy to spread the beams laterally. A single lead foil placed in the proton beam will result in a Gaussian intensity profile with a field diameter of only about 30 mm. This is too small, except possibly for treatment of eye lesions. To provide additional spreading, a second lead scatterer is introduced. The second scatterer is in the approximate shape of a Gaussian (it functions like a flattening filter in a linac). The thick portion in the center reduces the high-intensity central region by scattering protons to the periphery of the beam. This is illustrated in Figure 20.41. The second scatterer also includes a shaped piece of polycarbonate plastic to maintain uniform beam energy across the field, since it is desirable to maintain a uniform range laterally. With passive scattering, beams are shaped using either primary collimators with patient-specific secondary blocks, or with multileaf collimators. MLCs are clearly preferable, but these have proven difficult to fabricate for all but small fields. This is not a problem when active scanning is employed.

Figure 20.42 shows a photo of a patient specific beam aperture and compensator. Figure 20.43 shows the effect of the compensator. The compensator creates a dose distribution that conforms nicely to the distal boundary of the target. The drawback of this is that the SOBP shifts toward the surface, leading to an increase in the proximal dose.

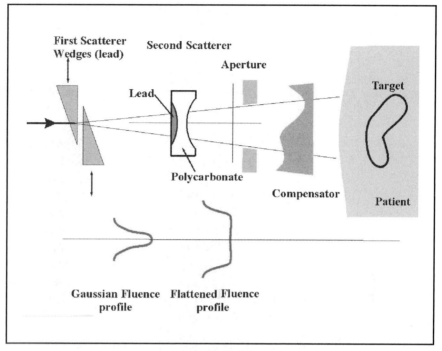

Figure 20.41: A passive scattering system for a proton beam. The first scatterer is a set of movable lead wedges. This creates a Gaussian beam profile. The second scatterer is thicker at the center than at the periphery and functions like a flattening filter. The lead provides the scattering and the polycarbonate is shaped to ensure that the beam energy does not vary laterally. Passage through the second scatterer results in a flattened beam profile and a uniform energy across the beam. The beam then traverses a patient-specific collimator and compensator. The compensator is designed so that the range of the protons corresponds to the location of the distal edge of the target (see Figure 20.43). See COLOR PLATE 32.

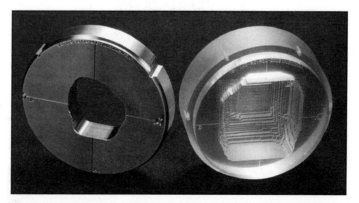

Figure 20.42: A patient-specific aperture and range compensator. The aperture shapes the beam laterally and the range compensator shapes the distal edge of the Bragg peak. The aperture is made of brass. These must be stored for a time after use because they become activated. They are then recycled. The compensators are made out of acrylic. (Courtesy of the.decimal point; http://www.thedotdecimal.com.). See COLOR PLATE 33.

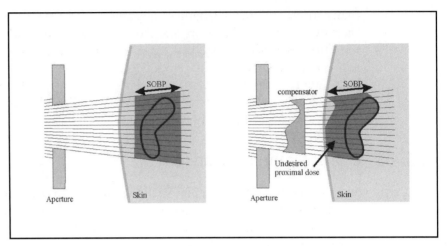

Figure 20.43: Customized patient proton treatment with a passive scattering system. The diagram on the left shows the spread-out Bragg peak (SOBP) prior to the insertion of a compensator. The diagram on the right shows the SOBP after the insertion of a customized compensator. The conformity with the distal edge of the tumor is excellent, but the shift in the SOBP produces unwanted dose proximal to the target. See COLOR PLATE 34.

Active Scanning

With active scanning, orthogonal magnets are used to deflect the proton pencil beam, as shown in Figure 20.44. The magnetic field is used to deflect the beam and "paint" the field. Simultaneously, the energy can be varied so that the depth of penetration can vary laterally. This has the advantage that no physical patient-specific beam modifiers are necessary. In addition, none of the protons are "wasted" by filters. This method clearly requires a sophisticated planning and delivery system; but since it enables simultaneous intensity *and* range modulation, it is

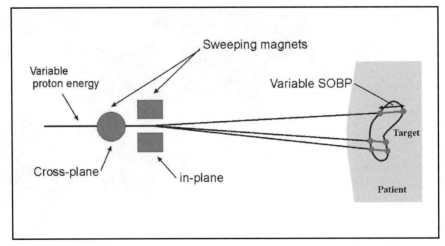

Figure 20.44: In proton active scanning, the target is "painted" with a pencil beam steered by a set of orthogonal magnets. The energy of the pencil beam is changed dynamically so that at any given lateral position the distal edge of the SOBP corresponds to the distal boundary of the target. See COLOR PLATE 35.

likely to become the scanning method of choice for most future proton therapy machines. There are serious safety and QA issues associated with this approach due to the intensity of the pencil beam. Because the whole energy of the beam is concentrated in a small spot, redundant fast beam abort systems are necessary. Tumor motion is also problematic with this technique. A future possibility is to follow the tumor motion in real-time and make scanning adjustments on the fly.

20.4.6   Beam Delivery/Transport

Most of the time that a patient spends in the treatment room is devoted to setup. To avoid wasting expensive beam time, the beam can be delivered to a number of treatment rooms sequentially so one patient can be treated while others are being set up.

One of the most difficult and complex aspects of proton therapy is beam delivery. The beam delivery system consists of the beam switchyard where the beam is diverted to various treatment rooms and beam gantries. There needs to be a system for selecting the appropriate room for beam delivery. It is necessary to develop rules for priority of beam switching. It must be verified that only one room can receive the beam. As the beam travels from the accelerator to the patient, it passes through many bending, focusing, and steering magnets; all must be monitored (interlocks) to ensure correct beam delivery to the patient (see Figures 20.45 and 20.46).

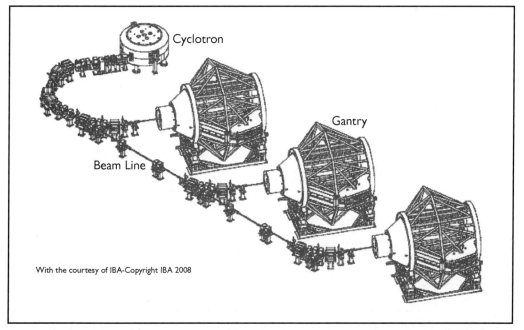

With the courtesy of IBA-Copyright IBA 2008

Figure 20.45: Beam line feeding three isocentric gantries. The beam line is a narrow evacuated pipe in which the beam travels. The magnets in the beam line are for steering and focusing. (Courtesy of Penn Medicine, Philadelphia, PA, and IBA, Louvain-la-Neuve, Belgium; www.iba-worldwide.com)

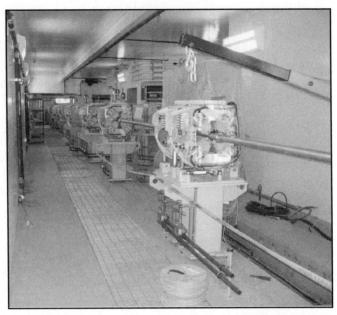

Figure 20.46: Photograph of a proton therapy beam line. Quadrupole magnets in the beam line provide focusing. (Courtesy of Penn Medicine, Philadelphia, PA, and IBA, Louvain-la-Neuve, Belgium; www.iba-worldwide.com). See COLOR PLATE 36.

A treatment room may have a fixed beam or an isocentric gantry. An eye beam room would use a fixed beam with a single scatterer to treat to a depth of about 35 mm or less. Rotating gantries are large; high-energy protons have a large radius of curvature in a magnetic field produced using room temperature magnets. Recall that $R = mv/QB$ and that the mass of a proton is about 2000 times larger than the mass of an electron. The large gantry necessary is one of the reasons for the high cost of proton therapy (see Figures 20.47 and 20.48). Fortunately, patients will not have to see these enormous gantries (see Figure 20.49), which they might find overwhelming.

20.4.7 Dose Calculations and Treatment Planning for Proton Therapy

Patient dose calculations and treatment planning procedures for proton therapy are similar to those for photons and electrons presented in chapters 14 and 15, respectively: doses and dose distributions measured in tissue-equivalent phantoms are used to calculate what happens in a patient. There is one major exception, however, and that relates to the effect of inhomogeneities.

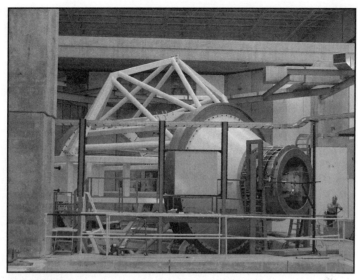

Figure 20.47: The gantry of an IBA proton therapy cyclotron. The entire structure rotates on the two rings shown. The beam enters from the right at the center of the gantry structure. To appreciate the scale, notice the man standing in the lower right. (Courtesy of Penn Medicine, Philadelphia, PA, and IBA, Louvain-la-Neuve, Belgium; www.iba-worldwide.com). See COLOR PLATE 37.

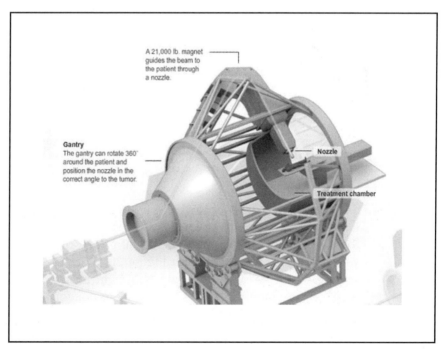

Figure 20.48: Diagram showing a drawing of the gantry in the photo in Figure 20.47. This illustrates the path of the beam and shows the treatment chamber with the beam nozzle. (Courtesy of IBA, Louvain-la-Neuve, Belgium; www.iba-worldwide.com). See COLOR PLATE 38.

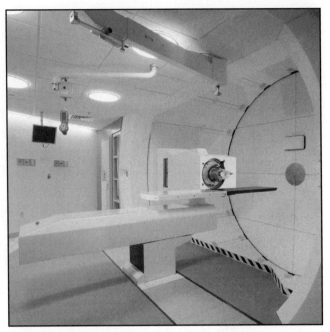

Figure 20.49: Treatment room at the University of Florida. The beam "nozzle" is visible near the center of the photo. (Courtesy of University of Florida, Gainesville, FL)

Effect of Inhomogeneities

With photons and electrons, the effect of an inhomogeneity in the beam is to modify the dose close to and beyond the inhomogeneity. The effect is typically small, and relatively simple calculational methods can be used to estimate the change in dose (see sections 14.13 and 15.7). For photons the intensity is changed by the presence of an inhomogeneity. For protons, however, the effect is quite different and often very significant. For protons the intensity stays roughly the same; rather it is the *range* that changes. This means that the depth of the Bragg peak is changed if the beam passes through an inhomogeneity. Since the dose beyond the Bragg peak is essentially zero, this can have a major impact on the dose distal to the Bragg peak. For example, if a proton beam is intercepted by a high-density inhomogeneity and this is not corrected for during treatment planning, the distal part of the tumor might receive zero dose. This is illustrated in Figure 20.50 for a sliver of bone intersecting the beam. With accurate treatment planning, this can be corrected for by modification of the compensator for a passive scattering system, as shown in the figure, or by adjustment of the scanning pattern of the proton pencil beam with active scanning. On the other hand, if a normal tissue that needs to be protected lies deeper than the tumor and the beam is intercepted by a *low*-density region, the depth of the Bragg peak is increased and the normal tissue might receive the full tumor dose. Clearly, determination of the distribution of proton stopping powers in and around the target is essential in proton therapy.

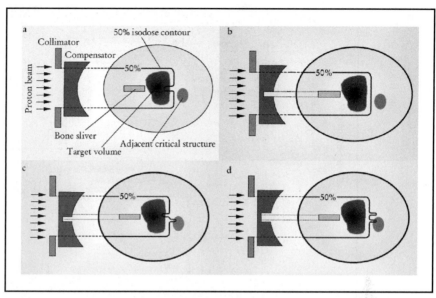

Figure 20.50: The effect of a thin sliver inhomogeneity for proton therapy. In (a) there has been no modification of the compensator to account for the inhomogeneity. As a result, there is a cold spot in the target volume. (b) The compensator has been modified to adjust for the presence of the bone sliver. (c) shows what can happen if there is even a slight misalignment of the compensator. In (d) we see what is called "opened" compensation. The target is fully covered in the event of a small misalignment but the critical structure receives some dose. (Reprinted from Goitein, M., A. J. Lomax, and E. S. Pedroni, Fig. 1, p. 46, "Treating Cancer with Protons." *Physics Today* 55(9):45–50, © 2002 with permission from the American Institute of Physics). See COLOR PLATE 39.

Determination of Stopping Powers

For proton therapy, proton stopping powers are determined from CT scans, much like electron densities are determined for photon and electron therapy. This is not as straightforward as is the determination of electron densities, however, since radiation used for CT scanning is x-rays, and x-ray attenuation is a simple function of electron density. Measured CT numbers in Hounsfield Units (HUs) can be readily converted to electron densities, as shown in chapter 19, section 19.4.3 and illustrated in Figure 19.15. Ideally, one would want to use a CT unit that employs protons instead of x-rays, but no such machine is currently in use for proton treatment planning. Consequently, it is necessary to convert CT numbers to proton stopping powers, which depend on both the electron density and the chemical composition of tissues. This can be done using a calibration curve similar to the one published by Schaffner and Pedroni,[19]

---

[19] Schaffner, B., and E. Pedroni, (1998), "The precision of proton range calculations in proton radiotherapy treament planning: Experimental verification of the relation between CT-HU and proton stopping power," *Phys Med Biol* 43(6):1579–1592.

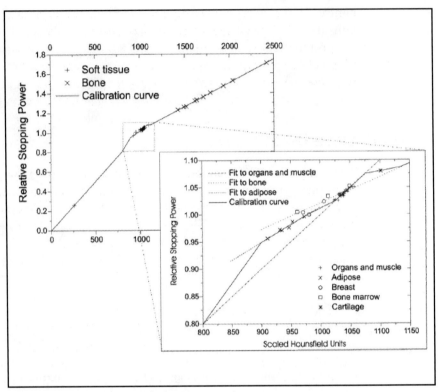

Figure 20.51: Relative stopping powers as a function of scaled HUs for biological tissues grouped into soft tissue and bone (behind) and, in the enlarged section of the graph (front), for specific soft tissues. The three broken lines show the three linear fits for soft tissue, adipose and bone, and the solid line is the chosen calibration curve. (Reprinted from *Physics in Medicine and Biology*, "The precision of proton range calculations in proton radiotherapy treatment planning: Experimental verification of the relation between CT-HU and proton stopping power." B. Schaffner and E. Pedroni, Fig. 1, p. 1582, vol. 43, issue 6, pp. 1579–1592, © 1998 with permission from IOP Publishing, Bristol, UK.)

shown in Figure 20.51. The authors of this paper state that use of this calibration curve should lead to errors in prediction of the range of protons no greater than about 1.8% for bone and 1.1% for soft tissue. Calibration curves, however, may be a unique property of the scanner and the kVp used, as was the case for the electron density/CT number calibration curves for photon and electron beam treatment planning shown in Figure 19.15.

Conventional treatment planning algorithms, such as those used for photons and electrons, cannot adequately handle correction for inhomogeneities with proton beams. The only recourse for the accurate dosimetry required for proton therapy inhomogeneity correction is to use Monte Carlo treatment planning (see chapter 7, section 7.10).

Monte Carlo Treatment Planning

As with photon and electron beams, Monte Carlo treatment planning has the potential to improve the accuracy of dose calculations significantly. Unfortunately, it is highly computationally intensive and takes considerably longer than conventional treatment planning. Nevertheless, for protons the benefits often outweigh the costs, so Monte Carlo planning is becoming quite common in proton therapy facilities. Fortunately, with computers getting faster and less expensive at a rapid rate, Monte Carlo treatment planning will soon become standard for proton therapy.

20.4.8 Dose Distributions

The integral dose (see chapter 14, section 14.7) is lower for proton treatment plans than for photon plans, although photon skin sparing is superior. The lower integral dose is due in part to the fact that there is almost no exit dose for protons. The lateral penumbra is generally smaller than for photon beams. This helps to make the plans more conformal. Proton plans generally use a smaller number of beams than photon plans. Very careful patient alignment is called for. An x-ray tube is often put in the beam line and on-line corrections are made to patient position.

The precipitous drop in dose beyond (distal to) the Bragg peak is sometimes referred to as "distal blocking." Distal blocking provides an extra degree of freedom and presents new options, such as the use of "patch" fields (see Figure 20.52).

Passive scattering provides poor conformity with the proximal edge of the target (see Figure 20.43). To improve this situation, multiple beams are used (see Figure 20.53).

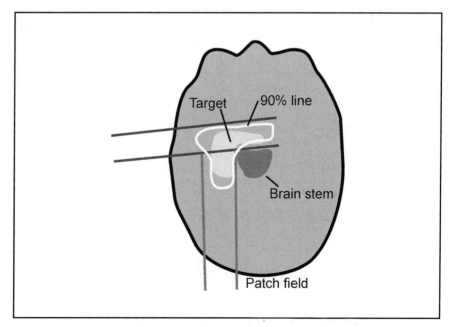

Figure 20.52: A proton therapy "patch" field is used in this illustration to fill in coverage of a tumor that wraps around the brain stem. The distal edge of the patch field is adjusted to coincide with the edge of the lateral beam. See COLOR PLATE 40.

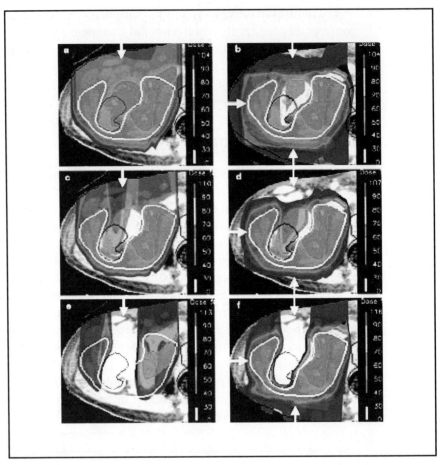

Figure 20.53: Treatment of Ewing's sarcoma with protons. The dose distribution is shown by a color-wash (see legend on the right of each frame). The target is the white contour. Critical structures are outlined in dark gray. The arrows show beam directions. In (a) a single passively scattered beam is used. Note the good conformity laterally and at the distal edge of the target but not at the proximal target border. In (b) we have a three-field dose distribution from passively scattered beams. (c) shows a single field delivered by an actively scanned beam. (d) shows three fields delivered by actively scanned beams. Each of these fields delivers a near uniform dose. (e) One of the intensity-modulated fields shown in panel (f). Panel (f) shows a three-field optimized IMPT plan. The dose distribution is extraordinarily conformal. (Reprinted from Goitein, M., A. J. Lomax, and E. S. Pedroni, Fig. 4, p. 50, "Treating Cancer with Protons." *Physics Today* 55(9):45–50, © 2002 with permission from the American Institute of Physics). See COLOR PLATE 41.

Intensity-modulated proton therapy (IMPT) offers the intriguing possibility of modulating both the intensity and the *energy* of the beam. For photon beam IMRT we can only modulate the intensity of the beam. IMPT implies the simultaneous optimization of all Bragg peaks from all fields to deliver the desired dose distribution to the target and organs at risk. See Figure 20.53 for an example of an IMPT dose distribution.

20.4.9   Calibration of Proton Beams and Routine Quality Assurance

For photons and electrons, ionization chambers are used as the standard method for calibration of machine outputs and the TG-51 protocol is used to convert ion chamber readings to absorbed dose (see chapter 11). A similar method is used to calibrate proton accelerators using the protocol published by the IAEA.[20] All the equations, ADCL ion chamber calibration, setup conditions, and steps in beam calibration are analogous to those for photon beams presented in the TG-51 protocol and described in chapter 11.

Quality assurance procedures are also similar to those applicable to linear accelerators (see chapter 18), and daily, weekly, monthly, and annual QA checks are analogous to those presented in the AAPM TG-40 Report.[21] No such report has been produced specifically for proton therapy, but a comprehensive QA program devised for the M.D. Anderson Cancer Center proton therapy synchrotron facility has been published.[22]

There is one major difference between the QA procedures for linear accelerators and those necessary for protons, and this relates to the depth and extent of the SOBP. With protons, any small change in the position of the SOBP can have a catastrophic effect if not detected: parts of the target might be grossly underdosed or normal tissues overdosed. At M.D. Anderson, for example, daily output and depth-dose measurements are made for 10×10 cm^2 beams for specific spread-out Bragg peaks at specified depths. Outputs are measured at the center of these SOBPs, and the distances between the proximal 95% and distal 90% depth-dose levels are determined to establish the width of the SOBP. Also measured on a daily basis is the falloff in dose at the distal edges of the proton beams, specifically the depths of the distal 90% and 10% dose levels, since this is a sensitive measure of beam quality.

20.4.10   Future Developments

The biggest drawback of proton therapy, and the reason it has been slow to develop, is cost. This has been dictated mostly by the sheer size and weight of conventional proton therapy machines and gantries, with current

---

[20] TRS-398: Absorbed Dose Determination in External Beam Radiotherapy, Technical Report Series No. 398, IAEA, pp. 135–150, 2000.

[21] Kutcher et al., (1994), "Comprehensive QA for Radiation Oncology: Report of AAPM Radiation Therapy Committee Task Group 40," *Med Phys* 21(6):581–618. AAPM Report No. 46.

[22] Arjomandy et al., (2009), "An overview of the comprehensive proton therapy machine quality assurance procedures implemented at The University of Texas M.D. Anderson Cancer Center Proton Therapy Center-Houston," *Med Phys* 36(6):2269–2282.

machines weighing in excess of about 100 tons. Considerable effort is being made to reduce this size, however, as shown below.

Superconducting Cyclotrons

Using superconducting technology to reduce the size and weight of magnets, it is possible to produce a compact proton therapy cyclotron that weighs about 20 tons. Not only is the weight reduced, but so is the size; and this makes it possible to rotate the entire cyclotron on a gantry, thus eliminating costly beam transport systems.

Proton Laser Accelerators

With very high-intensity short laser pulses it is possible to accelerate protons to energies sufficient for radiotherapy. Protons accelerated in this manner have a wide energy spectrum, however, so magnetic field energy separation is necessary to obtain the desired spread-out Bragg peak for therapy. This means that most of the protons have to be removed from the beam before use, which reduces the intensity of the useful beam considerably. Because of this lack of efficiency, laser beams of extremely high intensity are required. Such high intensities have not yet been achieved, but several groups in several countries are working to make such beams a reality.

Dielectric Wall Accelerators

Dielectric wall acceleration of protons is an outgrowth of nuclear weapons research at the Lawrence Livermore National Laboratory. This technology has been licensed to TomoTherapy® Inc. for development of a medical proton accelerator which will fit into an ordinary linac vault. The individual pulses from this accelerator can be varied in intensity, energy, and spot width making IMPT possible. The accelerator consists of a hollow tube with alternating rings of electrical insulators and conductors. A transmission line sends brief pulses to the conductors as the proton bunch travels down the tube. The insulator can withstand very high electrical fields for short periods of time without undergoing dielectric breakdown. It may be possible to accelerate protons to 200 MeV in a distance as short as 2 m, which would make proton tomotherapy a reality.

In the future it is possible that PET imaging will be used to validate proton treatment delivery. Small amounts of positron emitters are produced in tissue irradiated with protons such as ^{11}C, ^{15}O, and ^{10}C. There is apparently enough of this to perform imaging studies. The measured positron activity could be compared to the expected activity calculated by Monte Carlo techniques.

It may be possible to build accelerators that will deliver either a proton beam or a carbon ion beam. Carbon ions share the dose distribution advantage of protons. In addition, carbon ions have such a high LET that they maintain their biological advantage even in the SOBP. These particles may therefore be very useful for treating anoxic or hypoxic tumors. Carbon ion treatment centers in Japan and Germany have treated about 5000 patients. There are three factors which discourage the use of this modality in the United States: (1) no FDA clearance; (2) no procedure or reimbursement codes; and (3) much greater expense of carbon ion facilities compared to protons.

Chapter Summary

IMRT

- **Beamlets (bixels):** Square or rectangular regions over which the beam intensity is constant. For IMRT purposes a beam is divided up into beamlets; typical beamlet size is 1 cm by 1 cm.

- **Intensity Map:** A set of intensity values of the beamlets

- **IMRT dose distributions** tend to be more conformal and less uniform than conventional plans

- **Delivery Techniques** (all utilize an MLC)
  - Tomotherapy
    - Serial: One slice delivered at a time, couch indexed to deliver next slice
    - Helical: Beam rotates around the patient as couch moves continuously along the axis of the gantry

  - Cone Beam IMRT (uses a conventional linac, beam directions chosen by planner)
    - SMLC (segmental MLC): Intensity map for a given beam is delivered by a series of fixed MLC apertures. MLC leaves do not move when beam is on.
    - DMLC (dynamic MLC): Intensity map is delivered through a window which sweeps across the field while the beam is on (dose rate may also vary).
    - IMAT = intensity modulated arc therapy; gantry rotates while beam is on, MLC leaves move while beam is on

- **Leaf Sequencing Algorithm:** Calculates the sequence of leaf positions (segments), which when added results in a desired intensity map. May need to impose condition on MU (minimum value) and segment area size (larger than 3×3 cm^2)

- **Inverse Treatment Planning:** State planning goals at the beginning, usually in terms of DVH parameters
  - Optimization: Find intensity map that meets goals as closely as possible.

  - Cost/Objective function: Mathematical function of beamlet intensities that describes how close a plan is to the desired goals. Optimization algorithm finds beamlet weights that minimize the objective function.

  - Optimization algorithms:
    - Stochastic: has an element of probability or chance built in Simulated annealing is a stochastic method
    - Deterministic: does not have an element of chance built in. Gradient descent method is non-stochastic, can get stuck in local minimum

- **Inverse Planning Issues**
  - PTV should not extend to skin surface

  - Overlapping structures:
    - Define regions of overlap or
    - Set priority for one over the other

  - Use at least 5 to 7 beams; avoid parallel opposed beams; avoid beams entering through critical structures

  - For deep targets using 6 MV: use 9 or more beams

- **Aperture-based Optimization**
  - Sometimes called "field within a field"; often used for breast IMRT

  - Does not use inverse planning or leaf sequencing

  - Choose a number of beam segments that may only cover a portion of target as seen in beam's-eye view (BEV)

  - Sensitive structures are blocked in some segments

  - Isodose lines from open field often used to choose segment shapes

- **Plan Validation**
  - Hybrid phantom: Deliver patient beams to a phantom containing dosimeters (ion chamber, film); compare to treatment plan calculation of dose in the phantom

  - Dedicated check device using an array of diodes or ion chambers: check each beam individually

  - Criteria (common): In low-gradient regions dose agreement within 3%; in high-gradient regions, distance to agreement of 3 mm.

- **Whole-Body Dose and Shielding**
  - m = (MU for IMRT plan)/(MU for conventional plan)

  - m = 2 to 3 for SMLC, up to 10 for serial tomotherapy

  - At low energy (4–10 MV), whole-body dose due to leakage radiation is m times higher for IMRT than for conventional RT

  - At high energy (15–18 MV), whole-body dose much higher than at low energy because of neutron contamination (w_R) can be as high as 20

  - Greatest concern is for children who are an order of magnitude more sensitive to radiation-induced cancer than adults

Stereotactic Radiosurgery

- Single-fraction radiotherapy in which a stereotactic coordinate system is used for precise targeting; form of surgery in which radiation substitutes for a scalpel; usually intracranial

- Treatment machines: Modified conventional linacs, Gamma Knife (uses 201 Co-60 sources) and robotic linacs

- SRS usually restricted to targets with volume of less than about 35 cm^3 or diameter less than 3 cm

- Accuracy required: Dosimetric: ±5%; geometric: ±1 mm

- Rigid coordinate frame attached to patient's skull; attach localization box to frame for imaging to establish coordinate system

- **Linac-based SRS Methods:** Dynamic arc, static MLC, robotic linac
  - Dynamic arc: Circular beam aperture; beam is on while gantry rotates through series of arcs, each at different couch angle; usually 5 to 10 arcs; sometimes multiple isocenters
    - Temporary modifications:
      1. Tertiary cone containing circular apertures, aperture diameters: 5 mm to 40 mm
      2. Table brackets or floor stand to immobilize SRS frame during treatment
    - Strict mechanical tolerances on isocentricity; gantry and couch rotation axis must intersect within 1 mm throughout range of gantry and couch motion

  - Static MLC: Add on mini- or microMLC with small leaf width; use multiple non-coplanar beams; usually single isocenter
    - Leaf widths: 3–4 mm
    - BEV field shaping

- Robotic Linac (CyberKnife): 6 MV X-band linac mounted on robotic arm

  ○ X-band linac is compact (microwave frequency is 10,000 MHz)

  ○ Frameless treatment using orthogonal x-ray beams

  ○ Multiple non-coplanar beams

- **Gamma Stereotactic Units** (Gamma Knife – Model 4U)
  - 201 Co-60 sources, total activity about 6000 Ci; arranged in hemispherical shell 40 cm in diameter around unit center

  - Four helmets with collimator aperture diameters of 4, 8, 14, and 18 mm diameter

  - "Shot:" Treatment with a particular helmet and unit center at a specific anatomic location

- **Treatment Planning:** Considerations:
  1. Conformity
  2. Volume of normal tissue irradiated by prescription isodose surface
  3. Dose homogeneity inside target volume

  - SRS dose distribution highly conformal but usually also highly inhomogeneous

  - Prescribe to lowest isodose surface encompassing the target (100% is maximum)
    1. Linac prescription isodose surface: 80%–90%
    2. Gamma Knife prescription isodose surface: 50%

  - Linac: Dose distribution determined largely by location of isocenter and size of collimator
    1. Use one to a few isocenters, 5 to 10 arcs; avoid 180° arcs: do not want parallel opposed beams
    2. Avoid arcs crossing critical structures, weight arcs according to preference

  - Gamma Knife: Dose distribution from single shot approximately spherical
    1. Diameter of 50% surface approximately spherical, depends on helmet used
    2. Place shots of various diameters, locations, and weighting to achieve desired dose distribution; use one to ten shots (or more)

- **Evaluation of Dose Distribution**
  1. DVH
  2. PITV (prescription isodose to target volume) = (volume encompassed by prescription isodose surface)/(target volume)

~ $1.0 \leq PITV \leq 2$	Meets protocol
~ $2.0 < PITV < 2.5$ or $0.9 < PITV < 1.0$	Minor but acceptable deviation
~ $PITV > 2.5$	Unacceptable deviation

- **Dosimetry:** Complicated by small field sizes
  1. Measure: PDD or TMR, beam profiles, output factors $S_{c,p}$, absolute dose output
  2. Use film for beam profiles
  3. Use small volume (micro or pinpoint) ion chambers for PDD, $S_{c,p}$

- **Quality Assurance:** Routine equipment QA and patient treatment specific
  1. Equipment QA: isocentricity, lasers
  2. Patient Specific: requires checklist: e.g., jaw settings, collimator size, treatment coordinates, couch angle, etc.

Proton Radiotherapy

- The depth dose curve for protons is fairly flat until near the end of their range. The Bragg peak is a significant enhancement in dose near the end of the proton range. It occurs because the stopping power rises dramatically as the proton velocity declines.

- The width of the Bragg peak is only a few millimeters and therefore it must be spread-out by adding beams with different energies and intensities to get a spread-out Bragg peak (SOBP).

- The advantage of protons in comparison to photons is due to the dose distribution and not to radiobiology.

- Treatment of deep seated targets (30–40 cm) requires energies of up to 250 MeV.

- Proton therapy accelerators are circular machines that use electric fields to accelerate protons and a magnetic field to confine their motion to a circular or spiral path. There are two types of accelerators used: cyclotrons and synchrotrons.

- Motion of a charged particle in a magnetic field: A charged particle can move in a circle in the plane of this page provided that there is a magnetic field perpendicular to the page. The period of the particle is independent of the speed (or energy) and the radius of the circle for a non-relativistic particle.

- **Cyclotrons**

    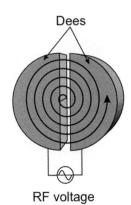

    Dees

    RF voltage

    – Has two hollow electrodes shaped like the letter "D" called *dees*

    – There is a high voltage between the dees; protons are accelerated in the gap between the dees

    – The potential difference between the dees oscillates with a period such that every time the proton finds itself between the dees, it is accelerated

    – Relativity causes a deviation from the independence of period on energy and radius; requires design modification for energies above about 10 MeV

    – One solution is to make magnetic field increase in strength with increasing distance from center of cyclotron to compensate for relativity. In this case, period remains independent of energy and radius. This design is called an *isochronous cyclotron*.

- **Synchrotrons**

    – Protons travel in a ring and have a fixed orbital radius. Protons are accelerated in RF cavities. Magnetic field has to increase as protons gain energy. Proton beam is pulsed.

- There are two methods for modulating the energy of the beam to produce the SOBP

    – Place variable thickness filter in the beam, e.g., a propellor (see Figure 20.40)

    – Electronically change beam energy; much more difficult, not yet common

- **Lateral Beam Spreading and Field Shaping:** Raw proton beam is only a few millimeters in diameter, beam has to be spread out. Two methods:

  – Passive scattering: Uses scattering foil. Spreads beam while maintaining constant energy across the beam. A patient-specific beam aperture is used (made out of brass).

  – Active scanning: Magnetic field used to deflect the pencil beam and "paint" the field. Possible to simultaneously vary beam energy for range modulation.

Problems

1. What is an IMRT fluence or intensity map?

2. Roughly how many intensity levels are typically used in an IMRT treatment plan?

3. What is the difference between SMLC and DMLC?

4. What is a cost or objective function? What is it a function of?

5. What are the two major categories of mathematical technique used for IMRT optimization? How do they differ?

6. What is a leaf sequencing algorithm?

7. Why is target and normal structure contouring/delineation crucial for IMRT?

8. Explain why an IMRT PTV should usually not extend close to the skin surface.

9. Common criteria for validation of patient specific IMRT dose distributions is _____% dose difference in high-dose low-gradient regions and _____ distance to agreement in high-dose gradient regions.

10. A patient receives a whole-body dose of 300 mSv from IMRT. What is the approximate lifetime risk of a second fatal cancer induced by this dose? See chapter 17.

11. How does IMRT change the shielding workload for primary barriers? For secondary barriers?

12. How does SRS differ from conventional fractionated radiation therapy?

13. What is the maximum diameter of targets usually treated with SRS?

14. What geometric accuracy is necessary for SRS?

15. Explain two methods of frameless stereotactic targeting.

16. Describe (a) treatment techniques used for linac based SRS and (b) the relative merits of these techniques.

17. What is the range in collimator aperture diameter used for linac-based dynamic SRS?

18. To what isodose line is the dose usually prescribed for (a) Gamma Knife (b) linac SRS?

19. How does the dose homogeneity of linac-based SRS compare to Gamma Knife SRS?

20. Compare the relative merits of CT and MRI in imaging for SRS.

21. What type of radiation detector has adequate spatial resolution for measuring SRS beam profiles?

22. Approximately what energy protons should be used to treat a target with a distal depth of 15 cm? Give the energy of the protons after they have passed through any scattering filters, compensators, etc.

23. What principle of the classical cyclotron allows the use of a constant RF frequency?

24. Define the following terms: dee, deflector, isochronous, magnet yoke.

25. How does a synchrotron differ from a cyclotron?

26. Explain the advantages and disadvantages of active scanning in comparison to passive scattering.

27. Why are proton gantries so large?

28. Why are the effects of inhomogeneities more critical for proton therapy than for photon therapy?

Bibliography

IMRT

"Algorithms: Business by Numbers." *The Economist*, September 15, 2007.

Ezzell, G. A., J. M. Galvin, D. Low, J. R. Palta, I. Rosen, M. B. Sharpe, P. Xia, Y. Xiao, L. Xing, C. X. Yu; IMRT subcommittee; AAPM Radiation Therapy committee. (2003). "Guidance document on delivery, treatment planning, and implementation of IMRT: Report of the IMRT Subcommittee of the AAPM Radiation Therapy Committee." *Med Phys* 30(8):2089–2115.

Goitein, M. *Radiation Oncology: A Physicist's-Eye View (Biological and Medical Physics, Biomedical Engineering)*. New York: Springer Science+Business Media LLC, 2008.

Hall, E. J. (2006). "The inaugural Frank Ellis lecture—Iatrogenic cancer: The impact of intensity-modulated radiotherapy." *Clin Oncol* 18:277–282.

Intensity Modulated Radiation Therapy Collaborative Working Group. (2001). "Intensity modulated radiotherapy: Current status and issues of interest." *Int J Radiat Oncol Biol Phys* 51(4):880–914.

Medical Dosimetry (2001). Official journal of the American Association of Medical Dosimetrists. Special issues on IMRT. Spring 26(1):1–110; Summer 26(1):111–242.

National Cancer Institute Guidelines for the Use of Intensity-Modulated Radiation Therapy in Clinical Trials. Bethesda, MD: NCI, 2005.

Palta, J. R., T. R. Mackie (eds.). *Intensity-Modulated Radiation Therapy: The State of the Art*. Proceedings of the AAPM 2003 Summer School. AAPM Medical Physics Monograph No. 29. Madison, WI: Medical Physics Publishing, 2003.

Pirzkall, A., M. P. Carol, B. Pickett, P. Xia, M. Roach 3rd, and L. J. Verhey. (2002). "The effect of beam energy and number of fields on photon-based IMRT for deep-seated targets." *Int J Radiat Biol Phys* 53:434–442.

Press, W. H., S. A. Teukolsky, W. T. Vetterling, and B. P. Flannery. *Numerical Recipes: The Art of Scientific Computing*, 3rd Edition. Cambridge, UK: Cambridge University Press, 2007.

Shepard, D. M., M. A. Earl, C. X. Yu, and Y. Xiao. "Aperture-Based Inverse Planning" in *Intensity-Modulated Radiation Therapy: The State of the Art*. J. R. Palta and T. R. Mackie (eds.). AAPM 2003 Summer School Proceedings. Medical Physics Monograph No. 29. Madison, WI: Medical Physics Publishing, 2003.

Sternick, E. S., M. P. Carol, and W. H. Grant III. "Intensity-Modulated Radiotherapy," Chapter 9 in *Treatment Planning in Radiation Oncology*. F. M. Khan and R. A. Potish (eds.). Baltimore, MD: Williams & Wilkins, 1998.

Van Dyk, J. (ed.). *The Modern Technology of Radiation Oncology*. Madison, WI: Medical Physics Publishing, 1999.

Van Dyk, J. (ed.). *The Modern Technology of Radiation Oncology, Volume 2*. Madison, WI: Medical Physics Publishing, 2005.

Webb, S. *Intensity-Modulated Radiation Therapy*. Bristol, UK: Institute of Physics Publishing, 2001.

Wu, Q., L. Xing, G. Ezzell, and R. Mohan. "Inverse Treatment Planning." Chapter 4 in *The Modern Technology of Radiation Oncology. Volume 2*, J. Van Dyk (ed.), pp. 133–183, 2005.

Stereotactic Radiosurgery

Bova, F. J., S. L. Meeks, and W. A. Friedman. "Linac Radiosurgery: System Requirements, Procedures and Testing" In: *Treatment Planning in Radiation Oncology*, 2nd Edition. F. M. Khan (ed.). Philadelphia: Lippincott Williams & Wilkins, p. 189, 2007.

Firlik, K. *Another Day in the Frontal Lobe*. New York: Random House, 2006. (The life of a neurosurgery resident; includes brief discussion of Gamma Knife).

Fishman, S. *Bomb in the Brain*. New York: Avon Books, 1990. (A fascinating description of the experience of an AVM patient).

Flickinger, J. C., D. Kondziolka, L. D. Lunsford, R. J. Coffey, M. L. Goodman, E. G. Shaw, W. R. Hudgins, R. Weiner, G. R. Harsh 4th, P. K. Sneed et al. (1994). "A multi-institutional experience with stereotactic radiosurgery for solitary brain metastasis." *Int J Radiat Oncol Biol Phys* 28:797–802.

Goetsch, S. J. "Stereotactic Radiosurgery Using the Gamma Knife" In: *Teletherapy: Present and Future*. Madison, WI: Advanced Medical Publishing, 1996.

Khan, F. M. *The Physics of Radiation Therapy*, Fourth Edition. Philadelphia: Lippincott Williams & Wilkins, 2009.

Leksell Society Report. Indications Treated. December 2008. Available on-line at http://www.elekta.com/healthcare_international_leksell_gamma_knife_society.php.

Lippitz, B. E. "Treatment of Brain Metastases Using Gamma Knife Radiosurgery – The Gold Standard" at www.elekta.com/assets/Elekta-Oncology/Image-Guided-Radiation-Therapy/case-studies/lippitz.pdf. Accessed April 12, 2010.

Metcalfe, P., T. Kron, and P. Hoban. *The Physics of Radiotherapy X-rays and Electrons*. Madison, WI: Medical Physics Publishing, 2007.

Niranjan, A., and L. D. Lunsford. (2000). "Radiosurgery: Where we were, are, and may be in the third millennium." *Neurosurgery* 46:531–543.

Podgorsak, E. B., and M. B. Podgorsak. "Stereotactic Irradiation." Chapter 16 in *The Modern Technology of Radiation Oncology*. J. Van Dyk (ed.). Madison, WI: Medical Physics Publishing, pp. 589–639, 1999.

Podgorsak, E.B., and M. B. Podgorsak. Special Procedures and Techniques in Radiotherapy (IAEA Slide Set based on Chapter 15 of *Radiation Oncology Physics: A Handbook for Teachers and Students*, IAEA, 2006).

Schell, M. C., F. J. Bova, D. A. Larson, D. D. Leavitt, W. R. Lutz, E. B. Podgorsak, and A. Wu. Stereotactic Radiosurgery, Report of Task Group 42, Radiation Therapy Committee. AAPM Report No. 54. Woodbury, NY: American Institute of Physics, Inc., 1995.

Webb, S. *The Physics of Three-Dimensional Radiation Therapy: Conformal Radiotherapy, Radiosurgery and Treatment*. Bristol, UK: Institute of Physics Publishing, 1993.

Proton Radiotherapy

Arjomandy, B., N. Sahoo, X. R. Zhu, J. R. Zullo, R. Y. Wu, X. Ding, C. Martin, G. Ciangaru, and M T. Gillin. (2009). "An overview of the comprehensive proton therapy machine quality assurance procedures implemented at The University of Texas M.D. Anderson Cancer Center Proton Therapy Center-Houston." *Med Phys* 36(6): 2269–2282.

Attix, F. H. *Introduction to Radiological Physics and Radiation Dosimetry*. New York: Wiley – Interscience, 1986.

Goitein, M. *Radiation Oncology: A Physicist's-Eye View (Biological and Medical Physics, Biomedical Engineering)*. New York: Springer Science+Business Media LLC, 2008.

Goitein, M., A. J. Lomax, and E. S. Pedroni. (2002). "Treating Cancer with Protons." *Physics Today* 55(9):45–50.

International Atomic Energy Agency (IAEA). Technical Report Series No. 398. Absorbed Dose Determination in External Beam Radiotherapy. Vienna, Austria: IAEA, pp. 135–150, 2000.

International Commission on Radiation Units and Measurements (ICRU). ICRU Report 78: Prescribing, Recording, and Reporting Proton-Beam Therapy. Bethesda, MD: ICRU, 2007.

Kutcher, G. J., L. Coia, M. Gillin, W. F. Hanson, S. Leibel, R. J. Morton, J. R. Palta, J. A. Purdy, L. L. Reinstein, G. K. Svensson, M. Weller, and L. Wingfield. (1994). "Comprehensive QA for Radiation Oncology: Report of AAPM Radiation Therapy Committee Task Group 40." *Med Phys* 21(6):581–618. AAPM Report No. 46.

Maughan, R. L., F. Van den Heuvel, and C. G. Orton. (2008). "Point/Counterpoint. Within the next 10–15 years protons will likely replace photons as the most common type of radiation for curative radiotherapy." *Med Phys* 35(10):4285–4288.

Schaffner, B., and E. Pedroni. (1998). "The precision of proton range calculations in proton radiotherapy treatment planning: Experimental verification of the relation between CT-HU and proton stopping power." *Phys Med Biol* 43(6):1579–1592.

Smith, A.R. (2009). "Vision 20/20: Proton therapy." *Med Phys* 36(2):556–568.

Van Dyk, J. (ed.). *The Modern Technology of Radiation Oncology.* Madison, WI: Medical Physics Publishing, 1999.

Webb, S. *The Physics of Three-Dimensional Radiation Therapy: Conformal Radiotherapy, Radiosurgery and Treatment.* Bristol, UK: Institute of Physics Publishing, 1993.

Webb, S., R. F. Mould, C. G. Orton, Jos A. E. Spaan, and J, G. Webster. *The Physics of Conformal Radiotherapy: Advances in Technology.* Bristol, UK: Institute of Physics Publishing, 1997.

Appendix A

Board Certification Exams in Radiation Therapy

The American Board of Radiology (ABR)[1]

Radiation Oncology Resident Training Guidelines for Radiological Physics

This is a listing of the topics covered on the physics portion of the American Board of Radiology (ABR) exam. References to the relevant section of the text appear after each topic. The reader is advised to check the ABR web site for any revisions to this list. A question mark indicates that we do not understand the intent of the listing and therefore cannot provide a reference.

	Section
I. Atomic and Nuclear Structure	
A. Bohr model of the atom	
1. Coulombic force and electron binding energy	*2.6*
2. Electron orbits (energy levels)	*2.6*
3. Electron transitions – absorption and emission of energy	*2.6*
4. Characteristic radiation and the Auger effect	*3.12 & 5.1*
B. Nuclear structure	
1. Nucleons – protons and neutrons	*2.6 & 3.1, Table 3.2*
2. Nuclear force	*3.2*
3. $E = mc^2$ and nuclear binding energy	*2.5 & 3.3*
C. Factors affecting nuclear stability	
1. Neutron-to-proton ratio	*3.4*
2. Average binding energy per nucleon	*3.4*
3. Pairing of similar nucleons in the nucleus	*3.4, Table 3.1*
D. Nuclear nomenclature	
1. The four iso's (isotopes, isotones, isobars, isomers)	*3.1*
2. Shorthand representation of isotopes	*3.1*
II. Radioactive Decay	
A. Modes of radioactive decay	
1. Beta (β)	*3.12.3*
a. β⁻ (negative beta, negatron)	*3.12.3*
b. β⁺ (positive beta, positron)	*3.12.3*
c. Electron capture	*3.12.3*
2. Alpha (α)	*3.12.1*
B. Other decay processes	
1. Gamma rays	*3.12.2*
2. Internal conversion	*3.12.2*

---

[1] Reproduced with permission from www.theabr.org. © 2010 American Board of Radiology. Accessed January 2010.

Section

V.   Interactions of Particulate Radiation with Matter
  A. Formalism
    1. W value   *6.2.4*
    2. Specific ionization   *Not covered*
                                                  (rarely used)
    3. Linear energy transfer   *6.2.2*
    4. Range   *6.2.3*
    5. Stopping power   *6.2.2*
  B. Types of interactions
    1. Heavy vs. light particles   *6.2, 6.2.5*
    2. Charged vs. uncharged particles   *Chapter 6,*
                                                  Introduction
    3. Elastic collisions   *6.2*
    4. Inelastic collisions   *6.2*
  C. Heavy charged particles   *6.2.5*
    1. Inelastic collisions with electrons   *6.2.5*
    2. Depth-dose characteristics (Bragg peak)   *6.2.5, 20.4.2*
  D. Light charged particles   *6.2.1*
    1. Elastic and inelastic collisions
       with electrons   *6.2.1*
    2. Inelastic collisions with nuclei   *6.2.1*
  E. Neutrons   *6.3*
    1. Elastic collisions with hydrogen nuclei   *6.3*
    2. Depth-dose characteristics vs. charged
       particles and photons   *Not covered*
  F. Biological implications of particle therapy *7.11, 20.4.2*

VI. Quantification and Measurement of Dose
       (including SI units)
  A. Exposure (air kerma)   *7.2, 7.4*
  B. Absorbed dose (kerma)   *7.4*
  C. Dose equivalent   *17.1 (dose*
                                                  equivalent
                                                  replaced by
                                                  equivalent dose)
  D. RBE dose   *20.4.2 for protons*
  E. Calculation of absorbed dose from exposure
     (e.g., f factor)   *7.7*
  F. Bragg-Gray cavity theory   *Not covered*
  G. Gas-filled detectors   *8.3*
    1. Principles of operation   *8.3*
    2. Uses   *8.3, 17.8.5*

Section

Section

Section

B. Factors affecting dose distributions (*continued*)
    7. Surface dose   *15.1*
    8. Inhomogeneities (e.g., CET)   *15.7*
    9. Other   *?*
C. Energy specification
    1. Most probable energy   *Not covered*
    2. Mean energy   *15.1*
    3. Energy at depth   *15.1*
    4. Ranges (extrapolated, practical, R50)   *15.1*
D. Choice of energy and field size   *15.1, 15.6*
E. Air gaps and oblique incidence   *15.4; oblique incidence is not covered*

F. Tissue inhomogeneities   *15.7*
G. Bolus, absorbers, and spoilers   *Not covered*
H. Matching adjacent fields   *15.8*
I. Point dose and treatment time calculations   *15.4*
J. Field shaping techniques   *15.3*
K. Electron arc   *Not covered*
L. Total skin electron therapy   *Not covered*

XI. Brachytherapy
A. Historical review – role of radium   *16.1, 16.3*
B. Calculation of dose from a point source   *16.6, 16.10.1*
C. Calculation of dose from a line source   *16.8, 16.10.2*
D. Physical and dosimetric properties of commercial
    sealed sources and applicators   *16.3, 16.4*
E. Implant instrumentation and techniques
    1. Low dose rate   *16.10–16.13*
    2. High dose rate (including PDR)   *16.14*
    3. Biological considerations of dose, dose rate,
       and fractionation   *Outside scope of this textbook; consult a book on radiobiology*
F. Calibration and specification of sources   *16.7*
G. Disseminated (unsealed) sources   *Not covered*
H. Acceptance testing and quality assurance   *18.2.2*
I. Dose specification, implantation dosimetry,
    and dosimetry systems   *16.10–16.13*
    1. Paterson-Parker   *16.10*
    2. Quimby   *16.10*
    3. Paris   *16.10*
    4. Other   *16.10*

Section

XII. Advanced Treatment Planning for EBRT

XIII. Quality Assurance   *Chapter 18*

XIV. Radiation Protection   *Chapter 17*

Section

XVI. Special Topics
A. Hyperthermia *Not covered*

B. Computers *Not covered*

The ARRT does not review, evaluate, or endorse publications. Permission to reproduce ARRT copyrighted materials within this publication should not be construed as an endorsement of the publication by ARRT.

The American Registry
of Radiologic Technologists® (ARRT)[2]

The American Registry of Radiologic Technologists (ARRT) administers certification exams to radiation therapy technologists. This exam covers five major content areas. This textbook is only relevant to three of these areas: radiation protection and quality assurance (17.5%), treatment planning (27.5%), and treatment delivery (12.5%). A listing of these topics appears below, keyed to the relevant section in the text that covers that subject matter. A question mark indicates that we do not understand the intent of the listing and therefore cannot provide a reference. The reader is urged to check the ARRT web site for updates.

A.   RADIATION PROTECTION AND QUALITY ASSURANCE

Section

1. Radiation Physics and Biology
   A. Sources of Radiation
      1. radioactive material — *Chapter 3, 16.3*
      2. machine-produced radiation — *Chapter 4, Chapter 9, 20.4.3*
   B. Basic Properties of Radiation
      1. wave characteristics — *2.4*
      2. exponential attenuation — *5.5.2*
      3. inverse-square law — *5.5.1*
      4. x-ray beam quality — *5.6*
   C. Interactions with Matter
      1. photon interactions (Compton, photoelectric effect, etc.) — *6.1*
      2. electron interactions — *6.2*
      3. particle interactions (proton, neutron, etc.) — *6.2, 6.3, 20.4.2*
   D. Biological Effects of Radiation
      1. radosensitivity — *7.11, 14.6*
      2. dose response relationships — *Not covered*
      3. somatic effects
         a. cellular — *7.11*
         b. tissue (hemopoietic, skin, reproductive organs, etc.) — *14.6*
         c. embryonic and fetal risks — *17.3.2*
         d. carcinogenesis — *17.3.1*
         e. early versus late effects — *Not covered*
         f. acute versus chronic effects — *Not covered*

---

[2] Reproduced with permission from http://www.arrt.org. © 2010 The American Registry of Radiologic Technologists. Accessed June 9, 2010.

Section

E. Measurement of Radiation
   1. units of measurement
      a. absorbed dose (gray)   *7.4*
      b. dose equivalent (rem)   *17.1 (equivalent dose)*
      c. exposure (Roentgen)   *7.2, 7.3*
   2. instrumentation
      a. ionization chamber   *8.3.1*
      b. Geiger-Müller detector   *8.3.5*
      c. TLD/OSL (Optically Stimulated
         Luminescence)   *8.4.1*
      d. diodes   *8.4.3, 18.3.4*
      e. neutron detectors   *Not covered*

2. Radiation Protection
  A. Fundamental Principles
    1. ALARA   *17.4*
    2. basic methods of protection (time, distance,
      shielding)   *17.4*
  B. Personnel Monitoring
    1. NCRP recommendations for personnel   *This text does not*
      monitoring (report #116)   *cover recommendations,*
                                             but instead covers
                                    requirements, see 17.6
      a. occupational exposure (sievert)   *17.5.1*
      b. public exposure   *17.5.1*
      c. embryo/fetus exposure   *17.5.1*
    2. maintenance and evaluation of personnel   *Not covered*
      dosimetry records
  C. Facilities and Area Monitoring
    1. NRC regulations (CFR 10, parts 20 and 35)   *17.5, 18.2.2*
      a. classification of areas (restricted, controlled,
        unrestricted)
      b. required postings (signs)   *17.5.5, 17.8.5*
      c. area monitoring devices   *17.5.6*
    2. barrier requirements
      a. primary   *17.8*
      b. secondary   *17.8*

3. Environmental Protection
  A. Toxic or Hazardous Material
    1. metals (shielding alloy, etc.)   *18.5*
    2. chemicals (film processing, etc.)   *Not covered*

Section

Section

C. TREATMENT PLANNING
  1. **Treatment Volume Localization**
     A. Treatment Techniques and Anatomic Relationships   *?*
        1. radiation therapy techniques
        2. sectional and topographic anatomy
        3. critical organs   *14.6*
        4. patient positioning and immobilization   *14.15*
     B. Fluoroscopic Simulation   *This text uses*
        1. image receptors   *term "conventional"*
        2. exposure factors   *simulation; see 19.3*
        3. image processing
        4. image labeling
        5. magnification factors
        6. contouring (purpose, devices, materials, technique, etc.)
        7. volume and isocenter determination
        8. image storage and retrieval
     C. CT Simulation   *19.4*
     D. Contrast Media   *Not covered*
     E. Contours   *Not covered*
     F. Documentation of Simulation Procedure   *Not covered*

  2. **Prescription and Dose Calculation**
     A. Treatment Prescription   *14.6*
        1. total tumor dose
        2. fractionation schedules   *Not covered*
        3. radiation energy
        4. types of radiation
        5. treatment volume (GTV, CTV, PTV, etc.)   *14.6*
        6. number of fields   *14.3–14.5*
        7. fixed versus rotational fields   *14.8*
        8. field weighting   *14.3.2*
        9. field orientation   *14.5*
        10. treatment unit capabilities and limitations
        11. modifications
     B. Geometric Parameters and Patient Measurements
        1. field size and shape
        2. tumor depth
        3. patient thickness
        4. SSD, SAD   *9.1*
        5. collimator setting   *9.1*
        6. abutting fields (gap calculations, etc.)   *14.14*

Section

C. Dose Calculation and Verification
1. selection of energy
2. equivalent square (open and blocked field)   *10.7*
3. scatter factors (collimator, phantom, etc.)   *12.3*
4. percentage depth dose   *10.2*
5. TAR, TMR   *10.4, 10.6*
6. SSD, SAD   *10.1, 12.4.2, 12.4.4*
7. inverse square   *5.5.1*
8. extended distance factor   *Mayneord's F factor,*
   see 10.2
9. wedges (wedge angle or factor, etc.)   *14.4*
10. off-axis calculation   *13.4*
11. isodose curves and their characteristics
    (penumbra, DVH, etc.)   *14.1, 14.2, 14.7*
12. factors for beam modifiers (tray factor,
    bolus, compensator, etc.)   *13.2.2, 14.10, 14.12*
13. inhomogeneity correction factors   *14.13*
14. rotational factors   *14.8*
15. machine output data (cGy/min, etc.)   *12.2, 12.3*
16. verification and documentation   *? ?*

3. **Treatment Accessories**
A. Types of Devices
1. immobilization   *14.15*
2. compensating filters   *14.12*
3. shielding (blocks, multileaf collimation,
   etc.)   *13.2.2, 13.2.3*
4. bolus   *14.10*
B. Design Methods and Materials
1. custom beam shaping devices
   a. photon   *13.2.2*
   b. electron   *15.3*
2. custom immobilization devices   *14.15*
3. bolus   *14.10*
C. Parameters
1. SSD, SAD   *9.1*
2. source-film distance (SFD)   *13.2.2*
3. image magnification factor   *Not covered*
4. collimator settings   *?*
5. source-to-block tray distance (STD)   *13.2.2*
6. patient thickness   *Not covered*

Section

7. block thickness, half-value layer (HVL),
    half-value thickness (HVT)   *13.2.2, 5.6*
8. beam energy and type

D. TREATMENT DELIVERY
1. Verification and Application of the Treatment Plan
A. Patient Position
B. Isocenter (x, y, z coordinates, etc.)
C. Treatment Parameters (beam orientation, energy, etc.)
D. Prescription
E. Modality
   1. 2D
   2. 3D
   3. 4D   *19.4.6*
   4. IMRT   *20.2*
   5. stereotactic   *20.3*

2. Treatment Machine Set-Up
A. Auxiliary Set-Up Devices
   1. couch indexing
   2. positioning aids   *14.15*
   3. alignment lasers   *18.2.1*
B. Machine Operation
   1. SSD, SAD   *9.1*
   2. collimator or cone settings   *9.2.2*
   3. optical or mechanical distance indicator   *9.2.2*
   4. gantry angle   *9.1*
   5. collimator angle   *9.1*
   6. field light   *9.2.2*
   7. treatment couch   *9.2.5*
   8. console controls
C. Beam Modifiers
   1. wedges (enhanced dynamic wedge,
      physical wedge)   *14.4*
   2. bolus   *14.10*
   3. compensators   *14.12*
   4. blocks   *13.2.2*
   5. multileaf collimation   *13.2.3*

Section

3. **Treatment Administration**
   A. Patient Monitoring Systems
      1. direct visual
      2. indirect visual (mirror; TV monitor)   *17.5.6, 18.2.1*
      3. two-way voice communication system   *17.5.6, 18.2.1*
      4. back-up systems
      5. monitoring regulations   *17.5.6*
      6. emergency situations   *17.5.6, 18.6*
   B. Record and Verify Systems   *18.3*
   C. Portal Imaging   *19.9*
   D. Site Verification
   E. Dose Verification (diodes, film, etc.)   *8.4.3, 8.4.4, 18.3.4,*
                                                      19.9, 19.10
   F. Equipment Malfunctions   *18.6, 18.7*
      1. types (radiation, electrical, mechanical, etc.)
      2. documentation and reporting

4. **Documentation**   *Not covered*

E. **PATIENT CARE AND EDUCATION**   *Not covered*

Reprinted with permission from
The American Registry of Radiologic Technologists®
1255 Northland Drive
St. Paul, MN 55120-1155
Phone: (651) 687-0048

Medical Dosimetrist Certification Board

The Medical Dosimetrist Certification Board (MDCB) administers a certification exam for medical dosimetrists. For an outline of the examination contents, visit their website (http://www.mdcb.org) to download the Exam Applicant's Handbook.

We wish we could provide you with a list of topics keyed to this text but our request to reproduce the exam content outline was denied by the MDCB.

Appendix B

Dosimetry Data

EQUIVALENT SQUARES FOR RECTANGULAR FIELDS

Long Axis (cm)	Short Axis (cm)																				
	0.5	1	2	3	4	5	6	7	8	9	10	11	12	13	14	15	16	17	18	19	20
0.5	0.5																				
1	0.7	1.0																			
2	0.9	1.4	2.0																		
3	1.0	1.6	2.4	3.0																	
4	1.1	1.7	2.7	3.4	4.0																
5	1.1	1.8	2.9	3.8	4.5	5.0															
6	1.2	1.9	3.1	4.1	4.8	5.5	6.0														
7	1.2	2.0	3.3	4.3	5.1	5.8	6.5	7.0													
8	1.2	2.1	3.4	4.5	5.4	6.2	6.9	7.5	8.0												
9	1.2	2.1	3.5	4.6	5.6	6.5	7.2	7.9	8.5	9.0											
10	1.3	2.2	3.6	4.8	5.8	6.7	7.5	8.2	8.9	9.5	10.0										
11	1.3	2.2	3.7	4.9	6.0	6.9	7.8	8.5	9.3	9.9	10.5	11.0									
12	1.3	2.2	3.7	5.0	6.1	7.1	8.0	8.8	9.6	10.3	10.9	11.5	12.0								
13	1.3	2.2	3.8	5.1	6.2	7.2	8.2	9.1	9.9	10.6	11.3	11.9	12.5	13.0							
14	1.3	2.3	3.8	5.1	6.3	7.4	8.4	9.3	10.1	10.9	11.6	12.3	12.9	13.5	14.0						
15	1.3	2.3	3.9	5.2	6.4	7.5	8.5	9.5	10.3	11.2	11.9	12.6	13.3	13.9	14.5	15.0					
16	1.3	2.3	3.9	5.3	6.5	7.6	8.6	9.6	10.5	11.4	12.2	12.9	13.7	14.3	14.9	15.5	16.0				
17	1.3	2.3	3.9	5.3	6.5	7.7	8.8	9.8	10.7	11.6	12.4	13.2	14.0	14.7	15.3	15.9	16.5	17.0			
18	1.3	2.3	3.9	5.3	6.6	7.8	8.9	9.9	10.9	11.8	12.6	13.5	14.3	15.0	15.7	16.3	16.9	17.5	18.0		
19	1.4	2.3	4.0	5.4	6.6	7.8	8.9	10.0	11.0	11.9	12.8	13.7	14.5	15.3	16.0	16.7	17.3	17.9	18.5	19.0	
20	1.4	2.3	4.0	5.4	6.7	7.9	9.0	10.1	11.1	12.1	13.0	13.9	14.7	15.5	16.3	17.0	17.7	18.3	18.9	19.5	20.0
22	1.4	2.4	4.0	5.5	6.8	8.0	9.1	10.2	11.3	12.3	13.3	14.2	15.1	16.0	16.8	17.6	18.3	19.0	19.7	20.3	20.9
24	1.4	2.4	4.0	5.5	6.8	8.1	9.2	10.4	11.4	12.5	13.5	14.5	15.4	16.3	17.2	18.0	18.8	19.6	20.3	21.0	21.7
26	1.4	2.4	4.1	5.5	6.9	8.1	9.3	10.5	11.6	12.6	13.7	14.7	15.7	16.6	17.5	18.4	19.3	20.1	20.9	21.6	22.4
28	1.4	2.4	4.1	5.5	6.9	8.2	9.4	10.5	11.7	12.7	13.8	14.8	15.8	16.8	17.8	18.7	19.6	20.5	21.3	22.1	22.9
30	1.4	2.4	4.1	5.6	6.9	8.2	9.4	10.6	11.7	12.8	13.9	15.0	16.0	17.0	18.0	18.9	19.9	20.8	21.6	22.5	23.3
32	1.4	2.4	4.1	5.6	6.9	8.2	9.4	10.6	11.8	12.9	14.0	15.0	16.1	17.1	18.1	19.1	20.1	21.0	21.9	22.8	23.7
34	1.4	2.4	4.1	5.6	6.9	8.2	9.5	10.7	11.8	12.9	14.0	15.1	16.2	17.2	18.2	19.2	20.2	21.2	22.1	23.1	24.0
36	1.4	2.4	4.1	5.6	7.0	8.2	9.5	10.7	11.8	13.0	14.1	15.2	16.2	17.3	18.3	19.3	20.4	21.3	22.3	23.3	24.2
38	1.4	2.4	4.1	5.6	7.0	8.3	9.5	10.7	11.9	13.0	14.1	15.2	16.3	17.4	18.4	19.4	20.5	21.5	22.4	23.4	24.4
40	1.4	2.4	4.1	5.6	7.0	8.3	9.5	10.7	11.9	13.0	14.1	15.2	16.3	17.4	18.5	19.5	20.5	21.5	22.6	23.5	24.5
45	1.4	2.4	4.1	5.6	7.0	8.3	9.5	10.7	11.9	13.1	14.2	15.3	16.4	17.5	18.5	19.6	20.7	21.7	22.7	23.7	24.8
50	1.4	2.4	4.1	5.6	7.0	8.3	9.5	10.7	11.9	13.1	14.2	15.3	16.4	17.5	18.6	19.7	20.7	21.8	22.8	23.8	24.9
55	1.4	2.4	4.1	5.6	7.0	8.3	9.5	10.8	11.9	13.1	14.2	15.3	16.4	17.5	18.6	19.7	20.8	21.8	22.9	23.9	24.9
60	1.4	2.4	4.1	5.6	7.0	8.3	9.5	10.8	11.9	13.1	14.2	15.4	16.5	17.6	18.6	19.7	20.8	21.8	22.9	23.9	25.0

(Reproduced with permission from Table A-2, p. 150, Central Axis Depth Dose Data for Use in Radiotherapy Departments: *British Journal of Radiology* Supplement No. 25. London, UK: British Institute of Radiology. © 1996 British Institute of Radiology)

PERCENT DEPTH DOSE DATA   4 MV

SSD = 100.0 cm
Normalized to depth d_0 = 1.2 cm
Field Size defined at 100.0 cm

Depth (cm)	Field Size (cm)						
	5	10	15	20	25	30	40
0.5	92.5	93.5	94.9	96.2	96.7	97.2	98.1
1.0	100.0	100.0	100.1	100.2	100.3	100.3	100.4
1.2	100.0	100.0	100.0	100.0	100.0	100.0	100.0
1.5	98.8	98.8	99.0	99.2	99.2	99.1	99.0
2.0	95.8	96.9	97.1	97.2	97.3	97.4	97.5
3.0	91.0	92.1	92.7	93.3	93.4	93.6	93.8
3.5	88.2	89.9	90.6	91.3	91.5	91.7	92.0
4.0	85.3	87.6	88.5	89.4	89.7	89.9	90.4
4.5	83.1	85.6	86.5	87.4	87.7	88.0	88.6
5.0	80.6	83.1	84.2	85.2	85.6	85.9	86.6
5.5	77.5	81.0	82.0	82.9	83.4	83.9	84.9
6.0	75.3	79.1	80.3	81.5	82.0	82.4	83.3
6.5	72.9	76.5	77.9	79.2	79.8	80.3	81.4
7.0	70.1	74.5	75.9	77.3	77.8	78.3	79.3
7.5	67.8	72.3	73.7	75.1	75.7	76.4	77.6
8.0	65.8	70.4	72.1	73.7	74.3	74.9	76.0
8.5	63.7	68.2	69.8	71.4	72.1	72.7	74.0
9.0	61.3	66.1	67.9	69.6	70.3	71.1	72.5
9.5	59.3	64.2	66.1	67.9	68.6	69.4	70.8
10.0	57.2	62.1	64.2	66.3	67.0	67.7	69.1
10.5	55.3	60.3	62.4	64.4	65.2	65.9	67.4
11.0	53.3	58.6	60.7	62.7	63.5	64.3	65.9
11.5	51.3	56.9	58.9	60.9	61.8	62.7	64.4
12.0	49.7	55.0	57.2	59.3	60.2	61.0	62.7
12.5	48.0	53.4	55.6	57.8	58.6	59.5	61.1
13.0	46.2	51.6	53.8	56.0	56.9	57.7	59.4
13.5	44.6	50.1	52.3	54.5	55.5	56.4	58.3
14.0	42.9	48.5	50.9	53.3	54.1	55.0	56.6
14.5	41.6	47.0	49.3	51.5	52.5	53.5	55.4
15.0	40.0	45.6	47.9	50.1	51.0	51.9	53.7
15.5	38.7	44.0	46.4	48.7	49.6	50.6	52.4
16.0	37.5	42.8	45.1	47.3	48.3	49.2	51.1
16.5	36.2	41.3	43.6	45.8	46.8	47.8	49.8
17.0	34.6	40.2	42.3	44.4	45.5	46.6	48.8
17.5	33.7	38.9	41.2	43.4	44.4	45.4	47.3
18.0	32.4	37.6	39.9	42.1	43.1	44.2	46.2
18.5	31.3	36.6	38.7	40.8	41.9	42.9	45.0
19.0	30.4	35.4	37.6	39.8	40.8	41.8	43.8
19.5	29.3	34.4	36.6	38.8	39.8	40.8	42.7
20.0	28.3	33.2	35.4	37.5	38.5	39.6	41.6
20.5	27.3	32.2	34.4	36.5	37.5	38.6	40.6
21.0	26.3	31.2	33.3	35.4	36.4	37.4	39.4
21.5	25.4	30.0	32.2	34.3	35.4	36.5	38.6
22.0	24.7	29.3	31.3	33.3	34.3	35.4	37.4
22.5	23.7	28.4	30.4	32.4	33.3	34.3	36.1
23.0	22.9	27.6	29.4	31.2	32.3	33.3	35.4
23.5	22.0	26.7	28.6	30.4	31.5	32.5	34.6
24.0	21.2	25.8	27.6	29.4	30.4	31.5	33.5
24.5	20.6	25.0	26.9	28.8	29.8	30.7	32.6
25.0	19.9	24.1	26.0	27.8	28.8	29.7	31.6

PERCENT DEPTH DOSE DATA   10 MV

SSD = 100.0 cm
Normalized to depth d_0 = 2.2 cm
Field Size defined at 100.0 cm

Depth (cm)	Field Size (cm)							
	5	10	15	20	25	30	35	40
0.5	68.7	73.8	78.3	82.8	84.1	85.4	86.8	88.1
1.0	89.1	92.2	94.4	96.5	97.0	97.4	97.8	98.2
1.5	97.2	98.8	99.7	100.5	100.6	100.6	100.6	100.6
2.0	100.0	100.3	100.4	100.5	100.5	100.5	100.5	100.5
2.2	100.0	100.0	100.0	100.0	100.0	100.0	100.0	100.0
2.5	99.7	99.4	99.2	99.0	99.1	99.2	99.2	99.3
3.0	98.1	97.9	97.8	97.7	97.8	97.8	97.8	97.8
3.5	96.1	96.0	96.0	95.9	96.0	96.0	96.0	96.0
4.0	93.7	94.2	94.2	94.1	94.3	94.4	94.5	94.6
4.5	91.6	92.1	92.2	92.3	92.4	92.6	92.8	93.0
5.0	89.5	90.2	90.4	90.5	90.6	90.7	90.8	90.9
5.5	87.3	88.0	88.3	88.6	88.8	89.0	89.1	89.3
6.0	85.1	86.1	86.5	86.9	87.1	87.3	87.4	87.6
6.5	83.1	84.4	84.9	85.3	85.5	85.7	85.9	86.0
7.0	80.9	82.5	83.1	83.8	83.9	84.1	84.3	84.4
7.5	78.6	80.9	81.6	82.2	82.4	82.6	82.7	82.9
8.0	77.0	79.1	79.6	80.1	80.5	80.9	81.3	81.6
8.5	74.9	77.1	78.1	79.0	79.3	79.7	80.0	80.3
9.0	73.0	75.4	76.6	77.9	78.2	78.5	78.8	79.1
9.5	71.1	73.8	75.0	76.2	76.6	77.0	77.4	77.7
10.0	69.3	72.0	73.3	74.6	75.1	75.5	75.9	76.3
11.0	65.7	68.5	70.0	71.5	71.9	72.3	72.6	73.0
12.0	62.5	65.4	66.9	68.5	69.0	69.4	69.9	70.4
13.0	59.4	62.5	63.9	65.2	65.9	66.5	67.1	67.7
14.0	56.5	59.6	61.0	62.5	63.2	63.9	64.6	65.3
15.0	53.7	56.8	58.5	60.1	60.8	61.5	62.2	62.9
16.0	51.0	54.0	55.8	57.7	58.4	59.0	59.7	60.3
17.0	48.4	51.4	53.5	55.5	56.0	56.6	57.2	57.8
18.0	46.0	49.1	51.1	53.2	53.8	54.3	54.9	55.4
19.0	43.8	46.6	48.7	50.7	51.4	52.1	52.9	53.6
20.0	41.6	44.6	46.6	48.7	49.4	50.1	50.8	51.5
21.0	39.5	42.4	44.5	46.7	47.3	48.0	48.7	49.4
22.0	37.6	40.4	42.5	44.6	45.4	46.1	46.9	47.6
23.0	35.7	38.7	40.7	42.7	43.4	44.2	44.9	45.6
24.0	34.1	36.9	38.9	40.9	41.7	42.4	43.2	44.0
25.0	32.3	35.2	37.2	39.3	40.0	40.8	41.6	42.3

PERCENT DEPTH DOSE DATA   15 MV

SSD = 100.0 cm
Normalized to depth d_0 = 2.8 cm
Field Size defined at 100.0 cm

Depth (cm)	Field Size (cm)							
	5	10	15	20	25	30	35	40
0.5	63.4	68.5	73.5	77.3	80.2	82.2	83.6	84.3
1.0	80.1	83.9	87.4	90.0	91.8	93.0	93.7	94.1
1.5	91.9	94.0	96.1	97.5	98.3	98.8	99.1	99.2
2.0	95.1	96.4	97.7	98.5	99.0	99.3	99.5	99.5
2.5	98.2	98.7	99.1	99.4	99.6	99.7	99.8	99.8
2.8	100.0	100.0	100.0	100.0	100.0	100.0	100.0	100.0
3.0	99.6	99.6	99.5	99.4	99.4	99.4	99.4	99.4
3.5	98.7	98.5	98.2	97.9	97.9	97.9	97.9	97.9
4.0	97.8	97.4	96.9	96.5	96.4	96.4	96.4	96.5
4.5	96.0	95.6	95.2	94.8	94.8	94.8	94.8	94.9
5.0	94.1	93.9	93.5	93.3	93.2	93.3	93.3	93.3
5.5	92.1	92.1	91.8	91.7	91.6	91.6	91.6	91.6
6.0	90.0	90.3	90.1	90.1	90.0	90.0	90.0	90.0
6.5	88.0	88.5	88.4	88.4	88.4	88.3	88.4	88.4
7.0	86.1	86.7	86.6	86.7	86.7	86.7	86.8	86.9
7.5	84.2	84.9	84.9	85.1	85.1	85.1	85.2	85.4
8.0	82.3	83.2	83.3	83.5	83.5	83.6	83.7	83.9
8.5	80.4	81.5	81.6	81.9	82.0	82.0	82.2	82.4
9.0	78.6	79.8	80.0	80.3	80.4	80.5	80.7	81.0
9.5	76.8	78.1	78.4	78.8	78.9	79.0	79.2	79.6
10.0	75.0	76.5	76.9	77.3	77.5	77.6	77.8	78.2
11.0	71.2	73.3	73.8	74.3	74.6	74.8	75.0	75.5
12.0	67.6	70.3	70.8	71.5	71.9	72.1	72.4	73.0
13.0	64.6	67.2	67.9	68.7	69.1	69.4	69.8	70.5
14.0	61.8	64.3	65.2	66.0	66.4	66.8	67.3	68.1
15.0	58.9	61.5	62.6	63.4	63.9	64.3	64.9	65.7
16.0	56.4	58.9	60.0	60.9	61.4	61.9	62.9	63.2
17.0	53.9	56.4	57.6	58.5	59.1	59.6	60.1	60.7
18.0	51.5	54.0	55.2	56.2	56.8	57.3	57.8	58.3
19.0	49.2	51.6	52.8	53.9	54.6	55.1	55.5	56.0
20.0	46.9	49.3	50.6	51.7	52.5	53.0	53.3	53.7
21.0	44.9	47.3	48.6	49.6	50.4	50.9	51.3	51.8
22.0	43.0	45.3	46.6	47.7	48.4	49.0	49.4	49.9
23.0	41.0	43.4	44.7	45.7	46.5	47.1	47.6	48.2
24.0	39.2	41.5	42.9	43.9	44.6	45.2	45.8	46.4
25.0	37.4	39.7	41.1	42.0	42.8	43.4	44.1	44.8

TISSUE-AIR RATIO (TAR) DATA   6 MV

Depth (cm)	Field Size (cm)							
	5	10	15	20	25	30	35	40
0.0	0.082	0.145	0.211	0.274	0.329	0.377	0.418	0.455
0.5	0.886	0.928	0.966	0.998	1.020	1.035	1.045	1.058
1.0	1.011	1.043	1.069	1.089	1.101	1.108	1.113	1.121
1.5	1.059	1.084	1.101	1.115	1.123	1.127	1.130	1.137
2.0	1.057	1.082	1.097	1.109	1.117	1.122	1.126	1.131
2.5	1.042	1.069	1.086	1.099	1.107	1.113	1.117	1.123
3.0	1.016	1.056	1.075	1.089	1.098	1.104	1.109	1.115
3.5	0.997	1.042	1.062	1.077	1.087	1.093	1.098	1.105
4.0	0.979	1.028	1.049	1.065	1.075	1.083	1.087	1.094
4.5	0.960	1.013	1.036	1.052	1.064	1.072	1.076	1.084
5.0	0.942	0.999	1.023	1.040	1.052	1.061	1.066	1.073
5.5	0.923	0.983	1.012	1.027	1.040	1.048	1.054	1.062
6.0	0.904	0.967	0.998	1.013	1.027	1.036	1.042	1.050
6.5	0.885	0.952	0.983	1.000	1.015	1.024	1.030	1.039
7.0	0.866	0.936	0.969	0.986	1.002	1.012	1.018	1.027
7.5	0.847	0.920	0.955	0.973	0.989	1.000	1.006	1.016
8.0	0.830	0.904	0.940	0.959	0.976	0.987	0.994	1.004
8.5	0.813	0.888	0.926	0.945	0.962	0.974	0.982	0.992
9.0	0.795	0.872	0.912	0.931	0.949	0.962	0.970	0.980
9.5	0.778	0.857	0.897	0.917	0.935	0.949	0.957	0.968
10.0	0.761	0.841	0.883	0.902	0.922	0.936	0.945	0.956
11.0	0.730	0.810	0.854	0.875	0.896	0.911	0.920	0.931
12.0	0.698	0.779	0.825	0.847	0.870	0.885	0.894	0.906
13.0	0.667	0.750	0.798	0.821	0.844	0.860	0.869	0.881
14.0	0.636	0.722	0.771	0.795	0.818	0.835	0.844	0.856
15.0	0.605	0.693	0.744	0.768	0.793	0.809	0.819	0.832
16.0	0.580	0.667	0.719	0.743	0.768	0.785	0.796	0.809
17.0	0.556	0.642	0.694	0.719	0.743	0.761	0.772	0.786
18.0	0.531	0.617	0.669	0.694	0.719	0.737	0.748	0.763
19.0	0.507	0.591	0.643	0.669	0.694	0.713	0.724	0.740
20.0	0.482	0.566	0.618	0.644	0.670	0.689	0.701	0.717
21.0	0.482	0.545	0.589	0.622	0.648	0.667	0.682	0.695
22.0	0.463	0.524	0.568	0.600	0.626	0.645	0.660	0.673
23.0	0.443	0.503	0.546	0.579	0.604	0.623	0.638	0.652
24.0	0.424	0.481	0.525	0.557	0.583	0.601	0.616	0.630
25.0	0.405	0.460	0.503	0.535	0.561	0.579	0.594	0.608

TISSUE-MAXIMUM RATIO (TMR) TABLE   10 MV

Depth (cm)	Field Size (cm)							
	5	10	15	20	25	30	35	40
0.5	0.664	0.713	0.756	0.800	0.813	0.826	0.839	0.851
1.0	0.870	0.900	0.921	0.942	0.947	0.951	0.955	0.958
1.5	0.959	0.974	0.983	0.991	0.992	0.992	0.992	0.992
2.0	0.996	0.999	1.000	1.001	1.001	1.001	1.001	1.001
2.2	1.000	1.000	1.000	1.000	1.000	1.000	1.000	1.000
2.5	1.002	1.000	0.998	0.996	0.997	0.997	0.998	0.998
3.0	0.996	0.994	0.993	0.993	0.993	0.993	0.993	0.993
3.5	0.986	0.985	0.984	0.984	0.984	0.984	0.985	0.985
4.0	0.970	0.975	0.975	0.975	0.976	0.977	0.978	0.980
4.5	0.957	0.962	0.964	0.964	0.966	0.968	0.970	0.972
5.0	0.945	0.951	0.953	0.955	0.956	0.957	0.958	0.959
5.5	0.930	0.937	0.941	0.944	0.946	0.947	0.949	0.951
6.0	0.915	0.925	0.930	0.934	0.936	0.938	0.940	0.941
6.5	0.901	0.915	0.921	0.925	0.928	0.930	0.932	0.933
7.0	0.885	0.902	0.910	0.916	0.919	0.921	0.923	0.924
7.5	0.868	0.892	0.901	0.908	0.911	0.913	0.914	0.916
8.0	0.858	0.880	0.888	0.893	0.898	0.901	0.905	0.909
8.5	0.842	0.865	0.877	0.887	0.893	0.896	0.900	0.903
9.0	0.828	0.853	0.868	0.881	0.888	0.891	0.895	0.898
9.5	0.813	0.841	0.857	0.870	0.877	0.881	0.885	0.889
10.0	0.801	0.828	0.845	0.859	0.867	0.872	0.876	0.880
11.0	0.772	0.802	0.821	0.836	0.846	0.850	0.854	0.858
12.0	0.747	0.778	0.798	0.814	0.825	0.830	0.835	0.840
13.0	0.721	0.756	0.775	0.790	0.801	0.807	0.814	0.820
14.0	0.698	0.732	0.753	0.768	0.780	0.788	0.796	0.803
15.0	0.674	0.709	0.732	0.750	0.764	0.771	0.779	0.787
16.0	0.651	0.684	0.709	0.730	0.746	0.753	0.761	0.768
17.0	0.628	0.662	0.689	0.712	0.729	0.735	0.742	0.748
18.0	0.607	0.642	0.669	0.692	0.711	0.717	0.723	0.730
19.0	0.588	0.620	0.647	0.670	0.690	0.698	0.706	0.714
20.0	0.567	0.601	0.629	0.652	0.673	0.681	0.689	0.697
21.0	0.547	0.581	0.609	0.633	0.655	0.663	0.671	0.679
22.0	0.529	0.562	0.590	0.614	0.637	0.646	0.654	0.663
23.0	0.509	0.544	0.573	0.596	0.619	0.627	0.636	0.645
24.0	0.494	0.527	0.555	0.579	0.602	0.611	0.621	0.630
25.0	0.475	0.509	0.539	0.563	0.588	0.597	0.606	0.615

Table 3.3: Commonly Used Isotopes in Radiation Therapy

Isotope	Half-Life	Therapeutic Radiation	Production
Co-60	5.26 years	1.25 MeV (average) γ	Neutron activation
Cs-137	30.0 years	0.662 MeV γ	Fission product
I-125	59.5 days	0.028 MeV (average) x-rays	Neutron activation
I-131	8.0 days	0.364 MeV γ	Fission product
Ir-192	73.8 days	0.38 MeV (average) γ	Neutron activation
Pd-103	17.0 days	0.021 MeV characteristic x-rays	Neutron activation
Sr-90	28.1 years	0.7 MeV β^- (average)	Fission product

Table 16.1: Brachytherapy Isotopes[a]

Isotope	Half-life	Mean energy (keV)	Maximum energy (keV)	HVL (mm-lead)	Γ[b] (R cm^2 h^{-1} mCi^{-1})	f (cGy/R)
Ra-226	1600 y	830	2450	16	8.25[c] (R cm^2 h^{-1} mg^{-1})	--
Cs-137	30.0 y	662	662	5.5	3.28	0.973
Ir-192	73.8 d	380	1060	2.5	4.69	0.970
I-125	59.5 d	28	35	0.025	1.51	0.910
Pd-103	17.0 d	21	23	0.008	1.48	0.886
Au-198	2.7 d	416	1090 (0.2%)	2.5	2.38	--

y = years; d = days
[a] Some of the values in this table were taken from the AAPM TG-43 report.[1]
[b] Ir-192, I-125, Pd-103, and Au-198 values are for an ideal unfiltered point source.
[c] For 0.5 mm platinum filtration.

[1] AAPM TG-43. (1995). Nath, R., L. L. Anderson, G. Luxton, K. A. Weaver, J. F. Williamson, and A. S. Meigooni. "Dosimetry of interstitial brachytherapy sources: Recommendations of the AAPM Radiation Therapy Committee Task Group No. 43." *Med Phys* 22:209–234. Also available as AAPM Report No. 51.

Appendix C

Mevalac* Beam Data

---

*The Mevalac is a fictitious linear accelerator.

Mevalac (SSD = 100 cm)

$\dot{D}_0 = 1.000$ cGy/MU for $f = 10 \times 10$ cm^2 field at depth d_0, SSD = 100 cm

6 MV: $d_0 = 1.5$ cm, $\dot{D}_{d_0}$ (100,10) = 1.030 cGy/MU, TF = 0.956

18 MV: $d_0 = 3.0$ cm, $\dot{D}_{d_0}$ (100,10) = 1.061 cGy/MU, TF = 0.970

Scatter Correction Factors

Field Size (cm)	6 MV			18 MV		
	$S_{c,p}$	S_c	S_p	$S_{c,p}$	S_c	S_p
3	0.919	0.954	0.963	0.881	0.946	0.931
4	0.939	0.963	0.975	0.919	0.956	0.961
5	0.949	0.969	0.979	0.936	0.962	0.973
6	0.964	0.979	0.984	0.955	0.973	0.982
7	0.974	0.985	0.989	0.968	0.980	0.987
8	0.984	0.991	0.993	0.980	0.988	0.992
9	0.992	0.995	0.997	0.990	0.994	0.996
10	1.000	1.000	1.000	1.000	1.000	1.000
11	1.007	1.004	1.003	1.008	1.006	1.002
12	1.014	1.007	1.007	1.016	1.013	1.003
13	1.019	1.010	1.010	1.022	1.016	1.006
14	1.025	1.012	1.012	1.029	1.019	1.009
15	1.030	1.015	1.015	1.035	1.023	1.012
16	1.035	1.018	1.017	1.040	1.026	1.013
17	1.040	1.022	1.018	1.045	1.029	1.015
18	1.045	1.025	1.019	1.049	1.033	1.016
19	1.050	1.029	1.021	1.054	1.036	1.017
20	1.055	1.032	1.022	1.059	1.040	1.018
21	1.058	1.035	1.022	1.062	1.042	1.019
22	1.061	1.037	1.022	1.064	1.044	1.019
23	1.063	1.040	1.023	1.067	1.046	1.020
24	1.066	1.042	1.023	1.069	1.048	1.020
25	1.069	1.045	1.023	1.072	1.050	1.021
30	1.080	1.053	1.026	1.081	1.058	1.021
35	1.084	1.058	1.025	1.084	1.062	1.021
40	1.087	1.061	1.025	1.084	1.066	1.017

Mevalac – 6 MV Percent Depth Dose

SSD = 100.0 cm – Normalized to depth d_0 = 1.5 cm – Field Size defined at 100.0 cm

Depth (cm)	3x3	4x4	5x5	6x6	7x7	8x8	9x9	10x10	11x11	12x12	13x13	14x14	15x15
0.5	82.0	82.1	82.6	83.1	83.5	84.0	84.4	84.8	85.2	85.6	86.1	86.6	87.1
1.0	97.2	96.9	97.2	97.3	97.2	97.2	97.6	98.0	97.9	97.8	98.0	98.3	98.6
1.5	100.0	100.0	100.0	100.0	100.0	100.0	100.0	100.0	100.0	100.0	100.0	100.0	100.0
2.0	98.4	98.8	99.2	98.8	98.9	99.1	98.9	98.7	98.7	98.8	98.8	98.7	98.7
2.5	96.6	96.3	96.7	96.8	97.1	97.3	97.5	97.6	97.4	97.2	97.2	97.2	97.2
3.0	93.7	94.1	94.3	94.7	94.8	95.0	94.9	94.9	94.9	94.8	95.0	95.2	95.4
3.5	91.3	91.6	92.2	92.3	92.5	92.8	92.8	92.9	93.0	93.2	93.3	93.4	93.5
4.0	88.8	89.3	89.8	90.0	90.4	90.7	90.7	90.7	90.9	91.0	91.2	91.5	91.7
4.5	86.2	86.8	87.4	87.8	88.3	88.7	88.9	89.0	89.1	89.1	89.3	89.5	89.7
5.0	83.6	84.3	84.9	85.5	85.8	86.0	86.4	86.9	86.8	86.8	87.2	87.5	87.9
5.5	81.1	82.2	82.7	83.2	83.7	84.1	84.5	84.9	85.0	85.1	85.4	85.6	85.9
6.0	78.7	79.4	80.5	81.1	81.7	82.2	82.5	82.7	82.9	83.1	83.4	83.7	84.0
6.5	76.3	77.2	78.3	79.2	79.7	80.2	80.6	81.0	81.3	81.5	81.7	81.8	81.9
7.0	74.2	75.3	75.9	76.8	77.6	78.3	78.7	79.1	79.3	79.4	79.7	79.9	80.2
7.5	71.8	72.9	74.2	74.7	75.3	76.0	76.4	76.9	77.3	77.7	78.0	78.3	78.7
8.0	69.5	70.8	71.8	72.8	73.5	74.2	74.5	74.9	75.3	74.1	74.5	74.9	75.3
8.5	67.7	68.5	69.8	70.7	71.4	72.1	72.6	73.1	73.6	71.8	72.3	72.8	73.3
9.0	65.4	66.6	68.0	68.4	69.3	70.3	70.8	71.3	71.6	70.3	70.8	71.2	71.7
9.5	63.3	64.7	65.6	66.8	67.5	68.2	68.8	69.4	69.9	70.3	70.8	71.2	71.7
10.0	61.7	62.7	63.9	64.9	65.8	66.6	67.1	67.6	68.1	68.5	69.0	69.5	70.0
10.5	59.6	61.0	62.3	63.1	63.8	64.6	65.3	66.1	66.5	67.0	67.4	67.8	68.2
11.0	58.0	59.1	60.4	61.5	62.3	63.1	63.7	64.3	64.7	65.1	65.6	66.1	66.6
11.5	56.1	57.4	58.6	59.7	60.5	61.3	61.9	62.4	62.9	63.4	64.0	64.5	65.0
12.0	54.3	55.6	56.9	58.0	58.9	59.8	60.3	60.9	61.5	62.0	62.4	62.9	63.3
12.5	52.9	53.9	55.3	56.2	57.2	58.3	58.9	59.5	60.0	60.4	61.0	61.6	62.2
13.0	51.2	52.5	53.5	54.7	55.6	56.5	57.2	57.9	58.4	58.9	59.5	60.0	60.6
13.5	49.5	50.9	52.1	53.0	54.0	55.0	55.7	56.4	56.9	57.4	57.9	58.4	59.0
14.0	48.0	49.3	50.6	51.6	52.5	53.3	54.1	55.0	55.4	55.9	56.5	57.2	57.8
14.5	46.7	48.0	49.2	50.1	51.0	52.0	52.6	53.3	53.9	54.6	55.2	55.7	56.3
15.0	45.5	46.5	47.7	48.7	49.6	50.4	51.1	51.8	52.5	53.2	53.7	54.2	54.7
15.5	44.1	45.3	46.4	47.3	48.3	49.4	50.0	50.6	51.2	51.8	52.4	53.0	53.6
16.0	42.7	43.9	45.3	46.2	47.1	48.0	48.6	49.2	49.9	50.6	51.0	51.5	52.0
16.5	41.6	42.5	43.6	44.7	45.6	46.6	47.3	48.0	48.5	49.1	49.6	50.2	50.8
17.0	40.3	41.4	42.4	43.5	44.4	45.4	46.0	46.6	47.3	48.0	48.5	49.1	49.6
17.5	39.1	40.2	41.2	42.2	43.2	44.1	44.8	45.5	46.0	46.5	47.1	47.6	48.2
18.0	37.8	39.0	40.1	41.1	41.9	42.7	43.5	44.2	44.7	45.3	45.9	46.5	47.1
18.5	36.8	37.9	38.9	40.0	40.9	41.8	42.5	43.2	43.7	44.2	44.8	45.3	45.9
19.0	35.7	36.8	37.7	38.9	39.7	40.6	41.3	41.9	42.5	43.2	43.7	44.3	44.9
19.5	34.6	35.6	36.7	37.6	38.6	39.5	40.1	40.7	41.3	42.0	42.5	43.1	43.6
20.0	33.6	34.6	35.6	36.6	37.5	38.3	39.0	39.7	40.3	41.0	41.5	42.0	42.6
20.5	32.6	33.5	34.7	35.7	36.5	37.2	37.9	38.6	39.3	40.0	40.5	41.0	41.4
21.0	31.5	32.7	33.7	34.6	35.4	36.3	36.9	37.5	38.2	38.9	39.4	39.9	40.4
21.5	30.7	31.8	32.7	33.9	34.6	35.2	35.9	36.6	37.3	37.9	38.4	39.0	39.5
22.0	30.0	30.8	31.7	32.8	33.5	34.2	35.0	35.8	36.3	36.9	37.4	37.9	38.5
22.5	29.0	29.8	30.8	31.9	32.7	33.4	34.0	34.6	35.3	36.0	36.4	36.9	37.4
23.0	28.2	29.0	30.0	30.9	31.7	32.4	33.1	33.8	34.3	34.9	35.4	35.9	36.4
23.5	27.3	28.2	29.1	30.0	30.7	31.5	32.2	32.9	33.5	34.2	34.6	35.1	35.6
24.0	26.6	27.4	28.4	29.3	30.0	30.8	31.4	32.0	32.7	33.3	33.8	34.3	34.8
24.5	25.8	26.6	27.4	28.3	29.1	29.9	30.4	31.0	31.6	32.3	32.8	33.2	33.7
25.0	25.0	25.7	26.8	27.6	28.3	28.9	29.7	30.4	30.8	31.3	31.9	32.5	33.1

Mevalac – 6 MV Percent Depth Dose (cont.)

SSD = 100.0 cm – Normalized to depth $d_0 = 1.5$ cm – Field Size defined at 100.0 cm

Depth (cm)	Field Size (cm)								
	16x16	17x17	18x18	19x19	20x20	25x25	30x30	35x35	40x40
0.5	87.5	87.9	88.3	88.8	89.2	90.1	91.3	91.8	92.3
1.0	98.7	98.8	98.9	99.0	99.1	99.0	99.4	99.4	99.5
1.5	100.0	100.0	100.0	100.0	100.0	100.0	100.0	100.0	100.0
2.0	98.8	98.9	98.9	99.0	99.1	98.4	98.5	99.0	98.9
2.5	97.3	97.3	97.3	97.3	97.3	96.9	97.3	97.3	97.6
3.0	95.5	95.5	95.5	95.5	95.6	95.2	95.6	96.0	95.8
3.5	93.6	93.6	93.7	93.7	93.8	94.0	94.0	94.3	94.5
4.0	91.8	91.9	92.0	92.1	92.2	92.2	92.4	92.6	93.2
4.5	89.8	89.9	90.0	90.2	90.3	90.4	90.7	91.1	91.2
5.0	88.0	88.1	88.1	88.2	88.3	88.7	89.1	89.4	89.9
5.5	86.0	86.1	86.2	86.3	86.5	86.8	87.4	87.8	88.4
6.0	84.1	84.2	84.4	84.5	84.7	85.1	85.9	86.4	86.9
6.5	82.2	82.5	82.7	83.0	83.3	84.0	84.3	84.8	85.5
7.0	80.4	80.6	80.9	81.1	81.3	82.0	82.8	83.3	83.9
7.5	78.9	79.0	79.2	79.4	79.6	80.5	81.0	81.8	82.6
8.0	77.0	77.3	77.5	77.7	77.9	78.6	79.6	80.1	80.7
8.5	75.5	75.7	75.9	76.1	76.3	77.2	78.0	78.6	79.3
9.0	73.6	73.8	74.1	74.4	74.6	75.5	76.3	77.2	77.7
9.5	72.0	72.2	72.5	72.8	73.0	73.8	75.0	75.6	76.2
10.0	70.3	70.7	71.0	71.3	71.6	72.2	73.6	74.0	74.6
10.5	68.6	69.0	69.3	69.7	70.0	70.6	71.9	72.7	73.5
11.0	67.0	67.3	67.6	67.9	68.2	69.2	70.3	71.3	72.0
11.5	65.4	65.7	66.1	66.5	66.8	67.8	68.8	69.9	70.6
12.0	63.7	64.1	64.6	65.0	65.4	66.4	67.5	68.3	69.1
12.5	62.5	62.9	63.2	63.5	63.9	64.9	66.3	67.0	67.7
13.0	60.9	61.3	61.6	61.9	62.3	63.6	64.9	65.7	66.5
13.5	59.3	59.7	60.1	60.4	60.8	62.0	63.3	64.3	65.1
14.0	58.0	58.3	58.6	58.9	59.2	60.7	62.0	63.1	63.6
14.5	56.6	56.9	57.2	57.6	57.9	59.3	60.6	61.6	62.4
15.0	55.1	55.6	56.0	56.4	56.9	58.0	59.5	60.3	61.0
15.5	53.9	54.3	54.7	55.0	55.4	57.0	57.9	59.0	59.9
16.0	52.4	52.8	53.2	53.6	54.0	55.5	56.8	57.9	58.5
16.5	51.2	51.6	52.0	52.4	52.8	54.2	55.5	56.8	57.2
17.0	50.0	50.5	50.9	51.3	51.8	53.3	54.5	55.3	56.1
17.5	48.7	49.1	49.5	50.0	50.4	51.8	53.3	54.2	55.0
18.0	47.5	47.9	48.4	48.8	49.2	50.7	52.0	52.9	53.9
18.5	46.3	46.7	47.1	47.6	48.0	49.5	50.7	51.7	52.7
19.0	45.3	45.7	46.1	46.5	46.9	48.3	49.7	50.5	51.6
19.5	44.0	44.4	44.8	45.2	45.6	47.3	48.8	49.6	50.6
20.0	43.0	43.4	43.8	44.2	44.6	46.1	47.4	48.6	49.2
20.5	41.8	42.2	42.6	43.0	43.4	44.9	46.3	47.3	48.3
21.0	40.8	41.2	41.6	42.0	42.4	44.0	45.3	46.3	47.2
21.5	39.9	40.3	40.7	41.1	41.6	43.0	44.4	45.3	46.1
22.0	38.8	39.2	39.6	40.0	40.4	41.9	43.3	44.3	45.1
22.5	37.8	38.3	38.7	39.2	39.6	40.9	42.3	43.2	44.1
23.0	36.8	37.3	37.7	38.1	38.6	40.1	41.4	42.3	43.2
23.5	36.0	36.4	36.8	37.3	37.7	39.1	40.4	41.5	42.3
24.0	35.2	35.5	35.9	36.3	36.7	38.4	39.6	40.5	41.3
24.5	34.1	34.6	35.0	35.4	35.8	37.2	38.6	39.6	40.2
25.0	33.5	33.8	34.2	34.6	35.0	36.3	37.7	38.6	39.5

Mevalac – 18 MV Percent Depth Dose

SSD = 100.0 cm – Normalized to depth d_0 = 3.0 cm – Field Size defined at 100.0 cm

Depth (cm)	Field Size (cm)												
	3x3	4x4	5x5	6x6	7x7	8x8	9x9	10x10	11x11	12x12	13x13	14x14	15x15
0.5	53.2	53.8	54.6	55.8	57.0	58.1	59.7	61.4	62.5	63.6	64.6	65.5	66.5
1.0	75.5	75.9	76.2	77.2	78.1	79.0	80.0	81.0	81.8	82.6	83.3	83.9	84.6
1.5	88.0	88.0	88.4	89.0	89.6	90.1	90.8	91.5	91.9	92.3	92.7	93.1	93.6
2.0	95.4	95.3	95.4	95.3	95.7	96.1	96.5	97.0	97.3	97.7	97.7	97.8	97.9
2.5	98.5	98.7	98.7	98.8	99.0	99.2	99.3	99.4	99.4	99.3	99.4	99.4	99.5
3.0	100.0	100.0	100.0	100.0	100.0	100.0	100.0	100.0	100.0	100.0	100.0	100.0	100.0
3.5	99.6	100.3	99.5	100.1	100.0	99.9	99.9	100.0	100.0	100.0	99.7	99.3	98.9
4.0	98.7	99.4	99.2	99.4	99.0	98.7	98.7	98.7	98.7	98.7	98.5	98.3	98.1
4.5	97.3	97.7	97.7	97.8	97.7	97.5	97.4	97.3	97.2	97.0	96.8	96.6	96.4
5.0	95.7	96.2	96.3	96.0	96.0	96.1	95.8	95.5	95.7	95.9	95.6	95.2	94.8
5.5	93.1	94.2	95.0	94.2	94.3	94.4	94.3	94.2	94.2	94.2	94.0	93.8	93.5
6.0	91.1	92.3	92.3	92.3	92.4	92.4	92.3	92.2	92.1	92.0	91.9	91.8	91.6
6.5	89.4	90.3	90.9	90.6	90.5	90.5	90.5	90.6	90.5	90.4	90.4	90.4	90.4
7.0	87.4	88.5	88.7	88.8	88.7	88.7	88.7	88.7	88.9	89.1	88.8	88.5	88.3
7.5	85.2	86.2	86.7	86.7	86.9	87.1	87.1	87.1	87.0	87.0	86.9	86.8	86.7
8.0	83.4	84.5	84.9	85.1	85.1	85.2	85.3	85.4	85.5	85.7	85.5	85.4	85.2
8.5	81.2	82.3	82.7	83.0	83.0	83.0	83.4	83.7	83.7	83.6	83.6	83.6	83.5
9.0	79.3	80.6	81.7	81.4	81.6	81.8	81.8	81.8	82.0	82.2	82.2	82.2	82.2
9.5	77.8	78.7	79.1	79.8	79.8	79.9	80.1	80.2	80.3	80.4	80.4	80.4	80.4
10.0	76.0	77.0	77.7	78.0	78.2	78.5	78.5	78.5	78.6	78.7	78.7	78.7	78.8
10.5	74.5	75.4	75.7	76.3	76.5	76.8	77.0	77.1	77.3	77.4	77.4	77.4	77.5
11.0	72.4	73.6	74.1	74.6	74.8	75.1	75.4	75.7	75.8	75.9	75.9	75.9	75.9
11.5	70.7	71.7	72.5	73.0	73.3	73.5	73.8	74.1	74.3	74.5	74.5	74.6	74.7
12.0	69.2	70.4	71.0	71.6	71.7	71.9	72.3	72.7	72.8	73.0	73.0	73.0	73.0
12.5	67.8	68.8	69.6	69.8	70.3	70.7	70.8	70.9	71.2	71.5	71.7	71.9	72.1
13.0	66.1	67.3	68.0	68.5	68.8	69.0	69.3	69.6	69.7	69.8	69.9	70.0	70.1
13.5	64.8	65.9	66.3	66.9	67.2	67.5	67.9	68.3	68.4	68.4	68.6	68.9	69.1
14.0	63.3	64.2	64.9	65.3	65.9	66.4	66.7	66.9	67.1	67.3	67.4	67.6	67.8
14.5	61.9	63.1	63.5	64.0	64.4	64.8	65.0	65.2	65.5	65.9	66.0	66.1	66.2
15.0	60.3	61.3	62.3	62.3	62.8	63.3	63.8	64.3	64.3	64.4	64.6	64.7	64.9
15.5	58.7	60.2	60.9	61.2	61.6	62.0	62.2	62.4	62.8	63.3	63.4	63.6	63.8
16.0	57.7	58.7	59.3	59.8	60.2	60.6	61.1	61.6	61.7	61.9	62.1	62.2	62.4
16.5	56.4	57.4	57.9	58.7	58.9	59.2	59.7	60.2	60.5	60.8	61.0	61.1	61.3
17.0	55.1	56.1	56.9	57.5	57.9	58.4	58.7	59.1	59.3	59.5	59.6	59.7	59.8
17.5	53.9	54.9	55.9	56.4	56.6	56.8	57.3	57.7	58.0	58.2	58.4	58.6	58.8
18.0	52.8	53.6	54.4	54.7	55.3	55.8	56.2	56.7	56.8	57.0	57.2	57.5	57.7
18.5	51.4	52.6	53.5	53.8	54.1	54.4	54.9	55.4	55.6	55.8	56.0	56.2	56.4
19.0	50.5	51.2	52.0	52.6	52.9	53.2	53.7	54.2	54.4	54.7	54.9	55.1	55.2
19.5	49.2	50.1	50.7	51.4	51.8	52.2	52.6	53.0	53.3	53.7	53.9	54.1	54.4
20.5	47.1	47.7	48.7	49.3	49.7	50.0	50.4	50.8	51.2	51.5	51.8	52.0	52.3
21.0	46.2	46.9	47.6	48.1	48.5	48.9	49.3	49.7	50.0	50.3	50.7	51.0	51.4
21.5	44.9	45.6	46.6	47.3	47.8	48.2	48.6	49.1	49.3	49.5	49.7	50.0	50.2
22.0	44.0	44.8	45.7	46.1	46.5	47.0	47.4	47.9	48.2	48.4	48.7	49.0	49.3
22.5	42.9	43.7	44.4	45.0	45.6	46.1	46.6	47.1	47.4	47.7	47.8	47.9	48.1
23.0	42.0	42.8	43.6	44.2	44.6	45.0	45.3	45.7	46.2	46.7	46.9	47.1	47.3
23.5	41.1	41.9	42.9	43.3	43.8	44.2	44.7	45.1	45.3	45.5	45.8	46.1	46.5
24.0	40.3	40.9	41.5	42.2	42.8	43.3	43.7	44.1	44.3	44.6	44.9	45.1	45.4
24.5	39.5	40.1	40.9	41.5	41.8	42.1	42.6	43.0	43.4	43.7	44.0	44.2	44.5
25.0	38.3	39.2	40.0	40.3	40.9	41.4	41.9	42.3	42.6	43.0	43.2	43.5	43.7

Mevalac – 18 MV Percent Depth Dose (cont.)

SSD = 100.0 cm – Normalized to depth d_0 = 3.0 cm – Field Size defined at 100.0 cm

Depth (cm)	Field Size (cm)								
	16x16	17x17	18x18	19x19	20x20	25x25	30x30	35x35	40x40
0.5	67.5	68.6	69.7	70.8	71.9	75.1	76.9	78.2	78.4
1.0	85.3	86.0	86.8	87.5	88.2	90.3	90.9	91.6	91.3
1.5	94.0	94.4	94.8	95.2	95.7	97.5	97.1	97.2	97.6
2.0	98.1	98.4	98.6	98.9	99.1	100.0	100.0	99.8	99.8
2.5	99.6	99.7	99.8	100.0	100.1	100.6	99.9	100.5	100.1
3.0	100.0	100.0	100.0	100.0	100.0	100.0	100.0	100.0	100.0
3.5	98.9	98.9	98.9	98.9	98.9	98.8	98.8	99.2	99.2
4.0	98.1	98.1	98.2	98.2	98.2	98.0	97.7	97.9	98.0
4.5	96.3	96.2	96.1	96.0	95.9	96.1	96.1	96.4	96.5
5.0	94.8	94.8	94.7	94.7	94.7	95.0	94.7	94.9	95.2
5.5	93.5	93.5	93.5	93.4	93.4	93.4	93.2	93.7	93.6
6.0	91.7	91.7	91.7	91.7	91.8	91.9	91.4	92.1	92.0
6.5	90.3	90.2	90.1	90.0	89.9	90.3	90.1	90.7	90.7
7.0	88.3	88.3	88.3	88.4	88.4	88.9	88.6	89.0	89.3
7.5	86.7	86.7	86.8	86.8	86.8	87.2	87.3	87.5	87.9
8.0	85.2	85.2	85.2	85.3	85.3	85.7	86.1	86.2	86.5
8.5	83.6	83.6	83.6	83.7	83.7	84.3	84.4	85.0	84.9
9.0	82.1	82.1	82.1	82.0	82.0	82.6	82.9	83.3	83.5
9.5	80.5	80.6	80.7	80.8	80.9	81.3	81.6	81.7	82.1
10.0	78.8	78.9	78.9	79.0	79.1	79.8	79.8	80.6	80.5
10.5	77.6	77.7	77.8	77.9	78.0	78.6	78.5	79.0	79.5
11.0	76.0	76.1	76.3	76.4	76.5	77.1	77.0	77.8	77.9
11.5	74.7	74.8	74.8	74.9	74.9	75.5	75.9	76.4	76.9
12.0	73.1	73.3	73.4	73.6	73.7	74.6	74.5	75.2	75.6
12.5	72.1	72.1	72.1	72.1	72.1	73.1	73.1	74.1	74.4
13.0	70.2	70.3	70.5	70.6	70.7	71.6	71.9	72.7	72.8
13.5	69.2	69.2	69.3	69.4	69.5	70.5	70.8	71.2	71.8
14.0	67.9	68.0	68.1	68.2	68.3	69.0	69.3	70.3	70.2
14.5	66.4	66.5	66.6	66.8	66.9	67.6	68.3	68.9	69.2
15.0	65.0	65.2	65.4	65.6	65.8	66.7	66.8	67.6	68.0
15.5	64.0	64.1	64.3	64.5	64.7	65.3	66.0	66.5	66.9
16.0	62.6	62.8	63.0	63.1	63.3	64.1	64.4	65.3	65.7
16.5	61.5	61.7	61.8	62.0	62.2	63.1	63.4	64.0	64.4
17.0	60.1	60.3	60.6	60.8	61.1	61.6	62.3	63.0	63.4
17.5	59.0	59.2	59.4	59.7	59.9	60.7	61.3	61.9	62.1
18.0	57.9	58.0	58.2	58.3	58.5	59.5	60.0	60.8	61.3
18.5	56.6	56.8	57.0	57.2	57.4	58.5	59.0	59.6	60.0
19.0	55.5	55.8	56.1	56.4	56.6	57.6	58.0	58.7	59.2
19.5	54.6	54.9	55.1	55.3	55.6	56.3	56.6	57.7	58.0
20.0	53.3	53.6	53.9	54.1	54.4	55.0	55.6	56.4	57.1
20.5	52.5	52.7	52.8	53.0	53.2	54.5	54.7	55.4	56.0
21.0	51.5	51.7	51.9	52.0	52.2	53.3	54.0	54.6	55.0
21.5	50.4	50.6	50.8	51.0	51.3	52.1	52.7	53.5	54.0
22.0	49.5	49.7	49.8	50.0	50.2	51.4	51.8	52.6	52.9
22.5	48.3	48.5	48.8	49.0	49.2	50.1	50.9	51.4	52.0
23.0	47.5	47.8	48.0	48.2	48.5	49.5	49.9	50.6	51.0
23.5	46.7	46.8	47.0	47.2	47.4	48.4	49.1	49.7	50.1
24.0	45.7	46.0	46.3	46.5	46.8	47.4	48.0	48.9	49.3
24.5	44.7	44.9	45.1	45.4	45.6	46.6	47.4	47.7	48.4
25.0	43.9	44.2	44.4	44.6	44.9	45.8	46.2	47.1	47.3

Mevalac – 6 MV TMR Data

$d_0 = 1.5$ cm

Depth (cm)	Field Size (cm)												
	3x3	4x4	5x5	6x6	7x7	8x8	9x9	10x10	11x11	12x12	13x13	14x14	15x15
0.5	0.797	0.798	0.815	0.819	0.824	0.829	0.833	0.836	0.840	0.844	0.849	0.853	0.858
1.0	0.959	0.957	0.961	0.960	0.960	0.960	0.964	0.967	0.967	0.966	0.968	0.970	0.972
1.5	1.000	1.000	1.000	1.000	1.000	1.000	1.000	1.000	1.000	1.000	1.000	1.000	1.000
2.0	0.993	0.997	1.001	0.997	0.999	1.000	0.999	0.997	0.997	0.997	0.996	0.996	0.995
2.5	0.984	0.982	0.985	0.987	0.989	0.991	0.993	0.994	0.993	0.992	0.991	0.991	0.990
3.0	0.964	0.968	0.970	0.974	0.976	0.977	0.977	0.977	0.977	0.976	0.977	0.979	0.980
3.5	0.948	0.952	0.957	0.959	0.961	0.963	0.965	0.966	0.967	0.967	0.968	0.968	0.969
4.0	0.930	0.936	0.941	0.945	0.948	0.950	0.951	0.952	0.953	0.954	0.956	0.957	0.959
4.5	0.912	0.920	0.924	0.929	0.933	0.937	0.940	0.943	0.943	0.943	0.944	0.945	0.946
5.0	0.892	0.901	0.907	0.913	0.916	0.919	0.923	0.927	0.928	0.928	0.930	0.933	0.935
5.5	0.872	0.885	0.891	0.897	0.901	0.905	0.910	0.914	0.916	0.917	0.919	0.921	0.923
6.0	0.855	0.864	0.874	0.881	0.887	0.893	0.897	0.900	0.902	0.903	0.906	0.908	0.911
6.5	0.836	0.847	0.857	0.867	0.873	0.879	0.884	0.889	0.892	0.894	0.895	0.897	0.898
7.0	0.820	0.833	0.840	0.848	0.856	0.864	0.870	0.876	0.878	0.880	0.882	0.884	0.886
7.5	0.802	0.815	0.826	0.835	0.841	0.846	0.853	0.859	0.863	0.866	0.869	0.873	0.876
8.0	0.782	0.797	0.808	0.818	0.826	0.833	0.839	0.844	0.848	0.851	0.855	0.859	0.863
8.5	0.768	0.780	0.791	0.802	0.810	0.817	0.824	0.831	0.835	0.839	0.843	0.848	0.852
9.0	0.750	0.763	0.776	0.786	0.794	0.802	0.810	0.817	0.820	0.823	0.827	0.832	0.836
9.5	0.733	0.747	0.758	0.769	0.778	0.786	0.794	0.801	0.806	0.810	0.815	0.819	0.824
10.0	0.718	0.731	0.742	0.755	0.764	0.773	0.781	0.788	0.792	0.796	0.801	0.806	0.811
10.5	0.702	0.716	0.729	0.741	0.749	0.757	0.766	0.774	0.780	0.785	0.790	0.794	0.799
11.0	0.688	0.701	0.713	0.726	0.736	0.745	0.753	0.761	0.766	0.770	0.775	0.780	0.785
11.5	0.671	0.686	0.698	0.711	0.720	0.729	0.737	0.745	0.750	0.755	0.761	0.766	0.772
12.0	0.656	0.670	0.683	0.697	0.707	0.716	0.725	0.734	0.739	0.744	0.749	0.754	0.759
12.5	0.644	0.656	0.669	0.682	0.692	0.702	0.712	0.721	0.726	0.731	0.737	0.743	0.749
13.0	0.628	0.642	0.654	0.666	0.677	0.688	0.698	0.707	0.713	0.718	0.724	0.730	0.736
13.5	0.613	0.627	0.640	0.653	0.663	0.673	0.684	0.694	0.700	0.705	0.711	0.716	0.722
14.0	0.599	0.613	0.626	0.640	0.650	0.659	0.669	0.679	0.686	0.693	0.699	0.705	0.711
14.5	0.588	0.602	0.614	0.627	0.637	0.646	0.656	0.666	0.672	0.678	0.685	0.692	0.699
15.0	0.576	0.589	0.600	0.614	0.624	0.633	0.643	0.652	0.659	0.665	0.672	0.679	0.686
15.5	0.563	0.577	0.589	0.602	0.612	0.622	0.633	0.643	0.649	0.654	0.661	0.668	0.675
16.0	0.551	0.564	0.577	0.592	0.602	0.611	0.621	0.631	0.637	0.642	0.649	0.656	0.663
16.5	0.539	0.552	0.562	0.575	0.586	0.597	0.607	0.617	0.624	0.631	0.637	0.644	0.650
17.0	0.527	0.541	0.552	0.564	0.575	0.585	0.596	0.606	0.612	0.618	0.625	0.633	0.640
17.5	0.513	0.529	0.540	0.552	0.563	0.573	0.584	0.594	0.601	0.608	0.614	0.620	0.626
18.0	0.502	0.516	0.529	0.541	0.551	0.561	0.571	0.581	0.588	0.595	0.601	0.608	0.614
18.5	0.491	0.506	0.517	0.530	0.541	0.551	0.562	0.572	0.579	0.585	0.591	0.598	0.604
19.0	0.480	0.496	0.506	0.517	0.529	0.540	0.550	0.560	0.567	0.573	0.580	0.588	0.595
19.5	0.471	0.484	0.495	0.508	0.518	0.528	0.539	0.549	0.555	0.561	0.568	0.576	0.583
20.0	0.461	0.474	0.485	0.497	0.507	0.517	0.527	0.537	0.544	0.551	0.558	0.566	0.573
20.5	0.450	0.463	0.473	0.487	0.497	0.507	0.517	0.526	0.533	0.540	0.548	0.555	0.563
21.0	0.440	0.453	0.465	0.476	0.486	0.496	0.506	0.516	0.523	0.529	0.537	0.544	0.552
21.5	0.431	0.444	0.455	0.466	0.477	0.488	0.497	0.505	0.513	0.520	0.527	0.535	0.542
22.0	0.422	0.436	0.444	0.456	0.466	0.476	0.485	0.494	0.503	0.511	0.518	0.525	0.532
22.5	0.412	0.425	0.433	0.446	0.457	0.468	0.477	0.486	0.492	0.498	0.506	0.514	0.522
23.0	0.403	0.417	0.425	0.437	0.447	0.457	0.467	0.476	0.483	0.490	0.497	0.504	0.511
23.5	0.394	0.407	0.416	0.428	0.438	0.447	0.457	0.466	0.474	0.481	0.488	0.496	0.503
24.0	0.385	0.399	0.408	0.420	0.430	0.439	0.449	0.458	0.465	0.472	0.479	0.487	0.494
24.5	0.377	0.389	0.398	0.408	0.419	0.429	0.439	0.448	0.454	0.460	0.467	0.475	0.482
25.0	0.370	0.381	0.388	0.402	0.411	0.420	0.429	0.437	0.446	0.454	0.460	0.465	0.471

Mevalac – 6 MV TMR Data (cont.)

$d_0 = 1.5$ cm

Depth (cm)	Field Size (cm)								
	16x16	17x17	18x18	19x19	20x20	25x25	30x30	35x35	40x40
0.5	0.862	0.866	0.870	0.875	0.879	0.887	0.899	0.904	0.909
1.0	0.974	0.975	0.976	0.978	0.979	0.978	0.982	0.982	0.983
1.5	1.000	1.000	1.000	1.000	1.000	0.999	0.999	1.000	0.999
2.0	0.996	0.997	0.998	0.999	1.000	0.995	0.995	0.998	0.998
2.5	0.990	0.990	0.991	0.991	0.992	0.989	0.991	0.992	0.995
3.0	0.980	0.981	0.982	0.982	0.983	0.980	0.984	0.987	0.986
3.5	0.970	0.971	0.972	0.972	0.973	0.976	0.977	0.979	0.981
4.0	0.960	0.962	0.963	0.964	0.966	0.967	0.969	0.971	0.976
4.5	0.948	0.950	0.951	0.953	0.955	0.957	0.960	0.964	0.966
5.0	0.937	0.938	0.940	0.941	0.943	0.947	0.952	0.955	0.959
5.5	0.924	0.926	0.928	0.930	0.931	0.936	0.942	0.945	0.951
6.0	0.912	0.914	0.916	0.918	0.920	0.925	0.933	0.938	0.944
6.5	0.901	0.903	0.906	0.909	0.911	0.921	0.926	0.930	0.936
7.0	0.888	0.891	0.893	0.896	0.898	0.908	0.916	0.921	0.928
7.5	0.878	0.881	0.883	0.885	0.888	0.898	0.905	0.911	0.920
8.0	0.865	0.868	0.871	0.874	0.876	0.886	0.896	0.902	0.908
8.5	0.855	0.857	0.860	0.863	0.865	0.876	0.886	0.892	0.899
9.0	0.839	0.842	0.846	0.849	0.853	0.864	0.875	0.882	0.891
9.5	0.827	0.831	0.835	0.838	0.842	0.853	0.865	0.874	0.880
10.0	0.815	0.819	0.823	0.827	0.831	0.843	0.855	0.864	0.870
10.5	0.803	0.807	0.811	0.815	0.819	0.831	0.842	0.853	0.862
11.0	0.789	0.793	0.797	0.801	0.806	0.820	0.833	0.842	0.853
11.5	0.776	0.781	0.786	0.790	0.795	0.810	0.822	0.832	0.844
12.0	0.764	0.768	0.773	0.778	0.782	0.800	0.813	0.822	0.832
12.5	0.753	0.758	0.763	0.767	0.772	0.788	0.802	0.814	0.823
13.0	0.740	0.745	0.750	0.754	0.759	0.776	0.792	0.803	0.813
13.5	0.727	0.732	0.736	0.741	0.746	0.764	0.780	0.791	0.802
14.0	0.716	0.721	0.725	0.730	0.734	0.752	0.769	0.781	0.793
14.5	0.704	0.709	0.713	0.718	0.723	0.741	0.758	0.769	0.782
15.0	0.691	0.696	0.701	0.707	0.712	0.732	0.748	0.761	0.771
15.5	0.680	0.685	0.690	0.696	0.701	0.721	0.739	0.747	0.761
16.0	0.668	0.672	0.677	0.682	0.687	0.709	0.727	0.739	0.753
16.5	0.655	0.660	0.666	0.671	0.677	0.698	0.716	0.728	0.743
17.0	0.645	0.651	0.656	0.662	0.667	0.690	0.708	0.720	0.730
17.5	0.632	0.637	0.643	0.649	0.654	0.678	0.696	0.710	0.721
18.0	0.620	0.626	0.632	0.638	0.643	0.667	0.685	0.699	0.709
18.5	0.610	0.615	0.621	0.626	0.632	0.656	0.675	0.686	0.699
19.0	0.600	0.606	0.612	0.617	0.623	0.646	0.663	0.678	0.689
19.5	0.589	0.594	0.600	0.605	0.611	0.634	0.654	0.670	0.681
20.0	0.578	0.584	0.589	0.594	0.600	0.623	0.644	0.657	0.671
20.5	0.568	0.573	0.579	0.584	0.589	0.611	0.631	0.647	0.659
21.0	0.557	0.563	0.568	0.573	0.579	0.602	0.622	0.636	0.650
21.5	0.548	0.553	0.559	0.565	0.570	0.595	0.614	0.628	0.640
22.0	0.537	0.543	0.548	0.554	0.559	0.582	0.602	0.617	0.631
22.5	0.528	0.533	0.538	0.543	0.549	0.575	0.593	0.608	0.621
23.0	0.516	0.522	0.527	0.533	0.538	0.565	0.585	0.599	0.611
23.5	0.509	0.514	0.519	0.525	0.530	0.556	0.574	0.589	0.603
24.0	0.500	0.505	0.511	0.516	0.521	0.545	0.567	0.582	0.594
24.5	0.488	0.494	0.499	0.505	0.510	0.535	0.555	0.570	0.584
25.0	0.477	0.484	0.490	0.497	0.503	0.528	0.545	0.560	0.574

Mevalac – 18 MV TMR Data

$d_0 = 3.0$ cm

Depth (cm)	Field Size (cm)									
	3x3	4x4	5x5	6x6	7x7	8x8	9x9	10x10	12x12	15x15
0.5	0.519	0.524	0.532	0.543	0.554	0.565	0.580	0.595	0.616	0.642
1.0	0.733	0.736	0.740	0.748	0.757	0.766	0.775	0.784	0.800	0.817
1.5	0.860	0.860	0.864	0.869	0.874	0.879	0.885	0.891	0.898	0.911
2.0	0.939	0.938	0.940	0.938	0.941	0.944	0.948	0.952	0.959	0.961
2.5	0.978	0.980	0.980	0.980	0.982	0.983	0.984	0.985	0.985	0.985
3.0	1.001	1.001	1.002	1.001	1.001	1.001	1.001	1.001	1.003	1.002
3.5	1.005	1.013	1.007	1.011	1.009	1.008	1.008	1.008	1.010	1.001
4.0	1.006	1.013	1.012	1.014	1.010	1.006	1.005	1.004	1.006	1.000
4.5	1.001	1.006	1.006	1.007	1.005	1.003	1.002	1.001	0.999	0.992
5.0	0.993	0.999	1.001	0.998	0.998	0.998	0.996	0.993	0.996	0.987
5.5	0.976	0.986	0.995	0.991	0.991	0.990	0.989	0.987	0.988	0.982
6.0	0.965	0.975	0.977	0.977	0.977	0.977	0.976	0.976	0.974	0.970
6.5	0.954	0.964	0.969	0.968	0.967	0.966	0.966	0.967	0.967	0.965
7.0	0.942	0.952	0.957	0.957	0.956	0.956	0.955	0.955	0.959	0.954
7.5	0.927	0.935	0.941	0.943	0.945	0.946	0.946	0.946	0.947	0.944
8.0	0.916	0.926	0.932	0.934	0.934	0.935	0.935	0.936	0.939	0.937
8.5	0.901	0.910	0.915	0.918	0.919	0.920	0.922	0.924	0.928	0.925
9.0	0.886	0.897	0.909	0.913	0.913	0.913	0.914	0.914	0.917	0.917
9.5	0.878	0.884	0.891	0.896	0.899	0.901	0.902	0.903	0.906	0.906
10.0	0.866	0.874	0.882	0.886	0.889	0.892	0.892	0.892	0.894	0.896
10.5	0.856	0.863	0.868	0.872	0.876	0.880	0.882	0.884	0.887	0.889
11.0	0.842	0.849	0.856	0.860	0.864	0.868	0.871	0.874	0.878	0.878
11.5	0.830	0.834	0.843	0.849	0.853	0.857	0.860	0.862	0.868	0.870
12.0	0.820	0.827	0.835	0.841	0.844	0.847	0.849	0.851	0.858	0.859
12.5	0.810	0.815	0.824	0.830	0.834	0.837	0.840	0.842	0.847	0.853
13.0	0.797	0.803	0.812	0.818	0.822	0.826	0.828	0.830	0.836	0.839
13.5	0.790	0.794	0.801	0.806	0.810	0.814	0.817	0.820	0.827	0.831
14.0	0.779	0.782	0.788	0.794	0.799	0.804	0.808	0.812	0.819	0.822
14.5	0.766	0.772	0.780	0.784	0.789	0.794	0.797	0.800	0.806	0.813
15.0	0.754	0.757	0.767	0.773	0.776	0.780	0.785	0.790	0.799	0.801
15.5	0.743	0.746	0.758	0.763	0.768	0.773	0.775	0.778	0.784	0.793
16.0	0.736	0.737	0.745	0.751	0.756	0.760	0.764	0.768	0.779	0.783
16.5	0.724	0.726	0.735	0.739	0.745	0.750	0.753	0.756	0.769	0.776
17.0	0.715	0.716	0.725	0.733	0.738	0.743	0.747	0.750	0.761	0.765
17.5	0.703	0.706	0.716	0.726	0.730	0.733	0.735	0.737	0.749	0.755
18.0	0.695	0.696	0.705	0.712	0.717	0.722	0.727	0.732	0.742	0.746
18.5	0.684	0.686	0.698	0.706	0.710	0.714	0.717	0.720	0.730	0.736
19.0	0.677	0.678	0.684	0.692	0.697	0.703	0.706	0.708	0.721	0.727
19.5	0.666	0.667	0.674	0.680	0.687	0.694	0.697	0.701	0.710	0.720
20.0	0.658	0.655	0.664	0.673	0.678	0.684	0.688	0.692	0.705	0.711
20.5	0.649	0.647	0.653	0.663	0.669	0.675	0.678	0.681	0.692	0.702
21.0	0.640	0.640	0.647	0.654	0.659	0.664	0.668	0.671	0.683	0.691
21.5	0.632	0.628	0.633	0.644	0.652	0.659	0.663	0.668	0.679	0.685
22.0	0.623	0.621	0.628	0.637	0.642	0.647	0.651	0.655	0.669	0.676
22.5	0.610	0.608	0.617	0.623	0.630	0.638	0.643	0.648	0.662	0.670
23.0	0.604	0.600	0.609	0.618	0.624	0.630	0.634	0.637	0.646	0.662
23.5	0.598	0.593	0.601	0.612	0.617	0.623	0.627	0.632	0.643	0.650
24.0	0.591	0.586	0.592	0.598	0.605	0.612	0.617	0.622	0.634	0.642
24.5	0.579	0.578	0.584	0.592	0.598	0.604	0.607	0.609	0.622	0.634
25.0	0.571	0.566	0.574	0.584	0.589	0.593	0.599	0.604	0.617	0.628

Mevalac – 18 MV TMR Data (cont.)

$d_0 = 3.0$ cm

Depth (cm)	Field Size (cm)				
	20x20	25x25	30x30	35x35	40x40
0.5	0.694	0.724	0.740	0.753	0.755
1.0	0.853	0.871	0.878	0.884	0.883
1.5	0.931	0.947	0.946	0.946	0.950
2.0	0.972	0.981	0.982	0.980	0.981
2.5	0.991	0.995	0.990	0.995	0.993
3.0	1.000	1.000	1.000	1.000	1.000
3.5	0.999	0.996	0.997	1.001	1.002
4.0	1.000	0.998	0.996	0.998	0.999
4.5	0.986	0.988	0.988	0.990	0.992
5.0	0.982	0.985	0.984	0.985	0.987
5.5	0.980	0.979	0.977	0.980	0.981
6.0	0.972	0.972	0.968	0.971	0.973
6.5	0.961	0.962	0.963	0.967	0.968
7.0	0.952	0.955	0.956	0.958	0.961
7.5	0.943	0.947	0.949	0.950	0.953
8.0	0.935	0.939	0.943	0.946	0.947
8.5	0.926	0.931	0.934	0.938	0.940
9.0	0.917	0.921	0.925	0.929	0.931
9.5	0.910	0.914	0.918	0.921	0.922
10.0	0.899	0.904	0.908	0.913	0.917
10.5	0.894	0.899	0.902	0.904	0.908
11.0	0.883	0.891	0.893	0.896	0.901
11.5	0.874	0.878	0.884	0.890	0.894
12.0	0.865	0.873	0.879	0.881	0.886
12.5	0.858	0.863	0.870	0.873	0.882
13.0	0.845	0.853	0.861	0.866	0.873
13.5	0.839	0.847	0.855	0.860	0.862
14.0	0.830	0.837	0.843	0.849	0.857
14.5	0.820	0.827	0.834	0.843	0.847
15.0	0.811	0.821	0.828	0.830	0.838
15.5	0.804	0.813	0.820	0.829	0.832
16.0	0.794	0.803	0.811	0.817	0.824
16.5	0.786	0.796	0.804	0.809	0.814
17.0	0.775	0.787	0.793	0.802	0.807
17.5	0.768	0.780	0.787	0.795	0.801
18.0	0.758	0.768	0.778	0.785	0.792
18.5	0.749	0.761	0.772	0.778	0.783
19.0	0.740	0.756	0.765	0.772	0.778
19.5	0.734	0.748	0.755	0.759	0.769
20.0	0.723	0.738	0.744	0.750	0.758
20.5	0.716	0.728	0.742	0.745	0.751
21.0	0.708	0.719	0.732	0.740	0.746
21.5	0.698	0.711	0.721	0.729	0.736
22.0	0.692	0.703	0.716	0.723	0.729
22.5	0.681	0.695	0.704	0.714	0.720
23.0	0.675	0.688	0.701	0.707	0.712
23.5	0.667	0.677	0.691	0.700	0.706
24.0	0.660	0.676	0.682	0.690	0.697
24.5	0.650	0.663	0.673	0.685	0.691
25.0	0.644	0.657	0.668	0.675	0.681

Mevalac – 6 MV SMR Data

$S_p(0) = 0.925$

$\text{TMR}(d,0) = e^{-\mu(d-d_0)}$ where $\mu = 0.0467$ cm^{-1} and $d_0 = 1.5$ cm

Depth (cm)	Square Field Size (cm)												
	3x3	4x4	5x5	6x6	8x8	10x10	12x12	15x15	20x20	25x25	30x30	35x35	40x40
	Radius												
	1.7	2.3	2.8	3.4	4.5	5.6	6.8	8.5	11.3	14.1	16.9	19.7	22.6
0.5	0.060	0.071	0.093	0.101	0.120	0.134	0.149	0.172	0.201	0.211	0.227	0.232	0.237
1.0	0.042	0.053	0.061	0.065	0.074	0.089	0.096	0.110	0.126	0.126	0.133	0.132	0.133
1.5	0.041	0.054	0.057	0.064	0.073	0.082	0.088	0.098	0.106	0.106	0.109	0.109	0.108
2.0	0.044	0.061	0.070	0.071	0.084	0.088	0.096	0.102	0.115	0.111	0.114	0.116	0.116
2.5	0.045	0.056	0.063	0.071	0.085	0.095	0.101	0.107	0.117	0.115	0.120	0.120	0.123
3.0	0.049	0.066	0.072	0.082	0.094	0.102	0.108	0.121	0.131	0.129	0.137	0.139	0.138
3.5	0.050	0.067	0.076	0.083	0.097	0.107	0.116	0.126	0.138	0.143	0.147	0.148	0.150
4.0	0.053	0.071	0.080	0.090	0.104	0.114	0.123	0.137	0.152	0.154	0.159	0.160	0.166
4.5	0.053	0.073	0.081	0.092	0.109	0.123	0.130	0.142	0.159	0.162	0.168	0.172	0.174
5.0	0.056	0.078	0.088	0.099	0.114	0.130	0.138	0.154	0.170	0.175	0.184	0.186	0.190
5.5	0.058	0.083	0.093	0.104	0.122	0.138	0.148	0.163	0.179	0.185	0.195	0.197	0.204
6.0	0.061	0.082	0.096	0.108	0.130	0.144	0.154	0.171	0.188	0.194	0.206	0.211	0.217
6.5	0.065	0.087	0.102	0.117	0.138	0.156	0.168	0.180	0.201	0.213	0.222	0.225	0.232
7.0	0.059	0.084	0.095	0.108	0.133	0.153	0.164	0.178	0.198	0.210	0.222	0.226	0.234
7.5	0.065	0.089	0.104	0.118	0.138	0.159	0.173	0.191	0.211	0.223	0.234	0.239	0.249
8.0	0.066	0.092	0.107	0.122	0.147	0.165	0.179	0.199	0.220	0.232	0.246	0.252	0.258
8.5	0.065	0.088	0.103	0.119	0.143	0.164	0.179	0.200	0.221	0.234	0.248	0.254	0.262
9.0	0.067	0.090	0.107	0.122	0.147	0.169	0.182	0.203	0.228	0.241	0.256	0.263	0.273
9.5	0.065	0.089	0.104	0.120	0.146	0.168	0.184	0.206	0.232	0.245	0.261	0.270	0.277
10.0	0.066	0.089	0.104	0.122	0.148	0.170	0.185	0.208	0.237	0.251	0.267	0.276	0.282
10.5	0.067	0.091	0.108	0.125	0.149	0.173	0.191	0.213	0.241	0.256	0.270	0.282	0.292
11.0	0.066	0.089	0.104	0.122	0.149	0.172	0.188	0.211	0.240	0.257	0.274	0.283	0.295
11.5	0.066	0.091	0.107	0.124	0.150	0.173	0.190	0.215	0.246	0.264	0.280	0.290	0.303
12.0	0.068	0.091	0.108	0.126	0.153	0.178	0.195	0.218	0.249	0.269	0.286	0.296	0.307
12.5	0.065	0.086	0.102	0.120	0.148	0.174	0.190	0.216	0.247	0.266	0.284	0.296	0.306
13.0	0.063	0.086	0.101	0.118	0.148	0.174	0.191	0.217	0.248	0.267	0.288	0.299	0.310
13.5	0.065	0.087	0.104	0.121	0.149	0.177	0.194	0.219	0.251	0.272	0.292	0.303	0.315
14.0	0.065	0.088	0.104	0.123	0.149	0.176	0.196	0.222	0.253	0.273	0.295	0.307	0.320
14.5	0.062	0.085	0.100	0.117	0.144	0.170	0.188	0.217	0.249	0.270	0.291	0.302	0.317
15.0	0.061	0.082	0.097	0.115	0.141	0.166	0.185	0.214	0.248	0.271	0.291	0.305	0.316
15.5	0.061	0.083	0.099	0.116	0.143	0.170	0.187	0.216	0.250	0.273	0.295	0.303	0.319
16.0	0.064	0.085	0.101	0.120	0.146	0.172	0.189	0.218	0.249	0.274	0.297	0.309	0.325
16.5	0.057	0.078	0.091	0.108	0.137	0.163	0.183	0.209	0.244	0.268	0.290	0.303	0.319
17.0	0.058	0.079	0.093	0.109	0.137	0.164	0.182	0.211	0.246	0.272	0.294	0.307	0.318
17.5	0.058	0.082	0.096	0.111	0.139	0.166	0.186	0.211	0.247	0.274	0.296	0.311	0.323
18.0	0.059	0.080	0.096	0.112	0.139	0.165	0.184	0.210	0.247	0.274	0.296	0.311	0.322
18.5	0.058	0.080	0.094	0.110	0.138	0.165	0.183	0.209	0.245	0.272	0.295	0.307	0.321
19.0	0.054	0.078	0.090	0.105	0.134	0.160	0.178	0.208	0.243	0.269	0.290	0.306	0.318
19.5	0.056	0.076	0.089	0.106	0.132	0.159	0.176	0.205	0.240	0.267	0.291	0.308	0.320

Mevalac – 6 MV SMR Data (cont.)

$S_p(0) = 0.925$

$\text{TMR}(d,0) = e^{-\mu(d-d_0)}$ where $\mu = 0.0467$ cm^{-1} and $d_0 = 1.5$ cm

Depth (cm)	Square Field Size (cm)												
	3x3	4x4	5x5	6x6	8x8	10x10	12x12	15x15	20x20	25x25	30x30	35x35	40x40
	Radius												
	1.7	2.3	2.8	3.4	4.5	5.6	6.8	8.5	11.3	14.1	16.9	19.7	22.6
20.0	0.054	0.074	0.088	0.103	0.129	0.155	0.174	0.203	0.237	0.263	0.289	0.302	0.318
20.5	0.055	0.074	0.087	0.104	0.130	0.155	0.174	0.204	0.237	0.262	0.286	0.303	0.316
21.0	0.054	0.073	0.088	0.102	0.128	0.153	0.171	0.201	0.235	0.261	0.285	0.300	0.316
21.5	0.052	0.071	0.085	0.099	0.127	0.149	0.169	0.198	0.233	0.261	0.284	0.299	0.312
22.0	0.049	0.070	0.080	0.095	0.121	0.144	0.166	0.194	0.228	0.254	0.278	0.294	0.309
22.5	0.049	0.068	0.079	0.095	0.123	0.146	0.163	0.193	0.227	0.256	0.278	0.294	0.309
23.0	0.049	0.069	0.079	0.094	0.120	0.144	0.162	0.190	0.223	0.254	0.278	0.293	0.306
23.5	0.049	0.068	0.079	0.094	0.119	0.142	0.162	0.191	0.224	0.254	0.275	0.291	0.307
24.0	0.049	0.069	0.080	0.095	0.120	0.143	0.162	0.190	0.224	0.251	0.277	0.293	0.307
24.5	0.045	0.063	0.074	0.087	0.113	0.137	0.154	0.182	0.216	0.245	0.268	0.285	0.300
25.0	0.046	0.063	0.072	0.089	0.112	0.134	0.155	0.178	0.217	0.245	0.266	0.282	0.297

Mevalac – 6 MV Off-Axis Ratios (OARs)

Depth d (cm)	Distance off axis u (cm)*					
	0	2	4	6	8	10
1.5	1.000	1.011	1.027	1.037	1.053	1.071
5.0	1.000	1.007	1.023	1.030	1.041	1.056
10.0	1.000	1.006	1.016	1.024	1.029	1.036
15.0	1.000	1.008	1.015	1.017	1.019	1.019

*The distance off axis, u, is measured on a plane perpendicular to the central axis at a source distance of 100 cm.

These are in-phantom off-axis ratios.

Mevalac – 18 MV Off-Axis Ratios (OARs)

Depth d (cm)	Distance off axis u (cm)*					
	0	2	4	6	8	10
3.0	1.000	1.012	1.036	1.042	1.050	1.050
5.0	1.000	1.011	1.030	1.033	1.039	1.038
10.0	1.000	1.011	1.024	1.026	1.029	1.024
20.0	1.000	1.000	1.009	1.003	0.992	0.977

*The distance off axis, u, is measured on a plane perpendicular to the central axis at a source distance of 100 cm.

These are in-phantom off-axis ratios.

6 MV Mevalac Wedge Factors $\mathrm{WF}(d, f_d')$

Maximum field size: 40 cm × 20 cm for 15°, 30°, and 45° and 40 cm × 15 cm for 60°

15°

Depth (cm)	Side of Equivalent Square f_d'				
	5	10	15	20	30
1.5	0.697	0.701	0.712	0.719	0.740
5.0	0.697	0.701	0.712	0.719	0.740
10.0	0.704	0.708	0.719	0.726	0.747
15.0	0.711	0.715	0.726	0.733	0.754
20.0	0.718	0.722	0.733	0.740	0.762
25.0	0.725	0.729	0.740	0.747	0.769

30°

Depth (cm)	Side of Equivalent Square f_d'				
	5	10	15	20	30
1.5	0.532	0.538	0.546	0.560	0.594
5.0	0.532	0.538	0.546	0.560	0.594
10.0	0.542	0.549	0.557	0.571	0.606
15.0	0.553	0.560	0.568	0.582	0.618
20.0	0.558	0.565	0.573	0.587	0.624
25.0	0.563	0.570	0.579	0.593	0.630

45°

Depth (cm)	Side of Equivalent Square f_d'			
	5	10	15	20
1.5	0.480	0.482	0.491	0.499
5.0	0.480	0.482	0.491	0.499
10.0	0.494	0.496	0.506	0.514
15.0	0.504	0.506	0.516	0.524
20.0	0.514	0.516	0.526	0.534
25.0	0.523	0.525	0.535	0.544

60°

Depth (cm)	Side of Equivalent Square f_d'			
	5	10	15	20
1.5	0.395	0.399	0.405	0.425
5.0	0.395	0.399	0.405	0.425
10.0	0.406	0.411	0.417	0.438
15.0	0.414	0.419	0.425	0.447
20.0	0.426	0.431	0.437	0.459
25.0	0.438	0.443	0.449	0.472

18 MV Mevalac Wedge Factors $\mathrm{WF}\left(d, f_d'\right)$

Maximum field size: 40 cm × 20 cm for 15°, 30°, and 45° and 40 cm × 15 cm for 60°

15°

Depth (cm)	Side of Equivalent Square f_d'				
	5	10	15	20	30
1.5	0.754	0.750	0.767	0.777	0.794
5.0	0.761	0.758	0.775	0.785	0.802
10.0	0.761	0.758	0.775	0.785	0.802
15.0	0.761	0.758	0.775	0.785	0.802
20.0	0.761	0.758	0.775	0.785	0.802
25.0	0.761	0.758	0.775	0.785	0.802

30°

Depth (cm)	Side of Equivalent Square f_d'				
	5	10	15	20	30
1.5	0.607	0.614	0.625	0.641	0.666
5.0	0.607	0.614	0.625	0.641	0.666
10.0	0.613	0.620	0.631	0.647	0.673
15.0	0.619	0.626	0.637	0.654	0.680
20.0	0.619	0.626	0.637	0.654	0.680
25.0	0.625	0.632	0.643	0.660	0.686

45°

Depth (cm)	Side of Equivalent Square f_d'			
	5	10	15	20
1.5	0.519	0.522	0.531	0.540
5.0	0.519	0.522	0.531	0.540
10.0	0.525	0.527	0.536	0.545
15.0	0.525	0.527	0.536	0.545
20.0	0.525	0.527	0.536	0.545
25.0	0.530	0.532	0.541	0.551

60°

Depth (cm)	Side of Equivalent Square f_d'			
	5	10	15	20
1.5	0.431	0.425	0.437	0.455
5.0	0.431	0.425	0.437	0.455
10.0	0.435	0.429	0.442	0.459
15.0	0.435	0.434	0.442	0.459
20.0	0.439	0.434	0.446	0.464
25.0	0.439	0.434	0.446	0.464

Percent Depth Dose for Mevalac Electron Beams

$(10 \times 10 \text{ cm}^2 \text{ fields and larger})$

Depth (cm)	Energy (MeV)				
	6	9	12	15	18
0.0	81.6	85.2	89.9	94.2	95.8
0.5	85.9	86.6	92.3	94.0	96.2
1.0	96.2	90.8	93.9	93.5	97.4
1.5	99.1	96.2	96.1	95.5	99.3
2.0	79.2	99.7	98.3	97.4	99.9
2.5	40	97.5	99.3	99.1	99.3
3.0	9	83.2	99.9	99.7	99.7
3.5	1.0	56.7	96.6	100.0	98.9
4.0	0.7	26.3	89.2	98.7	98.8
4.5	0.7	6.2	73.8	94.6	98.6
5.0	0.7	1.5	53.5	87.7	95.9
5.5	--	1.2	31.2	76.9	91.5
6.0	--	1.2	12.9	62.7	86.5
6.5	--	1.1	4.5	46.2	79.0
7.0	--	1.1	2.3	29.3	67.9
7.5	--	--	2.1	15.6	55.0
8.0	--	--	2.0	7.4	40.6
8.5	--	--	1.9	4.1	26.7
9.0	--	--	1.9	3.3	15.6
9.5	--	--	1.9	3.1	8.9
10.0	--	--	1.8	3.1	6.0
10.5	--	--	--	3.0	5.2
11.0	--	--	--	2.9	5.0
11.5	--	--	--	2.8	4.8
12.0	--	--	--	2.8	4.8
12.5	--	--	--	2.7	4.6
13.0	--	--	--	2.6	4.5
13.5	--	--	--	2.6	4.3

Mevalac Electron d_m Values

Energy (MeV)	6	9	12	15	18
d_m (cm)	1.3	2.2	2.8	3.4	1.8

$\dot{D}_d \left(100 + d_m, 10\right) = 1.000$ cGy/MU (normalization conditions)

Mevalac Electron Applicator Factors $S_e(f_a)$

E (MeV)	6 × 6	10 × 10	15 × 15	20 × 20	25 × 25
6	0.962	1.000	1.004	1.009	0.997
9	0.981	1.000	1.000	0.984	0.963
12	0.987	1.000	0.997	0.974	0.946
15	0.992	1.000	0.991	0.968	0.934
18	1.002	1.000	0.982	0.962	0.927

Appendix D

Answers to
Selected Problems

Chapter 2

2. 100 ms

3. 1.4 m/s

4. 1.0×10^3 kg/m^3

5. 10 μA

6. (a) 20 keV, 9.8×10^5 m/s
   (b) 10 keV, 5.9×10^7 m/s
   (c) in part (a) $v \ll c$, but not in part (b)

7. (a) 940 MeV
   (b) 1830

8. (a) 6.3×10^{10}
   (b) 0.17 nA

9. (c) 0.124 nm
   (d) same order of magnitude

11. (a) radio, microwave, infrared, visible, UV, x-rays
    (b) energy increases

12. (b) $\lambda = 1.24 \times 10^{-11}$ m, $\nu = 2.4 \times 10^{19}$ Hz

13. (a) 5000 MHz
    (b) microwaves

14. (a) 59 keV
    (b) 0.021 nm, x-ray

Chapter 3

3. (a) −28.3 MeV
   (b) 7.1 MeV, yes
   (c) 23.8 MeV released

5. (a) 8.05 nCi

6. 555 MBq

7. 1.1%

8. 3.2 d

9. 0.039 mCi

10. 0.1%

11. (a) 69 d
    (b) 0.58 d

12. (a) 9.88 mCi
    (b) 6.98 mCi

13. (a) 0.0231 y^{-1}
    (b) 955
    (c) −45

14. 490 MBq

15. 92%

16. August 31

17. 71.5 nCi

18. 0.379 mCi

Chapter 4

2. (a) 0.11
   (b) 0.29
   (c) 0.50

8. 250 mA

Chapter 5

1. 4 keV

3. 42.5 cGy/min

6. (a) 0.58 cm^{-1}
   (b) 5.6%

8. (a) 120 keV
   (b) 1%
   (c) heat
   (d) 120 keV
   (e) 0.010 nm

10. (a) 0.90 unit
    (b) 0.91 unit

11. 79%

Chapter 6

2. Factor of 8

3. (a) 12 keV
   (b) 73 keV

5. (a) 0.69 MeV
   (b) 0.35 cm

6. (a) 1.04 MeV
   (b) 0.52 cm

8. 3.98 MeV

12. 6 cm and 46 m

13. 3.5×10^5, no

Chapter 7

1. 109 R

2. 100 Gy

3. 1 cGy, the dose is uniform

4. (a) 3.38×10^3 J/m^2
   (b) 0.58 MeV
   (c) 1.26×10^{-3} MeV
   (d) 10 Gy
   (e) 10 Gy
   (f) 9.6 Gy

9. 4.97 MeV, yes, conservation of energy

Chapter 8

1. 2.69×10^{-2} cm^2/g

3. 0.187

4. Farmer/plane parallel = 15

7. 0.96

8. 17.7501 nC

11. 1.7

12. 0.1%

13. 2.4, 0.4%

17. 76.0 cGy

18. 1.17×10^{-8} J

20. 0.017 °C

Chapter 9

2. (a) 10 cm
   (b) 2.5 cm
   (c) 25 cm

5. 6.7 mm

6. 2.0 mm

10. (a) -8.9×10^{-3} min
    (b) 201.8 R/min

11. (a) 10.2 cm
    (b) 3.4%, no

12. 3.8 mm (lower), 5.3 mm (upper)

13. 37% by rule of thumb, actual value is 50%

Chapter 10

1. (a) 228 cGy
   (b) 139 cGy

2. 1.053

3. (a) 7.9, 8.0
   (b) 8.2, 8.6
   (c) 8.3, 9.2

8. TMR > DD

9. 66.8%

10. 0.776, 0.788

11. (a) 86.1%
    (b) 0.45
    (c) 87.4%
    (d) 0.47

Chapter 11

4. $\%dd(10)_x > \%dd(10)$

5. 1.000 by definition

6. 1.046

7. 0.1284 nC/MU

8. 5.282×10^7 Gy/C

9. 6.78×10^{-3} Gy/MU

10. 1.021 cGy/MU

11. 0.1536 nC/MU

12. 5.143×10^7 Gy/C

13. 0.791 cGy/MU

14. 0.995 cGy/MU

Chapter 12

1. (a) 111 cGy
   (b) 119 cGy

3. 246 MU

4. 250 MU

5. 163 MU

6. 200 MU

7. 131 MU

8. 226 cGy

9. 131 MU

10. 252 MU

11. 157 cGy

Chapter 13

2. 109 MU

3. 93 MU

4. (a) 0.11
   (b) 0.13

6. (a) 0.129
   (b) 6.5 cm
   (c) 6.7 cm

7. (a) 0.925 cGy/MU
   (b) 0.887 cGy/MU
   (c) 0.0823 cGy/MU
   (d) 16 cGy

8. 195 MU

Chapter 14

2. (a) 20.5 cm
   (b) 20.2 cm
   (c) in-plane = cross-plane = 0.7 cm

3. 103 cGy

4. 60 degrees

5. (a) 185 MU
   (b) 183 cGy

7. (a) 57%
   (b) 56%
   (c) 50%

9. Lateral beams: 63 MU;
   anterior/posterior beams: 54 MU

11. (a) 63 Gy
    (b) 165 cm^3

12. (a) $CF_A = 1.05$, $CF_B = 1.09$
    (b) $CF_A = 1.00$, $CF_B = 1.07$

14. 1.8 cm

15. 8.5 degrees

16. 303 degrees

Chapter 15

3. (a) 15 MeV (80%)
   (b) 15 cm by 15 cm
   (c) 182 MU

4. 227 MU

5. (a) 201 MU
   (b) 204 cGy

6. 4 mm

Chapter 16

1. Reduction of 99.9%

2. 54 mR/h

3. Low-energy radiation, along axis of tube sources

4. (a) 35.4 Gy/h
   (b) 5 min, 46 s

5. 23.4 Gy/h, 8 min 43 s

6. (a) 16.0 cGy/h
   (b) 14.9 cGy/h
   (c) Tube is not a point source

7. 4.9 cGy/h

9. (a) 55 cGy/h
   (b) 17.3 cGy/h

Chapter 17

1. 0.01 mSv

2. (a) 16.7 mSv
   (b) 8.4×10^{-4} Gy

3. (a) 1.2×10^{-5} Sv
   (b) $5 \times 10^{-7} = 5$ chances in 10 million

4. False

5. False

6. 400

7. 1.6

8. Radon

9. True

12. 400 Sv/wk

15. (a) 2.07×10^{-5}
    (b) 4.7
    (c) 2.3 m

16. $T = 1$, dose limits apply to individuals

Chapter 18

4. Daily: ±3%, monthly ±2%

6. Tolerance: 1 degree

Chapter 19

1. Pixel size 0.5 mm

2. 50 MB

3. 40 s

4. 914 HU

6. CT# < –50 are black, CT# > 250 are white

7. 1.4 mm

Index

Note: Page ranges are shown using longer dashes; an f denotes a figure; a t denotes a table.